Lessons from the ICU
Under the Auspices of the European Society
of Intensive Care Medicine

Series Editors
Maurizio Cecconi
Head Dept Anesthesia and ICU
Humanitas Research Hospital Head Dept Anesthesia and ICU
Rozzano, Milano, Milano, Italy

Daniel De Backer
Dept Intensive Care
Université Libre de Bruxelles Dept Intensive Care Erasme University
Bruxelles, Brussels Hoofdst.ge., Belgium

Hans Flaatten · Bertrand Guidet · Hélène Vallet

Editors

The Very Old Critically Ill Patients

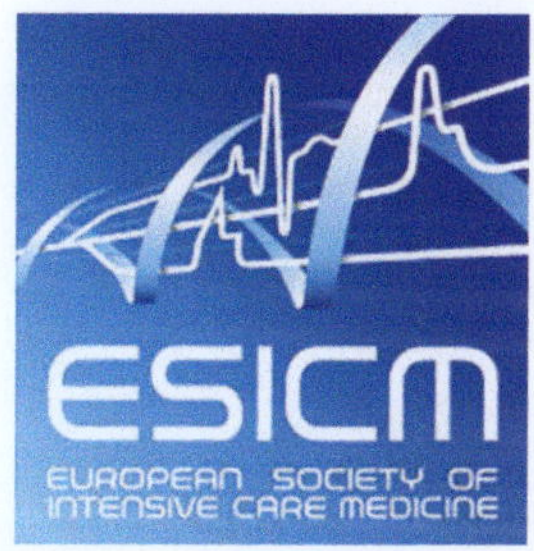

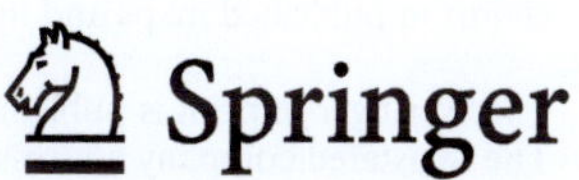

Editors
Hans Flaatten
Faculty of Medicine, Department of Clinical
Medicine and Department of Anaesthesia
and Intensive Care
University of Bergen and Haukeland
University Hospital
Bergen, Norway

Hélène Vallet
Sorbonne Université, Hôpital Saint Antoine
Unité de Gériatrie Aiguë, Assistance Publique
Hôpitaux de Paris
Paris, France

Bertrand Guidet
Sorbonne Université, INSERM
Institut Pierre Louis d'Epidémiologie et de
Santé Publique, AP-HP, Hôpital Saint
Antoine
Paris, France

ISSN 2522-5928   ISSN 2522-5936   (electronic)
Lessons from the ICU
ISBN 978-3-030-94135-2   ISBN 978-3-030-94133-8   (eBook)
https://doi.org/10.1007/978-3-030-94133-8

This Springer imprint is published by the registered company Springer Nature Switzerland AG
The registered company address is: Gewerbestrasse 11, 6330 Cham, Switzerland

Preface

Throughout history and even today, the elderly has been treated differently than the rest of the population. In some cultures, they are looked up to and honored both for their knowledge and skills, while in others they are considered of little value, like in the old Viking culture, and are expected to "disappear" when they are considered to be a burden for their tribe. Today, many modern societies practice another form for "disappearance," that is, the elderly are taken care of by the social welfare system in nursing homes and similar places, and this way, they are often separated from the rest of the family and are less visible to the society.

Cultural differences may also influence the way we meet critically ill elderly patients, and in our "modern world," it is easy for many to argue that large resources to increase life span in octogenarians could be used in better ways. We have recently observed what happened in the early phase of the COVID-19 pandemic where some countries overwhelmed with too many sick patients opted the "easy" way out: to use age alone as a criterion for ICU admission and treatment.

It is easy to understand why; when using a pure utility approach for ICU triage, the elderly will always loose. As a group, their expected life span will constantly be shorter than less-old patients. However, expanding these considerations into daily life without pandemic can be perilous.

We have written and edited this book since we hope to increase the awareness of a group within our ICUs that deserves to be taken seriously. The old patients will increase more than any other ICU sub-populations across the world in the coming 30–40 years. Without appropriate preparation now, we will end up with a constant "crisis" using ad hoc solution instead of doing some fundamental changes.

We sincerely believe that many critically ill old patients deserve to be given optimal care. There is no uniform evidence that intensive care is futile for the majority, although we also acknowledge that it is in many elderlies' interest to refrain from intensive care.

The target audience of this book is primarily the practicing intensivist who regularly sees elderly ICU patients admitted, which in fact is most of us. As with other patients, it is important to give timely and adequate care to the critically ill elderly patients, and we hope this book will give the reader new knowledge on how to provide such care. This may vary from full support, similar to most other ICU patients, but sometimes also to accept that offering palliative care is the best option. We believe that emergency physicians might be interested, since they propose old patients for an ICU admission. This is in fact the first triage step that is largely unknown to ICU physicians. Geriatricians might also be another target since they are involved in post-ICU care.

We wish to acknowledge our large group of authors that took on this assignment just prior to the pandemic and were able to write their chapters in spite of managing increased number of ICU patients and difficult working schedules. Thank you! We are also pleased that ESICM looked to this topic for its inclusion in the series Lessons from the ICU, and thanks a lot for the trust.

Hans Flaatten
Bergen, Norway

Bertrand Guidet
Paris, France

Hélène Vallet
Paris, France

Contents

I Introduction: The Very Old ICU Patients

II Age-Related Physiological Changes

III Geriatric Syndroms

Claire Roubaud-Baudron and Florent Guerville

Lozano Vicario Lucía, Gutiérrez-Valencia Marta,
and Martínez-Velilla Nicolas

22.7	**Refeeding Syndrome**	343
22.8	**Practical Issues**	343
22.9	**Monitoring Response to Feeding**	344
22.10	**The Post-ICU Period**	344
	References	345

VI Withhold and Withdraw Therapy

23 Limitation of Life-Sustaining Treatments ... 351
Bertrand Guidet and Hélène Vallet

23.1	**Introduction**	352
23.2	**General Consideration in Old Critically Ill Old Population**	352
23.3	**Limitation of Life-Sustaining Treatments**	353
23.4	**Reporting of Limitation of LST**	356
23.5	**Determinants of LLST**	356
23.6	**Implication of Patients and Caregivers in the Decision-Making Process**	358
23.7	**How**	358
23.8	**Treatment During the ICU Stay**	359
23.9	**Time-Limited Trial**	359
23.10	**Quality of Death**	361
	References	362

VII Outcomes After Intensive Care

24 Outcomes After Intensive Care: Survival ... 369
Hans Flaatten

24.1	**Introduction**	370
24.2	**Limitations of Crude Survival**	371
24.3	**Survival After a Defined Procedure or Admission**	371
24.4	**Survival After a Fixed Period**	371
24.5	**Survival in Specific Cohorts**	372
24.6	**The Effect of Age**	373
24.7	**The Effect of Gender**	375
24.8	**The Effect of Severity of Disease**	375
24.9	**The Effect of Frailty**	376
24.10	**The Effect of Limitation of Care**	376
24.11	**What Is the Reported Mortality of Elderly ICU Patients?**	378
24.12	**The Future of Reporting Mortality**	379
	References	379

25 Outcomes After Intensive Care: Functional Status ... 381
Sten M. Walther

25.1	**Introduction**	382
25.2	**Framing Functional Status**	382
25.3	**Instruments and Measures**	385

Contents

VIII   Specific Diseases and Conditions

IX   Future Developments

Contributors

Atul Anand   Royal Infirmary of Edinburgh, NHS Lothian, Edinburgh, UK
Centre for Cardiovascular Science, University of Edinburgh, Edinburgh, UK
atul.anand@ed.ac.uk

Antonio Artigas   CIBER de Enfermedades Respiratorias, Instituto de Salud Carlos III, Madrid, Spain
Critical Care Center, Corporació Sanitaria Universitaria Parc Tauli, and Autonomous University of Barcelona, Sabadell, Spain
aartigas@tauli.cat

Margaux Baqué   Sorbonne Université, Assistance Publique-Hôpitaux de Paris (APHP), Groupe Hospitalier Pitié-Salpêtrière-Charles Foix, Unit of Peri-Operative Geriatric Care (UPOG), Paris, France
margaux.baque@aphp.fr

Michael Beil   Department of Medical Intensive Care, Hadassah Medical Center and Faculty of Medicine, Hebrew University of Jerusalem, Jerusalem, Israel
beil@doctors.org.uk

Arie Ben-Yehuda   Department of Medical Intensive Care, Hadassah Medical Center and Faculty of Medicine, Hebrew University of Jerusalem, Jerusalem, Israel
BENYEHUDA@hadassah.org.il

Mette M. Berger   Service of Adult Intensive Care, Lausanne University Hospital (CHUV), Lausanne, Switzerland
Mette.Berger@chuv.ch

Gabriella Bettelli   2nd Level Master in Perioperative Geriatric Medicine, San Marino University, Città di San Marino, San Marino
gabriella.bettelli@unirsm.sm

Céline Bianco   Hôpital Saint Antoine, Unité de Gériatrie Aiguë, Assistance Publique Hôpitaux de Paris, Paris, France
celine.bianco@aphp.fr

Hubert Blain   Department of Internal Medicine and Geriatrics, University Hospital of Montpellier, Montpellier University, Centre Antonin Balmes, Montpellier, France
h-blain@chu-montpellier.fr

Jacques Boddaert   Sorbonne Université, Assistance Publique-Hôpitaux de Paris (APHP), Groupe Hospitalier Pitié-Salpêtrière-Charles Foix, Unit of Peri-Operative Geriatric Care (UPOG), Paris, France
jacques.boddaert@aphp.fr

Fabrizio Brau UOS Riabilitazione Post-acuzie, Fondazione Policlinico Universitario A. Gemelli IRCCS, Rome, Italy

Department of Geriatrics and Orthopaedics, Università Cattolica del Sacro Cuore, Rome, Italy

Matteo Cesari Department of Clinical Sciences and Community Health, University of Milan, Milan, Italy

Geriatric Unit, IRCCS Istituti Clinici Scientifici Maugeri, Milan, Italy

Raphaël Chancel Centre de Ressource Autisme Languedoc-Roussillon et Centre d'Excellence sur l'Autisme et les Troubles Neurodéveloppementaux, CHU Montpellier, Montpellier, France

Faculté de Médecine, Université de Montpellier, Montpellier, France

r-chancel@chu-montpellier.fr

Michelle Chew Department of Anaesthesia and Intensive Care, Biomedical and Clinical Sciences, Linköping University, Linköping, Sweden

michelle.chew@liu.se

Benjamin G. Chousterman AP-HP, CHU Lariboisière, Department of Anesthesia and Critical Care, DMU Parabol, FHU PROMICE, Paris, France

Université de Paris, INSERM U942 MASCOT, Inserm, Paris, France

benjamin.chousterman@aphp.fr

A. Clegg Bradford Teaching Hospitals NHS Foundation Trust, Leeds, UK

a.p.clegg@leeds.ac.uk

Lahaye Clement Université Clermont Auvergne, INRAE, Unité de Nutrition Humaine, CRNH Auvergne, CHU Clermont-Ferrand, service de Gériatrie, Clermont-Ferrand, France

Alan A. Cohen Department of Family Medicine, Research Center on Aging and Research Center of CHUS, Faculty of Medicine and Health Sciences, University of Sherbrooke, Sherbrooke, QC, Canada

Alan.cohen@usherbrooke.ca

Judith Cohen-Bittan Sorbonne Université, Assistance Publique-Hôpitaux de Paris (APHP), Groupe Hospitalier Pitié-Salpêtrière-Charles Foix, Unit of Peri-Operative Geriatric Care (UPOG), Paris, France

judith.cohen-bitan@aphp.fr

Dylan de Lange Intensive Care, University Medical Center Utrecht, Utrecht, The Netherlands

D.W.deLange-3@umcutrecht.nl

D.W.deLange@umcutrecht.nl

N. Efstathiou School of Nursing, University of Birmingham, Birmingham, UK

n.efstathiou@bham.ac.uk

H. Fanebust   Haukeland University Hospital, Bergen, Norway
runefane@online.no

Hans Flaatten   Faculty of Medicine, Department of Clinical Medicine and Department of Anaesthesia and Intensive Care, University of Bergen and Haukeland University Hospital, Bergen, Norway
Hans.Flaatten@uib.no

Tamas Fulop   Research Center on Aging, Division of Geriatrics, Department of Medicine, Faculty of Medicine and Health Sciences, University of Sherbrooke, Sherbrooke, QC, Canada
tamas.fulop@usherbrooke.ca

Vincenzo Galluzzo   UOS Riabilitazione Post-acuzie, Fondazione Policlinico Universitario A. Gemelli IRCCS, Rome, Italy

Department of Geriatrics and Orthopaedics, Università Cattolica del Sacro Cuore, Rome, Italy

Silvia Giovannini   UOS Riabilitazione Post-acuzie, Fondazione Policlinico Universitario A. Gemelli IRCCS, Rome, Italy

Department of Aging, Neurological, Orthopaedic and Head-Neck Sciences, Fondazione Policlinico Universitario A. Gemelli IRCCS, Rome, Italy

Department of Geriatrics and Orthopaedics, Università Cattolica del Sacro Cuore, Rome, Italy
silvia.giovannini@policlinicogemelli.it

Sandrine Greffard   Geriatric Center, Pitie Salpetriere Hospital (AP-PH, Medecine Sorbonne University), Paris, France
sandrine.greffard@aphp.fr

Florent Guerville   CHU de Bordeaux, Pôle de Gérontologie Clinique, Bordeaux, France
florent.guerville@chu-bordeaux.fr

Bertrand Guidet   Sorbonne Université, INSERM, Institut Pierre Louis d'Epidémiologie et de Santé Publique, AP-HP, Hôpital Saint Antoine, Paris, France
bertrand.guidet@aphp.fr

Katsuiku Hirokawa   Department of Diagnostic Pathology, Institute of Health and Life Science, Tokyo Medical and Dental University, Tokyo and Nitobe Memorial Nakanosogo Hospital, Tokyo, Japan
hirokawa@nakanosogo.or.jp

Claire Anne Hurni   Service of Adult Intensive Care, Lausanne University Hospital (CHUV), Lausanne, Switzerland
1unknown@meteor.com

Jeremy M. Jacobs   Department of Geriatric Rehabilitation, Hadassah Medical Center, Hebrew University of Jerusalem, Jerusalem, Israel
jacobsj@hadassah.org.il

Michael Joannidis   Division of Intensive Care and Emergency Medicine, Department of Internal Medicine, Medical University Innsbruck, Innsbruck, Austria
michael.joannidis@i-med.ac.at

Gavin M. Joynt   Department of Anaesthesia and Intensive Care, The Chinese University of Hong Kong, Hong Kong, China
gavinmjoynt@cuhk.edu.hk

Abdelouahed Khalil   Research Center on Aging, Division of Geriatrics, Department of Medicine, Faculty of Medicine and Health Sciences, University of Sherbrooke, Sherbrooke, QC, Canada
Abdelouahed.khalil@usherbrooke.ca

Antoine Lamblin   Anesthesiology and Critical Care Medicine, Edouard Herriot Hospital, Hospices Civils de Lyon, Lyon, France
unknwwn1@meteor.com

Anis Larbi   Singapore Immunology Network (SIgN), Agency for Science Technology and Research (A*STAR), Immunos Building, Biopolis, Singapore, Singapore

T. Lawton   Bradford Teaching Hospitals NHS Foundation Trust, Leeds, UK
Tom.Lawton@bthft.nhs.uk

Nazir I. Lone   Usher Institute, University of Edinburgh, Edinburgh, UK
Royal Infirmary of Edinburgh, NHS Lothian, Edinburgh, UK
nazir.lone@ed.ac.uk

José A. Lorente   CIBER de Enfermedades Respiratorias, Instituto de Salud Carlos III, Madrid, Spain
Servicio de Medicina Intensiva, Hospital Universitario de Getafe, Madrid, Spain
Universidad Europea, Madrid, Spain
joseangel.lorente@salud.madrid.org

Marta Lorente-Ros   Department of Medicine, Mount Sinai Morningside and Mount Sinai West, Icahn School of Medicine at Mount Sinai, New York, NY, USA

Lozano Vicario Lucia   Department of Geriatric Medicine, Complejo Hospitalario de Navarra, Pamplona, Spain
lucia.lozano.vicario@navarra.es

Gutiérrez-Valencia Marta   Servicio Navarro de Salud, Sección de Innovación y Organización, Pamplona, Spain
marta.gutierrez.valencia@navarra.es

I. Martin-Loeches   Saint James's Hospital, Intensive Care, Dublin, Ireland

Timo Mayerhöfer   Division of Intensive Care and Emergency Medicine, Department of Internal Medicine, Medical University Innsbruck, Innsbruck, Austria
timo.mayerhoefer@i-med.ac.at

J. Mellinghoff   School of Sport and Health Sciences, University of Brighton, Brighton, UK

Stéphanie Miot   Department of Internal Medicine and Geriatrics, University Hospital of Montpellier, Montpellier University, Centre Antonin Balmes, Montpellier, France
CESP, INSERM U1178, Centre de recherche en Epidemiologie et Santé des Populations, Paris, France
s-miot@chu-montpellier.fr

Rui Moreno   Hospital de São José, Centro Hospitalar Universitário de Lisboa Central E.P.E., Lisbon, Portugal
Faculdade de Ciências Médicas de Lisboa, Nova Medical School, Lisbon, Portugal
Faculdade de Ciências de Saúde, Universidade da Beira Interior, Covilhã, Portugal
r.moreno@mail.telepac.pt

Louis Morisson   AP-HP, CHU Lariboisière, Department of Anesthesia and Critical Care, DMU Parabol, FHU PROMICE, Paris, France
Université de Paris, INSERM U942 MASCOT, Inserm, Paris, France

Tiziano Nestola   ASP IMMeS Pio Albergo Trivulzio, Milan, Italy

Martínez-Velilla Nicolas   Department of Geriatric Medicine – Navarrabiomed, Complejo Hospitalario de Navarra, Pamplona, Spain
nicolas.martinez.velilla@navarra.es

Laura Orlandini   ASP IMMeS Pio Albergo Trivulzio, Milan, Italy

Olivier Pantet   Service of Adult Intensive Care, Lausanne University Hospital (CHUV), Lausanne, Switzerland
unknown2abc111@meteor.com

Fabian Perschinka   Division of Intensive Care and Emergency Medicine, Department of Internal Medicine, Medical University Innsbruck, Innsbruck, Austria
fabian.perschinka@student.i-med.ac.at

Carmen A. Pfortmueller   Department of Intensive Care Medicine, Inselspital, Bern University Hospital, University of Bern, Bern, Switzerland
carmen.pfortmueller@insel.ch

Saskia Rietjens   University Medical Center Utrecht, Dutch Poisons Information Center (DPIC), Utrecht, The Netherlands
S.Rietjens@umcutrecht.nl

Thomas Rimmele Anesthesiology and Critical Care Medicine, Edouard Herriot Hospital, Hospices Civils de Lyon, Lyon, France
thomas.rimmele@chu-lyon.fr

Claire Roubaud-Baudron CHU de Bordeaux, Pôle de Gérontologie Clinique, Bordeaux, France
claire.roubaud@chu-bordeaux.fr

Lisa Salisbury Queen Margaret University, Edinburgh, UK
LSalisbury@qmu.ac.uk

Joerg C. Schefold Department of Intensive Care Medicine, Inselspital, Bern University Hospital, University of Bern, Bern, Switzerland
joerg.schefold@insel.ch

G. Schwarz Anaesthesia and Intensive Care, Haukeland University Hospital, Bergen, Norway
gabriele.leonie.schwarz@helse-bergen.no

Florent Sigwalt Anesthesiology and Critical Care Medicine, Edouard Herriot Hospital, Hospices Civils de Lyon, Lyon, France
unknwwn2@meteor.com

E. Skaar Department of Heart Disease, Haukeland University Hospital, Bergen, Norway
elisabeth.skaar@helse-bergen.no

Jochanan Stessman Department of Geriatric Rehabilitation, Hadassah Medical Center, Hebrew University of Jerusalem, Jerusalem Institute for Aging Research, Jerusalem, Israel
jochanans@ekmd.huji.ac.il

Sigal Sviri Department of Medical Intensive Care, Hadassah Medical Center and Faculty of Medicine, Hebrew University of Jerusalem, Jerusalem, Israel
Sigals1@hadassah.org.il

Sara Thietart Geriatric Center, Pitie Salpetriere Hospital (AP-PH, Medecine Sorbonne University), Paris, France
Sorbonne Université, Assistance Publique-Hôpitaux de Paris (APHP), Groupe Hospitalier Pitié-Salpêtrière-Charles Foix, Unit of Peri-Operative Geriatric Care (UPOG), Paris, France
sara.thietart@aphp.fr

Caroline Thomas Hôpital Saint Antoine, Unité de Gériatrie Aiguë, Assistance Publique Hôpitaux de Paris, Paris, France
caroline.thomas@aphp.fr

Hélène Vallet Sorbonne Université, Hôpital Saint Antoine, Unité de Gériatrie Aiguë, Assistance Publique Hôpitaux de Paris, Paris, France
helene.vallet@aphp.fr

P. Vernon van Heerden   Department of Anesthesia, Intensive Care and Pain Medicine, Hadassah Medical Center and Faculty of Medicine, Hebrew University of Jerusalem, Jerusalem, Israel
veron@hadassah.org.il

Lenneke van Lelyveld-Haas   Intensive Care, Diakonessenhuis Utrecht, Utrecht, The Netherlands
lvlelyveld@diakhuis.nl

M. van Mol   Intensive Care Adults, Erasmus MC, Rotterdam, The Netherlands
m.vanmol@erasmusmc.nl

Marc Verny   Geriatric Center, Pitie Salpetriere Hospital (AP-PH, Medecine Sorbonne University), Paris, France
Geriatric Center, UMR8256 (CNRS), Team Neuronal Cell Biology & Pathology, Paris, France
marc.verny@aphp.fr

R. Walford   Bradford Teaching Hospitals NHS Foundation Trust, Leeds, UK
Rebecca.Walford@bthft.nhs.uk

Sten M. Walther   Department of Cardiovascular Anaesthesia and Intensive Care, Heart Centre, Linköping University Hospital, Linköping, Sweden
Department of Medical and Health Sciences, Faculty of Medicine and Health Sciences, Linköping University, Linköping, Sweden
sten.walther@telia.com

Yoram G. Weiss   Hadassah Medical Center and Faculty of Medicine, Hebrew University of Jerusalem, Jerusalem, Israel
weiss@hadassah.org.il

Jacek M. Witkowski   Department of Pathophysiology, Medical University of Gdansk, Gdansk, Poland
jacek.witkowski@gumed.edu.pl

Lorène Zerah   Sorbonne Université, Assistance Publique-Hôpitaux de Paris (APHP), Groupe Hospitalier Pitié-Salpêtrière-Charles Foix, Unit of Peri-Operative Geriatric Care (UPOG), Paris, France
lorene.zerah@aphp.fr

Patrick Zuercher   Department of Intensive Care Medicine, Inselspital, Bern University Hospital, University of Bern, Bern, Switzerland
patrick.zuercher@insel.ch

Abbreviations

ACP	Advance care planning
AF	Atrial fibrillation
AKI	Acute kidney injury
BIA	Bioimpedance analysis
BSI	Bloodstream infection
CIRCI	Critical illness-related cortico-steroid insufficiency
CO	Cardiac output
DRI	Daily recommended intakes
DVT	Deep vein thrombosis
EDV	End-diastolic volume
EE	Energy expenditure
EN	Enteral nutrition
ESICM	European Society of Intensive Care Medicine
GCP	Graduated compression stockings
GI	Gastrointestinal
H2EAs	Histamine-2 receptor antagonists
HB	Harris and Benedict equation
HES	Hydroxyethyl starch
HFNO	High flow nasal oxygen therapy
hMPV	Human metapneumovirus
ICU	Intensive care admission
IHD	Ischemic heart disease
IPC	Intermittent pneumatic compression
LBM	Lean body mass
LOS	Length of stay
LST	Life-sustaining treatment
MAP	Mean arterial pressure
MDRO	Multidrug-resistant organism
MNA-SF	Mini Nutritional Assessment-Short Form
NIV	Non-invasive mechanical ventilation
NRS	Nutritional Risk Screening score
ONS	Oral nutrition supplements
PCR-ESI-MS	Polymerase chain reaction/electrospray ionization-mass spectrometry
PD	Pharmacodynamics
PE	Pulmonary embolism
PICCO	Pulse Contour Cardiac Output
PK	Pharmacokinetics
PN	Parenteral nutrition
POC	Point of care
PPI	Proton-pump inhibitor
PPI	Proton pump inhibitors
PPV	Pulse pressure variation
RFS	Refeeding syndrome
SGA	Subjective Global Assessment
SIRS	Systemic inflammatory response syndrome
SOFA	Sequential (sepsis-related) Organ Failure Assessment
SSC	Surviving Sepsis Campaign
sTREM-1	soluble triggering receptor expressed on myeloid cells-1
TIA	Transient ischemic attack
TTE	Transthoracic echocardiography

Introduction: The Very Old ICU Patients

Contents

The Demography of Ageing and the Very Old Critical Ill Patients

Hans Flaatten, Bertrand Guidet, and Hélène Vallet

Contents

Learning Objectives

This introduction gives an overview of the demography of ageing in particular in a short (20–30-year) perspective. For this time period we already know a lot how the future populations will be composed, and the number of old and very old will increase considerably in most countries. In the developed countries this is accompanied by a decrease in the population below 20 years while this group will also increase in the less developed countries. In developed countries this will increase the burden by having a smaller workforce available.

In intensive care the increase in the number of patients >70 years, which soon is the median age of European ICU patients, will also rise absolutely but in some countries also more than the population increase in the same cohort.

The "normal" development in older persons is described and is accompanied by an increased prevalence in most chronic diseases, dementia and malnutrition with a decreased physical activity.

Last, the different options societies have to deal with the increase in old intensive care patients are shortly described.

1.1 Introduction: Demography of Ageing

In addition to global climate change, one of the major changes worldwide is the population ageing. This happens all over and in nearly all countries but is most visible in Europe and America.

Two important issues are worth discussing: the differences between high- and low-income countries and the differences within age cohorts. In low-income countries, the total population will most probably rise continuously towards 2100, mainly because of the growth in age groups 25–64 followed by a delayed growth in patients aged 65+ from 2050 and onwards. In the high-income countries, the picture is different, with a near zero overall growth from 2025 and a continuous growth in the age group 65+ in the whole period. This implies that the younger cohort shrinks; hence, we end up with an absolute and relative increase in the old population.

1.2 Diversity Within Europe

In Europe (2018) not only the life expectancy at the age of 60 varies from 26 years (France) to 17 in Turkmenistan, but also the healthy life expectancy at age 60 varies, from 21 years (France) to 14 years (Moldova). This, together with a decreased birth rate, gives profound changes in the so-called age pyramid and the composition of the population in different age groups (■ Fig. 1.1). We clearly see that the most pronounced changes in Europe will happen in the coming 30 years when the number of inhabitants above 65 years will represent 30% of the population. The absolute number of the very old (≥80) will in this period be doubled in 2050 compared with today.

The overall effects of such profound demographic changes are probably not completely revealed and although discussed have only superficially been planned or prepared for, in particular regarding health care. The consequences can be described as

Population pyramids, EU-27, 2019 and 2050
(% share of total population)

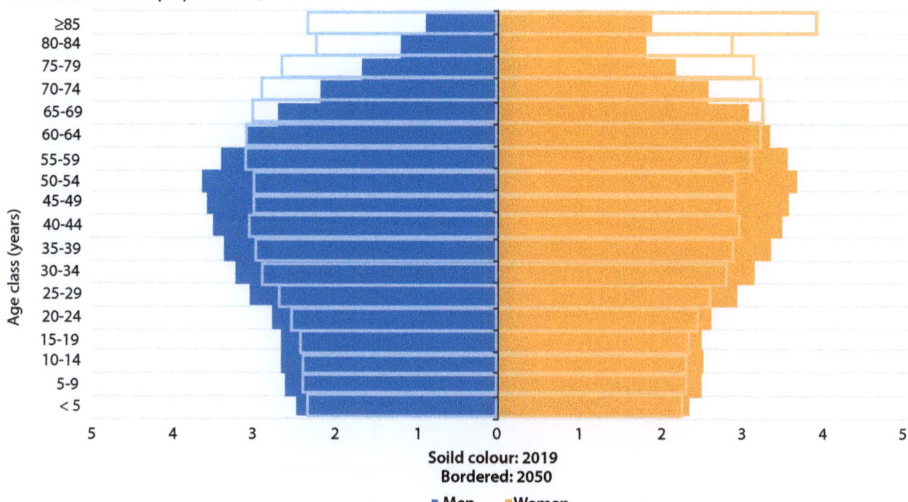

Note: all data as of 1 January. 2019: estimates and provisional. 2050: population according to the 2019 projections, baseline variant (EUROPOP2019).
Source: Eurostat (online data codes: demo_pjangroup and proj_19np)   eurostat

◘ Fig. 1.1 Population pyramid changes from 2019 to 2050 in Europe. (Published with permission for free use (▶ https://ec.europa.eu/eurostat/web/main/about/policies/copyright))

the age-dependency ratio, which is the ratio between the children (age 0–14) + older (age 65 and older) over the traditional working-age groups (age 15–64). In a recent study of different scenarios in the EU, this index will differ according to immigration policy and increase in the labour force by increasing the upper limit of working age, meaning a higher age before retiring from work [1]. If nothing is done, the productivity will be reduced with widespread consequences, not at least for health care. In a study from Norway, Gregersen published estimates for health-care expenditure in different age groups during two periods, and this study reveals both the high cost of health care to the old patients and the increase over time (◘ Fig. 1.2) from [2].

1.3 General Health Issues in the Very Old

Another major issue is obviously the health status in our aging populations. Seen from the health-care point of view, it would be fewer reasons for concern if an increasing part of the elderly had "healthy" lives and hence would not be in need of growing health-care resources. There is a lot of information about the health status, and what is familiar to most of us, "everything" seems to increase with age:

- The prevalence of most chronic diseases [3]
- Increased rates of dementia [4]
- Reduced physical activity [5]
- Malnutrition [6]

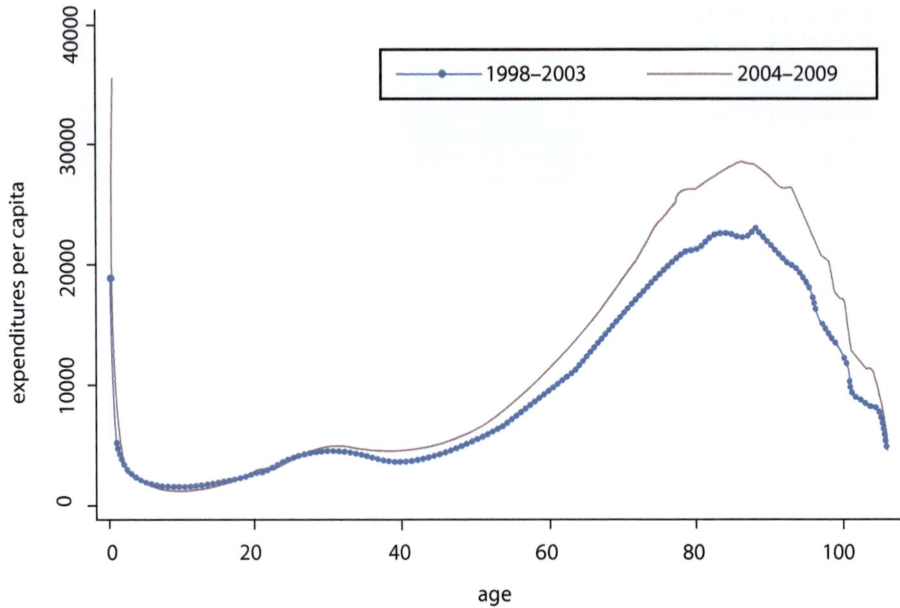

Fig. 1.2 Hospital expenditure per capita measured in NOK over age [2]. (Reproduced according to The Creative Commons CC BY)

Predictors of further survival after 90 years old are female gender, higher socio-economic status, better mobility and functional status, no frailty, fewer chronic condition and lower inflammation state [7–9].

The global objective for a successful aging is an increase of life without disability and without functional limitation. Life expectancy without disability increases since several years, but so is life expectancy with disability. In the UK, the projection is an increase of the total life expectancy at age of 65 years from 20.1 years in 2015 to 21.8 years in 2025 and an increase of the life expectancy without incapacity from 15.4 to 16.4 years. Unfortunately, the life expectancy with incapacity grows relatively more from 4.7 to 5.4 years [10]. In the oldest old population (>90 years old), women live longer than men (3.7 vs 3 years) but spend more time with disabilities and multi-morbidities (2 years vs 10 months) [11]. In sum, these developments probably absolutely and relatively will pose very large challenges for health care in the coming decades.

1.4 ICU Admission of the Very Old

A number of publications have specifically studied the very old patients admitted to intensive care, but not many have compared this cohort with data from the general population. We have already had an increase in the old population, although the large increase is yet to come. Still, it is of interest to find out if the number of old/very old in the ICU is increasing in parallel with aging of the population. Such an increase has been anticipated using data of expected increase and assume that the profile of ICU patients will be similar in the future [12]. In a recent study from France, ICU admissions in elderly with respiratory infections were compared from 2006 to 2016 [13]. They found in patients 85–89 and ≥90 years a 3.3- to 5.8-fold increase in the use of ICU resources. Similarly, a large study from the UK comparing ICU admissions in the period from 1997 to 2016 found a proportional increase of ICU bed days in the age group ≥75 years also when compared with the proportionally greater increase in the general population for the same group [14]. On the other hand, other studies from the USA and Scotland have demonstrated a relative decrease in ICU admissions for the elderly [15, 16], while a study from Denmark demonstrated a moderate increase in admission of patients ≥80 from 2005 to 2011 but with no corrections for demographic changes [17].

It is hence not evident how the increase in ICU admission of the elderly will look like in the next three decades, as this is a complex picture. As the experience shows, we might end up with different scenarios in different countries. In some countries we may have an "expected" increase proportional to the increase in the cohort of elderly; in some countries we may have an increase above the expected and in some below (◘ Fig. 1.3).

The bottom line is that all these scenarios will most likely increase the number of ICU patients, and if compensatory measures are not taken, there will be an increased strain to our ICUs. In particular this will be a challenge if we will experience a proportional increase as the figure shows.

To meet this increase countries do not have many choices, and these conceptually fall into three groups:

1. An overall increase in the number of ICU beds in order to cope with increased demand. An increase of intermediate care beds such as high dependency or step-up beds might be an option enabling to accommodate more patients together with avoiding the high financial burden of ICU bed mainly driven by the cost of personal.
2. A more efficient use of existing ICU beds. This may include shorter LOS made possible by more efficient treatment, stricter pre-ICU triage and increased use of time-limited ICU trials [18].
3. Rationing critical care beds by giving them only to those with a high probability of survival with an acceptable quality of life.

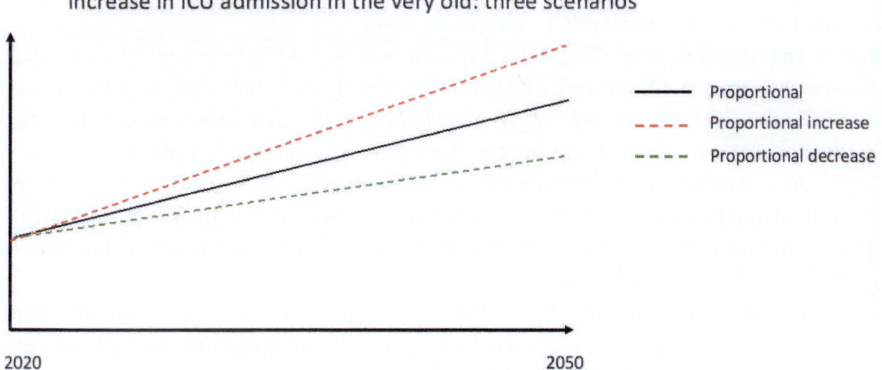

◘ **Fig. 1.3** Increase in ICU admission according to three different scenarios

Given the fact that the demographic changes not only increase the old population, but the young population will most likely decrease and hence less people will contribute to the workforce, This may hit the health sector in particular and probably render the first option of questionable value since there may not be enough skilled people. The projected need for health-care workers in Europe as elsewhere is discussed in several publications, and the conclusion is that this issue is extremely difficult to predict, since there are so many different factors, known and also probably also unknown. The effects of prophylactic measures in the population, the development of more effective treatments and medications and the increase of day-case surgery and mini-invasive procedures all may have an effect on hospital admissions in the future. The unknown issue of immigration is also a confounding factor. Will there be immigrants that readily can contribute in health-care service [19]?

1.5 The Very Old in the ICU

In addition to probably be the largest sub-group in the ICU, this group gives unique challenges to our ICU personnel. Some of them are related to medical issues like age-induced changes in normal physiology and its consequences for most acute diseases or trauma, but also regarding communication with family, most often from the next generation, and ethical issues with regard to admission and conduction of intensive care. A large number of the very old ICU patients have limitations of life sustaining treatments implemented during care, and such was recently found to affect more than one of four very old ICU patients in Europe [20]. We may expect this to increase in parallel with the shortage of ICU beds, a development that will require inclusion of many stakeholders in order to secure a firm fundament for end-of-life care in the ICU.

> **Conclusions**
>
> The above are considerations of large concern for us as intensive care physicians and nurses, but obviously there is very little we can do to influence it. One thing we can do with the increasing number of very old critical ill patients is to increase our knowledge about the specific characteristics of the critical ill elderly patients [20]. This is a task this book may contribute to, and with knowledge we can hopefully provide optimal care to these patients, be it ICU admission or not.
>
> The book has several sections, and each may be read independent of each other. The chapters are all written by recognized experts in their field and often by pairs of intensivists and geriatricians. We strongly believe in the interaction between these two medical fields as a way to improve care for the critically ill elderly patients.
>
> As a base for understanding diseases in the very old, we have to recognize the normal and pathological decline in body functions occurring with age. We will discuss this with regard to vital organ functions but also immune function and metabolism in ► Chaps. 3, 4, 5, 6, 7, 8, and 9.
>
> Further we will explore the so-called geriatric syndromes, which are ill defined. Both multimorbidity and multi-pharmacotherapy are closely related to age and can have impact during critical care, as well as frailty, sarcopenia, malnutrition and functional

status. This part ends with a discussion of the comprehensive geriatric assessment, also called the gold standard to assess geriatric patients.

We will further explore the complexity of triage, both before and during ICU admission, and the relevance of commonly used risk score in this population.

Most common ICU procedures may also be applied in the very old, but with some more concern. Ventilation, both invasive and non-invasive, is frequently used, as are vasoactive drugs. Renal replacement therapy (RRT) has not gained universal acceptance in this group even as we will see acute renal failure is not uncommon in the very old, and RRT is used less than in younger ICU patients. This will be discussed, as well as the state-of-the-art sedation and analgesia and nutritional support.

It is no secret that ICU procedures are withheld or withdrawn in many elderly patients, an important discussion given in ▶ Chap. 24.

Outcomes in terms of survival, functional status and cognition are discussed in a separate section that also includes the important aspect of specific rehabilitation, at present a large and unmet demand.

In the last section common acute diseases leading the elderly patients to the ICU are discussed, like acute respiratory failure, sepsis, kidney failure, trauma and postoperative care. A specific chapter on delirium is also included here with an update of the coronavirus pandemic and the very old.

We hope this book will be read and used throughout intensive care units across Europe and the rest of the world, and the users, the very old ICU patients, may be given even better care in our wards.

References

1. Guillaume M, Bélanger A, Lutz W. Population aging, migration, and productivity in Europe. Proc Natl Acad Sci. 2020;117(14):7690–5.
2. Gregersen FA. The impact of ageing on health care expenditures: a study of steepening. Eur J Health Econ. 2014;15(9):979–89.
3. Jaul E, Barron J. Age-related diseases and clinical and public health implications for the 85 years old and over population. Front Public Health. 2017;5:335.
4. Yang Z, Slavin MJ, Sachdev PS. Dementia in the oldest old. Nat Rev Neurol. 2013;9(7):382–93.
5. McPhee JS, French DP, Jackson D, et al. Physical activity in older age: perspectives for healthy ageing and frailty. Biogerontology. 2016;17(3):567–80.
6. Griffin A, O'Neill A, O'Connor M, et al. The prevalence of malnutrition and impact on patient outcomes among older adults presenting at an Irish emergency department: a secondary analysis of the OPTI-MEND trial. BMC Geriatr. 2020;20:455.
7. Tiainen K, Luukkaala T, Harvonen A, et al. Predictors of mortality in men and women aged 90 and older. Age Ageing. 2013;42(4):468–75.
8. Enroth L, Raitanen J, Hervonen A, et al. Is socioeconomic status a predictor of mortality in nonagenarians? Ageing. 2015;44(1):123–9.
9. Enroth L, Raitanen J, Hervonen A, et al. Cardiometabolic and inflammatory biomarkers as mediators between educational attainment and functioning at the age of 90 years. J Geront A Biol Sci Med Sci. 2016;71(3):412–9.
10. Guzman-Castillo M, Ahmadi-Abhari S, Bandosz P, et al. Forecasted trends in disability and life expectancy in England and Wales up to 2025: a modelling stud. Lancet Public Health. 2017;2(7):e307–13.
11. Hoogendijk EO, van der Noordt M, Onwuteaka-Philipsen BD, et al. Sex differences in healthy life expectancy among nonagenarians: a multistate survival model using data from the vitality 90+ study. Exp Gerontol. 2019;116:80–5.

12. Laake JH, Dybwik K, Flaatten HK, Fonneland I-L, Kvåle R, Strand K. Impact of the post-World War II generation on intensive care needs in Norway. Acta Anaesthesiol Scand. 2010;54(4):479–84.
13. Laporte L, Hermetet C, Jouan Y, et al. Ten-year trends in intensive care admissions for respiratory infections in the elderly. Ann Intensive Care. 2018;8(1):84.
14. Jones A, Toft-Petersen AP, Shankar-Hari M, Harrison DA, Rowan KM. Demographic shifts, case mix, activity, and outcome for elderly patients admitted to adult general ICUs in the United Kingdom, Wales, and Northern Ireland. Crit Care Med. 2020;48(4):466–74.
15. Weissman GE, Kerlin MP, Yuan Y, et al. Population trends in intensive care unit admissions in the United States among Medicare beneficiaries, 2006–2015. Ann Intern Med. 2019;170:213–5.
16. Docherty AB, Anderson NH, Walsh TS, et al. Equity of access to critical care among elderly patients in Scotland: a National Cohort Study. Crit Care Med. 2016;44(1):3–13.
17. Nielsson MS, Christiansen CF, Johansen MB, Rasmussen BS, Tønnesen E, Nørgaard M. Mortality in elderly ICU patients: a cohort study. Acta Anaesthesiol Scand. 2014;58(1):19–26.
18. Quill TE, Holloway R. Time-limited trials near the end of life. JAMA. 2011;306:1483–4.
19. Guidet B, Gerlach H, Rhodes A. Migrant crisis in Europe: implications for intensive care specialists. Intensive Care Med. 2016;42(2):249–51.
20. Guidet B, Flaatten H, Boumendil A, et al. Withholding or withdrawing of life-sustaining therapy in older adults (≥80 years) admitted to the intensive care unit. Intensive Care Med. 2018;44(7):1–12.

Objectives of ICU Management for Very Old Patients

Margaux Baqué, Sara Thietart, Judith Cohen-Bittan, Marc Verny, Lorène Zerah, and Jacques Boddaert

Contents

© The Author(s), under exclusive license to Springer Nature Switzerland AG 2022
H. Flaatten et al. (eds.), *The Very Old Critically Ill Patients*, Lessons from the ICU,
https://doi.org/10.1007/978-3-030-94133-8_2

2

> 🎓 **Learning Objectives**
> - The 1 + 2 + 3 model explains the concept of a geriatric syndrome and helps physicians to understand why older patients become frail and susceptible to diseases and organ failure.
> - Tools are needed to help admission decision, level of care adaptation, and ICU objectives, taken account on the old patient specificities.
> - Tight cooperation between intensivists, emergency physicians, and geriatricians is necessary.

2.1 Introduction

No clear cut-off age to define an old patient has been established. According to the World Health Organization (WHO) 2021 definitions, an old patient is defined a person aged 65 years or older. Studies evaluating older patients admitted in intensive care units (ICUs) use an age threshold which varied between 50 and over 90 years, although most papers included patients aged over 80 years. Geriatric management is proposed to patients aged over 75 years, although the weight of age is inferior to the weight of comorbidities and risk of loss of functional status.

The proportion of patients aged over 75 years is increasing, which is a great challenge for the healthcare system. In 2030, 12% of the French population will be over 75 years and is expected to continue increasing [1]. The impact of aging on healthcare resources is a major issue for the coming years.

2.2 Characteristics of Very Old Patients

There is not one unique "old patient" prototype. Some 80-year-old patients have the same physical and cognitive functions than a 20-year-old, whereas others have earlier functional decline. Each individual declines at a different rate, partially due to a decrease in physiological reserve, but mainly due to accumulation of comorbidities. Evolutionary biologists define aging as "an age-dependent or age-progressive decline in intrinsic physiological functions, leading to an increase in age-specific mortality rate and a decrease in age-specific reproductive rate." While aging seems to be a universal feature of life, there is a great variability of lifespan between human beings. There is a great heterogeneity in one's physiological reserve, mainly due the divergence between chronological and biological age with time. There have been attempts to describe and quantify biological age, but no quantitative evidence-based measures have yet been established for research or clinical purposes.

Homeostasis is the process through which the body maintains internal equilibrium. Aging is responsible for a progressive decrease in global functional and physiological reserve of each organ. This leads to a decreased resilience, when the patient is aggressed by an acute disorder. Homeostatic regulation of each system is slowly deregulated with time. In addition, when the body is submitted to a stress, such as exercise, trauma, an infection, or surgery, the body used its physiological reserve in order to maintain homeostasis. Therefore, more physiologic reserves are required to maintain homeostasis when the patient is exposed to an acute disorder, the body thus

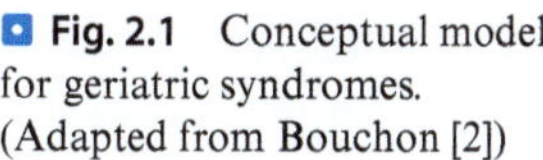

Fig. 2.1 Conceptual model for geriatric syndromes. (Adapted from Bouchon [2])

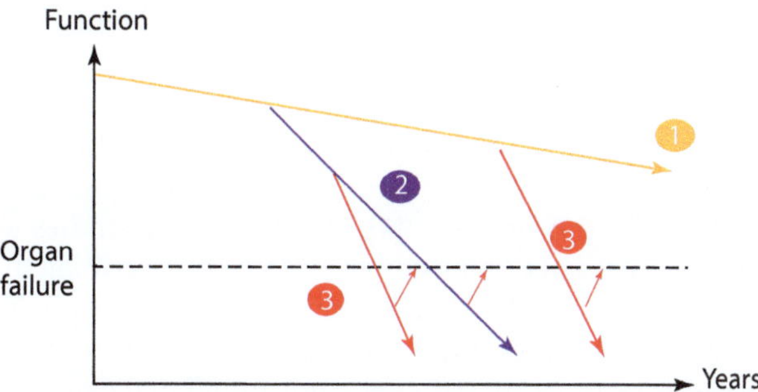

becoming less resistant. The greater the stress, the more physiological reserves are needed. As a result, an acute condition which could normally be easily overcome by a younger organ may overcome an older organ's physiological limit and lead to acute injury.

The 1 + 2 + 3 model (Fig. 2.1) summarizes the concept of decrease with age in physiological reserve. This model explains why older patients become frail, are susceptible to diseases and organ failure, and recover less from acute conditions. Bouchon defined in 1984 the concept of a geriatric syndrome using the 1 + 2 + 3 model (Fig. 2.1) representing three factors leading to a decline in an organ's reserve: physiological organ aging (1), pathological organ aging (2), and an acute stress factor (3). Only factors 2 and 3 can lead to organ failure.

All organs lose their functional reserve with age, but with different speed depending on the organ. The rapidity of its decline is variable and depends on patient's comorbidities, lifestyle, and hereditary background. Age-related physiological changes will be explained in the next chapter in detail.

When an older patient is hospitalized in an ICU, its baseline energy consumption is increased. Its energy reserves are thus diminished and are insufficient for other added stressful conditions, such as post-operative situations. The unbalance between energy needs and energy reserve increases with other factors: comorbidities, medication, social factors, and psychological conditions. For this reason, ICU admission was often refused to older patients, exclusively on the basis of their age. Aging of population has led to change this attitude, with an increase of ICU admissions of patients of 80 years or older. However, ICU admission in this population is burdened with high mortality, complications, and loss of functional status. Optimal triage and ICU care of older patient is therefore still a challenge.

2.3　ICU Admission of an Older Patient

2.3.1　Admission Criteria: What About Age?

No validated scale has been established to identify which patient should be admitted in an ICU. The intensivist who is considering admitting an older patient uses multiple criteria: comorbidities, organ dysfunctions requiring ICU admission, invasive procedures that are needed, and the patient's wish. Although the medical community agrees that age should not be the only criteria to be taken into consideration, a higher age was associated with an increased risk of refusing ICU admission. A prospective study, performed on 1009 patients in 25 centers, found that admission was refused to 283 patients (28%). Refusal of admission was independently associated with older age (>65 years) and poor health conditions [3]. Similar results were found in a monocentric prospective study, with 38% of non-admissions, age over 65 years being associated with this outcome [4]. However, these studies were not specifically performed on older patients. In a study prospectively describing the triage process of 180 patients aged >80 years, 26% were admitted in an ICU [5]. The reasons of refusal of ICU admission were refusal expressed by patient directives or by family and patient being too sick or too well. Another study found that causes of denial were an age >65 years and unavailability of ICU beds, using multivariate analysis [6]. Among them, 1981 were refused ICU admission because they were considered too well or too sick. Hospital mortality was 8% for patients considered as being "too well", 33% for those admitted in the ICU, and 68% for those considered "too sick." A 6-month mortality of patients considered as being "too well" for ICU stay was similar to those which were admitted in an ICU (41% vs. 48%) [7].

Other factors have to be taken into account in the triage process. In a prospective study following 2646 patients over 80 years with an acute condition theoretically needing ICU admission, patients were proposed to the intensivist by the emergency physician in only 31% of them. Among them, 16% were finally admitted to the ICU. Factors associated with the absence of proposal to the intensivist were age, active cancer, lack of information regarding way of living, a recent hospitalization, baseline functional status, and use of psychotropic drugs [8]. There is a high variability of admission of older patients in ICUs depending on hospital and ward policies and habits. One study found that admission of older patients varied between 30% and 6%, without finding any organizational reasons to explain these differences [8].

The proportion of older patients hospitalized in ICUs is increasing. Haas and colleagues have observed an increase in the proportion of patients aged >80 years in ICUs in the Netherlands, with a rise from 13.4% to 13.9% between 2005 and 2009 [9]. Other similar results were found in other countries: a rise from 11.7 to 13.8% between 2005 and 2011 in Denmark [10], from 11.5% to 15.3% from 1998 to 2008 in Austria [11], and an annual rise of 5.6% from 2000 to 2005 in Australia and New Zealand [12]. The only study finding a decrease was by Docherty and colleagues [13], with a decrease from 10% to 8.4% from 2005 to 2009. Another cohort of patients hospitalized in ICUs showed that in 10 years the median age of patients admitted in ICUs has increased by 5 years, whereas life expectancy has increased by 2.5 years [14]. In this cohort, 12% of admitted patients were older than 80 years. However, an important heterogeneity was observed from one center to another, which could be due to geographical specifities or to different admission policies.

2.3.2 Prognostic Tools for Older ICU Patients

Recent progress has been made on knowledge concerning factors associated with poor outcome such as mortality and morbidity in older patients. The weight of age and pre-existing diseases has reached 50% in the most recent severity of illness scoring systems. However, vulnerability of patients, which could be defined as the ability for an aged patient to face an acute and severe condition, should also be taken into account to predict outcome, in order to add the influence of physiological age rather than biological age. This vulnerability may be approached by the geriatric concept of frailty [15]. The gold standard for diagnosis of frailty is to consider it as a part of the comprehensive geriatric assessment (CGA), based on specific domains including physical, functional, cognitive, mobility, emotional, social, nutritional, and sarcopenia components. But this is complex and inadequate for emergency situations. For acute and emergency conditions, some tools have been used and validated [16–18] despite the best remains to be determined. Haas et al. [19] have found in a prospective cohort of very old patient admitted in ICU that age (5 years increase) but also frailty and severity of organ dysfunction are independently associated with 6-month mortality. But for ICU management of elderly patients, there is still a need to develop a reliable bedside tool to assess frailty, which could also be integrated in a prognostic model to predict outcome. It is not sure whether this tool will have enough discriminating power to be used for triage of older patients. Today, only multidisciplinary decision-making processes which integrate multiple variables (age, functional ability, comorbidities, acute disease) should be done by the intensivists for triage.

2.3.3 Admission Criteria and Pre-ICU Triage

Limited availability of ICU beds requires that triage should be performed before ICU admission: by the emergency physician, which decides or not to propose the patient to the intensivist, and by the intensivist himself. The Eldicus study [20] has found a dose-effect relation between age and non-admission in ICU (12% of non-admission under 45 years old, 36% over 85 years old), whereas survival of patients admitted in the ICU increases with age. Even though age is a key feature to take into account when performing triage, it is also important to determine what the expected benefit of admitting the patient in the ICU is. A French study did not find any benefit of admitting patients >75 years in an ICU, in comparison with those which were refused admission [21].

For older patients, triage process is based on the physician's ability to estimate the patient's capacity to survive, avoid severe functional decline, and maintain a correct quality of life. One must also take into consideration the patient's will. It is actually based on acute condition, comorbidities, and functional status determination. One can also be helped by scales predictive of mortality, such as the Acute Physiology and Chronic Health Evaluation (APACHE), the Simplified Acute Physiology Score (SAPS), and the Mortality Probability Model (MPM), although theses scales were not specifically designed for older patients. Other scores assess the presence of organ dysfunction during the ICU stay and its severity, such as the Sequential Organ Failure Assessment (SOFA) and the Multiple Organ Dysfunction Score (MODS). While these scores are widely used for patients hospitalized in an ICU, they are not designed for triage before ICU admission [22]. Frailty assessment could also help the intensivist in the triage process, but data are still lacking for ICU admission, as it is an important marker of biological age and an important predictor of outcome. The concept has been described in 1994 by Fried [15] but has been used by ICU physicians fairly recently. Although frailty is associated with increased age, not all of the older population is frail. It is defined as a clinical state of increased susceptibility to age-associated decline of reserve and function of a wide range of physiological systems [23].

2.4 What Are the Objectives of ICU Care in Older Patients?

Survivors of critical diseases suffer from long-term sequelae, with an increased risk of mortality, cognitive impairment, and functional disability [24, 25], with a lower quality-adjusted survival [26], independently of age at admission. Older patients also suffer from these long-term consequences, and its impact on this population can be heavier than the younger patients, due to heavy sedation, prolonged ventilation, immobilization, malnutrition, and more. An older ICU patient is at high risk of vulnerability and functional decline. A French cohort of patients >80 years admitted in an ICU showed that 63% either died or experienced functional decline [27]. A Canadian cohort study following up 610 older patients hospitalized at least 24 hours in an ICU reported an increased functional decline after 3 and 12 months, in comparison with an age- and gender-matched control group [28]. In this study 1-year mortality was similar between patients whom admission in an ICU was accepted or refused. However, Hoffman and colleagues [29] observed that long-term quality of life was poor in both studies but was similar to an age-matched population, thus suggesting a benefit of ICU admission in older patients. An important unachieved goal is to predict which older patient will have a high long-term survival rate and good quality of life after ICU discharge. In ICU patients of all age, factors associated with outcome are disease severity, socio-economic status, comorbidities, frailty at admission, and limitations in life-sustaining therapy [30]. In older ICU patients, baseline functional status and frailty weigh more on outcome than disease severity [31]. In this study, age also appeared to be independently associated with poor outcome. In a study evaluating 30-day mortality of 6205 patients with community-acquired pneumonia [32], the overall mortality rate was 8% and it increased with age. In this study, in the subgroup of patients with one comorbidity or none, mortality was similar between patients <65 years and those 65–79 years. However, in this subgroup, mortality was still higher among patients >80 years. These results suggest that when evaluating the risk of poor outcome, the cut-off of 80 years seems more appropriate than 65 years.

2.4.1 Time for Post ICU Geriatric Units?

Mortality 1 year after ICU admission varies from 40% to 70% among patients aged over 75 years [33]. Age is associated with 1-year mortality, independently of the reason of ICU admission (infection, respiratory failure, shock). Today, an older patient hospitalized in an ICU is managed by the intensivist, in cooperation with the referring geriatrician or physician. Specific geriatric ICUs are scarce [34] and most of these patients have never been evaluated by a geriatrician. In the presence of multimorbidity and functional risk, the geriatrician will have to play a crucial and additional role. First, before admission in the ICU there is a collegial discussion. Second, the geriatrician is involved in the level of care adaptation during ICU stay. Last, after ICU management, the geriatrician provides care for patients in dedicated acute geriatric units. This type of units, called geriatric post-ICU care units and requiring intermediate level of care, may also be used as alternative to ICU. As well, a care pathway approach may be the next cornerstone and challenge in management of elderly patients through ICU considerations. Considering care pathway from emergency department or direct

ICU admission, to geriatric unit and rehab units, and through geriatric post-ICU care unit stay will allow continuity of management, with special consideration for comorbidities, drug-related problems, and functional prognosis. The use of dedicated geriatric units to perioperative care was associated with better outcome in old patients after hip fracture surgery [35, 36]. For these reasons, projects of creating geriatric post-ICU care units are in progress, which will manage multimorbidity, prevent and treat further complications, and propose early rehabilitation [37]. A tight cooperation between intensivists, emergency physicians, and geriatricians is necessary. The aims of this cooperation are to optimize patient triage using validated prognostic tools specific to the older population, adapt critical care in older patients using adapted hypnotic medication, and improve rehabilitation immediately after ICU stay.

Practical Implications

- The population is aging due to decreased mortality as well as aging of the baby-boomer generation. Consequently, the amount of older patients admitted in ICUs is expected to continue increasing.
- Older patients have biological and functional specificities, with a decreased effectiveness in the response of an acute situation. So, ICU healthcare might find their place for old patient than might benefit the most of their specific treatment.
- There is no validated score for the triage process of older patients with a critical disease. Most decisions are taken based on age. There is a need for tools based on functional status and biological age.
- ICU stay is burdened by increased mortality, and specific integrated geriatric care should be proposed, before, during, and after ICU stay.

Conclusion

There is no one unique old patient prototype. Admission with needed tools, level of care, and objectives during ICU stay must be taken into account on each patient. Even after ICU, post-ICU care units are in development to optimize critically ill old patient management and improve their outcome.

Take-Home Messages

- The increase in demand of intensive care and shortage of ICU beds puts the intensivist in a difficult situation when making triage decisions. This is particularly true when facing an older patient requiring critical care, as its life expectancy is limited. Many countries are facing the problem of determining whether ICU care will ameliorate long-term survival.
- The triage process before admitting a patient in an ICU is different between younger and older patients. There is no ideal prognostic tool specific to older age, to predict the benefit of an ICU stay.
- Geriatric syndromes, such as frailty, sarcopenia, delirium, and cognitive disorders, probably play a major role on outcome.

References

1. Nathalie Blanpain et Guillemette Buisson, division Enquêtes et études démographiques, Insee. Projections de population à l'horizon 2070: Deux fois plus de personnes de 75 ans ou plus qu'en 2013. https://www.insee.fr/fr/statistiques

2. Bouchon JP. 1+2+3 ou comment tenter d'être efficace en gériatrie ? Rev Prat. 1984;34:888–92.

3. Azoulay E, Pochard F, Chevret S, Vinsonneau C, Garrouste M , Cohen Y et al.; PROTOCETIC Group. Compliance with triage to intensive care recommendations. Crit Care Med. 2001; 29: 2132–6.

4. Joynt GM, Gomersall CD, Tan P, Lee A, Cheng CA, Wong EL. Prospective evaluation of patients refused admission to an intensive care unit: triage, futility and outcome. Intensive Care Med. 2001;27:1459–65.

5. Garrouste-Orgeas M, Tabah A, Vesin A, Philippart F, Kpodji A, Bruel C, Grégoire C, Max A, Timsit JF, Misset B. The ETHICA study (part II): simulation study of determinants and variability of ICU physician decisions in patients aged 80 or over. Intensive Care Med. 2013;39:1574–83.

6. Garrouste-Orgeas M, Timsit JF, Montuclard L, Colvez A, Gattolliat O, Philippart F, Rigal G, Misset B, Carlet J. Decision-making process, outcome, and 1-year quality of life of octogenarians referred for intensive care unit admission. Intensive Care Med. 2006;32:1045–51.

7. Boumendil A, Angus DC, Guitonneau AL, Menn AM, Ginsburg C, Takun K, et al. Variability of intensive care admission decisions for the very elderly. PLoS One. 2012;7(4):e34387.

8. Garrouste-Orgeas M, Boumendil A, Pateron D, Aergerter P, Somme D, Simon T, Guidet B. Selection of intensive care unit admission criteria for patients aged 80 years and over and compliance of emergency and intensive care unit physicians with the selected criteria: an observational, multicenter, prospective study. Crit Care Med. 2009;37:2919–28.

9. Haas LEM, Karakus A, Holman R, Cihangir S, Reidinga AC, de Keizer NF. Trends in hospital and intensive care admissions in the Netherlands attributable to the very elderly in an ageing population. Crit Care. 2015;19:353.

10. Nielsson MS, Christiansen CF, Johansen MB, Rasmussen BS, Tønnesen E, Nørgaard M. Mortality in elderly ICU patients: a cohort study. Acta Anaesthesiol Scand. 2014;58(1):19–26.

11. Ihra GC, Lehberger J, Hochrieser H, Bauer P, Schmutz R, Metnitz B, et al. Development of demographics and outcome of very old critically ill patients admitted to intensive care units. Intensive Care Med. 2012;38(4):620–6.

12. Bagshaw SM, Webb SA, Delaney A, George C, Pilcher D, Hart GK, Bellomo R. Very old patients admitted to intensive care in Australia and New Zealand: a multi-centre cohort analysis. Crit Care. 2009;13(2):R45.

13. Docherty AB, Anderson NH, Walsh TS, Lone NI. Equity of access to critical care among elderly patients in Scotland: a national cohort study. Crit Care Med. 2016;44(1):3–13.

14. Guidet B, Boumendila A, Garrouste-Orgeas M, Pateron D. Admission en réanimation du sujet âgé à partir du service des urgences État des lieux Admitting elderly patients in intensive-care unit An emergency-department perspective. Réanimation. 2008;17(8):790–801.

15. Fried LP. Frailty. In: Hazzard WR, Bierman EL, Blass JP, Ettinger WH, Halter JB, editors. Principles of geriatric medicine and gerontology. 3rd ed. New York: McGraw-Hill, Inc; 1994. p. 1149–56.

16. Rockwood K, Song X, MacKnight C, et al. A global clinical measure of fitness and frailty in elderly people. CMAJ. 2005;173(5):489–95.

17. Le Manach Y, Collins G, Rodseth R, Le Bihan-Benjamin C, Biccard B, Riou B, Devereaux PJ, Landais P. Preoperative score to predict postoperative mortality (POSPOM): derivation and validation. Anesthesiology. 2016;124(3):570–9.

18. Moppett IK, Parker M, Griffiths R, Bowers T, White SM, Moran CG. Nottingham hip fracture score: longitudinal and multi-centre assessment. Br J Anaesth. 2012;109:546–50.

19. Haas LEM, Boumendil A, Flaatten H, Guidet B, Ibarz M, Jung C, Moreno R, Morandi A, Andersen FH, Zafeiridis T, Walther S, Oeyen S, Leaver S, Watson X, Boulanger C, Szczeklik W, Schefold JC, Cecconi M, Marsh B, Joannidis M, Nalapko Y, Elhadi M, Fjølner J, Artigas A, de Lange DW, VIP2 study group. Frailty is associated with long-term outcome in patients with sepsis who are over 80 years old: results from an observational study in 241 European ICUs. Age Ageing. 2021;50(5):1719–27.

20. Sprung CL, Artigas A, Kesecioglu J, Pezzi A, Wiis J, Pirracchio R, et al. The Eldicus prospective, observational study of triage decision making in European intensive care units. Part II: intensive care benefit for the elderly. Crit Care Med. 2012;40:132–8.

21. Le Guen J, Boumendil A, Guidet B, Corvol A, Saint-Jean O, Somme D. Are elderly patients' opinions sought before admission to an intensive care unit? Results of the ICE-CUB study. Age Ageing. 2016;45(2):303–9.

22. Guidet B, Thomas C, Leblanc G, Boumendil A, Pateron D. Postoperative admission to the intensive care unit. Perioperative care of the elderly. Cambridge University Press; 2018. p. 277–82.

23. Qian-Li X. The frailty syndrome: definition and natural history. Clin Geriatr Med. 2011;27(1): 1–15.

24. Pandharipande PP, Girard TD, Jackson JC, Morandi A, Thompson JL, Pun BT, Brummel NE, Hughes CG, Vasilevskis EE, Shintani AK, Moons KG, Geevarghese SK, Canonico A, Hopkins RO, Bernard GR, Dittus RS, Ely EW, The BRAIN-ICU Study Investigators. Long-term cognitive impairment after critical illness. N Engl J Med. 2013;369:1306–16.

25. Iwashyna TJ, Ely EW, Smith DM, Langa KM. Long-term cognitive impairment and functional disability among survivors of severe sepsis. JAMA. 2010;304:1787–94.

26. Angus DC, Musthafa AA, Clermont G, Griffin MF, Linde-Zwirble WT, Dremsizov TT, Pinsky MR. Quality-adjusted survival in the first year after the acute respiratory distress syndrome. Am J Respir Crit Care Med. 2001;163:1389–94.

27. Boumendil A, Aegerter P, Guidet B, CUB-Rea Network. Treatment intensity and outcome of patients aged 80 and older in intensive care units: a multicenter matched-cohort study. J Am Geriatr Soc. 2005;53:88–93.

28. Heyland DK, Garland A, Bagshaw SM, Cook D, Rockwood K, Stelfox HT, et al. Recovery after critical illness in patients aged 80 years or older: a multi-center prospective observational cohort study. Intensive Care Med. 2015;41:1911–20.

29. Hoffman KR, Loong B, Haren FV. Very old patients urgently referred to the intensive care unit: long-term outcomes for admitted and declined patients. Crit Care Resusc. 2016;

30. Flaatten H, de Lange DW, Artigas A, et al. The status of intensive care medicine research and a future agenda for very old patients in the ICU. Intensive Care Med. 2017;43:1319–28. https://doi. org/10.1007/s00134-017-4718-z.

31. Boumendil A, Somme D, Garrouste-Orgeas M, Guidet B. Should elderly patients be admitted to the intensive care unit? Intensive Care Med. 2007;33:1252–62.

32. Kaplan V, Clermont G, Griffin MF, Kasal J, Watson RS, Linde-Zwirble WT, Angus DC. Pneumonia: still the old man's friend? Arch Intern Med. 2003;163(3):317–23.

33. Boumendil A, Latouche A, Guidet B, ICE-CUB Study Group. On the benefit of intensive care for very old patients. Arch Intern Med. 2011;171:1116–7.

34. Zeng A, Song X, Dong J, Mitnitski A, Liu J, Guo Z, et al. Mortality in relation to frailty in patients admitted to a specialized geriatric intensive care unit. J Gerontol A Biol Sci Med Sci. 2015;70:1586–94.

35. Boddaert J, Cohen-Bittan J, Khiami F, Le Manach Y, Raux M, Beinis J-Y, et al. Postoperative admission to a dedicated geriatric unit decreases mortality in elderly patients with hip fracture. PLoS One. 2014;9(1):e83795.

36. Moyet J, Deschasse G, Marquant B, et al. Which is the optimal orthogeriatric care model to prevent mortality of elderly subjects post hip fractures? A systematic review and meta-analysis based on current clinical practice. Int Orthop (SICOT). 2019;43:1449–54.

37. Vallet H, Cohen-Biitan J, Boddaert J. Lifelines of intensive care medicine in elderly patients. Reanimation. 2015;24:351–3.

Age-Related Physiological Changes

Contents

Aged-Related Physiological Changes: CNS Function

Stéphanie Miot, Raphaël Chancel, and Hubert Blain

Contents

> **ℹ Learning Objectives**
>
> The central nervous system (CNS) is a complex entity characterised by lots of cells organised in networks, and has various functions. In this chapter, we will expose CNS normal ageing at a molecular, cellular, and functional level, in order to better understand the interdependence of CNS age-related changes. It will highlight intensive care issues in older people from the point of view of our brain.

3.1 Introduction

There is no one but a multitude of ageing. Phenotype is the result of interactions between our genes (genome) and our lifelong exposures (exposome). If our genome is inborn, our exposome depends on our life. The more we live, the more we are exposed. So the human phenotype heterogeneity is even more visible in older people because ageing implies longer and more various environmental exposures. The central nervous system (CNS) exposure to environment is complex because of its brain-blood barrier (BBB) selectivity, the prolonged survival of neurons even more chronically exposed, and its high sensitivity to low-level chronic exposures [1]. This specificity participates in the heterogeneity of CNS ageing.

CNS functioning can be considered at different levels: molecular, histological, neuroanatomical, etc. focusing on one element or on networks. This multimodal and integrative functioning can also explain that normal CNS ageing in older people is not uniform. Furthermore, CNS is involved not only in cognitive functions but also in motility, affective processes, or stress regulations.

So normal CNS ageing encompasses a range of processes and clinical presentations. Here the question will be explored artificially to make matters clearer, in addressing first ageing of CNS (at cellular and neuroanatomical levels) and second consequences of normal ageing for CNS functions (cognitive, movement, and affective aspects) considering the underlying physiological processes.

3.2 CNS Ageing

3.2.1 General Cellular Age-Related Changes in the Brain

Senescence and some molecular processes due to ageing affect the whole brain.

3.2.1.1 β-Amyloid and Tau Protein Accumulation

CNS ageing is characterised by β-amyloid deposition and Tau aggregation in brain tissue.

Aβ(1–40) and Aβ(1–42/43) peptides are produced by secretases' action on β-amyloid precursor protein. These Aβ proteins are enriched in β sheets, which confer to them a higher tendency to self-aggregate, leading to extracellular β-amyloid deposits. These amyloid plaques are more frequent in oldest old and even those who have intact cognitive functioning [2]. Neurofibrillary tangles (NFT) are intracellular hyperphosphorylated Tau protein accumulation, inducing cytoskeletal structure weakening [3]. NFT can be observed in normal ageing, but its number is correlated with cognitive decline, in particular in hippocampus, entorhinal cortex, and area 9 [4]. Furthermore, β-amyloid aggregates potentiate NFT and participate in neural hypoactivity during ageing [5]. Clearance of β-amyloid aggregates and NFT is provided by microglia and astrocytes [6], and their accumulation seems to follow a continuum between normal and pathological brain ageing.

3.2.1.2 Autophagia

Cellular wastes' recycling is also essential for cell survival. This turnover is provided by lysosomes into the autophagic process, which decreases in normal ageing [7]. This leads to aggregation of altered proteins as Lewy bodies or neurofibrillary, and impaired lipids as lipofuscin commonly names intracellular pigments [8]. This autophagy dysregulation affects neurons but also microglia and is involved in neuroinflammation [9].

3.2.1.3 Oxidative Stress

Oxidative stress is common in ageing [10]. In the brain, oxidative damages induce high mitochondrial DNA mutation accumulation [11], lipid peroxidation correlated with cognitive decline [12], and protein oxidation as carbonyl accumulation in hippocampus associated with memory impairment [13]. Furthermore, this oxidative stress plays a key role in neuroinflammation and microglia activation in a bidirectional process. Chronic reactive oxygen species production induces microglia activation, and prolonged inflammation induces exhaustion of antioxidant defences reserved in microglia [14].

3.2.1.4 Neuroinflammation

Another challenge for ageing CNS is the neuroinflammation process. Acute inflammatory response produces some pro-inflammatory cytokines as Il-1β, TNF-α, or Il-6 at the peripheral level but also into the brain, leading to microglia activation. In young individuals, this pro-inflammatory response is modest and short, while it is higher and longer in older people [15]. At a steady state, we can observe pro-inflammatory cytokine over-expression (IL-1β and IL-6) [16], decrease of anti-inflammatory cytokines (e.g. IL-4 or IL-10) [17], and a microglia sensitisation in the ageing brain, inducing a hyper-reactivity to peripheral or central injury. While various molecular processes (e.g. autophagy or oxidative stress) are involved in neuroinflammation, lot of brain cells participate in neuroinflammation. During acute or chronic neuroinflammation, neurons, astrocytes, or microglia are indeed acting in a complex interaction and balance between these three cellular types. Because brain cells have a long lifespan, this neuroinflammation seems to have a cumulative effect inducing senescence and loss of function [18].

3.2.2 Specific Cellular Type Age-Related Changes in the Brain

The human brain is composed of billions of neurons and non-neural cells [19], diversely impacted by ageing processes.

3.2.2.1 Neurone

Considered for a long time as the principal component of the brain, neurons are affected by ageing at a cellular and network level.

Intraneuronal injection of current induces an action potential characterised by depolarisation followed by afterhyperpolarisation (AHP), when membrane potential is under the resting potential, before a new increase to resting state. The larger the AHP is, the longer the refractory period is. So this AHP amplitude determines the neuron ability to have a firing activity. In old neurons, AHP amplitude increases, in particular in hippocampus neurons [20], leading to a decreased neuron excitability and plasticity in vitro. Even if this reduced firing is not observed in vivo, or only if rodents are exposed to a novel environment [21], it could reduce neuron plasticity when exposed to extreme stimuli. Lower synaptic plasticity is also observed in senescent neurons, with higher long-term potentiation (LTP) activation thresholds due to longer and larger AHP [22] but also to post-synaptic receptor (e.g. NMDA) activation reduction [23].

These age-related changes can affect neuron connectivity and increase neurotoxicity [24]. Neurogenesis decreases with age [25] and takes also part in this neuron loss. This slowing of neuronal production is drastic and early in hippocampus [26] and can be observed less or more in all neurogenesis area in adult (subventricular zone and olfactory epithelium) [27, 28]. This brain senescence is influenced by stress and glucocorticoids [29] but also by some neurotransmitters as glutamate [30] and inflammation [31] in a complex balance and threshold effects. Nevertheless, exercise and enriched environment upregulate neurogenesis even in the aged brain [32, 33].

All of these senescent mechanisms in neurons have been studied largely in hippocampus and have memory effects. This neuron loss seems to be brain region dependent and localised in the cortex [34], while the subcortical atrophy is essentially due to axonal impairment due to neuroglia ageing.

3.2.2.2 Neuroglia

In the CNS, myelin from oligodendrocytes isolate axons for faster depolarisation transmission. In transmission electronic microscopy, ageing myelin shows cytoplasmic electron-dense pockets corresponding to proteasome accumulation [35] and is correlated with cognitive decline [36]. A loss of nerve fibres is observed in the ageing brain [37]. But the upregulation of genes implicated in oligodendrocytes activity is in favour of a compensation of this myelin degeneration by a remyelination process [38]. Nevertheless, this continuous production of myelin by oligodendrocytes is less efficient with thinner myelin layers, aberrant paranodal loops, and increased internodal length [39], leading to a myelin plasticity decrease [40].

Neuron microenvironment is also composed of astrocytes, in contact with synapses and blood capillaries. Astrocytes are hypertrophic with age, and inclusions of myelin are observed in their cytoplasm, indicating a phagocytosis activity [41]. They also play an essential role in oxidative stress and neuroinflammation response during ageing, in particular though glutathione production [42] and autophagy activity [43]. Astrocytes are also immune cells releasing cytokines. They prevent neurodegeneration thanks to neurotrophic factors release as GDNF [44], control microglia trafficking, and are able to activate microglia to promote inflammatory response [45].

3.2.2.3 **Microglia**

Microglia activity is modulated by astrocytes but is also able to regulate astrocyte activity [46]. Microglia have, as astrocyte, a phagocytosis function in the CNS increasing with age [47]. Microglial cells are activated by brain injury, stroke, trauma, neurotoxic protein, or pro-inflammatory cytokines. They have a lifelong evolving specific profile [48, 49], and play a key role in immune response and brain homeostasis. In normal adult brain of mice, microglial disappearance does not affect behavioural and cognitive task [50]. Nevertheless, microglia can modulate glutamate transporter expression in response to excitotoxicity [51] and influence synaptic activity [52], while neurons produce some neurotransmitters, purines, or cytokines acting as activator or inhibitor of the microglia phenotype [53, 54]. And disruption of this *on-off balance* between microglia and neurons induces cognitive impairment [54, 55]. Furthermore, ageing induces a translation of microglia from a "non-inflammatory" state to an activated or "primed" state, reducing neuroprotection and increasing neuroinflammation [56]. Aged brain microglia are more sensitive to pro-inflammatory stimuli so that chronic neuroinflammation is maintained longer and higher [42].

Microglia play also a role in neurogenesis. As discussed above, neurogenesis consists in the production of new neurons but also in their integration into an already existing neuron network without dying [57]. Astrocytes are essential to include new neurons in synaptic circuit [58], but microglia are also important to favour neuron survival by releasing growth factors [59] and regulating neuroinflammation in a complex balance with not too much [60] but not too less activation [61].

3.2.2.4 **Vascular Unit**

The brain is principally composed of neurons, glial cells (oligodendrocytes, astrocytes, and microglia), and vessels. Microvascular density, plasticity, and integrity decrease with age, inducing lower perfusion and higher permeability [62]. Age-related microvessel impairment is associated with β-amyloid aggregates [63], oxidative stress [64], and neuroinflammation [65]. Astrocytes are essential for the communication between neurons and vascular cells, so that their senescence could also have an impact on vascular unit functioning in the ageing CNS [66]. The aged-related adaptation loss of vascular response to neuronal activity, called neurovascular uncoupling, is indeed correlated with cognitive decline [67]. Furthermore, the brain-blood barrier permeability increases with age and is associated with neuroinflammation [68].

Thus, various molecular and cellular age-related changes are observed in CNS ageing and are closely interdependent with over-activation loops.

3.2.3 **Specific Anatomical Age-Related Changes in the Brain**

These molecular and cellular age-related changes are ubiquitous in the brain, so that we can observe some global anatomical modifications during ageing as cortical atrophy and connectivity decrease. Nevertheless, some areas are more affected by ageing, due to their energy or neurogenesis dependence.

3.2.3.1 Global Age-Related Variations

Functional MRI studies have shown a significant effect of age on the decrease of cortical grey matter and white matter volume [69].

The grey matter becomes thinner with age, with greater ventricular and cerebrospinal fluid volume [70]. This grey matter atrophy is more pronounced in the frontal and temporal cortex and in the striatum and thalamus [71]. The primary motor cortex and somatosensory cortex seem also to be affected [70]. This grey matter impairment seems to be more due to dendritic arborisation and synapse reduction than to neuron loss itself [72].

The loss of white matter is observed in all brain area [73] and is later but faster than grey matter decline [74]. This is due to a length of nerve fibre reduction from 10% to 45% [75], in particular in the frontal lobe [76] and corpus callosum [77], following an anterior to posterior gradient [78, 79]. This leads to brain disconnectivity [80] associated with cognitive decline [81]. This white matter impairment reflects the myelin impairment in older brain [79].

Some brain areas are more vulnerable to ageing, or their age-related activity decrease is more clinically noisy.

3.2.3.2 PFC and Dopamine System

The prefrontal cortex (PFC) and the reward circuit are the most affected brain areas of ageing. A structural decline is observed with the highest decrease of grey matter volume [82] estimated at about 5% per decade after 20 years old [83]. Striatum, which projects dopamine afferences on the PFC, shows also an age-related decrease of its grey matter volume around 3% per decade [84]. The white matter is also altered in the PFC and anterior corpus callosum, more than the other brain regions [85]. A functional decline of PFC is also observed in older adults when they are submitted to a complex cognitive task. For example, during a simple working memory task, older adults require more PFC activation than younger adults to obtain the same performance level [86]. But this compensatory phenomenon is no more sufficient for difficult working memory tasks [87]. Concurrently, a dopamine system decline is observed in older adults, with a continuous decrease of dopamine transporter (DAT) and D2 receptor expressions in the reward circuit – including striatum and PFC – after 40 years old [88–90]. Finally, this is the structural, functional, and connectivity of the whole fronto-striato-thalamic circuit that seems to be impaired in older people and could be a biomarker of cognitive decline in the future [91].

3.2.3.3 Hippocampus and Cholinergic System

The hippocampus is another brain area essential for cognition. If its volume decreases significantly in Alzheimer's disease, most of studies did not reveal a hippocampal volume impairment in healthy older adults [92]. Age-related changes in the hippocampus seem to affect especially its functioning. Thus, hippocampus cerebrovascular reactivity decreases with age and is associated with cognitive complaints in older adults [93]. In a more comprehensive way, the cholinergic system, including hippocampus, is modified in the ageing brain.

Cholinergic afferences from the basal forebrain modulate cognition in the hippocampus [94], and waking state and behaviour (in particular anxiety) in the thalamus and central tegmental area (VTA) [95]. These cholinergic neurons seem to be more sensitive to age-related energy deprivation [96], partially explaining memory impairment during ageing. Indeed, the cholinergic system implies also non-neuronal cells which express cholinergic receptors: microglia and astrocytes [97]. There is a bidirectional relationship between cholinergic neurons and these glial cells: loss of cholinergic neurons overactivates microglia and induces chronic inflammation, while acetylcholine release has an anti-inflammatory effect through activation of α7nAChR, a cholinergic receptor expressed by astrocytes and microglia [98]. So age-related impairment of the cholinergic pathway has a direct impact on cognition and emotion but also has a more global effect by over-activating neuroinflammation. The disruption of the homeostasis between the pro- and anti-inflammatory role of the cholinergic system and the vicious circle induced by loss of cholinergic afferences could explain the growing neurodegenerative disease emergence with age.

Thus, global and specific anatomical age-related changes are observed in CNS ageing. Functional systems are more affected, than specific regions, following an anterior to posterior gradient. And here again underlying molecular and cellular processes involve neuroinflammation.

3.3 Ageing Consequences for CNS Functions

3.3.1 Cognitive Profile

Because brain structure and function vary according to brain area and individuals, age-related cognitive function changes are not uniform. Some cognitive functions are more impacted by ageing, as attention or memory, but ageing tends to affect the whole brain functions.

3.3.1.1 Attention

We can describe several attention subtypes.

Selective attention refers to the ability to treat effectively and fast one relevant information to perform a task. The subject needs to discriminate targets and distractors. This selective attention can be intentional when we are looking for a specific object in a complex environment (e.g. your pink sock in the laundry hamper), or non-intentional when our attention capture is activated by an external stimulus (e.g. the shout of your son in the hubbub of his birthday party). In research, selective attention can be assessed using visual search, in particular with letters or words. Rather than looking for socks, participants have to identify one letter or word among distractors (with close physical or conceptual similarities). Latency and error number are collected and are significantly higher in older people [99]. But this difference could be due to perception impairment or cognitive and motor slowdown, so that selective attention could be intact in older people.

Furthermore, older people are able to anticipate the selection of stimuli if they have been informed before the task, as well as younger participants [100]. The information accumulation between the tests can also increase performances, and this perceptual priming is also preserved in healthy older people [101]. Finally, inhibition – that is to say the ability to exclude distractors, also called Stroop effect – is less efficient in older people [102]. But differences between younger and older people disappear when participants' attention is guided by environmental input [103]. So processes modulating selective attention seem to be largely preserved in older people.

Divided attention is the ability to pay attention to several information at the same time, for example, when you are looking for your pink socks and your green T-shirt in the laundry hamper. Older people can integrate several objects in their environment, even if these objects are in movement, but they do it slower and they need to be focused on fewer objects than younger adults [104].

Sustained attention depends essentially on vigilance to capture rare event during an attention task. Almost all studies have showed a decrease of sustained attention in older people [105].

If attention is more or less impaired by ageing, it is also essential for other cognitive function, as memory or decision making.

3.3.1.2 Memory

There are several memories: working memory, episodic memory, semantic memory, implicit memory, and procedural memory. Working memory is characterised by the ability to store and treat some information to realise a current task, for example, when you have to remember to buy new pink socks during your shopping. The four other memories are long-term memories: declarative for episodic memory (related to personal experience) and semantic memory (corresponding to knowledge storage), non-declarative for implicit memory (non-intentional), and procedural memory (perceptive, motor, and cognitive skills) which facilitates a performance. Ageing of these different memories is differential and heterogeneous.

Working memory is impaired in older adults [106] but the mechanism of this decline is controversial, probably because cognitive tasks used in previous studies are very diverse and assess different modulators of working memory. Attention impairment can explain encoding difficulties [107]. As for attention, age-related general slowing can affect working memory [108], in particular for inhibitory control decrease [109]. But external support remains able to improve working memory performances in older people [110].

Episodic memory is the frailest memory during ageing. It depends on encoding and storage, so it is affected as working memory. But it implies also retrieval processes, which decline with age [111]. This episodic memory impairment plays a role in false recognitions [112], even more when older people are exposed to perceptual similarities [113].

Semantic memory remains intact in ageing, even if older people have a significant higher latency during tests [114].

Implicit memory and ***procedural memory*** act as priming for other cognitive or motor tasks. Their exploration is various so that results of studies are conflicting [101, 115, 116], but implicit learning, influenced by implicit memory, largely remains intact in older people [117].

3.3.1.3 Decision Making

At a higher level of complexity, decision making can be affected by cognitive ageing. This cognitive process involves attention, working memory, but also episodic memory, flexibility, and emotional aspects. Experiments in decision making show an aged-related decline in performances associated with heterogeneous changes in strategy selection [118]. Here again modulators remain efficient in healthy older people, in particular attention training [119].

All of these cognitive functions depend essentially on the most brain regions affected by ageing: prefrontal cortex in its structural and functional decline and hippocampus in its functional decline [111]. They depend also on the age-related connectivity impairment [120]. PFC white matter integrity disruption is indeed associated with processing speed, attention control (in particular in Stroop task), and memory decline in healthy older people [121, 122]. Furthermore, most of these cognitive functions depend on pre-existing expertise level for a specific task, cognitive reserve [123, 124], and physical activity [125, 126], probably at the origin of the clinical heterogeneity in healthy older adults.

3.3.2 Movement

Movement is another CNS function that can be damaged by ageing. Mild motor signs are described in healthy ageing: gait and movement coordination decrease or movement slowing down. Furthermore, older people show less efficient movements with more variability [127]. Besides peripheral processes involving peripheral nervous and neuromuscular systems, ageing can also affect the central control of movement.

3.3.2.1 Functional Dispersion of Motor CNS Activity

A structural impairment of the CNS motor system is observed in healthy ageing with the atrophy of motor cortex and striatum (▶ Sect. 3.2.3). White matter reduction could also have consequences on movement in older people. For example, motor-skills learning seems to depend on new oligodendrocyte production [128], so that myelin plasticity reduction by ageing could reduce this motor ability.

At a functional level, older people have a higher activity in some motor brain areas during motor task compared to younger people. For example, when they move their right hand, their left motor cortex is more activated than in younger adults [129]. During more complex motor tasks, activation of non-motor systems is also observed in older people in comparison to younger people [130]. This over-activation and over-recruitment can be explained by two theories: the de-differentiation and the compensation. First, older people could have less abilities to use relevant neuronal networks for motor task [131]. This over-recruitment would be a kind of background noise of their non-specific response. Second, the connectivity between motor networks increases in healthy older people [132]. The recruitment of areas spanning motor and cognitive functions as prefrontal and sensorimotor cortex [133, 134] could also lead to an equal performance in older people by improving attention and integrative functions [135, 136]. These phenomena could compensate for the impairment of peripheral and primary central motor systems, as far as homeostasis is disrupted.

3.3.2.2 Movement and Cognition

If cholinergic system is especially involved in cognition, dopamine is essential for movement. Balance and fine motor decrease is associated with striatal dopamine system impairment in older people [137, 138]. Furthermore, emotional status can impact movement, by affecting motivation, such as in psychomotor slowing induced by depression [139]. Cognition is also closely associated with dopamine thought executive functions and movement.

In fact movement is not only a question of motor control. Dual tasks implicating motor and cognitive activity are harder to perform for healthy older people, because of neural resource availability reduction, when some brain areas are already over-recruited for by a single task [140], in particular for prefrontal cortex [141].

Embodiment is an emergent concept, which converges movement and cognition. Embodiment refers to cognitive processes, emotions, body perception, and movement relationships. Current evidences show that embodiment seems to be affected by ageing [142]. This embodiment impairment can affect movement, orientation, attention, but also empathy and social abilities. Motor impairment, processing speed, attention, and multisensory integration decline are some explanations of this embodiment age-related impairment [143]. Mirror neurons, which are essential for embodiment, show an anterior to posterior degeneration that could also affect embodiment [144].

Thus, the anterior to posterior gradient and dopamine system impairment in ageing are here central in the movement and more globally embodiment age-related decline.

3.3.3 Affective and Emotional Aspects

The CNS is involved in an even more complex function, among others related to movement and cognition thought embodiment: affective and emotional phenotype.

3.3.3.1 Late-Onset Disorders

Inter-individual heterogeneity in cognitive ageing trajectories can be explained by the concept of cognitive reserve. Indeed, only 50% of cognitive decline degree differences in older people are explained by neuropathology [145]. The other half is probably associated with the cognitive reserve, resulting in the interaction between exposome (from environment to lifelong experiences) and genome [146]. This individual predisposition controls brain resistance or maintenance, that is to say the ability of the brain to repair to an insult. It controls also brain resilience, that is to say the ability of the brain to adapt to an engaged pathological process. Furthermore, this cognitive reserve is closely related to prefrontal cortex activity [147].

In psychiatry, lots of diseases are associated with prefrontal cortex hypomyelinisation and dysfunction and neuroinflammation [148, 149]. Patients suffering from early-onset bipolar disorders or schizophrenia are at high risk to develop neurocognitive disorders [150], in particular frontotemporal dementia [148], because ageing processes are cumulated with this frontal fragility and inflammageing. Besides, some patients without any psychiatric history have late-onset psychiatric disorders, with a frontal fragility [148]. Moreover, it is sometimes difficult to determine if these late-onset psychiatric disorders are only prodromal symptoms of neurocognitive disorders [151, 152], in particular of frontotemporal dementia. Thus, cognitive reserve and pre-existing PFC plasticity could modulate the pathological ageing in early-onset psychiatric disorders and the late-onset psychiatric disorder emergence: the less the older people have a cognitive reserve, the less they have the ability to adapt on a cognitive but also emotional level during ageing. One more time, anterior to posterior neurodegeneration gradient and neuroinflammation seem to have a key role. When ageing progresses, homeostasis can be disrupted and the older people can "fall over" into the disease.

3.3.3.2 **Personality**

When the frontier between normal and pathological is not easy to define, a dimensional approach can be performed, what is particularly relevant in personality studies. Personality is a combination of patterns determining emotional, interpersonal experience, attitude, and motivation of a subject [153]. Personality traits can be defined by the five theory models, including five factors of personality: neuroticism (tendency to experience negative emotions), extraversion (tendency to experience positive emotion and to be involved in social communication), openness to experience, agreeableness (tendency to be empathic and pleasant), and conscientiousness (tendency to be careful, perfectionist, far-sighted, but also more compulsive and less cognitive flexible) [154]. Personality traits tend to change with age, and older people have higher conscientiousness and agreeableness, and less extraversion [155]. Neuroticism seems to be more stable but is predictive for late-onset depression [156] and neurocognitive disorders [157]. These personality traits are associated with structural and functional brain patterns, involving in particular the grey and white matter volume and the activity of the prefrontal cortex [158–160]. This PFC implication in extraversion and neuroticism seems to be specific of older people [161] [158, 160], and it could be at least in part the modulator of personality age-related changes.

3.3.3.3 **Well-Being Paradox**

Personality traits are also associated with well-being feeling [162]. Paradoxically, even if ageing is the time of decline and bereavement, stressors have less impact on older people than younger people [163], thanks to more resilience and less negative affects in healthy older people [164, 165]. Because of a change of time perspective in old age, the motivation to increase positive affects and reduce negative affects is improved. This well-being paradox depends on coping strategies [166], on cultural models [167], but also on semantic autobiographical memory cognitive functions most preserved during healthy ageing [168]. Other cognitive functions do not influence subjective well-being, leading to its stability in older people [169]. Another explanation could be a survival bias, because well-being improves life expectancy [170] so that oldest old people expressing a high life satisfactory could have been selected in studies.

Thus, frontal age-related changes and neuroinflammation are key to understand some affective and emotional particularities in older people.

Practical Implications

- CNS ageing embodies more than other system the difficulty to define a frontier between normal and pathology in older people. It has to be considered as a continuum, with a frailest homeostasis in older people due to brain reserve decline. Older brain is in a hypersensitivity state so that its vulnerability to stress is higher.
- Because of the cholinergic system impairment, anticholinergic drugs have to be carefully used.
- Longer time laps, higher fatigue, and cognitive over-recruitment have to be considered when caring for healthy older people.

- Frontal vulnerability can produce specific disorders when brain reserve is over-requested, with, for example, more frequently manic, catatonic, or dysexecutive symptom emergence.
- Resilience of older people and their environment have also to be assessed in order to better address them after an acute event, because it could be a source of rehabilitation.

Conclusion

An intensive care hospitalisation is an acute stress for patients and is a strong challenge for the ageing CNS. Microglia are already sub-activated in older people and are over-reactive. Furthermore, the high rates of glucocorticoids due to chronic stress induce oxidative stress, which increase dramatically brain vulnerability in ageing [171]. Some cumulative exposures can also induce pressure on our genes' expression and accelerate epigenetic ageing [172]. Thus, an over-request of older CNS could disrupt its homeostasis and cause more severe and faster decline due to a kind of racing of the ageing processes.

Moreover, this higher vulnerability depends on interdependent processes, with complex interactions between neurons, glia, and vascular unit, but also an adaptability loss at cellular (e.g. as neuron firing decreases), network (as cholinergic, dopamine, or frontal systems decline), and finally functional (as cognitive or affective reserve) levels.

Finally, CNS ageing reveals the lifelong and normal to pathological continuum in humans. If the frontal system is more sensitive to ageing because of its phylogenetically more recent status [173], it is also more sensitive to environmental exposures [174]. Environment can also be helpful to reduce the ageing impact on this CNS frailty, because it can improve lots of processes involved in ageing, as neuronal firing, neurogenesis, attention abilities, working memory, or well-being. It could support the maintenance of a sub-threshold CNS recruitment to allow older people to access resilience and what developmental psychologists name "gerotranscendence" [175].

Take-Home Messages

- A complex synergy between molecular, cellular, and functional processes is observed in CNS normal ageing, with a particular key role of neuroinflammation and antero-posterior impairment gradient.
- This normal ageing has cognitive but also motor and affective consequences, in a multimodal and interdependence perspective.
- Brain reserve can be an explanation of heterogeneity in CNS ageing but also of emergence of late-onset disorders and brain vulnerability to acute and chronic stress.

Conflict of Interest   None

References

1. Heffernan AL, Hare DJ. Tracing environmental exposure from neurodevelopment to neurodegeneration. Trends Neurosci. 2018;41(8):496–501.
2. Gold G, Bouras C, Kovari E, Canuto A, Glaria BG, Malky A, et al. Clinical validity of Braak neuropathological staging in the oldest-old. Acta Neuropathol. 2000;99(5):579–82; discussion 83–4.
3. Maccioni RB, Cambiazo V. Role of microtubule-associated proteins in the control of microtubule assembly. Physiol Rev. 1995;75(4):835–64.
4. Bouras C, Hof PR, Morrison JH. Neurofibrillary tangle densities in the hippocampal formation in a non-demented population define subgroups of patients with differential early pathologic changes. Neurosci Lett. 1993;153(2):131–5.
5. Zhang K, Mizuma H, Zhang X, Takahashi K, Jin C, Song F, et al. PET imaging of neural activity, beta-amyloid, and tau in normal brain aging. Eur J Nucl Med Mol Imaging. 2021;
6. Clayton KA, Van Enoo AA, Ikezu T. Alzheimer's disease: the role of microglia in brain homeostasis and proteopathy. Front Neurosci. 2017;11:680.
7. Wong SQ, Kumar AV, Mills J, Lapierre LR. Autophagy in aging and longevity. Hum Genet. 2020;139(3):277–90.
8. Keller JN, Dimayuga E, Chen Q, Thorpe J, Gee J, Ding Q. Autophagy, proteasomes, lipofuscin, and oxidative stress in the aging brain. Int J Biochem Cell Biol. 2004;36(12):2376–91.
9. Plaza-Zabala A, Sierra-Torre V, Sierra A. Autophagy and microglia: novel partners in neurodegeneration and aging. Int J Mol Sci. 2017;18(3)
10. Harman D. Aging: a theory based on free radical and radiation chemistry. J Gerontol. 1956;11(3):298–300.
11. Santos RX, Correia SC, Zhu X, Smith MA, Moreira PI, Castellani RJ, et al. Mitochondrial DNA oxidative damage and repair in aging and Alzheimer's disease. Antioxid Redox Signal. 2013;18(18):2444–57.
12. Pratico D, Sung S. Lipid peroxidation and oxidative imbalance: early functional events in Alzheimer's disease. J Alzheimers Dis. 2004;6(2):171–5.
13. Nicolle MM, Gonzalez J, Sugaya K, Baskerville KA, Bryan D, Lund K, et al. Signatures of hippocampal oxidative stress in aged spatial learning-impaired rodents. Neuroscience. 2001;107(3): 415–31.
14. Gemma C, Vila J, Bachstetter A, Bickford PC. Oxidative stress and the aging brain: from theory to prevention. In: Riddle DR, editor. Brain aging: models, methods, and mechanisms. Frontiers in neuroscience. Boca Raton (FL); 2007.
15. Barrientos RM, Kitt MM, Watkins LR, Maier SF. Neuroinflammation in the normal aging hippocampus. Neuroscience. 2015;309:84–99.
16. Kuzumaki N, Ikegami D, Imai S, Narita M, Tamura R, Yajima M, et al. Enhanced IL-1beta production in response to the activation of hippocampal glial cells impairs neurogenesis in aged mice. Synapse. 2010;64(9):721–8.
17. Nolan Y, Maher FO, Martin DS, Clarke RM, Brady MT, Bolton AE, et al. Role of interleukin-4 in regulation of age-related inflammatory changes in the hippocampus. J Biol Chem. 2005;280(10):9354–62.
18. Desplats P, Gutierrez AM, Antonelli MC, Frasch MG. Microglial memory of early life stress and inflammation: susceptibility to neurodegeneration in adulthood. Neurosci Biobehav Rev. 2020;117:232–42.
19. Azevedo FA, Carvalho LR, Grinberg LT, Farfel JM, Ferretti RE, Leite RE, et al. Equal numbers of neuronal and nonneuronal cells make the human brain an isometrically scaled-up primate brain. J Comp Neurol. 2009;513(5):532–41.
20. Turner DA, Deupree DL. Functional elongation of CA1 hippocampal neurons with aging in Fischer 344 rats. Neurobiol Aging. 1991;12(3):201–10.
21. Wilson IA, Ikonen S, Gallagher M, Eichenbaum H, Tanila H. Age-associated alterations of hippocampal place cells are subregion specific. J Neurosci. 2005;25(29):6877–86.
22. Kumar A, Foster TC. Enhanced long-term potentiation during aging is masked by processes involving intracellular calcium stores. J Neurophysiol. 2004;91(6):2437–44.

23. Barnes CA, Rao G, McNaughton BL. Functional integrity of NMDA-dependent LTP induction mechanisms across the lifespan of F-344 rats. Learn Mem. 1996;3(2–3):124–37.

24. Kelly KM, Nadon NL, Morrison JH, Thibault O, Barnes CA, Blalock EM. The neurobiology of aging. Epilepsy Res. 2006;68 Suppl 1:S5–20.

25. Kaplan MS. Formation and turnover of neurons in young and senescent animals: an electronmicroscopic and morphometric analysis. Ann N Y Acad Sci. 1985;457:173–92.

26. Gould E, Reeves AJ, Fallah M, Tanapat P, Gross CG, Fuchs E. Hippocampal neurogenesis in adult Old World primates. Proc Natl Acad Sci U S A. 1999;96(9):5263–7.

27. Freundlieb N, Francois C, Tande D, Oertel WH, Hirsch EC, Hoglinger GU. Dopaminergic substantia nigra neurons project topographically organized to the subventricular zone and stimulate precursor cell proliferation in aged primates. J Neurosci. 2006;26(8):2321–5.

28. Nibu K, Kondo K, Ohta Y, Ishibashi T, Rothstein JL, Kaga K. Expression of NeuroD and TrkB in developing and aged mouse olfactory epithelium. Neuroreport. 2001;12(8):1615–9.

29. Saaltink DJ, Vreugdenhil E. Stress, glucocorticoid receptors, and adult neurogenesis: a balance between excitation and inhibition? Cell Mol Life Sci. 2014;71(13):2499–515.

30. Nacher J, Alonso-Llosa G, Rosell DR, McEwen BS. NMDA receptor antagonist treatment increases the production of new neurons in the aged rat hippocampus. Neurobiol Aging. 2003;24(2):273–84.

31. Conde JR, Streit WJ. Microglia in the aging brain. J Neuropathol Exp Neurol. 2006;65(3):199–203.

32. van Praag H, Christie BR, Sejnowski TJ, Gage FH. Running enhances neurogenesis, learning, and long-term potentiation in mice. Proc Natl Acad Sci U S A. 1999;96(23):13427–31.

33. Speisman RB, Kumar A, Rani A, Pastoriza JM, Severance JE, Foster TC, et al. Environmental enrichment restores neurogenesis and rapid acquisition in aged rats. Neurobiol Aging. 2013;34(1):263–74.

34. Smith DE, Rapp PR, McKay HM, Roberts JA, Tuszynski MH. Memory impairment in aged primates is associated with focal death of cortical neurons and atrophy of subcortical neurons. J Neurosci. 2004;24(18):4373–81.

35. Dickson DW, Crystal HA, Mattiace LA, Masur DM, Blau AD, Davies P, et al. Identification of normal and pathological aging in prospectively studied nondemented elderly humans. Neurobiol Aging. 1992;13(1):179–89.

36. Wang DS, Bennett DA, Mufson EJ, Mattila P, Cochran E, Dickson DW. Contribution of changes in ubiquitin and myelin basic protein to age-related cognitive decline. Neurosci Res. 2004;48(1):93–100.

37. Peters A, Sethares C. Aging and the myelinated fibers in prefrontal cortex and corpus callosum of the monkey. J Comp Neurol. 2002;442(3):277–91.

38. Blalock EM, Chen KC, Sharrow K, Herman JP, Porter NM, Foster TC, et al. Gene microarrays in hippocampal aging: statistical profiling identifies novel processes correlated with cognitive impairment. J Neurosci. 2003;23(9):3807–19.

39. Sugiyama I, Tanaka K, Akita M, Yoshida K, Kawase T, Asou H. Ultrastructural analysis of the paranodal junction of myelinated fibers in 31-month-old-rats. J Neurosci Res. 2002;70(3):309–17.

40. Chen D, Huang Y, Shi Z, Li J, Zhang Y, Wang K, et al. Demyelinating processes in aging and stroke in the central nervous system and the prospect of treatment strategy. CNS Neurosci Ther. 2020;26(12):1219–29.

41. Peters A, Sethares C. Is there remyelination during aging of the primate central nervous system? J Comp Neurol. 2003;460(2):238–54.

42. Wolf SA, Boddeke HW, Kettenmann H. Microglia in physiology and disease. Annu Rev Physiol. 2017;79:619–43.

43. Wang JL, Xu CJ. Astrocytes autophagy in aging and neurodegenerative disorders. Biomed Pharmacother. 2020;122:109691.

44. Rocha SM, Cristovao AC, Campos FL, Fonseca CP, Baltazar G. Astrocyte-derived GDNF is a potent inhibitor of microglial activation. Neurobiol Dis. 2012;47(3):407–15.

45. Farina C, Aloisi F, Meinl E. Astrocytes are active players in cerebral innate immunity. Trends Immunol. 2007;28(3):138–45.

46. Jha MK, Jo M, Kim JH, Suk K. Microglia-astrocyte crosstalk: an intimate molecular conversation. Neuroscientist. 2019;25(3):227–40.

47. Streit WJ, Sammons NW, Kuhns AJ, Sparks DL. Dystrophic microglia in the aging human brain. Glia. 2004;45(2):208–12.
48. Matcovitch-Natan O, Winter DR, Giladi A, Vargas Aguilar S, Spinrad A, Sarrazin S, et al. Microglia development follows a stepwise program to regulate brain homeostasis. Science. 2016;353(6301):aad8670.
49. Benmamar-Badel A, Owens T, Wlodarczyk A. Protective microglial subset in development, aging, and disease: lessons from transcriptomic studies. Front Immunol. 2020;11:430.
50. Elmore MR, Najafi AR, Koike MA, Dagher NN, Spangenberg EE, Rice RA, et al. Colony-stimulating factor 1 receptor signaling is necessary for microglia viability, unmasking a microglia progenitor cell in the adult brain. Neuron. 2014;82(2):380–97.
51. Lopez-Redondo F, Nakajima K, Honda S, Kohsaka S. Glutamate transporter GLT-1 is highly expressed in activated microglia following facial nerve axotomy. Brain Res Mol Brain Res. 2000;76(2):429–35.
52. Akiyoshi R, Wake H, Kato D, Horiuchi H, Ono R, Ikegami A, et al. Microglia enhance synapse activity to promote local network synchronization. eNeuro. 2018;5(5)
53. Biber K, Neumann H, Inoue K, Boddeke HW. Neuronal 'On' and 'Off' signals control microglia. Trends Neurosci. 2007;30(11):596–602.
54. Cox FF, Carney D, Miller AM, Lynch MA. CD200 fusion protein decreases microglial activation in the hippocampus of aged rats. Brain Behav Immun. 2012;26(5):789–96.
55. Sheridan GK, Wdowicz A, Pickering M, Watters O, Halley P, O'Sullivan NC, et al. CX3CL1 is up-regulated in the rat hippocampus during memory-associated synaptic plasticity. Front Cell Neurosci. 2014;8:233.
56. Deczkowska A, Keren-Shaul H, Weiner A, Colonna M, Schwartz M, Amit I. Disease-associated microglia: a universal immune sensor of neurodegeneration. Cell. 2018;173(5):1073–81.
57. Vivar C, van Praag H. Functional circuits of new neurons in the dentate gyrus. Front Neural Circ. 2013;7:15.
58. Sultan S, Li L, Moss J, Petrelli F, Casse F, Gebara E, et al. Synaptic integration of adult-born hippocampal neurons is locally controlled by astrocytes. Neuron. 2015;88(5):957–72.
59. Kreisel T, Wolf B, Keshet E, Licht T. Unique role for dentate gyrus microglia in neuroblast survival and in VEGF-induced activation. Glia. 2019;67(4):594–618.
60. Monje ML, Toda H, Palmer TD. Inflammatory blockade restores adult hippocampal neurogenesis. Science. 2003;302(5651):1760–5.
61. Ziv Y, Ron N, Butovsky O, Landa G, Sudai E, Greenberg N, et al. Immune cells contribute to the maintenance of neurogenesis and spatial learning abilities in adulthood. Nat Neurosci. 2006;9(2):268–75.
62. Kalaria RN, Hase Y. Neurovascular ageing and age-related diseases. Subcell Biochem. 2019;91:477–99.
63. del Zoppo GJ. Aging and the neurovascular unit. Ann N Y Acad Sci. 2012;1268:127–33.
64. Toth P, Tarantini S, Tucsek Z, Ashpole NM, Sosnowska D, Gautam T, et al. Resveratrol treatment rescues neurovascular coupling in aged mice: role of improved cerebromicrovascular endothelial function and downregulation of NADPH oxidase. Am J Physiol Heart Circ Physiol. 2014;306(3):H299–308.
65. Meszaros A, Molnar K, Nogradi B, Hernadi Z, Nyul-Toth A, Wilhelm I, et al. Neurovascular Inflammaging in health and disease. Cell. 2020;9(7)
66. Tarantini S, Tran CHT, Gordon GR, Ungvari Z, Csiszar A. Impaired neurovascular coupling in aging and Alzheimer's disease: contribution of astrocyte dysfunction and endothelial impairment to cognitive decline. Exp Gerontol. 2017;94:52–8.
67. Sorond FA, Kiely DK, Galica A, Moscufo N, Serrador JM, Iloputaife I, et al. Neurovascular coupling is impaired in slow walkers: the MOBILIZE Boston Study. Ann Neurol. 2011;70(2):213–20.
68. Elahy M, Jackaman C, Mamo JC, Lam V, Dhaliwal SS, Giles C, et al. Blood-brain barrier dysfunction developed during normal aging is associated with inflammation and loss of tight junctions but not with leukocyte recruitment. Immun Ageing. 2015;12:2.
69. Haeger A, Mangin JF, Vignaud A, Poupon C, Grigis A, Boumezbeur F, et al. Imaging the aging brain: study design and baseline findings of the SENIOR cohort. Alzheimers Res Ther. 2020;12(1):77.
70. Salat DH, Buckner RL, Snyder AZ, Greve DN, Desikan RS, Busa E, et al. Thinning of the cerebral cortex in aging. Cereb Cortex. 2004;14(7):721–30.

71. Fjell AM, Walhovd KB. Structural brain changes in aging: courses, causes and cognitive consequences. Rev Neurosci. 2010;21(3):187–221.
72. Jacobs B, Driscoll L, Schall M. Life-span dendritic and spine changes in areas 10 and 18 of human cortex: a quantitative Golgi study. J Comp Neurol. 1997;386(4):661–80.
73. Pakkenberg B, Gundersen HJ. Neocortical neuron number in humans: effect of sex and age. J Comp Neurol. 1997;384(2):312–20.
74. Ge Y, Grossman RI, Babb JS, Rabin ML, Mannon LJ, Kolson DL. Age-related total gray matter and white matter changes in normal adult brain. Part I: volumetric MR imaging analysis. AJNR Am J Neuroradiol. 2002;23(8):1327–33.
75. Marner L, Nyengaard JR, Tang Y, Pakkenberg B. Marked loss of myelinated nerve fibers in the human brain with age. J Comp Neurol. 2003;462(2):144–52.
76. Takahashi T, Murata T, Omori M, Kosaka H, Takahashi K, Yonekura Y, et al. Quantitative evaluation of age-related white matter microstructural changes on MRI by multifractal analysis. J Neurol Sci. 2004;225(1–2):33–7.
77. Ota M, Obata T, Akine Y, Ito H, Ikehira H, Asada T, et al. Age-related degeneration of corpus callosum measured with diffusion tensor imaging. NeuroImage. 2006;31(4):1445–52.
78. Davis SW, Dennis NA, Buchler NG, White LE, Madden DJ, Cabeza R. Assessing the effects of age on long white matter tracts using diffusion tensor tractography. NeuroImage. 2009;46(2):530–41.
79. Zahr NM, Rohlfing T, Pfefferbaum A, Sullivan EV. Problem solving, working memory, and motor correlates of association and commissural fiber bundles in normal aging: a quantitative fiber tracking study. NeuroImage. 2009;44(3):1050–62.
80. Dennis EL, Thompson PM. Functional brain connectivity using fMRI in aging and Alzheimer's disease. Neuropsychol Rev. 2014;24(1):49–62.
81. de Groot JC, de Leeuw FE, Oudkerk M, van Gijn J, Hofman A, Jolles J, et al. Cerebral white matter lesions and cognitive function: the Rotterdam Scan Study. Ann Neurol. 2000;47(2):145–51.
82. Resnick SM, Pham DL, Kraut MA, Zonderman AB, Davatzikos C. Longitudinal magnetic resonance imaging studies of older adults: a shrinking brain. J Neurosci. 2003;23(8):3295–301.
83. Raz N, Gunning-Dixon F, Head D, Rodrigue KM, Williamson A, Acker JD. Aging, sexual dimorphism, and hemispheric asymmetry of the cerebral cortex: replicability of regional differences in volume. Neurobiol Aging. 2004;25(3):377–96.
84. Gunning-Dixon FM, Head D, McQuain J, Acker JD, Raz N. Differential aging of the human striatum: a prospective MR imaging study. AJNR Am J Neuroradiol. 1998;19(8):1501–7.
85. Pfefferbaum A, Adalsteinsson E, Sullivan EV. Frontal circuitry degradation marks healthy adult aging: evidence from diffusion tensor imaging. NeuroImage. 2005;26(3):891–9.
86. Rypma B, D'Esposito M. Isolating the neural mechanisms of age-related changes in human working memory. Nat Neurosci. 2000;3(5):509–15.
87. Rypma B, Berger JS, Genova HM, Rebbechi D, D'Esposito M. Dissociating age-related changes in cognitive strategy and neural efficiency using event-related fMRI. Cortex. 2005;41(4):582–94.
88. Volkow ND, Logan J, Fowler JS, Wang GJ, Gur RC, Wong C, et al. Association between age-related decline in brain dopamine activity and impairment in frontal and cingulate metabolism. Am J Psychiatry. 2000;157(1):75–80.
89. Kaasinen V, Kemppainen N, Nagren K, Helenius H, Kurki T, Rinne JO. Age-related loss of extrastriatal dopamine D(2)-like receptors in women. J Neurochem. 2002;81(5):1005–10.
90. Chen PS, Yang YK, Lee YS, Yeh TL, Lee IH, Chiu NT, et al. Correlation between different memory systems and striatal dopamine D2/D3 receptor density: a single photon emission computed tomography study. Psychol Med. 2005;35(2):197–204.
91. Bonifazi P, Erramuzpe A, Diez I, Gabilondo I, Boisgontier MP, Pauwels L, et al. Structure-function multi-scale connectomics reveals a major role of the fronto-striato-thalamic circuit in brain aging. Hum Brain Mapp. 2018;39(12):4663–77.
92. Sullivan EV, Marsh L, Pfefferbaum A. Preservation of hippocampal volume throughout adulthood in healthy men and women. Neurobiol Aging. 2005;26(7):1093–8.
93. Catchlove SJ, Parrish TB, Chen Y, Macpherson H, Hughes ME, Pipingas A. Regional cerebrovascular reactivity and cognitive performance in healthy aging. J Exp Neurosci. 2018;12:1179069518785151.

94. Boskovic Z, Meier S, Wang Y, Milne MR, Onraet T, Tedoldi A, et al. Regulation of cholinergic basal forebrain development, connectivity, and function by neurotrophin receptors. Neuronal Signals. 2019;3(1):NS20180066.

95. Mena-Segovia J. Structural and functional considerations of the cholinergic brainstem. J Neural Transm (Vienna). 2016;123(7):731–6.

96. Szutowicz A, Bielarczyk H, Jankowska-Kulawy A, Pawelczyk T, Ronowska A. Acetyl-CoA the key factor for survival or death of cholinergic neurons in course of neurodegenerative diseases. Neurochem Res. 2013;38(8):1523–42.

97. Maurer SV, Williams CL. The cholinergic system modulates memory and hippocampal plasticity via its interactions with non-neuronal cells. Front Immunol. 2017;8:1489.

98. Gamage R, Wagnon I, Rossetti I, Childs R, Niedermayer G, Chesworth R, et al. Cholinergic modulation of glial function during aging and chronic neuroinflammation. Front Cell Neurosci. 2020;14:577912.

99. Hommel B, Li KZ, Li SC. Visual search across the life span. Dev Psychol. 2004;40(4):545–58.

100. Madden DJ, Whiting WL, Cabeza R, Huettel SA. Age-related preservation of top-down attentional guidance during visual search. Psychol Aging. 2004;19(2):304–9.

101. Zhivago KA, Shashidhara S, Garani R, Purokayastha S, Rao NP, Murthy A, et al. Perceptual priming can increase or decrease with aging. Front Aging Neurosci. 2020;12:576922.

102. Belanger S, Belleville S, Gauthier S. Inhibition impairments in Alzheimer's disease, mild cognitive impairment and healthy aging: effect of congruency proportion in a Stroop task. Neuropsychologia. 2010;48(2):581–90.

103. Cohen-Shikora ER, Diede NT, Bugg JM. The flexibility of cognitive control: age equivalence with experience guiding the way. Psychol Aging. 2018;33(6):924–39.

104. Trick LM, Perl T, Sethi N. Age-related differences in multiple-object tracking. J Gerontol B Psychol Sci Soc Sci. 2005;60(2):P102–5.

105. Vallesi A, Tronelli V, Lomi F, Pezzetta R. Age differences in sustained attention tasks: a meta-analysis. Psychon Bull Rev. 2021;

106. Spencer WD, Raz N. Differential effects of aging on memory for content and context: a meta-analysis. Psychol Aging. 1995;10(4):527–39.

107. Brown LA, Brockmole JR. The role of attention in binding visual features in working memory: evidence from cognitive ageing. Q J Exp Psychol (Hove). 2010;63(10):2067–79.

108. Salthouse TA. The processing-speed theory of adult age differences in cognition. Psychol Rev. 1996;103(3):403–28.

109. Crawford TJ, Higham S, Mayes J, Dale M, Shaunak S, Lekwuwa G. The role of working memory and attentional disengagement on inhibitory control: effects of aging and Alzheimer's disease. Age (Dordr). 2013;35(5):1637–50.

110. Cheke LG. What-where-when memory and encoding strategies in healthy aging. Learn Mem. 2016;23(3):121–6.

111. Koen JD, Yonelinas AP. The effects of healthy aging, amnestic mild cognitive impairment, and Alzheimer's disease on recollection and familiarity: a meta-analytic review. Neuropsychol Rev. 2014;24(3):332–54.

112. Sauzeon H, N'Kaoua B, Pala PA, Taillade M, Auriacombe S, Guitton P. Everyday-like memory for objects in ageing and Alzheimer's disease assessed in a visually complex environment: the role of executive functioning and episodic memory. J Neuropsychol. 2016;10(1):33–58.

113. Burnside K, Hope C, Gill E, Morcom AM. Effects of perceptual similarity but not semantic association on false recognition in aging. PeerJ. 2017;5:e4184.

114. Heine MK, Ober BA, Shenaut GK. Naturally occurring and experimentally induced tip-of-the-tongue experiences in three adult age groups. Psychol Aging. 1999;14(3):445–57.

115. Ward EV, Berry CJ, Shanks DR, Moller PL, Czsiser E. Aging predicts decline in explicit and implicit memory: a life-span study. Psychol Sci. 2020;31(9):1071–83.

116. Davis EE, Foy EA, Giovanello KS, Campbell KL. Implicit associative memory remains intact with age and extends to target-distractor pairs. Neuropsychol Dev Cogn B Aging Neuropsychol Cogn. 2021;28(3):455–71.

117. Schwab JF, Schuler KD, Stillman CM, Newport EL, Howard JH, Howard DV. Aging and the statistical learning of grammatical form classes. Psychol Aging. 2016;31(5):481–7.

118. Duverne S, Lemaire P. Arithmetic split effects reflect strategy selection: an adult age comparative study in addition comparison and verification tasks. Can J Exp Psychol. 2005;59(4):262–78.

119. Schmicker M, Menze I, Koch D, Rumpf U, Muller P, Pelzer L, et al. Decision-making deficits in elderly can be alleviated by attention training. J Clin Med. 2019;8(8)
120. Duchek JM, Balota DA, Thomas JB, Snyder AZ, Rich P, Benzinger TL, et al. Relationship between Stroop performance and resting state functional connectivity in cognitively normal older adults. Neuropsychology. 2013;27(5):516–28.
121. Gunning-Dixon FM, Raz N. The cognitive correlates of white matter abnormalities in normal aging: a quantitative review. Neuropsychology. 2000;14(2):224–32.
122. Soderlund H, Nilsson LG, Berger K, Breteler MM, Dufouil C, Fuhrer R, et al. Cerebral changes on MRI and cognitive function: the CASCADE study. Neurobiol Aging. 2006;27(1):16–23.
123. Lavrencic LM, Richardson C, Harrison SL, Muniz-Terrera G, Keage HAD, Brittain K, et al. Is there a link between cognitive reserve and cognitive function in the oldest-old? J Gerontol A Biol Sci Med Sci. 2018;73(4):499–505.
124. Lavrencic LM, Churches OF, Keage HAD. Cognitive reserve is not associated with improved performance in all cognitive domains. Appl Neuropsychol Adult. 2018;25(5):473–85.
125. Arida RM, Teixeira-Machado L. The contribution of physical exercise to brain resilience. Front Behav Neurosci. 2020;14:626769.
126. Blanchet S, Chikhi S, Maltais D. The benefits of physical activities on cognitive and mental health in healthy and pathological aging. Geriatr Psychol Neuropsychiatr Vieil. 2018;16(2): 197–205.
127. Contreras-Vidal JL, Teulings HL, Stelmach GE. Elderly subjects are impaired in spatial coordination in fine motor control. Acta Psychol. 1998;100(1–2):25–35.
128. Xiao L, Ohayon D, McKenzie IA, Sinclair-Wilson A, Wright JL, Fudge AD, et al. Rapid production of new oligodendrocytes is required in the earliest stages of motor-skill learning. Nat Neurosci. 2016;19(9):1210–7.
129. Carp J, Park J, Hebrank A, Park DC, Polk TA. Age-related neural dedifferentiation in the motor system. PLoS One. 2011;6(12):e29411.
130. Mattay VS, Fera F, Tessitore A, Hariri AR, Das S, Callicott JH, et al. Neurophysiological correlates of age-related changes in human motor function. Neurology. 2002;58(4):630–5.
131. Ward NS, Swayne OB, Newton JM. Age-dependent changes in the neural correlates of force modulation: an fMRI study. Neurobiol Aging. 2008;29(9):1434–46.
132. Wang L, Zhang Y, Zhang J, Sang L, Li P, Yan R, et al. Aging changes effective connectivity of motor networks during motor execution and motor imagery. Front Aging Neurosci. 2019;11:312.
133. Li SC, Brehmer Y, Shing YL, Werkle-Bergner M, Lindenberger U. Neuromodulation of associative and organizational plasticity across the life span: empirical evidence and neurocomputational modeling. Neurosci Biobehav Rev. 2006;30(6):775–90.
134. Heuninckx S, Wenderoth N, Swinnen SP. Systems neuroplasticity in the aging brain: recruiting additional neural resources for successful motor performance in elderly persons. J Neurosci. 2008;28(1):91–9.
135. Heuninckx S, Wenderoth N, Debaere F, Peeters R, Swinnen SP. Neural basis of aging: the penetration of cognition into action control. J Neurosci. 2005;25(29):6787–96.
136. Li KZ, Lindenberger U. Relations between aging sensory/sensorimotor and cognitive functions. Neurosci Biobehav Rev. 2002;26(7):777–83.
137. Cham R, Perera S, Studenski SA, Bohnen NI. Striatal dopamine denervation and sensory integration for balance in middle-aged and older adults. Gait Posture. 2007;26(4):516–25.
138. Emborg ME, Ma SY, Mufson EJ, Levey AI, Taylor MD, Brown WD, et al. Age-related declines in nigral neuronal function correlate with motor impairments in rhesus monkeys. J Comp Neurol. 1998;401(2):253–65.
139. Bonin-Guillaume S, Hasbroucq T, Blin O. [Psychomotor retardation associated to depression differs from that of normal aging]. Psychol Neuropsychiatr Vieil. 2008;6(2):137–44.
140. Reuter-Lorenz PA, Lustig C. Brain aging: reorganizing discoveries about the aging mind. Curr Opin Neurobiol. 2005;15(2):245–51.
141. Harada T, Miyai I, Suzuki M, Kubota K. Gait capacity affects cortical activation patterns related to speed control in the elderly. Exp Brain Res. 2009;193(3):445–54.
142. Costello MC, Bloesch EK. Are older adults less embodied? A review of age effects through the lens of embodied cognition. Front Psychol. 2017;8:267.
143. Kuehn E, Perez-Lopez MB, Diersch N, Dohler J, Wolbers T, Riemer M. Embodiment in the aging mind. Neurosci Biobehav Rev. 2018;86:207–25.

144. Farina E, Baglio F, Pomati S, D'Amico A, Campini IC, Di Tella S, et al. The mirror neurons network in aging, mild cognitive impairment, and Alzheimer disease: a functional MRI study. Front Aging Neurosci. 2017;9:371.
145. Boyle PA, Yu L, Wilson RS, Leurgans SE, Schneider JA, Bennett DA. Person-specific contribution of neuropathologies to cognitive loss in old age. Ann Neurol. 2018;83(1):74–83.
146. Stern Y, Arenaza-Urquijo EM, Bartres-Faz D, Belleville S, Cantilon M, Chetelat G, et al. Whitepaper: defining and investigating cognitive reserve, brain reserve, and brain maintenance. Alzheimers Dement. 2020;16(9):1305–11.
147. Colangeli S, Boccia M, Verde P, Guariglia P, Bianchini F, Piccardi L. Cognitive reserve in healthy aging and Alzheimer's disease: a meta-analysis of fMRI studies. Am J Alzheimers Dis Other Dement. 2016;31(5):443–9.
148. Maas DA, Valles A, Martens GJM. Oxidative stress, prefrontal cortex hypomyelination and cognitive symptoms in schizophrenia. Transl Psychiatry. 2017;7(7):e1171.
149. Jackowski AP, Araujo Filho GM, Almeida AG, Araujo CM, Reis M, Nery F, et al. The involvement of the orbitofrontal cortex in psychiatric disorders: an update of neuroimaging findings. Braz J Psychiatry. 2012;34(2):207–12.
150. Fischer CE, Aguera-Ortiz L. Psychosis and dementia: risk factor, prodrome, or cause? Int Psychogeriatr. 2018;30(2):209–19.
151. Gossink FT, Vijverberg E, Krudop W, Scheltens P, Stek ML, Pijnenburg YAL, et al. Predicting progression in the late onset frontal lobe syndrome. Int Psychogeriatr. 2019;31(5):743–8.
152. Mendez MF, Parand L, Akhlaghipour G. Bipolar disorder among patients diagnosed with frontotemporal dementia. J Neuropsychiatry Clin Neurosci. 2020;32(4):376–84.
153. Mischel W. Toward an integrative science of the person. Annu Rev Psychol. 2004;55:1–22.
154. Goldberg LR. An alternative "description of personality": the big-five factor structure. J Pers Soc Psychol. 1990;59(6):1216–29.
155. Roberts BW, Walton KE, Viechtbauer W. Patterns of mean-level change in personality traits across the life course: a meta-analysis of longitudinal studies. Psychol Bull. 2006;132(1):1–25.
156. Sadeq NA, Molinari V. Personality and its relationship to depression and cognition in older adults: implications for practice. Clin Gerontol. 2018;41(5):385–98.
157. Wilson RS, Fleischman DA, Myers RA, Bennett DA, Bienias JL, Gilley DW, et al. Premorbid proneness to distress and episodic memory impairment in Alzheimer's disease. J Neurol Neurosurg Psychiatry. 2004;75(2):191–5.
158. Wright CI, Feczko E, Dickerson B, Williams D. Neuroanatomical correlates of personality in the elderly. NeuroImage. 2007;35(1):263–72.
159. DeYoung CG, Hirsh JB, Shane MS, Papademetris X, Rajeevan N, Gray JR. Testing predictions from personality neuroscience. Brain structure and the big five. Psychol Sci. 2010;21(6):820–8.
160. Kapogiannis D, Sutin A, Davatzikos C, Costa P Jr, Resnick S. The five factors of personality and regional cortical variability in the Baltimore longitudinal study of aging. Hum Brain Mapp. 2013;34(11):2829–40.
161. Wright CI, Williams D, Feczko E, Barrett LF, Dickerson BC, Schwartz CE, et al. Neuroanatomical correlates of extraversion and neuroticism. Cereb Cortex. 2006;16(12):1809–19.
162. Anglim J, Horwood S, Smillie LD, Marrero RJ, Wood JK. Predicting psychological and subjective well-being from personality: a meta-analysis. Psychol Bull. 2020;146(4):279–323.
163. Jeste DV, Oswald AJ. Individual and societal wisdom: explaining the paradox of human aging and high well-being. Psychiatry. 2014;77(4):317–30.
164. Kunzmann U, Little TD, Smith J. Is age-related stability of subjective well-being a paradox? Cross-sectional and longitudinal evidence from the Berlin Aging Study. Psychol Aging. 2000;15(3):511–26.
165. Windsor TD, Anstey KJ. Age differences in psychosocial predictors of positive and negative affect: a longitudinal investigation of young, midlife, and older adults. Psychol Aging. 2010;25(3):641–52.
166. Mayordomo T, Viguer P, Sales A, Satorres E, Melendez JC. Resilience and coping as predictors of well-being in adults. J Psychol. 2016;150(7):809–21.
167. Blanco-Molina M, Pinazo-Hernandis S, Tomas JM. Subjective Well-being key elements of successful aging: a study with lifelong learners older adults from Costa Rica and Spain. Arch Gerontol Geriatr. 2019;85:103897.

168. Rathbone CJ, Holmes EA, Murphy SE, Ellis JA. Autobiographical memory and well-being in aging: the central role of semantic self-images. Conscious Cogn. 2015;33:422–31.
169. Braun T, Schmukle SC, Kunzmann U. Stability and change in subjective well-being: the role of performance-based and self-rated cognition. Psychol Aging. 2017;32(2):105–17.
170. Zaninotto P, Steptoe A. Association between subjective well-being and living longer without disability or illness. JAMA Netw Open. 2019;2(7):e196870.
171. Costantini D, Marasco V, Moller AP. A meta-analysis of glucocorticoids as modulators of oxidative stress in vertebrates. J Comp Physiol B. 2011;181(4):447–56.
172. Zannas AS, Arloth J, Carrillo-Roa T, Iurato S, Roh S, Ressler KJ, et al. Lifetime stress accelerates epigenetic aging in an urban, African American cohort: relevance of glucocorticoid signaling. Genome Biol. 2015;16:266.
173. Rapoport SI. Integrated phylogeny of the primate brain, with special reference to humans and their diseases. Brain Res Brain Res Rev. 1990;15(3):267–94.
174. Dong BE, Chen H, Sakata K. BDNF deficiency and enriched environment treatment affect neurotransmitter gene expression differently across ages. J Neurochem. 2020;154(1):41–55.
175. Wong GH, Yap PL. Active ageing to gerotranscendence. Ann Acad Med Singap. 2016;45(2): 41–3.

Age-Related Physiology Changes: Cardiovascular Function in the Very Old Critically Ill Patient

E. Skaar, H. Fanebust, and G. Schwarz

Contents

© The Author(s), under exclusive license to Springer Nature Switzerland AG 2022
H. Flaatten et al. (eds.), *The Very Old Critically Ill Patients*, Lessons from the ICU,
https://doi.org/10.1007/978-3-030-94133-8_4

> **Learning Objectives**
>
> Physiological changes associated with cardiovascular ageing impact on the presentation of both cardiovascular failure and other conditions warranting admission to intensive care. In the very elderly patient different types of shock frequently occur simultaneously, since it is common that cardiac involvement accompanies other organ failure. Cardiovascular pathophysiology has also a wide range of implications for the diagnosis of shock and monitoring in the circulatory unstable elderly patient.
>
> In this chapter, we will describe the most common physiological changes of the ageing cardiovascular system.
>
> Furthermore, we will give advice for clinical practice, wherever these changes may influence on diagnostic approach and haemodynamic monitoring in elderly patients presenting with circulatory compromise.

4.1 Introduction

In the process of ageing, the heart undergoes changes that might not affect older adults in daily life; however, in the critically ill elderly patient, age-related decline in organ reserves is of major impact. Ageing may lead to a functional deterioration in multiple organs even in the absence of a specific disease. Functional and structural alterations in the atria, myocardium, valves and vasculature (including coronary arteries) and the cardiac conduction system contribute to reduced cardiovascular reserve. There is a gradual transition between normal ageing and pathology. Older adults admitted to intensive care due to non-cardiac causes may decompensate and/ or develop cardiac disease on top of their index disease. Atypical presentation is common. In this chapter, we will give an overview of the most important age-related changes in the cardiovascular system and practical advice how to diagnose and monitor shock in the elderly intensive care patient.

4.2 Physiology of Cardiovascular Ageing with Clinical Relevance for Intensive Care

4.2.1 Atria

The atrial chambers are highly compliant and allow for blood flow between the atrial and ventricular chambers at low venous blood pressures [1]. The major age-related change in the left atrium is an increase in diameter (volume). Age-related fibrosis in the atria is associated with impaired conduction and contractility [2]. The atrial enlargement increases the risk of atrial fibrillation. Older adults with atrial fibrillation are likely to suffer from reduced cardiac output and dyspnoea [3]. At rest the quantitative contribution of the atrial systole to filling of the ventricles is relatively low, with the left atrium contributing 10–20% to the effective stroke volume of the left ventricle, rising to 20–30% during physical exercise or stress [4], like high metabolic demands during critical illness. Increased age is associated with reduced left atrium filling and emptying [2] due to decreased compliance (increased left atrial stiffness). The atria have also endocrine secretory function which is essential to fluid homeostasis, most importantly the secretion of atrial natriuretic peptide (ANP). With advanced age, the level of serum ANP increases [5]. During haemodynamic stress, secretory ANP granules are released in response to increased atrial cell stretch. ANP acts as a potent hormone that inhibits renal salt and water excretion and regulates smooth muscle tone in vessels and blood pressure [1].

4.2.2 Ventricles

During the physiological process of ageing, the left ventricle hypertrophies; however, the interventricular septum increases in thickness more than the free wall and there is a change in LV shape (■ Fig. 4.1). The shift from an elongated ellipsoid geometry to a more spherical shape of the left ventricle reduces the contractile efficiency due to higher wall tension which translates into higher afterload [3].

4.2.3 Myocardium

Ageing has been associated with low-grade systemic inflammation "inflammaging" closely linked to interstitial fibrosis and cardiomyocyte stiffness [6]. Progressive loss of myocytes due to necrotic and apoptotic cell death decreases the absolute number of myocytes in ageing hearts, and the remaining cardiomyocytes undergo hypertrophy and myocardial fibrosis [5]. Ageing cardiomyocytes have prolonged contraction and relaxation times caused by changes in calcium homeostasis. The increased stiffness of the myocardium leads to reduced cardiac filling during the early diastolic phase and to overall slower filling of the ventricle, leaving the heart more dependent on the atrial contribution to ventricular filling. Early diastolic filling rate decreases 30–50% between the third and ninth decades [3]. Hence, tachycardia or atrial fibrillation may lead to reduced ventricular filling and decompensation with heart failure. Systolic function is less affected by normal ageing, and the heart retains a normal ejection fraction at rest. There is a shift from normal ageing to diastolic dysfunction. Diastolic ventricular failure is related to reduced ventricular filling caused by hypertrophied (less compliant) ventricles and by impaired ventricular relaxation. The pathophysiology is heterogeneous and may include age-dependent interstitial fibrosis, hypertension, atrial fibrillation, aortic stenosis, coronary artery disease, diabetes, chronic kidney disease, obesity and chronic obstructive pulmonary disease. This type of heart failure with preserved ejection fraction is more prevalent in older adults and more common in women. End-diastolic pressure increases, and the end-diastolic volume is reduced due to decreased ventricular compliance [6]. In conclusion, the ability of the ageing heart to increase ventricular contractile function under high demand situations is impaired [7].

4.2.4 Valves

During ageing, the valves become stiffer as there is decreased matrix turnover and regeneration. Therefore, valvular degeneration accompanied by calcification is more common in older adults [8]. This process involves endothelial

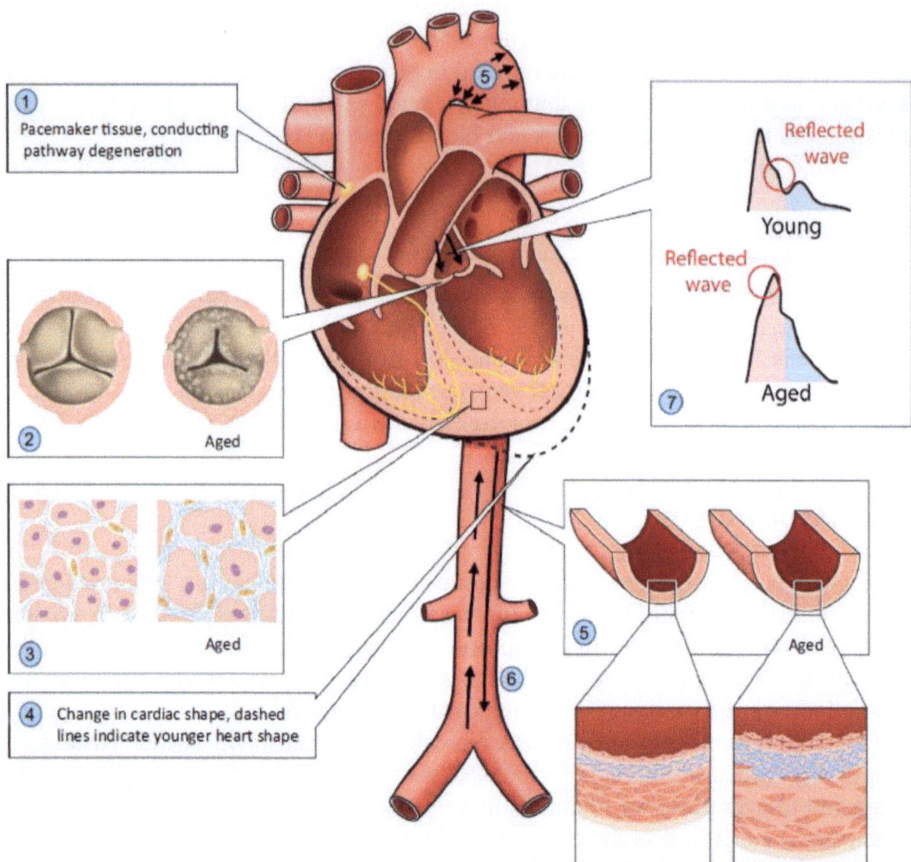

Fig. 4.1 Cardiovascular changes with ageing as a consequence of the complex process of senescence, apoptosis and autophagy linked to decreases in sirtuins (SIRT 1), cell cycle regulators, mitochondrial dysfunction, activation of inflammatory genes, alterations in nitric oxide production and other factors [14, 15]. (1) Pacemaker and conducting pathways degenerate, slowing heart rate response to stress and increasing the risk of arrhythmias. (2) Valve stiffening and calcification, increasing afterload, turbulence and risk of valvular incompetence; murmurs are common. (3) Myocyte hypertrophy and increase in fibrinous matrix reduce plasticity and ability to respond to stress. (4) Altered cardiac shape, e.g. septal hypertrophy, is common reducing efficiency. (5) Vascular changes affect the intima and media leading to increasing thickness, fibrosis and loss of elasticity, resulting in a stiffer vascular system. Endothelial inflammatory tendency and changes in endothelial signalling, e.g. altered nitric oxide-mediated responses, contribute to dysfunction. (6) and (7) Increased pulse wave velocity results in reflected waves arriving in the central arteries during systole rather than diastole, increasing systolic pressure and increasing afterload, while resulting in the loss of augmented diastolic filling. Permission granted to use the figure from the BASIC website of the ICU, PWH, Medical Faculty, Chinese University of Hong Kong. Cardiovascular failure is the second most common reason for admission of octogenarians to intensive care units in Europe [16]

dysfunction, lipid accumulation, inflammation and changes in the extracellular matrix resulting in irreversible calcification of the valve leaflets. The most common valve disease in the Western aging population is mitral regurgitation and aortic stenosis [8, 9].

4.2.5 **The Conduction System**

The elastic and collagenous tissue increases with advancing age in all parts of the conduction system. Fat accumulates around the sinoatrial node (SA) and a marked decrease in the number of pacemaker cells in the SA node commonly occurs after age 60. By the age of 75, the number of pacemaker cells is reduced to less than 10% compared to the young adult. These changes predispose the older heart to sick sinus syndrome. With aging, the aortic and mitral annuli are subject to a variable degree of calcification. AV or intraventricular block may develop if the atrioventricular (AV) node, AV bundle, bifurcation and proximal left and right bundle branches are involved in this process [3].

4.2.6 **Vascular**

The arterial system consists of the large elastic arteries and the small muscular peripheral arteries. Large arteries are rich in collagen and elastin and small muscular arteries are rich in vascular smooth muscle [10]. Vascular ageing is a process of endothelial dysfunction, vascular remodelling, plaque formation and increased arterial stiffness, resulting in higher systolic arterial pressure and pulse pressure (◘ Fig. 4.1). Through its secretion of nitric oxide (vasodilator) and endothelin (vasoconstrictor), the endothelium is a potent regulator of arterial tone. Ageing is associated with reduced endothelial-dependent vasodilation. Furthermore, there is a marked increase in angiotensin II concentration, a potent vasopressor, in aged arterial walls [3]. Endothelial senescence and inflammation are mediated through oxidative stress, telomere shortening and mitochondrial dysfunction [2]. Ageing increases arterial stiffness also by increasing the thickness of the arterial wall as the intimal layer increases 2–3 folds between the age of 20 and 90 years [2]. Central arterial stiffening follows aging even in the absence of clinical hypertension. However, in patients with hypertension there is an accelerated increase in arterial stiffness [11]. Systolic blood pressure (SBP) is determined by both arterial stiffness and cardiac function and increases with age even in normotensive cohorts. In contrast, diastolic blood pressure (DBP) typically rises until the sixth decade and declines in later years [11]. Thus, isolated or predominant SBP elevation is typically for hypertension in older adults. Thus, pulse pressure width is a useful clinical marker of arterial stiffness and the pulsatile load on the arterial tree [3]. Large arterial stiffness rather than peripheral vascular resistance becomes the central haemodynamic factor in both normotensive and hypertensive persons from age 50 onwards [11].

4.2.7 **Coronary Arteries**

Atherosclerotic plaque accumulation in the epicardial arteries increases with age disposing for coronary artery disease. The disease can have long, stable periods; however, it can become unstable at any time, typically due to an acute atherotrombotic event caused by plaque rupture or erosion [12]. Myocardial infarction due to plaque rupture or erosion is classified as type 1. Myocardial infarction type 2 is a mismatch between oxygen supply and demand by a pathophysiological mechanism other than acute coronary atherothrombosis. Type 2 is common in older adults and associated with hypertension, arrhythmia, severe anaemia, surgery, renal failure and heart failure [13].

4.3 Circulatory Failure: Types of Shock

Shock is the state of insufficient oxygen delivery to the body's tissues due to reduced blood flow. To date there is no measure of tissue blood flow established in clinical practice.

The classical clinical signs of hypoperfusion are:

- Hypotension.
- Tachycardia.
- Tachypnoea.
- Confusion.
- Oliguria.
- Weak peripheral pulses.
- Cool peripheries.
- Impaired capillary refill.
- Skin mottling.

The presence of several of these clinical signs makes systemic hypoperfusion likely, but the absence of any of them, especially a normal blood pressure, does not exclude a state of shock. In many elderly patients, physiological compensatory mechanisms are blunted, and heart rate may not rise as expected to maintain cardiac output, owing to pharmacological beta-blockade and age-related changes in adrenergic responsiveness. Both beta-receptor density and beta-receptor sensitivity have been shown to gradually decrease with increasing age [17]. Likewise, cognitive reserves are reduced in the advanced age groups, and acute confusion warrants a high level of attention; the patient should be monitored closely and carefully examined for further signs and possible causes of reduced tissue perfusion. High lactate, when haemoglobin concentration and arterial oxygen saturations are adequate, is highly suggestive of either regional or global tissue hypoperfusion.

In elderly critically ill patients, frequent combinations of different types of shock occur, as myocardial depression and/or arrhythmia often accompanies other types of shock; such cardiac involvement may be caused by ischaemia, hypothermia, medication discontinuation, metabolic derangement or other circulating toxic factors [18].

Complications of circulatory instability frequently occur at an earlier stage than in younger patients due to reduced overall physiologic reserve. In particular, attention should be paid to escalation of cognitive impairment and occurrence of delirium, as well as secondary organ failure caused by regional hypoperfusion like stroke, myocardial ischaemia, mesenteric ischaemia, acute kidney injury and ischaemic hepatitis.

Circulatory failure upon admission has been shown to independently and negatively affect the prognosis in elderly patients regardless of the underlying cause of shock [19]. In cases with premorbid conditions involving several organ systems and higher frailty scores, the prospects of survival in the oldest patients presenting with shock are reduced to a degree that warrants a thorough consideration of the expected benefits of intensive care admission [16].

Type of shock	Heart rate (Caveat: beta-blockade)	JVP or CVP	Peripheries	Common causes in elderly ICU patients
Cardiac	↑↑ ↓↓↓ or ↑↑↑ in arrhythmia-induced cardiac shock	↑ or normal	Cold	Myocardial infarction (type II > type I) Pre-existing heart failure Arrhythmia Pre-existing valvular heart disease Acute valvular lesion Septic myocardial dysfunction Post-cardiotomy
Hypovolaemic	↑↑	↓	Cold	Dehydration Haemorrhage (GI tractus, post-operative, trauma)
Distributive	↑↑	↓	Warm	Sepsis Inflammatory response Anaphylaxis
Obstructive	↑↑	↑↑↑	Cold	Pulmonary embolus Tension pneumothorax SVC/IVC obstruction (malignant masses) Cardiac tamponade

Types of shock, clinical features and common causes in elderly ICU patients

Practical Implications

Circulatory Monitoring: Particular Aspects in the Elderly

1. Cannulation

Arteriosclerotic disease carries increasing prevalence with increasing age affecting target vessels with implications for both arterial and central venous cannulation. Altered anatomy may cause technical difficulties, and restricted flow results in higher risk of complications, namely: Arterial cannulation of a narrow artery may cause arterial ischaemia distal to the cannulation site either due to plaque injury resulting in embolization or by the catheter narrowing the lumen of the vessel to such a degree that flow becomes critically low. Cannulation of a vein draining from the territory of a narrow artery may be poorly filled resulting in technical difficulties, and the catheter will be more prone to catheter-related thrombosis due to low flow. Peripheral vascular disease is often unequally distributed and physical examination alone does usually not aid the selection of the best cannulation site. Therefore, ultrasound assessment of all eligible puncture sites is recommended for both arterial and central venous cannulations, so the approach which is technically most suitable and carries the least risk of complications can be chosen [20, 21]. No firm recommendations regarding the size of the cannula in the presence of arteriosclerosis can be made, but a small study (N = 30) from Turkey showed that, when cannulating an arteriosclerotic radial artery, a larger cannula (22G) was easier to insert and caused less complications than a smaller cannula (20 G) [22].

2. Invasive and Non-invasive Blood Pressure Measurement

Indications and contraindications for each form of blood pressure measurement in the elderly ICU patient remain the same as in the general ICU population. Non-invasive blood pressure (NIBP) measurement in general is with a 95% CI of approx. 15 mmHg within the normal range for systolic NIBP and approximately 10 mmHg for diastolic NIBP markedly less reliable than invasive arterial blood pressure (IABP) measurement, which remains the golden standard of blood pressure measurement in intensive care [23]. With increasing age, the NIBP measurements become even more unreliable compared to the pressures measured in the aortic root, because systolic blood pressure and pulse pressure are increasingly underestimated and diastolic blood pressure overestimated by NIBP measurements [24]. However, in severe hypotension and septic shock NIBP tends to overestimate systolic blood pressure throughout all age groups [25]. Accuracy of NIBP readings is also negatively affected by several patient factors as movement, arrhythmia and shivering which are more common among the elderly. Choice of proper cuff size is crucial in order to produce reliable measurements and may be challenging in the extremes of body weight. In hemiplegic patients the NIBP should be measured on the unaffected limb, as there is some evidence that changes in muscle tone may alter the readings on the affected limb [26]. In conclusion, both patient and procedural factors are frequent sources of NIBP inaccuracy in elderly ICU patients warranting low threshold for IABP monitoring. Still physiological changes and chronic conditions in elderly ICU patients also result frequently in artefacts on IABP traces. Altered blood viscosity, arterial stiffness and tachyarrhythmia increase the natural frequency of the IABP system resulting in an underdamped arterial pressure trace with systolic overshoot [27]. Underdamping can be proven by a fast-flush test, but is hard to abolish in clinical practice. Hence, the charted systolic blood pressure needs to be corrected manually, while the mean and diastolic IABP readings usually are less affected by underdamping [28].

3. Central Venous Pressure (CVP) Measurement

CVP traces and automatically calculated CVP values may be affected by various conditions frequently occurring in elderly ICU patients, namely: tricuspid regurgitation causing increased CVP readings by allowing retrograde transmission of right ventricular systolic pressure, absence of atrial contractions in atrial fibrillation resulting in decreased mean CVP values and asynchronous atrial contractions, e.g. during ventricular pacing, resulting in cannon A waves and increased mean CVP readings. The normal CVP trace pattern may not always be obvious and its absence does not necessarily equal pathology, though an altered CVP trace morphology may give a clue to underlying abnormalities [29] (◘ Fig. 4.2).

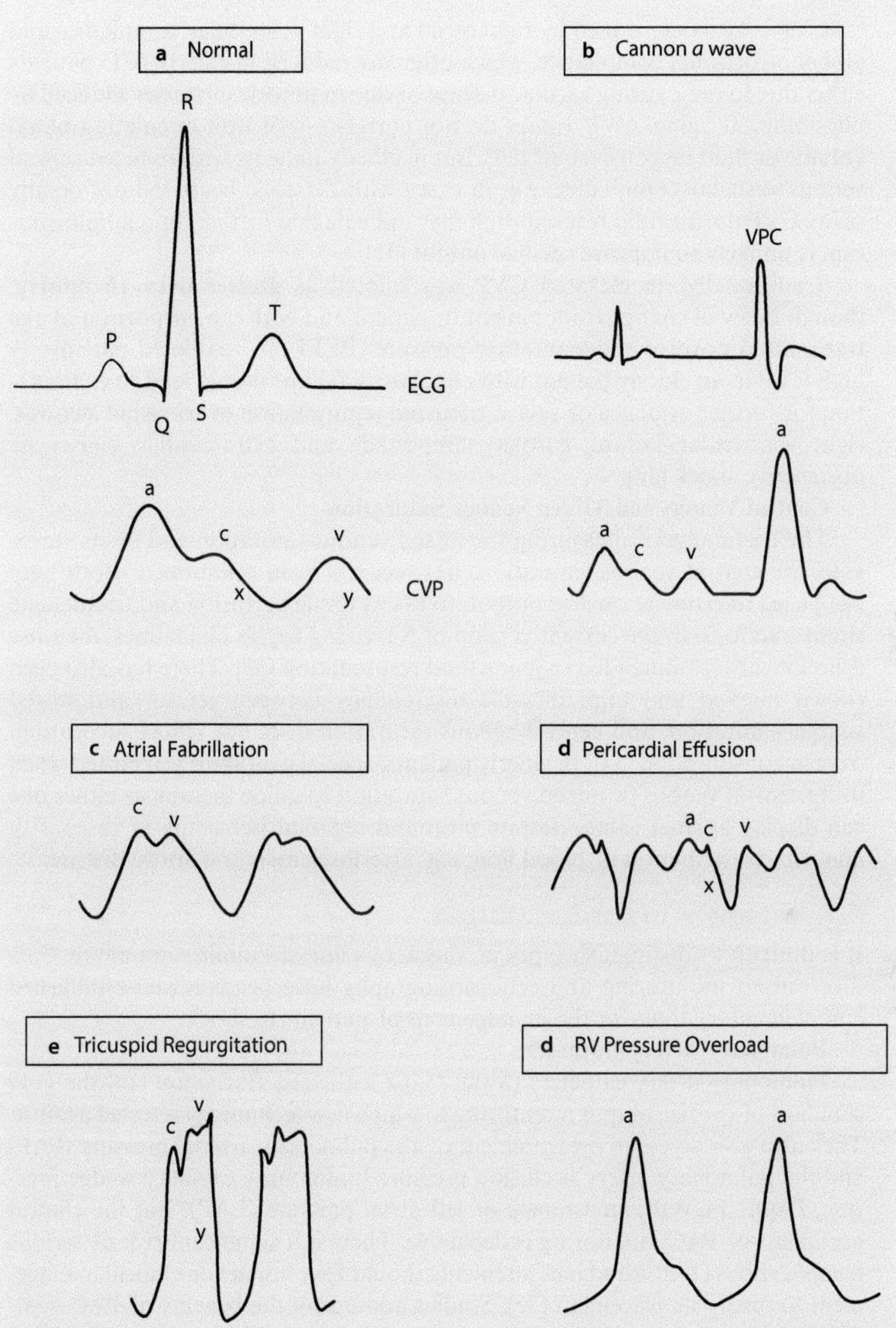

Fig. 4.2 Normal CVP wave form (upper left) and altered CVP trace as expected in certain pathologies

CVP is also determined by right atrial and right ventricular compliance and global myocardial compliance, which often are reduced in elderly ICU patients either due to pre-existing cardiac disease or due to fibrotic processes induced by physiological aging. CVP values do not correlate well with circulating blood volume or fluid responsiveness [30]. But in elderly patients with reduced central venous vascular compliance, e.g. in cases with diastolic heart failure, rapidly rising CVP during fluid resuscitation may indicate that further fluid administration is unlikely to improve cardiac output [31].

Traditionally, an elevated CVP was quoted as greater than 15 mmHg, though this will change from patient to patient and with the proportion of the transmitted positive end-expiratory pressure (PEEP) in ventilated patients. A high CVP in an elderly patient with circulatory failure should lead to examination for further evidence of severe tricuspid regurgitation or tricuspid stenosis, right ventricular failure, cardiac tamponade and extra-cardiac causes of obstructive shock [32].

Central Venous and Mixed Venous Saturation

The usefulness of measuring the mixed venous saturation and of its surrogate, the central venous saturation, has recently been questioned. Both have been used to estimate cardiac output, to assess tissue perfusion and to calculate shunt fractions. In the current version of Surviving Sepsis Guidelines, their use is no longer recommended to guide fluid resuscitation [33]. There has also been shown marked and unpredictable discrepancy between central and mixed venous saturation, and central venous saturation does not reflect myocardial oxygen consumption [34]. In elderly patients, special caution is warranted when using central venous or mixed venous saturation to guide therapy as either one can display normal values despite profound regional ischaemia in cases with abnormal distribution of blood flow, e.g. arteriosclerosis and aortic disease.

4. Assessment of Cardiac Output

It is difficult to distinguish types of shock by clinical examination alone. Cardiac output monitoring and echocardiography have become well-established complementary tools for the management of patients in shock.

Pulmonary Artery Catheter

Pulmonary artery catheters (Swan-Ganz catheters, PACs) are still the gold standard of cardiac output monitoring to which new technology is tested against. They also give access to measurement of the pulmonary arterial pressure (PAP) and the pulmonary artery occlusion pressure (pulmonary capillary wedge pressure, PAOP, PCWP), an estimate of left atrial pressure (LAP). But the clinical usefulness of PAC monitoring is debatable. There is a significant risk of serious complications (2–9%) and measurements should have impact on clinical management to justify its placement [35]. Studies addressing the benefits of PAC goal-directed intensive care in elderly are scarce. One large multicentre study of 1994 ICU patients after major elective or urgent surgery aged 65 years or older (mean 72 years) did neither show any clinical benefit nor increased mortality compared to standard care, but morbidity (i.e. pulmonary embolism) and catheter-related complications were more frequent in the PAC group [36].

Acknowledged Indications for PAC Insertion Are [35, 37]
- Shock with evidence of tissue hypoperfusion not responding to conventional therapy (especially cardiogenic or combination of shock forms).
- RV infarct – acute RV failure.
- Management of refractory pulmonary oedema.
- Cardiac output monitoring with IABP in situ.
- Patients with pulmonary hypertension (PHT) undergoing open heart surgery.

Parameter	Normal	Cardiogenic shock	RV infarct or failure	Septic shock	Cardiac tamponade
Directly measured:					
RAP [mmHg]	0–8	↑↑	↑↑↑	N	Equalization of RAP, RVEDP, PA diastolic and PAOP: 12–18 mmHg
RV systolic diastolic (mmHg)	15–28 0–12	↑↑	EDP ↑↑↑	N or ↓	
PA systolic diastolic mean (mmHg)	15–28 5–15 10–22	↑↑	N or ↑	N or ↓	
PAOP (mmHg)	5–12	↑↑	N	N	
CO (L/min)	4–6	↓↓	↓↓	↑↑	↓↓↓
Derived:					
Stroke volume (ml/beat)	70–130	↓↓	↓↓	N or ↑	↓↓↓
Cardiac index (l/min/m^2)	2.5–4.2	↓↓	↓↓	↑↑	↓↓↓
Systemic vascular resistance (dynes.s/cm^5)	900–1500	↑↑	N or ↑	↓↓↓	N
Pulmonary vascular resistance (dynes.s/cm^5)	120–250	↑↑	N or ↑	N or ↓	N
Left ventricular stroke work index (g/m/beat/m^2)	45–60	↓↓↓	↓↓	↓↓	↓↓↓

Haemodynamic parameters available from a PAC – normal values in recumbent adults, and alterations to expect in common pathologies among elderly ICU patients

Measurement of Cardiac Output

The thermodilution method by a PAC is well validated and remains the gold standard to which other systems are tested against. It is based on the injection of an indicator substance (usually 10 ml of cold dextrose or saline) into the bloodstream at the proximal port of the PAC and the measurement of its dilution in the blood downstream at the distal port of the PAC in the PA. The lowering of the blood temperature over time is recorded as a temperature-time curve. The area under the curve is inversely proportional to the flow rate, and hence an estimate of CO, as long as there is no intra-cardiac shunt (overestimation of the CO) or tricuspid regurgitation (underestimation of the CO).

Modern PACs have an integrated heating filament that warms the blood flowing past it. A thermistor near the tip of the catheter measures temperature changes of the blood and uses the data to average CO over time, providing continuous readings.

Several non-invasive CO measurement technologies have been developed and they may be categorized into calibrated and non-calibrated systems [38]. Calibrated systems use intermittent dilutional CO data (transpulmonary thermodilution or lithium dilution) to calibrate the pulse waveform data. Both PiCCO® and LiDCO® are validated against PAC, but very elderly patients are not addressed in a majority of validation studies [39]. CO measurement with the PiCCO® system is achieved by transpulmonary thermodilution, when 20 ml of cold dextrose or saline is injected on a CVC port, and the temperature drop is measured at the PiCCO® catheter, an arterial cannula with thermistor, usually placed in the femoral artery, where also the IABP trace is recorded for continuous pulse contour analysis. Hence, in contrary to the PAC, the PiCCO® system does not impose invasive procedures exceeding standard monitoring devices and frequently an already placed central venous catheter can be used. CO measurements obtained by transpulmonary thermodilution are likely reliable also in elderly individuals, as long as the pulmonary vasculature is not severely altered and there is no intra-cardiac shunt or tricuspid regurgitation. Whether age-related physiological changes impact on the numerous derived volume parameters provided by PiCCO® is still unknown. Continuous cardiac output measurement by pulse contour analysis is inaccurate, hence limiting its usefulness in several conditions which occur frequently among elderly ICU patients, namely, aortic disease, severe arteriosclerosis, atrial and ventricular arrhythmia causing irregular pulse curve, under- and overdamping of the IABP trace and in cases where mechanical circulatory assist is provided.

Non-calibrated systems use patient data such as sex, height and weight to derive CO from measurement data alone. Calibrated non-invasive CO monitoring systems are more reliable in patients on vasopressor/inotrope therapy than the non-calibrated pulse contour systems or the oesophageal Doppler systems. Furthermore, the non-calibrated systems rely on trending responses to fluid challenges that may be detrimental to very elderly critically ill patients with significant pre-existing impairment of cardiac function [38].

Method	Device	Precision	Features
Pulmonary thermodilution	PAC	+/−20%	Gold standard, but invasive
Echo	TTE/TOE	Operator dependent	Allows additional assessment of contractility and structural features
Transpulmonary Thermodilution	PiCCO™, VolumeView™	Good agreement with PAC	Calibrated, less invasive (CVC + arterial cannula)

Method	Device	Precision	Features
Transpulmonary indicator dilution	LiDCO™	Good agreement with PAC	Calibrated, less invasive (PVC and arterial cannula)
Arterial pressure waveform derived	PiCCO™, LiDCO (*rapide*)™ FloTrac/ Vigileo™ Finapres™, Nexfin™	Variable, depending on reliable waveform	Non-calibrated, continuous, measurement, does not work with irregular HR or IABP
Oesophageal Doppler	CardioQ™	Variable, depending on probe position	Non-calibrated, continuous measurement, minimally invasive, but requires some sedation

Methods of measuring or estimating the cardiac output

5. Assessment of Fluid Responsiveness

Fluid responsiveness is asking the question whether a patient's cardiac output will increase on fluid administration. But it is important to remember that in healthy individuals the heart usually still is fluid responsive; therefore, fluid therapy should only be given to the patient if there is evidence of fluid responsiveness *and* organ hypoperfusion at the same time [40, 41].

Fluid challenge: The easiest way of answering this question is to give a fluid bolus – in patients with impaired systolic or diastolic function, smaller fluid boluses should be given over a longer period of time (e.g. 100 ml crystalloid over 15 minutes).

A subsequent 15% increase of cardiac output from baseline is usually considered proof of fluid responsiveness. Notwithstanding, in elderly patients already the first fluid challenge might be harmful, when hypotension is not attributable to hypovolaemia, and the heart already is operating on the horizontal limb of the Frank-Starling curve.

Leg raise test: A proper conducted leg raise test resulting in "auto-transfusion" from the patient's lower limbs has the advantage of reversibility compared to the fluid challenge. To obtain reliable test results, several factors are important:
- The patient should be informed, if awake, and not be in any apparent distress.
- The patient's bed is moved from semirecumbent position to leg raise position.
- Preferably, cardiac output should be assessed for at least 1 minute.
- If no CO measure is available, a 10–15% increase in mean arterial pulse pressure can be regarded as a sign of fluid responsiveness.

There are also several other surrogate measures of fluid responsiveness. They all have specific limitations, but may give additional information to enhance the clinical picture.

		Measure	Method/device
Static measures	Pressure	Jugular vein pressure (JVP)	Visualization
		Central venous pressure (CVP)	Central venous catheter
		Pulmonary artery occlusion pressure (PAOP)	Pulmonary artery catheter
	Volume	Global end- diastolic volume (GEDV)	Transpulmonary thermodilution (PiCCO™, VolumeView™)
		Left ventricular end-diastolic volume	Echocardiography
Dynamic measures		Pulse pressure variation (PPV)	(PiCCO™, LiDCO plus™, Most care™)
		Stroke volume variation (SVV)	Arterial pulse contour analysis (PiCCO™, LiDCO Plus™, Most care™, FloTrac/Vigileo™), volume clamp method (Finapres™, Nexfin™), assessment of superior vena cava (SVC) and inferior vena cava (IVC), echo Doppler

Static and dynamic measures of fluid responsiveness

Measuring venous pressures and end-diastolic volumes of the heart chambers results in static surrogate estimates of RV preload and LV preload. They all are poorly correlated to fluid responsiveness since the relationship of preload and stroke volume depends on ventricular contractility and the compliance of the venous system.

There are also limitations of dynamic measures in the mechanically ventilated patients. These methods rely on the concept that the variations in intrathoracic pressure imposed by the cycle of positive pressure ventilation affect venous return and subsequently cardiac output. These variations are exaggerated in hypovolaemia, indicating that the heart currently is operating on the ascending limb of the Frank-Starling curve. The major drawback with all respiratory cycle-related measurements estimating LV preload is that they are only validated in paralyzed patients receiving a tidal volume of at least 8–10 ml/kg, who also must have a regular heart rate. In elderly ICU patients with a regular heart rate, these tests still can be performed, as long as they are sedated and paralyzed, by transiently increasing the TV to 10 ml/kg, even though in general a more lung protective ventilator setting is preferred. Under these circumstances a pulse pressure or stroke volume variation of more than 10–15% is regarded as a reliable predictor of fluid responsiveness.

> ## Conclusion
>
> Age alone is an important prognostic factor in critically ill elderly patients due to the continuous decline in cardiovascular reserves. This process may be without any implications for daily life, but becomes apparent during critical illness and affects the course and outcome of intensive care also for non-cardiac conditions. Age-related structural and functional changes of the heart and the large vessels need to be taken into account in intensive care diagnostic approach and monitoring.

> ### Take-Home Messages
>
> - Investigate for multiple forms of shock and multiple underlying causes in the elderly patient presenting with circulatory compromise.
> - Remember high prevalence of altered heart and vascular anatomy and function, when cannulating, monitoring and interpreting measured values.
> - Consider the additional effects of comorbidity and frailty on the prognosis of shock.

References

1. Brandenburg S, Arakel EC, Schwappach B, Lehnart SE. The molecular and functional identities of atrial cardiomyocytes in health and disease. Biochim Biophys Acta. 2016;1863(7 Pt B):1882–93.
2. Obas V, Vasan RS. The aging heart. Clin Sci (Lond). 2018;132(13):1367–82.
3. Fleg JL, Strait J. Age-associated changes in cardiovascular structure and function: a fertile milieu for future disease. Heart Fail Rev. 2012;17(4–5):545–54.
4. Rahimtoola SH, Ehsani A, Sinno MZ, Loeb HS, Rosen KM, Gunnar RM. Left atrial transport function in myocardial infarction. Importance of its booster pump function. Am J Med. 1975;59(5):686–94.
5. Lu L, Guo J, Hua Y, Huang K, Magaye R, Cornell J, et al. Cardiac fibrosis in the ageing heart: contributors and mechanisms. Clin Exp Pharmacol Physiol. 2017;44(Suppl 1):55–63.
6. Loffredo FS, Nikolova AP, Pancoast JR, Lee RT. Heart failure with preserved ejection fraction: molecular pathways of the aging myocardium. Circ Res. 2014;115(1):97–107.
7. Ruiz-Meana M, Bou-Teen D, Ferdinandy P, Gyongyosi M, Pesce M, Perrino C, et al. Cardiomyocyte ageing and cardioprotection: consensus document from the ESC working groups cell biology of the heart and myocardial function. Cardiovasc Res. 2020;116(11):1835–49.
8. Baumgartner H, Falk V, Bax JJ, De Bonis M, Hamm C, Holm PJ, et al. 2017 ESC/EACTS guidelines for the management of valvular heart disease. Eur Heart J. 2017;38(36):2739–91.
9. Iung B, Vahanian A. Epidemiology of acquired valvular heart disease. Can J Cardiol. 2014;30(9):962–70.
10. Jani B, Rajkumar C. Ageing and vascular ageing. Postgrad Med J. 2006;82(968):357–62.
11. Nilsson PM, Khalili P, Franklin SS. Blood pressure and pulse wave velocity as metrics for evaluating pathologic ageing of the cardiovascular system. Blood Press. 2014;23(1):17–30.
12. Knuuti J, Wijns W, Saraste A, Capodanno D, Barbato E, Funck-Brentano C, et al. 2019 ESC guidelines for the diagnosis and management of chronic coronary syndromes. Eur Heart J. 2020;41(3):407–77.
13. DeFilippis AP, Chapman AR, Mills NL, de Lemos JA, Arbab-Zadeh A, Newby LK, et al. Assessment and treatment of patients with type 2 myocardial infarction and acute nonischemic myocardial injury. Circulation. 2019;140(20):1661–78.
14. Olivetti G, Melissari M, Capasso JM, Anversa P. Cardiomyopathy of the aging human heart. Myocyte loss and reactive cellular hypertrophy. Circ Res. 1991;68(6):1560–8.
15. Strait JB, Lakatta EG. Aging-associated cardiovascular changes and their relationship to heart failure. Heart Fail Clin. 2012;8(1):143–64.

16. Guidet B, de Lange DW, Boumendil A, Leaver S, Watson X, Boulanger C, et al. The contribution of frailty, cognition, activity of daily life and comorbidities on outcome in acutely admitted patients over 80 years in European ICUs: the VIP2 study. Intensive Care Med. 2020;46(1):57–69.
17. Ferrara N, Komici K, Corbi G, Pagano G, Furgi G, Rengo C, et al. Beta-adrenergic receptor responsiveness in aging heart and clinical implications. Front Physiol. 2014;4:396.
18. Merx MW, Weber C. Sepsis and the heart. Circulation. 2007;116(7):793–802.
19. Biston P, Aldecoa C, Devriendt J, Madl C, Chochrad D, Vincent JL, et al. Outcome of elderly patients with circulatory failure. Intensive Care Med. 2014;40(1):50–6.
20. Troianos CA, Hartman GS, Glas KE, Skubas NJ, Eberhardt RT, Walker JD, et al. Guidelines for performing ultrasound guided vascular cannulation: recommendations of the American Society of Echocardiography and the Society of Cardiovascular Anesthesiologists. J Am Soc Echocardiogr. 2011;24(12):1291–318.
21. Franco-Sadud R, Schnobrich D, Mathews BK, Candotti C, Abdel-Ghani S, Perez MG, et al. Recommendations on the use of ultrasound guidance for central and peripheral vascular access in adults: a position statement of the Society of Hospital Medicine. J Hosp Med. 2019;14:E1–E22.
22. Eker HE, Tuzuner A, Yilmaz AA, Alanoglu Z, Ates Y. The impact of two arterial catheters, different in diameter and length, on postcannulation radial artery diameter, blood flow, and occlusion in atherosclerotic patients. J Anesth. 2009;23(3):347–52.
23. Kallioinen N, Hill A, Horswill MS, Ward HE, Watson MO. Sources of inaccuracy in the measurement of adult patients' resting blood pressure in clinical settings: a systematic review. J Hypertens. 2017;35(3):421–41.
24. Picone DS, Schultz MG, Otahal P, Black JA, Bos WJ, Chen CH, et al. Influence of age on upper arm cuff blood pressure measurement. Hypertension. 2020;75(3):844–50.
25. Lehman LW, Saeed M, Talmor D, Mark R, Malhotra A. Methods of blood pressure measurement in the ICU. Crit Care Med. 2013;41(1):34–40.
26. Dewar R, Sykes D, Mulkerrin E, Nicklason F, Thomas D, Seymour R. The effect of hemiplegia on blood pressure measurement in the elderly. Postgrad Med J. 1992;68(805):888–91.
27. Romagnoli S, Ricci Z, Quattrone D, Tofani L, Tujjar O, Villa G, et al. Accuracy of invasive arterial pressure monitoring in cardiovascular patients: an observational study. Crit Care. 2014;18(6):644.
28. Moxham IM. Physics of invasive blood pressure monitoring. South Afr J Anaesth Analg. 2003;9(1):33–8.
29. Pittman JA, Ping JS, Mark JB. Arterial and central venous pressure monitoring. Int Anesthesiol Clin. 2004;42(1):13–30.
30. Marik PE, Baram M, Vahid B. Does central venous pressure predict fluid responsiveness? A systematic review of the literature and the tale of seven mares. Chest. 2008;134(1):172–8.
31. Pinsky MR, Kellum JA, Bellomo R. Central venous pressure is a stopping rule, not a target of fluid resuscitation. Crit Care Resusc. 2014;16(4):245–6.
32. Magder S. Understanding central venous pressure: not a preload index? Curr Opin Crit Care. 2015;21(5):369–75.
33. Howell MD, Davis AM. Management of sepsis and septic shock. JAMA. 2017;317(8):847–8.
34. Chawla LS, Zia H, Gutierrez G, Katz NM, Seneff MG, Shah M. Lack of equivalence between central and mixed venous oxygen saturation. Chest. 2004;126(6):1891–6.
35. Practice guidelines for pulmonary artery catheterization: an updated report by the American Society of Anesthesiologists Task Force on pulmonary artery catheterization. Anesthesiology. 2003;99(4):988–1014.
36. Sandham JD, Hull RD, Brant RF, Knox L, Pineo GF, Doig CJ, et al. A randomized, controlled trial of the use of pulmonary-artery catheters in high-risk surgical patients. N Engl J Med. 2003;348(1):5–14.
37. Chatterjee K. The Swan-Ganz catheters: past, present, and future. A viewpoint. Circulation. 2009;119(1):147–52.
38. Vincent JL, Rhodes A, Perel A, Martin GS, Della Rocca G, Vallet B, et al. Clinical review: update on hemodynamic monitoring–a consensus of 16. Crit Care. 2011;15(4):229.
39. Litton E, Morgan M. The PiCCO monitor: a review. Anaesth Intensive Care. 2012;40(3):393–409.
40. Marik PE, Lemson J. Fluid responsiveness: an evolution of our understanding. Br J Anaesth. 2014;112(4):617–20.
41. Marik PE, Monnet X, Teboul JL. Hemodynamic parameters to guide fluid therapy. Ann Intensive Care. 2011;1(1):1.

Age-Related Changes of the Kidneys and their Physiological Consequences

Fabian Perschinka, Timo Mayerhöfer, and Michael Joannidis

Contents

Introduction

The kidneys are among the most vulnerable organs when it comes to critical illness and its consequences such as haemodynamic alterations, inflammation or mechanical ventilation. This applies in particular to very old critically ill, who have less reserves to respond to homeostatic disturbances.

According to demographic changes in nearly all Western societies, very old patients represent an increasing proportion of the total community and therefore become more present at the intensive care units (ICU). Ageing is associated with a decline in organ function including the kidneys and the immune system. Changes in kidney histology as well as kidney function, a moderate decrease in glomerular filtration (GFR) and the reduction of the number of nephrons throughout the life cycle may be considered normal. In addition, variations regarding sodium, potassium as well as water balance have to be taken into account when treating very old critically ill patients. In order to understand the full range of the complex renal situation in elderly patients, including various alterations and interactions with other comorbidities, it is necessary to deal with the pathophysiological mechanisms behind these changes and the clinical aspects accompanying them. Their understanding might be helpful to distinguish disease from normal features of renal ageing.

This chapter provides an overview of the pathophysiological as well as histological and morphological changes of the ageing kidney. Furthermore, functional changes and their diagnostic and therapeutic implications for very old critically ill patients will be discussed.

5.1   (Patho)Physiology of Renal Ageing

Mechanisms of renal ageing are manifold, ranging from epigenetic and molecular processes to immunological alterations, and often associated with comorbidities like diabetes and hypertension [1–3]. These transitions lead to limited glomerular regeneration as well as single nephron hyperfiltration (in very high age) and inflammation.

Epigenetics seems to have significant impact on cellular ageing of kidney tissue, which is affected by methylation and mutation of genes expressed primarily in kidneys. Of particular note is the Klotho gene, which is reduced in its expression through hypermethylation in the presence of uraemic toxins [4]. This gene affects ageing via various mechanisms. Additionally, Klotho influences inflammatory pathways by inhibiting NF-KB translocating to the nucleus, which has an anti-inflammatory effect. Polymorphisms in this gene are correlated with healthy ageing [5] and methylation of the Klotho promotor gene is one attribute of chronic kidney disease (CKD) [1].

So-called inflammageing is a continuous moderate inflammatory process, which is more activated in the elderly, and contributes to changes in tissue structure characterised by fibrotic changes. Uraemic inflammation shows important parallels, especially in kidneys, and may be an accelerating factor in CKD [6]. Inflammation triggered by uraemia leads to premature ageing in kidneys and alterations in both, the innate and the adaptive immune system [7]. Age-associated alterations of the immune system result in systemic inflammation. The fact that 30–50% of patients with predialysis, haemodialysis and peritoneal dialysis show signs of active inflammatory response demonstrates the importance of this chronic pro-inflammatory state in the context of renal ageing. The inflammation is both the cause and consequence of (renal) ageing. A link between inflammatory markers and shortened telomere has been demonstrated. Furthermore, genome regulation, concerning inflammation-associated genes, changes in very old patients, which correlates with reduced expression of Sirtuin 1 and Sirtuin 3. These genes are connected to acute kidney insufficiency in animal models [6]. Inflammation affects renal ageing at multiple pathways and is connected with uraemic inflammation in the kidney.

5.2 Histological and Morphologic Aspects

Changes in cellular structures are observed in endothelial and epithelial renal cells and podocytes. They may be considered a consequence of autoimmunologic "injuries" leading to alterations in glomerular basal membrane thickness and podocyte hypertrophy as well as permeability of the capillary wall. Resulting proteinuria and increased filtration lead to changes in tubular function and further trigger an inflammatory process [8].

In addition to "normal" age-related loss of functional nephrons, decline from 990,000 in young adults to 520,000 in 70–75-year-olds (6200 nephrons per year) [9], pathological processes like nephrosclerosis, vasculitis or diabetic nephropathy may contribute to a reduction of working glomeruli in very old patients and thus a decreased glomerular filtration rate (GFR).

Nephrosclerosis, associated with hypertension [10], is characterised by interstitial fibrosis, global glomerulosclerosis, atrophic tubules and arteriosclerosis resulting in ischaemic injury to nephrons. Ischaemic changes like a thickened basement membrane, wrinkled capillary tufts and pericapsular fibrosis are the consequence. Additionally, due to deposition of hyaline material in the Bowman's space, globally sclerotic glomeruli (GSG) develop [8] and lead to higher prevalence of GSG in very old patients. Whereas the prevalence of nephrosclerosis is 2.7% in the 18–29 age group, it rises to 73% in the 70–77-year-olds. However, increased prevalence of nephrosclerosis with age seems to be independent of age-related decreasing GFR in elderly patients [11]. Distinction between age-associated nephrosclerosis and alterations due to specific kidney diseases is difficult. Common comorbidities contributing to glomerular sclerosis are diabetes mellitus and hypertension, which show an increased prevalence in the elderly population [11, 12].

Whether decline in kidney parameters is associated with concomitant comorbidities or part of a physiological ageing progress has not been finally clarified. Several studies suggested no correlation of age and kidney parenchymal volume in patients <65 years of age followed by successive decrease [13]. Considering the cortex, medulla and parenchyma separately, a decline in cortical volume, an increase in medullary volume and stable parenchyma volume can be observed with age until the age of 50. All three compartments decline after the age of 50 years [14]. These changes may be observed with ultrasound diagnostic during acute kidney injury or CKD in very old patients, whereby a physiological volume reduction of 16–22 cm^3 per decade has to be taken into account [14, 15].

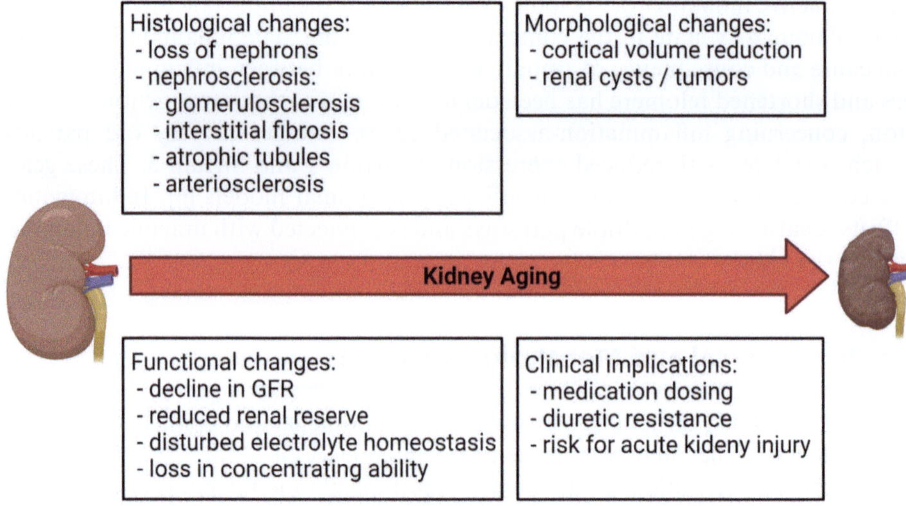

Fig. 5.1 Overview of the process of kidney ageing and clinical aspects. (Created with ▶ BioRender. com)

Another aspect of the ageing kidney is an increased number of cysts. The cysts are more common in men and often asymptomatic. However, they may indicate an underlying pathology and should be distinguished from malignancies and tumours [16] (■ Fig. 5.1).

5.3 Renal Function/Functional Alterations

Similar to ageing in other organs, the ageing of kidney cells also leads to a decline in kidney function. An ongoing matter of discussion when it comes to the alterations of kidney function in the elderly is the differentiation between a physiological decline and disease. The kidney has many different functions. One way to determine the kidney function is the measurement or estimation of the GFR.

5.3.1 Determination of GFR in the Elderly

5.3.1.1 Estimation of GFR

A direct measurement of GFR is difficult to assess especially in daily clinical routine. Therefore, estimation of glomerular filtration rate by different formulas is well established and superior to creatinine levels alone. The most commonly used equations are the Cockcroft-Gault (CG), the Modification of Diet in Renal Disease (MDRD) and the Chronic Kidney Disease Epidemiology Collaboration (CKD-EPI). The CG equation takes a back seat due to some limitation, as it relies on body weight rather than body surface, leading to inaccuracies in obese patients. Furthermore, the performance of MDRD seems better in the context of very old patients [17]. Besides serum creatinine, it also includes sex, ethnicity and age. Another commonly used equation is the CKD-EPI, with advantages especially in patients with normal GFR. It is calculated with serum creatinine or serum cystatin C or the combination of both. Cystatin C is less influenced by muscle mass and may therefore be better in the very old patient and some studies indicate a slightly better performance in older patients [18, 19].

5.3.1.2 Measurement of GFR

Another possibility to determine GFR is the creatinine clearance from 24 h urine collection. The collecting time may be reduced up to 2 h almost without loss in accuracy [20]. However, due to tubular secretion of creatinine, this method tends to overestimate real GFR. This problem becomes manifest when GFR is declining to values below 20 ml/kg/1.73 m^2, when an accurate determination would be most important [21].

Although the MDRD and CKD-EPI equations seem to have limitations in the very old patient, the estimation of GFR is the best available tool for daily clinical practice.

Recently developed methods for real-time GFR measurements are currently under clinical investigation and may improve accuracy as well as time required for GFR determination.

5.3.2 Changing GFR in the Elderly

The decline in GFR is part of the natural processes of ageing and confirmed by many studies for healthy individuals. These physiological changes with ageing are often difficult to distinguish from decline in GFR caused by various diseases and comorbidities. A remarkable difference between healthy ageing and different states of diseases may be seen in single nephron GFR (snGFR). While the number of nephrons decreases with age, snGFR remains unchanged unless alterations beyond physiological ageing are present [9].

In this context, the definition of CKD by the KDIGO guidelines with a threshold of <60 ml/min 1.72 m^2 has been repeatedly discussed. The cut-off is defined as 50% of renal function of young and healthy individuals [22]. However, this approach may be insufficient for older patients and lead to overdiagnosis of CKD. According to a recent cohort study (2017), these criteria are met by approximately 38–62% of patients over the age of 70 [23].

This is especially relevant for patients with GFR of 45–59 and without albuminuria. Albuminuria must be considered separately, as it should not be a part of healthy ageing and may therefore serve as an instrument to identify patients with a decline in GFR beyond healthy ageing [9]. This is important, since very old critically ill suffer more frequently from comorbidities with negative impact on the kidney function. If a decline in GFR is recognized, a differentiation between a normal age-related decline and a decline caused by comorbidities or other underlying diseases may help to treat and prevent a further deterioration.

The definitions play an important role especially for the epidemiology of CKD. With the current threshold, otherwise healthy individuals may meet the criteria of CKD.

However, the discussion about defining CKD should not obscure the fact that the reduction in GFR has important implications for the clinician regarding, e.g. medication dosing and an increased risk of acute kidney injury (see below).

An important aspect of the decline in GFR by age is reduced renal reserve [24]. While younger patients with more functioning nephrons can more easily adapt to all kinds of stress on the kidney (e.g. various diseases, nephrotoxic medication or haemodynamic alterations), older patients with a reduced renal reserve are more vulnerable.

The reason for the decline, whether healthy ageing or not, is initially of limited relevance for the treatment of the very old critically ill patient.

5.3.3 Renal Tubular Function in the Elderly

Another important task of the kidney is the maintenance of electrolyte homeostasis, including tubular reabsorption and secretion as well as hormonal activity. These transport mechanisms are changing in very old patients. While sodium reabsorption is increased in proximal parts of the nephron, it is lower in distal parts compared to younger individuals. This leads to a more unstable equilibrium and a limited response to varying sodium load.

Regarding potassium balance in very old patients, endocrine changes in addition to prescribed medications, especially angiotensin-converting-enzyme inhibitors or diuretics, may facilitate an imbalance in potassium homeostasis. Potassium secretion by tubular cells diminishes with increasing age, because of lower renin and aldosterone levels. These changes result in an increased risk for hyperkalemia and are related to a predisposition to metabolic disturbances, especially metabolic acidosis [25].

Furthermore, the ability of the kidney to concentrate urine declines with advanced age [26]. This may be due to reduction of urea transporters and aquaporins and leads to an impaired response to different amounts of fluid intake. This is especially important, because very old patients are susceptible to dehydration. On top of this, very old critically ill patients often take many medications with the potential to affect tubular secretion [9].

5.4 Consequences on Drug Therapy

5.4.1 Dosing

An important aspect when it comes to drug administration in very old critically ill is nephrotoxicity. In general, nephrotoxic medications and procedures should be reduced to the minimum in the elderly with reduced GFR.

Furthermore, as GFR and tubular function change with age, the dosage of drugs excreted through the kidneys must be adjusted. These adjustments depend on the GFR. However, it should be noted that the information on dose adaptions is mostly based on GFR in ml/min and not normalized to 1.73 m^2 body surface area.

5.4.2 Diuretic Resistance

In very old critically ill patients, treatment with diuretics is often required because of comorbidities such as chronic heart failure accompanied by fluid overload/oedema. The treatment of choice are loop diuretics (LD). These patients occasionally show a phenomenon called diuretic resistance, which is characterized by fluid overload despite diuretic use [27]. Diuretic resistance in the elderly has various causes.

Pharmacodynamic and pharmacokinetic changes affecting diuretic effectiveness have to be taken into consideration. In the case of oral administration, bioavailability may range from 10% to 80% of furosemide dose applied, especially in the elderly. Thus, an intravenous administration should be preferred [28]. Additionally, a continuous administration results in a more constant weight reduction and increase in total urine output as compared to bolus administration [29] and does not exacerbate post-diuretic sodium retention, which is boosted by drug-free interval longer than four half-lives [27]. Torasemide or bumetanide show a more consistent bioavailability and may be considered as an alternative in diuretic resistance [28].

Chloride as essential electrolyte for salt sensing influences the potency of LD [30]. The link between the effectiveness of LD and hypochloremia has been shown in a study, in which one cohort got chloride lysine orally administrated, followed by improving cardio-renal parameters such as NT-proBNP and weight loss [31].

While extended renal hypoperfusion results in lower diuretic concentration in the kidneys, lower GFR reduces necessary sodium delivery [28, 32]. Furosemide needs albumin to reach the kidneys [28]. As a result, hypoproteinemia causes a reduction of effective furosemide levels in the kidneys [33].

There are different options to overcome diuretic resistance or at least to improve the LD effect. While sodium restriction in the course of very low sodium diet achieved consensus to be the therapy for fluid overload, it is now being questioned due to poorer outcomes and occasionally resulting in hyponatraemia and hypochloremia leading to diuretic resistance themselves. Other approaches to handle diuretic resistance are using various combinations of diuretics to overcome the sodium reabsorption in distal tubules, but randomized controlled trials (RTC) to investigate effects and side effects are rare. Different studies investigating the addition of hypertonic saline infusion to furosemide showed conflicting results [34, 35].

Another aspect to consider is increased susceptibility of elderly patients to develop hyponatraemia after administration of thiazide diuretics or diuretics affecting the distal tubule like xipamide. This may result in severe complication when used in combination with LD [36].

5.5 AKI – Aspects when Treating Very Old Patients

Acute kidney injury (AKI), defined by KDIGO as increased creatinine levels ≥ 1.5 times within the previous 7 days or ≥ 0.3 mg/dL within 48 h or decreased urine volume <0.5 ml/kg for 6 h [37], varies regarding its pathophysiological causes (infections of kidney parenchyma, hypovolaemia, nephrotoxins as well as sepsis). This definition is considered age independent. However, lack of muscle mass may lead to concealed changes in renal function, which are not represented by an increase in serum creatinine. On the other hand, age is an independent risk factor for AKI. Therefore, very old critically ill patients with multiple comorbidities need special attention regarding preventive measures. Optimising the haemodynamic status (administration of fluids, vasopressor drugs and inotropics) to ensure renal perfusion is the first-line intervention to prevent AKI. Considering the cardiovascular comorbidities in geriatric patients, close observation and experience are needed to prevent fluid overload [38].

In very old patients prescribed medications, like angiotensin-converting-enzyme inhibitors or angiotensin II receptor blockers (ACEI/ARB), are often accused to be responsible for AKI. Various observational studies showed no increased rate of AKI when the patients were medicated with ACEI/ARB during hospital admission [39, 40]. In every age group the absolute rate of AKI was higher when ACEI/ARB was combined with LDs up to a difference of 33.4/1000 person years in the group 85 years and older (60.1 vs. 26.7) [40], but not when ACEI/ARB was the only prescribed "nephrotoxic" drug. The common practice of discontinuing ACEI/ARB during intercurrent illness to prevent AKI could be questioned [41]. However, discontinuation can be indicated in the setting of an acute disease associated with dehydration and/or hypovolaemia, e.g. diarrhoea or sepsis.

> **Take-Home Message**
> - Nephron loss and renal downsizing are aspects of healthy ageing.
> - GFR declines with age, resulting in a reduced renal reserve.
> - Because of these changes we should be cautious about nephrotoxic drugs and the risk of acute kidney injury in elderly patients.
> - Due to comorbidities, very old patients need special attention for AKI; however, obligatory discontinuing of medication should be questioned and decided in the context of clinical presentation.

References

1. Shiels PG, McGuinness D, Eriksson M, Kooman JP, Stenvinkel P. The role of epigenetics in renal ageing. Nat Rev Nephrol. 2017;13(8):471–82.
2. Fang Y, Gong AY, Haller ST, Dworkin LD, Liu Z, Gong R. The ageing kidney: molecular mechanisms and clinical implications. Ageing Res Rev. 2020;63:101151.
3. Sato Y, Yanagita M. Immunology of the ageing kidney. Nat Rev Nephrol. 2019;15(10):625–40.
4. Sun CY, Chang SC, Wu MS. Suppression of Klotho expression by protein-bound uremic toxins is associated with increased DNA methyltransferase expression and DNA hypermethylation. Kidney Int. 2012;81(7):640–50.
5. Di Bona D, Accardi G, Virruso C, Candore G, Caruso C. Association of Klotho polymorphisms with healthy aging: a systematic review and meta-analysis. Rejuvenation Res. 2014;17(2):212–6.
6. Kooman JP, Dekker MJ, Usvyat LA, Kotanko P, van der Sande FM, Schalkwijk CG, et al. Inflammation and premature aging in advanced chronic kidney disease. Am J Physiol Renal Physiol. 2017;313(4):F938–F50.
7. Ebert T, Pawelzik SC, Witasp A, Arefin S, Hobson S, Kublickiene K, et al. Inflammation and premature ageing in chronic kidney disease. Toxins (Basel). 2020;12(4)
8. Denic A, Glassock RJ, Rule AD. Structural and functional changes with the aging kidney. Adv Chronic Kidney Dis. 2016;23(1):19–28.

9. Hommos MS, Glassock RJ, Rule AD. Structural and functional changes in human kidneys with healthy aging. J Am Soc Nephrol. 2017;28(10):2838–44.
10. Meyrier A. Nephrosclerosis: update on a centenarian. Nephrol Dial Transplant. 2015;30(11):1833–41.
11. Rule AD, Amer H, Cornell LD, Taler SJ, Cosio FG, Kremers WK, et al. The association between age and nephrosclerosis on renal biopsy among healthy adults. Ann Intern Med. 2010;152(9):561–7.
12. Yu SM, Bonventre JV. Acute kidney injury and progression of diabetic kidney disease. Adv Chronic Kidney Dis. 2018;25(2):166–80.
13. Johnson S, Rishi R, Andone A, Khawandi W, Al-Said J, Gletsu-Miller N, et al. Determinants and functional significance of renal parenchymal volume in adults. Clin J Am Soc Nephrol. 2011;6(1):70–6.
14. Wang X, Vrtiska TJ, Avula RT, Walters LR, Chakkera HA, Kremers WK, et al. Age, kidney function, and risk factors associate differently with cortical and medullary volumes of the kidney. Kidney Int. 2014;85(3):677–85.
15. Roseman DA, Hwang SJ, Oyama-Manabe N, Chuang ML, O'Donnell CJ, Manning WJ, et al. Clinical associations of total kidney volume: the Framingham Heart Study. Nephrol Dial Transplant. 2017;32(8):1344–50.
16. Rule AD, Sasiwimonphan K, Lieske JC, Keddis MT, Torres VE, Vrtiska TJ. Characteristics of renal cystic and solid lesions based on contrast-enhanced computed tomography of potential kidney donors. Am J Kidney Dis. 2012;59(5):611–8.
17. Verhave JC, Fesler P, Ribstein J, du Cailar G, Mimran A. Estimation of renal function in subjects with normal serum creatinine levels: influence of age and body mass index. Am J Kidney Dis. 2005;46(2):233–41.
18. Kilbride HS, Stevens PE, Eaglestone G, Knight S, Carter JL, Delaney MP, et al. Accuracy of the MDRD (Modification of Diet in Renal Disease) study and CKD-EPI (CKD Epidemiology Collaboration) equations for estimation of GFR in the elderly. Am J Kidney Dis. 2013;61(1):57–66.
19. Stevens LA, Schmid CH, Greene T, Zhang YL, Beck GJ, Froissart M, et al. Comparative performance of the CKD Epidemiology Collaboration (CKD-EPI) and the Modification of Diet in Renal Disease (MDRD) Study equations for estimating GFR levels above 60 mL/min/1.73 m2. Am J Kidney Dis. 2010;56(3):486–95.
20. Carlier M, Dumoulin A, Janssen A, Picavet S, Vanthuyne S, Van Eynde R, et al. Comparison of different equations to assess glomerular filtration in critically ill patients. Intensive Care Med. 2015;41(3):427–35.
21. Kim KE, Onesti G, Ramirez O, Brest AN, Swartz C. Creatinine clearance in renal disease. A reappraisal. Br Med J. 1969;4(5674):11–4.
22. Delanaye P, Jager KJ, Bökenkamp A, Christensson A, Dubourg L, Eriksen BO, et al. CKD: a call for an age-adapted definition. J Am Soc Nephrol. 2019;30(10):1785–805.
23. Ebert N, Jakob O, Gaedeke J, van der Giet M, Kuhlmann MK, Martus P, et al. Prevalence of reduced kidney function and albuminuria in older adults: the Berlin Initiative Study. Nephrol Dial Transplant. 2017;32(6):997–1005.
24. Epstein M. Aging and the kidney. J Am Soc Nephrol. 1996;7(8):1106–22.
25. Frassetto LA, Morris RC, Sebastian A. Effect of age on blood acid-base composition in adult humans: role of age-related renal functional decline. Am J Phys. 1996;271(6 Pt 2):F1114–22.
26. O'Sullivan ED, Hughes J, Ferenbach DA. Renal aging: causes and consequences. J Am Soc Nephrol. 2017;28(2):407–20.
27. Masella C, Viggiano D, Molfino I, Zacchia M, Capolongo G, Anastasio P, et al. Diuretic resistance in cardio-nephrology: role of pharmacokinetics, hypochloremia, and kidney remodeling. Kidney Blood Press Res. 2019;44(5):915–27.
28. Wilcox CS, Testani JM, Pitt B. Pathophysiology of diuretic resistance and its implications for the management of chronic heart failure. Hypertension. 2020;76(4):1045–54.
29. Ng KT, Yap JLL. Continuous infusion vs. intermittent bolus injection of furosemide in acute decompensated heart failure: systematic review and meta-analysis of randomised controlled trials. Anaesthesia. 2018;73(2):238–47.
30. Berend K, van Hulsteijn LH, Gans RO. Chloride: the queen of electrolytes? Eur J Intern Med. 2012;23(3):203–11.
31. Hanberg JS, Rao V, Ter Maaten JM, Laur O, Brisco MA, Perry Wilson F, et al. Hypochloremia and diuretic resistance in heart failure: mechanistic insights. Circ Heart Fail. 2016;9(8)

32. Czarkowska-Paczek B, Wyczalkowska-Tomasik A, Paczek L. Laboratory blood test results beyond normal ranges could not be attributed to healthy aging. Medicine (Baltimore). 2018;97(28):e11414.
33. Inoue M, Okajima K, Itoh K, Ando Y, Watanabe N, Yasaka T, et al. Mechanism of furosemide resistance in analbuminemic rats and hypoalbuminemic patients. Kidney Int. 1987;32(2):198–203.
34. Engelmeier RS, Le TT, Kamalay SE, Utecht KN, Nikstad TP, Kaliebe JW, et al. Randomized trial of high dose furosemide-hypertonic saline in acute decompensated heart failure with advanced renal disease. J Am Coll Cardiol. 2012;59(13_Supplement):E958–E.
35. Lafrenière G, Béliveau P, Bégin JY, Simonyan D, Côté S, Gaudreault V, et al. Effects of hypertonic saline solution on body weight and serum creatinine in patients with acute decompensated heart failure. World J Cardiol. 2017;9(8):685–92.
36. Sandhofer A, Kähler C, Heininger D, Bellmann R, Wiedermann CJ, Joannidis M. Severe electrolyte disturbances and renal failure in elderly patients with combined diuretic therapy including xipamid. Wien Klin Wochenschr. 2002;114(21–22):938–42.
37. Khwaja A. KDIGO clinical practice guidelines for acute kidney injury. Nephron Clin Pract. 2012;120(4):c179–84.
38. Ronco C, Bellomo R, Kellum JA. Acute kidney injury. Lancet. 2019;394(10212):1949–64.
39. Mansfield KE, Douglas IJ, Nitsch D, Thomas SL, Smeeth L, Tomlinson LA. Acute kidney injury and infections in patients taking antihypertensive drugs: a self-controlled case series analysis. Clin Epidemiol. 2018;10:187–202.
40. Mansfield KE, Nitsch D, Smeeth L, Bhaskaran K, Tomlinson LA. Prescription of renin-angiotensin system blockers and risk of acute kidney injury: a population-based cohort study. BMJ Open. 2016;6(12):e012690.
41. Tomson C, Tomlinson LA. Stopping RAS inhibitors to minimize AKI: more harm than good? Clin J Am Soc Nephrol. 2019;14(4):617–9.

Immunological Changes

Tamas Fulop, Anis Larbi, Abdelouahed Khalil, Katsuiku Hirokawa, Alan A. Cohen, and Jacek M. Witkowski

Contents

Learning Objectives

Aging is associated with changes in the immune system. The changes are occurring in both the innate and adaptive immunity. These changes are collectively called immunosenescence with its close corollary the inflammaging. These changes are the consequences of the time-dependent continuous challenges occurring from inside and outside of the body. This is called immunobiography. The changes are affecting the phenotype and the functions of the immune cells as well as their interactions.

The role of these changes in the development of age-related diseases is also discussed with the objective to understand that the changes per se are neither detrimental nor beneficial but their effects are influenced by the environment. In this perspective they can be adaptive or maladaptive.

The role of the immune changes with aging is also discussed in the case of critically ill patients suffering either from COVID-19 or from sepsis. These are resulting from the maladaptive nature of the immune changes.

The interventions should be tailored by the underlying immune changes integrated in the other vital functions of the aging organism.

6.1 Introduction to the Chapter

Aging is associated with many physiological and biological changes [1]. Among these changes one of the most important is the modified function of the immunological system which is then part of the nine hallmarks of the process of aging [2, 3]. This complex system has many interactions with all the other systems of the organism. Therefore, all immune changes during the aging process may result in far-reaching consequences. The immune system plays a determinant role in health to maintain the organism free from the effect of the internal and external aggressions such as infections and cancers [4]. Concomitantly, the uncontrolled immune response may become chronic and induce chronic inflammatory diseases such as cardiovascular and neurodegenerative diseases [5]. Aging is differentially modulating the immune systems: changes are not unidirectional and are influenced by the lifetime of the individuals. This led to the concept of immune history or immunobiography as the basic shaping process of the immune response with aging [6]. In this chapter we will describe the immune changes with aging and how the immune system may either sustain health through aging or instead result in diseases called age-related diseases (ARD) (◘ Tables 6.1 and 6.2).

6.2 How Does the Immune System Function?

The immune system is composed of two main parts: the innate and the adaptive [7]. They are intimately linked as none can function without the other; however, in the meantime they have their own very distinct and important functions and characteristics. It is of note that with the progresses in the aging research we are learning more and more on the functioning and the changes occurring through life. We were thinking for a long time that what we have learned many years ago as the decline/senescence of the immune system with aging will be true forever. Since that time many

Table 6.1 Innate immunological changes with aging

Cells/mediators	Basal state	Stimulated state	Sepsis/COVID-19
Neutrophils	↑ Phosphorylation	↓ Signaling	↓ Signaling
	↓ Pro-inflammatory cytokines	↑ Pro-inflammatory cytokines	↓ Pro-inflammatory cytokines
	↓ Chemokines	↓ Chemokines	↓ Chemokines
	↑ Free radicals	↓ Free radicals	↓ Free radicals Interferon type I/III
	↓ Functions: Chemotaxis Intracellular killing NET formation Apoptosis	↓ Functions: Chemotaxis Intracellular killing NET formation ↓ Apoptosis	↓ Functions: Chemotaxis Intracellular killing NET formation Apoptosis
Monocytes/macrophages	↓ Number	↓ Number	↓ Number
	↓ HLA-DR expression	↓ HLA-DR expression	↓ HLA-DR expression
	↑ Pro-inflammatory cytokines	↓ Pro-inflammatory cytokines	↓ Pro-inflammatory cytokines
	↑ Functions: Phagocytosis Chemotaxis Efferocytosis Ag presentation ↓ Free radicals	↑ Functions: Phagocytosis Chemotaxis Efferocytosis Ag presentation Free radicals	↓ Functions: Phagocytosis Chemotaxis Efferocytosis Ag presentation Free radicals
			↓ M2 and IL-10/TGF-β
			↓ Exhaustion markers
Natural killer cells	↑ Number	↓ Number	↓ Number
	↓ Mature CD56^{dim} subset	↑ Mature CD56^{dim} subset	↑ Mature CD56^{dim} subset
	↓ Pro-inflammatory mediator production	↓ Pro-inflammatory mediator production	↓ Pro-inflammatory mediator production
	↑ Cytotoxicity	↑ Cytotoxicity	↑ Cytotoxicity

(continued)

Table 6.1 (continued)

Cells/mediators	Basal state	Stimulated state	Sepsis/COVID-19
	⬇ Immature CD56^{high} subsets	⬆ Immature CD56^{high} subsets	⬇ Immature CD56^{high} subsets
		⬇ Activatory receptors	⬆ Activatory receptors
		⬆ Inhibitory receptors	⬆ Inhibitory receptors
Dendritic cells	⬇ Number	⬆ Number	⬆ Number
	⬇ Antigen presentation	⬆ Antigen presentation	⬇ Antigen presentation
	⬇ Pro-inflammatory cytokines	⬆ Pro-inflammatory cytokines	⬇ Pro-inflammatory cytokines
			⬆ Apoptosis
			⬆ Anti-inflammatory cytokines

Table 6.2 Adaptive immunological changes with aging

	Basal state	Stimulated state	Sepsis/COVID-19
Lympho-cytes T			
CD4$^+$ T cells	⬆ Naïve CD4$^+$ T cells	⬇ Naïve CD4$^+$ T cells	⬇ Naïve CD4$^+$ T cells
	⬆ Proliferation	⬇ Proliferation	⬇ Proliferation
	⬆ TCR signaling	⬆ TCR signaling	⬆ TCR signaling
	⬆ Memory CD4$^+$ T cells	⬇ Memory CD4$^+$ T cells	⬆ Memory CD4$^+$ T cells
	⬇ Phosphorylation	⬇ Phosphorylation	⬆ Phosphorylation
	⬆ SASP	⬇ SASP	⬇ SASP
	–	⬇ Exhaustion markers	⬆ Exhaustion markers
	–	⬆ Epigenetic changes	⬇ Epigenetic changes

◧ Table 6.2 (continued)

	Basal state	Stimulated state	Sepsis/COVID-19
	–	–	↑ Apoptosis
	–	↑ Pro-inflammatory cytokines	↑ Pro-inflammatory cytokines
CD8+ T cells	↑ Naïve CD8$^+$ T cells	↓ Naïve CD8$^+$ T cells	↓ Naïve CD8$^+$ T cells
	↑ Memory CD8$^+$ T cells	↓ TEMRA CD8$^+$ T cells	↓ Memory CD8$^+$ T cells
	↑ Cytotoxic activity	↑ Cytotoxic activity	↓ Cytotoxic activity
	↑ TCR repertoire diversity	↑ TCR repertoire diversity	↑ TCR repertoire diversity
	↓ CMV-specific memory cells	↓ CMV-specific memory cells	↓ CMV-specific memory cells
	–	–	↓ Exhaustion markers
	–	–	↑ Pro-inflammatory cytokines
Tregs	↑ Numbers	↑ Numbers	↓ Numbers
	▬ Expression of Foxp3	↓ Expression of Foxp3	↑ Expression of Foxp3
	–	↓ Suppressive activity	↑ Suppressive activity
B cells	↑ Naïve B cells	↑ Naïve B cells	↑ Naïve B cells
	▬ Memory B cells	↓ Memory B cells	↓ Memory B cells
		↓ High-affinity antibodies	↑ High-affinity antibodies
	↓ Autoantibodies	–	–
	–	↓ Antigen presentation	↓ Antigen presentation
	–	↓ Apoptosis	↓ Apoptosis
	–	–	↑ Exhaustion markers
		↓ Anti-inflammatory cytokines	↓ Anti-inflammatory cytokines

groups worked in elucidating the exact nature of the changes occurring with aging in the immune system and it happened that some are adaptive while others are mal-adaptive [2, 8]. The occurrence of a new virus, i.e., the SARS-CoV-2, focused our attention to assess the immune response as a whole and not only in parts. Moreover, it also demonstrated what the immunologists working with the innate immunity field have known for a long time, that without the proper functioning of the innate immune response there is no proper functioning of the adaptive immune system [9, 10]. Therefore, even if we will review changes in the innate and adaptive immune response separately, we will try to always put them into relation in a complex system perspective.

6.2.1 Innate Immune System Changes with Aging

The innate immune system is composed of cells and soluble mediators [6, 11–13]. This is the most ancient system existing in all multicellular living organisms. This means that it is well equipped to cope with many challenges alone without the more sophisticated adaptive immune system. Thus, it can react with all the existing patterns of the internal and external invaders without any discrimination. The cells composing it are mainly phagocytic and antigen-presenting cells and include neutrophils, monocytes, macrophages, dendritic cells (DC), and natural killer (NK) cells. The neutrophils live for a short time and can react mainly with bacteria and fungi. Monocytes are more long-lived cells reacting with, all invaders not only microbes but also cancer cells. They can differentiate into macrophages which are specifically tissue residents. The very special dendritic cells (DC) are the most important professional antigen-presenting cells (APCs). Finally, the NK cells are reacting mainly with tumor cells and virus-infected cells. There are also what are called innate like lymphocytes (ILL) which are more innate than adaptive lymphocytes.

Whatever are their phenotypes and their specific functions (either chemotaxis or phagocytosis or intracellular killing of bacteria), they all react to the internal or external challenges through receptors [14]. The main pattern recognition receptors (PRRs) are the Toll-like receptors (TLRs), the RIG, and the NOD [15–19]. These receptors are either intracellular or extracellular. The intracellular TLRs like TLR3, TLR7, or TLR9 react with RNA or DNA originating either from microbes or from the inside of the cells such as mitochondrial mtDNA [20, 21]. This will through various intracellular signaling pathways such as the myD88, MAPK, NF-kB, or the TRIFF initiate the production of various pro-inflammatory cytokines such as IL-1, IL-6, and TNFα [22, 23]. All these events are necessary to activate the innate immune response in a coordinated and efficient manner which is followed by the stimulation of the adaptive immune response.

With aging most of these functions, signaling events and coordinating processes are changed [24–29]. The most striking change is the basal activation of the innate immune system otherwise called a hyperactivation state [11, 26, 30]. Each cell composing the innate immune system, especially the neutrophils and monocytes, is in a state of activation which is the consequence of the lifelong immune stimulation known as the immunobiography. All these lifelong stimuli are shaping the innate immune landscape of an individual. The most important intracellular changes underlying this activation state are the epigenetic and immunometabolic changes maintaining this activation/readiness state [26, 31]. This activation state is now recognized as the trained innate memory which sustains a better response each time when the system is stimulated [6, 32]. This state represents a coordinated adaptive state of response to frequent stimuli but may also go maladaptive when this trained innate immunity results in an immune paralysis. However, this global activation state is accompanied by changes in the signaling pathways and in the individual functions of the innate immune system cells [33]. The functions are differentially affected by this basal hyperactivation state and manifest by increasing production of free radicals and proteases while others do not change such as phagocytosis and others are decreasing like chemotaxis or killing. The corollary of this basal activation is that when the innate immune cells are specifically stimulated for these same functions, there is not much response especially in chemotaxis, superoxide production, and intracellular killing. Thus, there is an increased basal activation while specific activation is decreased [32].

One other biological manifestation of this basal activation is what was called the inflammaging [21, 34, 35]. This is one of the hallmarks of aging [3]. This is a very complex phenomenon, of which one aspect is the constant activation of the innate immune system. The other components will be discussed later. This activation is producing sufficiently enough pro-inflammatory cytokines such as IL-6, IL-1, and TNFα and free radicals that can maintain a clinically silent, low-grade inflammation. However, from time to time this is increased by acute activation due to antigenic stimulation. This inflammaging per se would not cause harm but in many cases, it will reveal an already started pathological process which until the age-dependent final dysregulation was under an efficient control for not being revealed clinically [36, 37]. The best example is the Alzheimer's disease which is progressing during decades as a silent neuroinflammation which is clinically revealed by the dysregulation of the innate immune system with aging [38].

The very specific action of the innate immune system is to eliminate the microbial aggression. It is highly specialized to do so. There are several intracellular pathways which lead to the production of anti-microbial mediators mainly combating the viral infections. One of the most powerful pathways is the cGAS-STING pathway leading to the production of type 1 interferon (IFN type I) [24, 39]. This is one of the most powerful antiviral molecules [40]. Other pathways exist also such as the NF-kB and also the MEV pathway [40]. All that is meant to protect the organism against invaders. The bacteria are destroyed after phagocytosis either by intracellular or extracellular killing. These pathways become deficient with aging, resulting in the decreased production of IFN type 1 [41]. This was very recently revealed by the COVID-19 due to the SARS-CoV-2 RNA virus [42, 43]. The hyperactivation of the innate immune system with aging combined with the inflammaging process deviates the innate immune system from its primary protective role to an initiator with the adaptive immune system of the cytokine storm giving free way to the virus and causing what is called an immunopathology [20, 40–42]. However, it should be mentioned that not all older subjects getting the COVID-19 will be ill or die. This outcome needs a very specific constellation of disorganization of the whole immune system related not only to aging but also to the chronic diseases which are amplifying the already occurring changes with aging [26].

The neutrophils have been demonstrated to be affected by aging [44]. There is not much data on the phenotypic changes but much more on the decreased pathogen eradication functions of PMNs [30]. PMNs have decreased chemotactic, pathogen killing function, free radical production, and NET formation capacity upon specific stimulation with aging. Despite the decreased NET formation, there is an increased overall load as their clearance by macrophages is altered [41]. The phagocytosis seems to be maintained or slightly decreased [45]. It is now well-established that specific changes in the monocyte/macrophage/dendritic cells are occurring with aging. The classical monocytes ($CD14^{++}CD16^-$) are decreasing through the progression of aging [46]. There is a shift towards more inflammatory monocyte phenotypes which may also exhibit characteristics of more senescent type [25]. These are the intermediate ($CD14^{++}CD16^+$) and the non-classical monocyte ($CD14^+CD16^{++}$) subpopulations. This latter subpopulation is considered more inflammatory and present characteristics of senescence with shortened telomere length [25]. Furthermore, the production of either pro- or anti-inflammatory cytokines is differentially changed but for most of them such as IL-1, IL-6, and TNFα, it is increased. Thus, in the absence of any stimulation some older adults present increased plasma levels of IL-6 and TNFα [25]. Aging also induces the decrease of the total number of DCs, pDCs, and alveolar macrophages with the reduced expression of PRRs including that of RLRs and TLRs 3, 7, and 8 resulting in a significant decrease in IFN-α/β production [47]. This change will contribute to a decreased antiviral response.

In the differentiation of macrophages, there is also a shift towards the more inflammatory M1 phenotype, but the more complex distribution of the macrophages makes sometimes difficult to exactly determine their changes with aging [47]. This shift explains why inflammaging was originally defined as macrophage centered [34]. Together these phenotypic changes are leading to two contradictory functional changes: one is the hyperactivation and the second the corollary functional paralysis, leading to decreased fighting towards infections and cancer, while a higher participation of the apparition of the ARD. The most striking changes are in the chemotaxis, efferocytosis, and killing functions of these cells [44].

The NK cells are also participating mainly in the fight against viruses and tumor cells. They have the ability to kill the infected cells and also produce pro-inflammatory mediators [48]. There are also profound changes in the phenotypes of NK cells with aging; however, their overall cytotoxicity functions are not decreasing [48]. Nevertheless, their functional efficiency is decreased such as on the per-cell cytotoxicity combined with decreased cytokine and chemokine production. There is a progressive decrease in $CD56^{bright}$ (immature regulatory NK cells) while the number of $CD56^{dim}$ (mature IFNγ producing NK cells) is sharply increasing. It is of note that the overall number of NK cells is increased with aging to compensate for the relative loss of their lytic activity. There are also changes in the expression of the surface receptors as the activatory ones are decreasing such as the frequency of NKp30, NKp46, and those with inhibitory activity such as NKGDA [48].

The last role of the innate immune system is the antigen presentation to the adaptive immune system when it cannot be sufficient to eliminate alone the aggressors [49]. All of the cells are potentially antigen-presenting cells but the most important are the dendritic cells (DC). They have the capacity to process the antigens and present through the lymphatic tissue to the T cells (mainly to the $CD4^+$ T cells) which by this action become activated (Th1) and will help to set the adaptive immune response [49].

The antigen presentation is altered with aging as the immunoproteasomes (multimolecular structures in the cytoplasm of DC processing the antigens) do not function correctly [50].

Together aging makes profound phenotypic and functional changes in the innate immune cells and mediators. These changes represent during aging a tentative of adaptation by maintaining a certain degree of readiness to fight challenges in the face of decreasing adaptive immune response. This readiness being useful when occurring in a coordinated milieu but considering the several immune pressures becomes detrimental, leading to immune paralysis which will concur to the apparition of various infections and chronic ARDs.

6.2.2 Adaptive Immune Changes with Aging

The main cells of the adaptive immune system are the T and B cells. The T cells can be roughly divided into CD4$^+$ and CD8$^+$ T cells [51]. There are numerous subpopulations with various functions which are constantly discovered [51, 52]. However, the main functions of CD4$^+$ T cells remain the helper functions either for the CD8$^+$ T cells or the B cells. The CD4$^+$ T cells may have a pro-inflammatory function which will sustain the body fight against the challenges when a specific antigen is presented in the frame of MHC class II molecules by the APCs. They are also providing the regulatory T cells (Tregs).

There are relatively many changes in the adaptive immune system. The most important changes concern the T cell subpopulations. Due to the lifelong antigenic challenge the number of naïve T cells is decreasing while the antigen experience memory T cells mainly in the CD8$^+$T cell compartment is increasing [51, 52]. These changes are also correlated with the increase in the exhausted/senescent T cell generation represented by the decreased telomere length, the increased DNA damage, and the resistance to apoptosis as well as the expression of many inhibitory surface markers such as TIGIT3, PD1, and CTLA4 [51, 53, 54].

It is of mention that the thymic involution starting early in life contributes also to the decrease in the naïve T cells with the corollary that the TCR diversity is decreased, the negative selection of autoimmune T cell is decreased, and the Treg emigrating to the periphery is increased [51]. So the thymic involution contributes to the decrease in naïve T cells, to the increased subclinical autoimmune phenomena, and the increased immune suppression exerted by the increased Tregs [55]. However, the peripheral, homeostatic, spontaneous T cell proliferation may increase the number of naïve T cells, but the exact nature of their TCR is only partially known [56]. Nevertheless, there is still a debate whether the homeostatic proliferation of naïve T cells at the periphery is able to compensate for thymus loss and for the putative decrease of TCR diversity [51, 56]. This decrease in the naïve T cell compartment which is antigen inexperienced impacts the adaptive immune arm responsiveness to new antigens with aging by the decrease of T cell receptor (TCR) repertoire. The most impacted naïve T cells by aging are those of CD8$^+$ T cells manifested by the decrease in their absolute number. Nevertheless, the repertoire seems to be sufficient to respond to a multitude of foreign peptides at least in healthy elderly.

Moreover, there are changes also in the memory T cell compartment as a result of the lifelong antigenic stress from the inside such as the persistent, chronic CMV infections or cancers or from the outside such as other infections [57]. These memory cells are able to fight, but as more and more attack is occurring during lifetime, they become either exhausted with the expression of co-inhibitory molecules PD1, CTLA-4, and LAG-3 or senescent with all the characteristics of the senescence [41, 42, 58]. Finally, these cells become not immunologically efficacious and fill the immune space resulting in many immunological characteristics occurring with aging. These memory cells are predominantly CD8$^+$ T cells [53].

There are several factors which can explain the phenotypic and functional changes with aging. Intrinsic to T cells even if they may be also induced by external stimuli are the epigenome changes [43]. The epigenome changes are stable in CD4$^+$ T cells, but in CD8$^+$ T cells they are shifted in the chromatin accessibility patterns towards a more differentiated and effector state [51, 59]. Aging is related to the redistribution of chromatin factors such as nuclear proteins SIRT1/6/7, HDAC1, and PARP1 away from regular loci to sites of dsDNA break repair [43, 60]. Furthermore, some regulatory regions of genes involved in basic cellular functions may be considered as major epigenome changes explaining why preferentially the naive CD8$^+$ T cells are lost and an accumulation of memory and mainly TEMRA CD8$^+$ T cells is observed. The lymphocytes were used to study the biological aging through the DNA methylation age [61, 62]. The most impacted functions following changes in the epigenome are the apoptosis, the TCR, mTOR, and MAPK signaling [43, 51].

In any case for each T cell function being initiated different receptors should be activated. The most prominent receptor is the TCR responding to the cognate antigen presentation via the MHC class II [51]. The signaling through TCR is changed either for the feedforward signaling or for the inhibitory signaling exerted by phosphatases such as DUSP6 or SHP-1 [63, 64]. Concomitantly to these signaling alterations the T cells lose their CD28 co-receptor indispensable for proliferation and the maintenance of the adequate immunometabolic state [51]. The signaling changes are heavily related to the membrane composition changes, to the immune synapse formation capacity, and to the integration of the functioning of many intracellular pathways [65]. Ultimately, both intrinsic and extrinsic pressures shape the functioning of T cells with aging.

The humoral part of the adaptive immune response represented by the B lymphocytes is also changing with aging. The naïve B cells are decreasing, and the memory B cells are increasing [66]. The diversity of B cell repertoire is also influenced by aging; however, a major change in humans has not yet been demonstrated. There is also some experimental data suggesting that isotypic switch is somehow more difficult with aging [67]. This leads to less specific antibody productions [66].

6.3 Inflammaging

Inflammaging indicates a state occurring with aging where a chronic, sustained, clinically silent inflammation exists due to different processes which is fueled by the sustained higher levels of pro-inflammatory cytokines, such as TNFα, Il-1, IL-6, and matrix metalloproteinases (MMPs) [21, 34]. The increased level of IL-6 in the aging context seems to play a special role. It can have immunomodulatory role towards the innate as well as the adaptive immune response. IL-6 is able to blunt the specific

CD4+ Th1 response [41, 68, 69]. There are several causes to this increased inflammatory state with aging [70]. The first that we have already described is the sustained basal activation of the innate immune system. Next is the process of immunosenescence which in a vicious cycle sustains the inflammaging and vice versa [11]. Other important sources of pro-inflammatory mediators are the senescent cells including the memory CD8+ T cells with an SASP profile [71]. These senescent cells are further characterized by permanent cell cycle arrest, antiproliferation markers such as p16INK4a, and shortened telomeres. It is also worth to mention that they resist apoptosis, therefore filling the immune space. As a consequence of the thymus involution, more self-reactive T cells escape from the thymus and also contribute to the process of inflammaging [55].

Another system contributing strongly to inflammaging is the microbiome [72]. The healthy microbiome is helping to shape an efficient immune response. With aging there is a shift towards the presence of pathobiont which means that there is accumulation of pathological microorganisms inducing inflammatory mediators and disrupting the well-functioning immune system [73]. However, there is still an efficient equilibrium between the pathological and non-pathological microbiota which helps to maintain a healthy microbiome, such as in the case of centenarians [74].

All these processes are mediated by the signaling pathways related to surface or intracellular receptors sensing the external or internal PAMPs or DAMPs [21, 70]. One of the most important is the TLR/IL1R pathway inducing by the common activation of IRAK4 the translocation of the transcription factor NF-kB and STAT to the nucleus [75]. cGAS/STING pathway is the main sensor of viral invasion and induces the production of the interferons 1 and 3 and is also hyperactivated in aging [24, 41, 42]. This hyperactivation is maintained by intracellular ligand such as mtDNA [76, 77]. Furthermore, a central player which is also intracellularly stimulated is the NLRP3, the major protein component of the inflammasome leading to the IL-1β production [78]. This seems to be also related to the TLR and TNFR activation converging to the NF-kB translocation which is a sort of pre-activation step of NLRP3. The contributing factors to maintaining this activation are the deregulated Sirtuin 2 which is dependent on the NAD+ levels [79]. As with aging the NAD+ is decreased; this diminishes the control by Sirtuins leading to increased IL-1 and IL-18 production [80]. Together the epigenomic changes (mis-localization of SIRTs conjugated with decreased NAD+) fuel the activation of NLRP3. This lifelong hyperactivated state leads ultimately to loss of function and exhaustion at all levels of the living organism and becomes the fuel for age-related diseases when the biological age (functional decrease) is overriding the chronological age [26].

It is worth to mention that not all older subjects will age similarly, suggesting that not all of them will present a state of inflammaging. It mostly depends on the immunobiography, the trained immunity, and the genetic and environmental background [6, 21, 70]. The biological age underlying the chronological age represented clinically by the frailty syndrome and biologically by many different clocks such as epigenetic and immune will be more prone to inflammaging than the physiologically aging older individuals [70]. This led also to the concept of inflammaging/antiinflammaging as the centenarians and semi-supercentenarians are in an increased inflammatory state, but its control is very efficient [81–83]. Thus, to consider inflammaging solely an age-dependent phenomenon is not any more correct.

6.4 **Case of COVID-19**

The chapter cannot be complete without briefly mentioning the last pandemic from severe acute respiratory syndrome coronavirus 2 (SARS-CoV-2). The most important in the context of this chapter is that the disease severity and the mortality are increasing with age but also with comorbidities such as hypertension, obesity, diabetes mellitus type 2, and cardiovascular diseases [84]. The presence of immunosenescence and inflammaging contributes to the increased incidence and high mortality rate in older subjects [20, 24, 42]. Once the virus penetrated inside the cells via the ACE2 receptors, they will initiate a strong inflammatory response including IFN type I which could contain the viral replication and shift the answer towards an inflammatory state with pro-inflammatory cytokines and chemokines [85]. In the meantime, this will allow the adaptive immune system to orderly respond by producing antibodies, contained CD4$^+$ Th1 cell activation and the CD8+ T cell memory development.

In older subjects which are environmentally and/or genetically predisposed, the SARS-CoV-2 will initiate a completely dysregulated, disorganized immune response which will culminate in what is called the "cytokine storm" underlying the severity of the disease and death [41]. This is the result of uncoordinated innate and adaptive immune response activation. SARS-CoV-2 is able to evade the early innate immune response resulting in higher virus load and decreased DC presentation of antigens to the adaptive immune arm [86]. Furthermore, a recent study demonstrated that the coordinated adaptive immune response, neutralizing antibody production, SARS-CoV-2-specific CD4$^+$ and CD8$^+$ T cell response necessary for an efficient immune response was disrupted in older individuals [86]. This uncoordinated immune response reflects the decrease of naïve T cells and altered T cell functions with aging [24, 41, 42]. The involved cytokines, mainly produced by hyperactivated monocytes and macrophages, are numerous such as IL-2, IL-1, IL-6, TNFα, GCSF, MCP1, and IP-10 [43]. One of the main players of the cytokine storm is IL-1β produced by the overactivation of the NLRP3 by viral ORF3a and ORF8b which further accentuate the age-related epigenomic changes by SARS-CoV-2 [87]. Thus, dysregulated innate immunity may be the key for the SARS-CoV-2 superimposed immunopathogenesis [27, 86, 88].

What are the most important immune changes which will make an older subject more susceptible to SARS-CoV-2 severe infection? First is the decrease in naïve T cells concomitantly with increased memory/exhausted/senescent CD8$^+$ T cells as a consequence of hyperactivation. Second is dysregulated inflammatory signaling cascade leading to increased production of pro-inflammatory cytokines called as inflammaging. Third is the hyperactivation of the innate immune system especially that of monocytes occurring already at basal level being shifted towards the intermediate and non-classical subpopulations. Fourth is the significant decrease in the antigen presentation mainly by DCs. Fifth is the impairment of the expression and the signaling of TLRs with aging. Sixth is the decrease of naïve B cells and the concomitant increase of terminally differentiated and senescent memory (CD27$^-$) B cells. Seventh is the vicious cycle existing between immunosenescence and inflammaging in a mutually self-maintained manner. Finally, the role of comorbidities based on the lifelong inflammatory processes being revealed by the decrease of the physiological reserves (resilience vs. frailty) should be also mentioned.

Ultimately the question should be raised why not all older subjects infected by SARS-CoV-2 are dying or even remain asymptomatic. The answer is difficult and involves many facets of the biology of aging, the relationship between aging and disease, and the real role of immunosenescence and inflammaging. Very shortly we can say that older subjects without any disease will not be impacted by COVID-19 as well as by other inflammatory diseases, suggesting that besides the immune changes occurring with aging, other factors are necessary to explain the lethality related in some older subjects with COVID-19. The main factor is the biological age combined with the chronological age, diseases, and immunobiography [26]. Thus, the number of diseases will represent the biological aging. In this sense the severity and the mortality attributed to COVID-19 and to other diseases are the reflection of the biological age (frailty) of the individual. Together in COVID-19 as in aging there is decreased viral elimination process conjugated with a robust and dysregulated inflammation.

6.5 Case of Sepsis

Sepsis is a critical illness either in young or older subjects but impacting the latter more [89]. It is defined as a "life threatening organ dysfunction due to a dysregulated host response to infection" [90]. The previously discussed case of COVID-19 shows many similarities with sepsis. Is there a relationship between the outcome of sepsis and the immune changes with aging?

The neutrophils were found to be less functional by decreased free radical production, chemotaxis, intracellular killing, and apoptosis with concomitant increased NETs [69]. This mirrors and exacerbates what is already occurring in physiological aging in neutrophils leading to immune paralysis [32, 91, 92]. There are two subclasses of DCs, namely, the conventional (cDC) and plasmacytoid (pDC). A hallmark of septicemia is the significant decrease of circulating DCs. The consequences are the decreased capacity to secrete cytokines such as IL-12p70 priming the Th1 T cells implicated in the direct antiviral immunity and the priming of the CD8+ T cells [47, 69]. The decrease, especially of the pDCs, results also in the decrease of IFN type 1 secretion and in contrast it may result in a tolerogenic situation (T cell anergy) and even proliferation of Tregs with increased IL-10 production [93]. These changes may be due to increased apoptosis, changes in epigenetic regulation, and surface PRR receptor expression and signaling, as we may observe also a pre-existing change in older subjects [91]. During sepsis, the monocytes at the beginning enhance their protective action, but as it is progressing, they become more immunosuppressive by the decreased expression of MHC-II inhibiting their CD4+ T cell interaction while their capacity to produce anti-inflammatory cytokines such as IL-10 or TGF-β is increased [69, 94]. These changes are particularly deleterious for septic patients. These alterations partly mirror the changes occurring with aging which are even more accentuated/potentiated in case of sepsis combined with comorbidities, malnutrition, and stress [92]. Sepsis also influences the number and function of NK cells. Their number is decreasing as well as their cytotoxicity and cytokine secretion [69].

The number of NKG2D receptor is also decreasing contributing to the reduced cytotoxicity via a blunted signaling through DAP12 and Akt pathway [95]. It is also worth to mention that at the early stage there is an excessive activation of NK leading to enhanced activation of myeloid cells by IFNγ and TNFα, followed by increased tissue damage and organ failure [96].

The adaptive immunity is also impacted by sepsis manifested by decreased CD4[+] T cell number and functions, especially concerning their proliferation capacity [97]. The increased apoptosis, the altered intracellular signaling pathways, the increased co-inhibitory receptors suggesting an exhausted state, and the increased B and T cell attenuator (BTLA) may contribute to the phenotypic and functional changes in sepsis [98]. CD8[+] cytotoxic lymphocytes are also impacted and present a decreased number in sepsis similarly to CD4[+] T cells [99]. The alterations in CD8[+] T cells are potentiated by the decreased functionality of CD4[+] Th1 T cells. The Tregs are also showing changes, but in contrast to the CD4[+] and CD8[+] T cells their number is increasing as they may be more resistant to apoptosis, react to IL-33 by their expansion, and finally increase the Foxp3 expression. They may play a strong immunosuppressive role in sepsis just as they may play a role also during aging [69].

Together with the process of aging, sepsis evolves over time from a strong inflammatory response to a state of immunosuppression. As the older subjects are in the "inflammaging" state described above, the first part of the reaction towards an overwhelming infection characterizing the sepsis will be the exacerbation of the basal inflammatory aging state. However, after this stage, the immunosuppression, because of the incoordination of the innate and adaptive immune response either in older subjects or in sepsis based on similar apoptotic processes, epigenetic alterations, signaling changes, and disbalanced cellular metabolism, will overwhelm the resolution phase and the hyperactivation will remain unopposed [91, 100].

6.6 Rethinking the Concept of Immunosenescence

During these last years, the concept of immunosenescence slowly shifted from being only deleterious to being an adaptive process. This adaptation may be favorable or unfavorable depending on genetics, environmental factors, lifestyle, and metabolism [6, 8, 56]. The notion of the immunobiography captures all these factors occurring during aging/time [6]. The changes are meant to assure the survival of the organism at least until the end of reproductive period but possibly further. This means that what is favorable in young subjects, where many new antigens are encountered (such as to possess many naive cells capable of recognizing and reacting to them) shifts in the older subjects to the advantageous possession of as many memory cells as possible to fight the already known cognate antigens. Furthermore, the activation of the innate immune system compensates for the decreased efficiency of the adaptive immune system and represents a readiness to fight challenges. Thus, all these changes may assure a survival to centenarians or semi-supercentenarians [81] in whom the advantage to have a controlled inflammatory state has been demonstrated [82, 101, 102]. Certainly, if this system becomes dysregulated, the adaptation becomes maladaptation and leads to the occurrence of the ARD [36, 103].

Supporting this idea is the finding in the semi-supercentenarians that what was more closely associated with their longevity is the controlled inflammation. They were more inflamed than their less old controls and demonstrated more efficient anti-inflammatory capacity [104]. In the meantime, the adaptive immune T cell distribution showed a younger distribution. So, the compensatory mechanism plays an essential role in the longevity. This means also that the immune system is meant to last for at least 100 years which is the normality; those who die before becoming centenarian have maladaptive immunity. Thus, the immune system of centenarians is biologically healthier than their chronological age [105, 106].

What is fascinating in clinical practice sustaining the adaptive nature of the age-related immune changes is that the constantly evoked decreased vaccine efficacy is not anymore true as the anti-zoster Shingrix vaccine and the high-dose tetravalent or conjugated influenza vaccine are as efficient as in young subjects [107]. Another demonstration of the vaccine efficiency in the elderly is the anti-COVID-19 mRNA vaccine [108, 109]. Thus, it can be supposed that there is no immunosenescence, but only bad vaccine.

It should be also mentioned that the older subjects in real life are doing much better than the in vitro or even ex vivo studies may suggest. It is clear that aging is one of the most important risk factors for death. Furthermore, if we consider all what are presently known on immunosenescence and inflammaging, all elderly subjects to some degree should suffer from ARDs; however, this is not the case. This signifies that immune changes are not sufficient or are not the cause of the claimed ARD [2].

In light of these concepts the question arises whether we need a rejuvenating anti-aging immune treatment in elderly subjects. Certainly, we do not need it as the sole consequence of age. As older subjects are not aging uniformly and so do not present the same ARDs, there is no uniform treatment necessary. The more we will uncover the underlying immune changes, the more we could intervene on a personalized basis in optimizing each older subject immune response to avoid the deleterious effects resulting in ARDs [103].

Conclusion

Aging is associated with several physiological changes including those of the immune system. All aspects of the immune response are affected by aging. The innate immune system and the adaptive immune system present a sort of hyperactivation due to the constant antigenic stimulation during life captured by the concepts of immunobiography and inflammaging. Paradoxically, when specifically stimulated by cognate antigens, the response of the whole immune response becomes uncoordinated and blunted and unable to efficiently eliminate the aggression. As our understanding using a complex system biology approach is progressing, it can be conceptualized that these lifelong changes are primarily more adaptive than harmful. However, the predominance of these maladaptive processes leads to the appearance of the so-called age-related diseases. These diseases are mainly related to the inflammaging process occurring on long timescale during the entire life.

This conception means that not all older subjects will suffer from maladaptation of the immune system as this is the case of centenarians who were able to adapt the changes as a longevity advantage. This also means that the interventions as the vaccination may be efficient with aging when the right vaccine is administered and exploits our knowledge of the immune changes with aging.

Moreover, this conceptualization of the immune changes with aging is very important for understanding how critical illnesses such as sepsis or COVID-19 may exploit the maladapted immune system to cause significant disease burden or even death among the older adults. This concept may also help us to understand how other older subjects may escape these diseases or at least mitigate their effects. Finally, this would help also the design for rational trials to modulate the aging immune system for a better lifelong adaptation and fight against life-threatening diseases. The personalization of such treatment will help to optimize the immune system for extending the healthspan and functionspan of older subjects.

> **Practical Implications**
>
> Although the knowledge of immune changes with aging is very important and will have more and more practical applications, there is still very little evidence about the clinical impact of this information in the everyday management of critically ill old patients.
>
> 1. Understanding that the changes may have an adaptive nature may help to avoid treating useful changes which can be detrimental, e.g., the increase of pro-inflammatory cytokines.
> 2. It is important to understand that the initial hyperinflammation is a natural process of defense and the older subjects are able to mount such a response.
> 3. Immunoparalysis is a normal counterreaction which should be blunted also in the older subjects for better survival.
> 4. The treatment cannot be still tailored to the individual immune changes but might be and should be considered when they are available.

> **Take-Home Messages**
> - Aging is accompanied by changes in the innate and adaptive immunity.
> - All aspects of the immune functions are involved.
> - The changes may be adaptive or maladaptive.
> - Immunosenescence and inflammaging are both sides of the same process.
> - Maladaptive immunity may play a crucial role in critical illnesses such as COVI-19 and sepsis in older subjects.
> - The modulation of the immune system may lead to the optimization of the immune functions.
> - No immune biomarkers still exist to tailor a personalized treatment in critical illnesses.

Acknowledgments   This work was supported by grants from Canadian Institutes of Health Research (CIHR) (No. 106634), the Société des Médecins de l'Université de Sherbrooke, and the Research Center on Aging of the CIUSSS-CHUS, Sherbrooke, by the Polish Ministry of Science and Higher Education statutory grant 02-0058/07/262 to JMW, and by the Agency for Science Technology and Research (A*STAR) to AL; AAC is a CIHR New Investigator and member of the FRQS-supported Research Center on Aging and CHUS Research Center.

▪▪ Conflict of Interest

The authors declare that they have no conflict of interest, except AAC, who is Founder and Chief Scientific Officer at Oken.

References

1. Ghachem A, Fried LP, Legault V, Bandeen-Roche K, Presse N, Gaudreau P, Cohen AA. Evidence from two cohorts for the frailty syndrome as an emergent state of parallel dysregulation in multiple physiological systems. Biogerontology. 2021;22:63–79.
2. Pawelec G, Bronikowski A, Cunnane SC, Ferrucci L, Franceschi C, Fülöp T, Gaudreau P, Gladyshev VN, Gonos ES, Gorbunova V, Kennedy BK, Larbi A, Lemaître JF, Liu GH, Maier AB, Morais JA, Nóbrega OT, Moskalev A, Rikkert MO, Seluanov A, Senior AM, Ukraintseva S, Vanhaelen Q, Witkowski J, Cohen AA. The conundrum of human immune system "senescence". Mech Ageing Dev. 2020;192:111357.
3. López-Otín C, Blasco MA, Partridge L, Serrano M, Kroemer G. The hallmarks of aging. Cell. 2013;153:1194–217.
4. Müller L, Di Benedetto S, Pawelec G. The immune system and its dysregulation with aging. Subcell Biochem. 2019;91:21–43.
5. Fülöp T, Dupuis G, Witkowski JM, Larbi A. The role of immunosenescence in the development of age-related diseases. Rev Investig Clin. 2016;68:84–91.
6. Franceschi C, Salvioli S, Garagnani P, de Eguileor M, Monti D, Capri M. Immunobiography and the heterogeneity of immune responses in the elderly: a focus on inflammaging and trained immunity. Front Immunol. 2017;8:982.
7. McComb S, Thiriot A, Akache B, Krishnan L, Stark F. Introduction to the immune system. Methods Mol Biol. 2019;2024:1–24.
8. Fulop T, Larbi A, Hirokawa K, Cohen AA, Witkowski JM. Immunosenescence is both functional/adaptive and dysfunctional/maladaptive. Semin Immunopathol. 2020;42:521–36.
9. Wu Z, Mc Googan JM. Characteristics of and important lessons from the coronavirus disease 2019 (COVID-19) outbreak in China: summary of a report of 72 314 cases from the Chinese Center for Disease Control and Prevention. JAMA. 2020;323:1239–42.
10. Paces J, Strizova Z, Smrz D, Cerny J. COVID-19 and the immune system. Physiol Res. 2020;69:379–88.
11. Fulop T, Larbi A, Dupuis G, Le Page A, Frost EH, Cohen AA, Witkowski JM, Franceschi C. Immunosenescence and inflamm-aging as two sides of the same coin: friends or foes? Front Immunol. 2018;8:1960.
12. Medzhitov R, Janeway CA Jr. Innate immunity: impact on the adaptive immune response. Curr Opin Immunol. 1997;9:4–9.
13. Kennedy MA. A brief review of the basics of immunology: the innate and adaptive response. Vet Clin North Am Small Anim Pract. 2010;40:369–79.
14. Kaufmann SHE, Dorhoi A. Molecular determinants in phagocyte-bacteria interactions. Immunity. 2016;44:476–91.
15. Vidya MK, Kumar VG, Sejian V, Bagath M, Krishnan G, Bhatta R. Toll-like receptors: significance, ligands, signaling pathways, and functions in mammals. Int Rev Immunol. 2018;37:20–36.
16. Kufer TA, Nigro G, Sansonetti PJ. Multifaceted functions of NOD-like receptor proteins in myeloid cells at the intersection of innate and adaptive immunity. Microbiol Spectr. 2016;4(4)
17. Barik S. What really rigs up RIG-I? J Innate Immun. 2016;8:429–36.

18. Xu W, Wong G, Hwang YY, Larbi A. The untwining of immunosenescence and aging. Semin Immunopathol. 2020;42:559–72.
19. De la Fuente M. Where could research on immunosenescence lead? Int J Mol Sci. 2019;20:5906.
20. Bajaj V, Gadi N, Spihlman AP, Wu SC, Choi CH, Moulton VR. Aging, immunity, and COVID-19: how age influences the host immune response to coronavirus infections? Front Physiol. 2021;11:571416.
21. Franceschi C, Garagnani P, Vitale G, Capri M, Salvioli S. Inflammaging and "garb-aging". Trends Endocrinol Metab. 2017;28:199–212.
22. Fulop T, Le Page A, Fortin C, Witkowski JM, Dupuis G, Larbi A. Cellular signaling in the aging immune system. Curr Opin Immunol. 2014;29:105–11.
23. Fitzgerald KA, Kagan JC. Toll-like receptors and the control of immunity. Cell. 2020;180:1044–66.
24. Moskalev A, Stambler I, Caruso C. Innate and adaptive immunity in aging and longevity: the Foundation of Resilience. Aging Dis. 2020;11:1363–73.
25. De Maeyer RPH, Chambers ES. The impact of ageing on monocytes and macrophages. Immunol Lett. 2021;230:1–10.
26. Blagosklonny MV. From causes of aging to death from COVID-19. Aging (Albany NY). 2020;12:10004–21.
27. Zheng Y, Liu X, Le W, Xie L, Li H, Wen W, Wang S, Ma S, Huang Z, Ye J, Shi W, Ye Y, Liu Z, Song M, Zhang W, Han JJ, Belmonte JCI, Xiao C, Qu J, Wang H, Liu GH, Su W. A human circulating immune cell landscape in aging and COVID-19. Protein Cell. 2020;11:740–70.
28. Golubev AG. COVID-19: a challenge to physiology of aging. Front Physiol. 2020;11:584248.
29. Channappanavar R, Perlman S. Age-related susceptibility to coronavirus infections: role of impaired and dysregulated host immunity. J Clin Invest. 2020;130:6204–13.
30. Bandaranayake T, Shaw AC. Host resistance and immune aging. Clin Geriatr Med. 2016;32:415–32.
31. Omarjee L, Perrot F, Meilhac O, Mahe G, Bousquet G, Janin A. Immunometabolism at the cornerstone of inflammaging, immunosenescence, and autoimmunity in COVID-19. Aging (Albany NY). 2020;12:26263–78.
32. Fulop T, Dupuis G, Baehl S, Le Page A, Bourgade K, Frost E, Witkowski JM, Pawelec G, Larbi A, Cunnane S. From inflamm-aging to immune-paralysis: a slippery slope during aging for immune-adaptation. Biogerontology. 2016;1:147–57; Netea MG, Domínguez-Andrés J, Barreiro LB, Chavakis T, Divangahi M, Fuchs E, Joosten LAB, van der Meer JWM, Mhlanga MM, Mulder WJM, Riksen NP, Schlitzer A, Schultze JL, Stabell Benn C, Sun JC, Xavier RJ, Latz E. Defining trained immunity and its role in health and disease. Nat Rev Immunol. 2020;20:375–88.
33. Fulop T, Larbi A, Douziech N, Fortin C, Guérard KP, Lesur O, Khalil A, Dupuis G. Signal transduction and functional changes in neutrophils with aging. Aging Cell. 2004;3:217–26.
34. Franceschi C, Bonafè M, Valensin S, Olivieri F, De Luca M, Ottaviani E, De Benedictis G. Inflamm-aging. An evolutionary perspective on immunosenescence. Ann N Y Acad Sci. 2000;908:244–54.
35. Monti D, Ostan R, Borelli V, Castellani G, Franceschi C. Inflammaging and human longevity in the omics era. Mech Ageing Dev. 2017;165(Pt B):129–38.
36. Fulop T, Witkowski JM, Olivieri F, Larbi A. The integration of inflammaging in age-related diseases. Semin Immunol. 2018;40:17–35.
37. Barbé-Tuana F, Funchal G, Schmitz CRR, Maurmann RM, Bauer ME. The interplay between immunosenescence and age-related diseases. Semin Immunopathol. 2020;42:545–57.
38. Le Page A, Dupuis G, Frost EH, Larbi A, Pawelec G, Witkowski JM, Fulop T. Role of the peripheral innate immune system in the development of Alzheimer's disease. Exp Gerontol. 2018;107:59–66.
39. Vabret N, Britton GJ, Gruber C, Hegde S, Kim J, Kuksin M, Levantovsky R, Malle L, Moreira A, Park MD, Pia L, Risson E, Saffern M, Salomé B, Esai Selvan M, Spindler MP, Tan J, van der Heide V, Gregory JK, Alexandropoulos K, Bhardwaj N, Brown BD, Greenbaum B, Gümüş ZH, Homann D, Horowitz A, Kamphorst AO, Curotto de Lafaille MA, Mehandru S, Merad M, Samstein RM, Sinai Immunology Review Project. Immunology of COVID-19: current state of the science. Immunity. 2020;52:910–41.
40. Nikolich-Zugich J, Knox KS, Rios CT, Natt B, Bhattacharya D, Fain MJ. SARS-CoV-2 and COVID-19 in older adults: what we may expect regarding pathogenesis, immune responses, and outcomes. Geroscience. 2020;42:505–14.

41. Hazeldine J, Lord JM. Immunesenescence: a predisposing risk factor for the development of COVID-19? Front Immunol. 2020;11:573662.
42. Cunha LL, Perazzio SF, Azzi J, Cravedi P, Riella LV. Remodeling of the immune response with aging: immunosenescence and its potential impact on COVID-19 immune response. Front Immunol. 2020;11:1748.
43. Mueller AL, McNamara MS, Sinclair DA. Why does COVID-19 disproportionately affect older people? Aging (Albany NY). 2020;12:9959–81.
44. Solana R, Tarazona R, Gayoso I, Lesur O, Dupuis G, Fulop T. Innate immunosenescence: effect of aging on cells and receptors of the innate immune system in humans. Semin Immunol. 2012;24:331–41.
45. Fülöp T, Fóris G, Leövey A. Age-related changes in cAMP and cGMP levels during phagocytosis in human polymorphonuclear leukocytes. Mech Ageing Dev. 1984;27:233–7.
46. Metcalf TU, Wilkinson PA, Cameron MJ, Ghneim K, Chiang C, Wertheimer AM, Hiscott JB, Nikolich-Zugich J, Haddad EK. Human monocyte subsets are transcriptionally and functionally altered in aging in response to pattern recognition receptor agonists. J Immunol. 2017;199:1405–17.
47. Poulin LF, Lasseaux C, Chamaillard M. Understanding the cellular origin of the mononuclear phagocyte system sheds light on the myeloid postulate of immune paralysis in sepsis. Front Immunol. 2018;9:823.
48. Tarazona R, Campos C, Pera A, Sanchez-Correa B, Solana R. Flow cytometry analysis of NK cell phenotype and function in aging. Methods Mol Biol. 2015;1343:9–18.
49. Agrawal A, Agrawal S, Gupta S. Role of dendritic cells in inflammation and loss of tolerance in the elderly. Front Immunol. 2017;8:896.
50. Johnston-Carey HK, Pomatto LC, Davies KJ. The immunoproteasome in oxidative stress, aging, and disease. Crit Rev Biochem Mol Biol. 2015;51:268–81.
51. Zhang H, Weyand CM, Goronzy JJ. Hallmarks of the aging T-cell system. FEBS J. 2021;
52. Pawelec G. Does the human immune system ever really become "senescent"? F1000Res. 2017;6. pii: F1000 Faculty Rev-1323.
53. Effros RB, Dagarag M, Spaulding C, Man J. The role of CD8+ T-cell replicative senescence in human aging. Immunol Rev. 2005;205:147–57.
54. Wherry EJ, Kurachi M. Molecular and cellular insights into T cell exhaustion. Nat Rev Immunol. 2015;15:486–99.
55. Thomas R, Wang W, Su DM. Contributions of age-related thymic involution to immunosenescence and inflammaging. Immun Ageing. 2020;17:2.
56. Goronzy JJ, Weyand CM. Successful and maladaptive T cell aging. Immunity. 2017;46:364–78.
57. Pawelec G. Immunosenenescence: role of cytomegalovirus. Exp Gerontol. 2014;54:1–5.
58. Minato N, Hattori M, Hamazaki Y. Physiology and pathology of T-cell aging. Int Immunol. 2020;32:223–31.
59. Moskowitz DM, Zhang DW, Hu B, Le Saux S, Yanes RE, Ye Z, Buenrostro JD, Weyand CM, Greenleaf WJ, Goronzy JJ. Epigenomics of human CD8 T cell differentiation and aging. Sci Immunol. 2017;2:eaag0192.
60. Kugel S, Mostoslavsky R. Chromatin and beyond: the multitasking roles for SIRT6. Trends Biochem Sci. 2014;39:72–81.
61. Horvath S, Pirazzini C, Bacalini MG, Gentilini D, Di Blasio AM, Delledonne M, Mari D, Arosio B, Monti D, Passarino G, De Rango F, D'Aquila P, Giuliani C, Marasco E, Collino S, Descombes P, Garagnani P, Franceschi C. Decreased epigenetic age of PBMCs from Italian semi-supercentenarians and their offspring. Aging (Albany NY). 2015;7:1159–70.
62. Goel N, Karir P, Garg VK. Role of DNA methylation in human age prediction. Mech Ageing Dev. 2017;166:33–41.
63. Li G, Yu M, Lee WW, Tsang M, Krishnan E, Weyand CM, Goronzy JJ. Decline in miR-181a expression with age impairs T cell receptor sensitivity by increasing DUSP6 activity. Nat Med. 2012;18:1518–24.
64. Le Page A, Fortin C, Garneau H, Allard N, Tsvetkova K, Tan CT, Larbi A, Dupuis G, Fülöp T. Downregulation of inhibitory SRC homology 2 domain-containing phosphatase-1 (SHP-1) leads to recovery of T cell responses in elderly. Cell Commun Signal. 2014;12:2.

65. Larbi A, Dupuis G, Khalil A, Douziech N, Fortin C, Fülöp T Jr. Differential role of lipid rafts in the functions of CD4+ and CD8+ human T lymphocytes with aging. Cell Signal. 2006;18:1017–30.

66. Frasca D. Senescent B cells in aging and age-related diseases: their role in the regulation of antibody responses. Exp Gerontol. 2018;107:55–8.

67. Hagen M, Derudder E. Inflammation and the alteration of B-cell physiology in aging. Gerontology. 2020;66:105–13.

68. Bektas A, Zhang Y, Wood WH 3rd, Becker KG, Madara K, Ferrucci L, Sen R. Age-associated alterations in inducible gene transcription in human CD4+ T lymphocytes. Aging (Albany NY). 2013;5:18–36.

69. He W, Xiao K, Fang M, Xie L. Immune cell number, phenotype, and function in the elderly with sepsis. Aging Dis. 2021;12:277–96.

70. Fülöp T, Larbi A, Witkowski JM. Human inflammaging. Gerontology. 2019;65:495–504.

71. Callender LA, Carroll EC, Beal RWJ, Chambers ES, Nourshargh S, Akbar AN, Henson SM. Human CD8 + EMRA T cells display a senescence-associated secretory phenotype regulated by p38 MAPK. Aging Cell. 2018;17:e12675.

72. Santoro A, Zhao J, Wu L, Carru C, Biagi E, Franceschi C. Microbiomes other than the gut: inflammaging and age-related diseases. Semin Immunopathol. 2020;42:589–605.

73. Biagi E, Candela M, Fairweather-Tait S, Franceschi C, Brigidi P. Aging of the human metaorganism: the microbial counterpart. Age (Dordr). 2012;34:247–67.

74. Biagi E, Franceschi C, Rampelli S, Severgnini M, Ostan R, Turroni S, Consolandi C, Quercia S, Scurti M, Monti D, Capri M, Brigidi P, Candela M. Gut microbiota and extreme longevity. Curr Biol. 2016;26:1480–5.

75. Lin SC, Lo YC, Wu H. Helical assembly in the MyD88-IRAK4-IRAK2 complex in TLR/IL-1R signalling. Nature. 2010;465:885–90.

76. Vizioli MG, Liu T, Miller KN, Robertson NA, Gilroy K, Lagnado AB, Perez-Garcia A, Kiourtis C, Dasgupta N, Lei X, Kruger PJ, Nixon C, Clark W, Jurk D, Bird TG, Passos JF, Berger SL, Dou Z, Adams PD. Mitochondria-to-nucleus retrograde signaling drives formation of cytoplasmic chromatin and inflammation in senescence. Genes Dev. 2020;34:428–45.

77. Lan YY, Heather JM, Eisenhaure T, Garris CS, Lieb D, Raychowdhury R, Hacohen N. Extranuclear DNA accumulates in aged cells and contributes to senescence and inflammation. Aging Cell. 2019;18:e12901.

78. Kelley N, Jeltema D, Duan Y, He Y. The NLRP3 inflammasome: an overview of mechanisms of activation and regulation. Int J Mol Sci. 2019;20:3328.

79. He M, Chiang HH, Luo H, Zheng Z, Qiao Q, Wang L, Tan M, Ohkubo R, Mu WC, Zhao S, Wu H, Chen D. An acetylation switch of the NLRP3 inflammasome regulates aging-associated chronic inflammation and insulin resistance. Cell Metab. 2020;31:580–591.e5.

80. Massudi H, Grant R, Braidy N, Guest J, Farnsworth B, Guillemin GJ. Age-associated changes in oxidative stress and NAD+ metabolism in human tissue. PLoS One. 2012;7:e42357.

81. Arai Y, Martin-Ruiz CM, Takayama M, Abe Y, Takebayashi T, Koyasu S, Suematsu M, Hirose N, von Zglinicki T. Inflammation, but not telomere length, predicts successful ageing at extreme old age: a longitudinal study of semi-supercentenarians. EBioMedicine. 2015;2:1549–58.

82. Franceschi C, Capri M, Monti D, Giunta S, Olivieri F, Sevini F, Panourgia MP, Invidia L, Celani L, Scurti M, Cevenini E, Castellani GC, Salvioli S. Inflammaging and anti-inflammaging: a systemic perspective on aging and longevity emerged from studies in humans. Mech Ageing Dev. 2007;128(1):92–105.

83. Morrisette-Thomas V, Cohen AA, Fülöp T, Riesco É, Legault V, Li Q, Milot E, Dusseault-Bélanger F, Ferrucci L. Inflamm-aging does not simply reflect increases in pro-inflammatory markers. Mech Ageing Dev. 2014;139:49–57.

84. Chen Y, Klein SL, Garibaldi BT, Li H, Wu C, Osevala NM, Li T, Margolick JB, Pawelec G, Leng SX. Aging in COVID-19: vulnerability, immunity and intervention. Ageing Res Rev. 2021;65:101205.

85. Vetter P, Eberhardt CS, Meyer B, Martinez Murillo PA, Torriani G, Pigny F, Lemeille S, Cordey S, Laubscher F, Vu DL, Calame A, Schibler M, Jacquerioz F, Blanchard-Rohner G, Siegrist CA, Kaiser L, Didierlaurent AM, Eckerle I. Daily viral kinetics and innate and adaptive immune response assessment in COVID-19: a case series. mSphere. 2020;5:e00827-20.

86. Rydyznski Moderbacher C, Ramirez SI, Dan JM, Grifoni A, Hastie KM, Weiskopf D, Belanger S, Abbott RK, Kim C, Choi J, Kato Y, Crotty EG, Kim C, Rawlings SA, Mateus J, Tse LPV, Frazier A, Baric R, Peters B, Greenbaum J, Ollmann Saphire E, Smith DM, Sette A, Crotty S. Antigen-specific adaptive immunity to SARS-CoV-2 in acute COVID-19 and ssociations with age and disease severity. Cell. 2020;183:996–1012.e19.

87. Shi CS, Nabar NR, Huang NN, Kehrl JH. SARS-coronavirus open reading frame-8b triggers intracellular stress pathways and activates NLRP3 inflammasomes. Cell Death Discov. 2019;5:101.

88. Pence BD. Severe COVID-19 and aging: are monocytes the key? Geroscience. 2020;42:1051–61.

89. Rowe TA, McKoy JM. Sepsis in older adults. Infect Dis Clin N Am. 2017;31:731–42.

90. Seymour CW, Liu VX, Iwashyna TJ, Brunkhorst FM, Rea TD, Scherag A, Rubenfeld G, Kahn JM, Shankar-Hari M, Singer M, Deutschman CS, Escobar GJ, Angus DC. Assessment of clinical criteria for sepsis: for the third international consensus definitions for sepsis and septic shock (Sepsis-3). JAMA. 2016;315:762–74.

91. Martín S, Pérez A, Aldecoa C. Sepsis and immunosenescence in the elderly patient: a review. Front Med (Lausanne). 2017;4:20.

92. Monneret G, Gossez M, Venet F. Sepsis and immunosenescence: closely associated in a vicious circle. Aging Clin Exp Res. 2021;33:729–32.

93. Faivre V, Lukaszewicz AC, Alves A, Charron D, Payen D, Haziot A. Human monocytes differentiate into dendritic cells subsets that induce anergic and regulatory T cells in sepsis. PLoS One. 2012;7:e47209.

94. Cazalis MA, Friggeri A, Cavé L, Demaret J, Barbalat V, Cerrato E, Lepape A, Pachot A, Monneret G, Venet F. Decreased HLA-DR antigen-associated invariant chain (CD74) mRNA expression predicts mortality after septic shock. Crit Care. 2013;17:R287.

95. Kjaergaard AG, Nielsen JS, Tønnesen E, Krog J. Expression of NK cell and monocyte receptors in critically ill patients–potential biomarkers of sepsis. Scand J Immunol. 2015;81:249–58.

96. Guo Y, Patil NK, Luan L, Bohannon JK, Sherwood ER. The biology of natural killer cells during sepsis. Immunology. 2018;153:190–202.

97. Aziz M, Yang WL, Matsuo S, Sharma A, Zhou M, Wang P. Upregulation of GRAIL is associated with impaired CD4 T cell proliferation in sepsis. J Immunol. 2014;192:2305–14.

98. Boomer JS, Shuherk-Shaffer J, Hotchkiss RS, Green JM. A prospective analysis of lymphocyte phenotype and function over the course of acute sepsis. Crit Care. 2012;16:R112.

99. Condotta SA, Khan SH, Rai D, Griffith TS, Badovinac VP. Polymicrobial sepsis increases susceptibility to chronic viral infection and exacerbates CD8+ T cell exhaustion. J Immunol. 2015;195:116–25.

100. Delano MJ, Ward PA. The immune system's role in sepsis progression, resolution, and long-term outcome. Immunol Rev. 2016;274:330–53.

101. Alberro A, Osorio-Querejeta I, Sepúlveda L, Fernández-Eulate G, Mateo-Abad M, Muñoz-Culla M, Carregal-Romero S, Matheu A, Vergara I, López de Munain A, Sáenz-Cuesta M, Otaegui D. T cells and immune functions of plasma extracellular vesicles are differentially modulated from adults to centenarians. Aging (Albany NY). 2019;11:10723–41.

102. Franceschi C, Ostan R, Santoro A. Nutrition and inflammation: are centenarians similar to individuals on calorie-restricted diets? Annu Rev Nutr. 2018;38:329–56.

103. Fulop T, Larbi A, Khalil A, Cohen AA, Witkowski JM. Are we ill because we age? Front Physiol. 2019;10:1508.

104. Sansoni P, Vescovini R, Fagnoni F, Biasini C, Zanni F, Zanlari L, Telera A, Lucchini G, Passeri G, Monti D, Franceschi C, Passeri M. The immune system in extreme longevity. Exp Gerontol. 2008;43:61–5.

105. Minciullo PL, Catalano A, Mandraffino G, Casciaro M, Crucitti A, Maltese G, Morabito N, Lasco A, Gangemi S, Basile G. Inflammaging and anti-inflammaging: the role of cytokines in extreme longevity. Arch Immunol Ther Exp. 2016;64:111–26.

106. Franceschi C, Garagnani P, Morsiani C, Conte M, Santoro A, Grignolio A, Monti D, Capri M, Salvioli S. The continuum of aging and age-related diseases: common mechanisms but different rates. Front Med (Lausanne). 2018;5:61.

107. Lal H, Cunningham AL, Godeaux O, Chlibek R, Diez-Domingo J, Hwang SJ, Levin MJ, McElhaney JE, Poder A, Puig-Barberà J, Vesikari T, Watanabe D, Weckx L, Zahaf T, Heineman TC, ZOE-50 Study Group. Efficacy of an adjuvanted herpes zoster subunit vaccine in older adults. N Engl J Med. 2015;372:2087–96.

108. Polack FP, Thomas SJ, Kitchin N, Absalon J, Gurtman A, Lockhart S, Perez JL, Pérez Marc G, Moreira ED, Zerbini C, Bailey R, Swanson KA, Roychoudhury S, Koury K, Li P, Kalina WV, Cooper D, Frenck RW Jr, Hammitt LL, Türeci Ö, Nell H, Schaefer A, Ünal S, Tresnan DB, Mather S, Dormitzer PR, Şahin U, Jansen KU, Gruber WC, C4591001 Clinical Trial Group. Safety and efficacy of the BNT162b2 mRNA covid-19 vaccine. N Engl J Med. 2020;383:2603–15.
109. Walsh EE, Frenck RW Jr, Falsey AR, Kitchin N, Absalon J, Gurtman A, Lockhart S, Neuzil K, Mulligan MJ, Bailey R, Swanson KA, Li P, Koury K, Kalina W, Cooper D, Fontes-Garfias C, Shi PY, Türeci Ö, Tompkins KR, Lyke KE, Raabe V, Dormitzer PR, Jansen KU, Şahin U, Gruber WC. Safety and immunogenicity of two RNA-based covid-19 vaccine candidates. N Engl J Med. 2020;383:2439–50.

Drug Metabolism

Saskia Rietjens and Dylan de Lange

Contents

Learning Objectives

With advancing age, various anatomical and physiological changes in several organ systems take place, which may influence drug pharmacokinetics and pharmacodynamics. Elderly patients might have alterations in various pharmacokinetic processes in such a way that drugs need to be dosed differently. Understanding the physiological changes of organ systems that occur with ageing, and consequently the changes in pharmacokinetics and pharmacodynamics, will improve drug therapy in the elderly. Prescribing medication for older people is challenging, as the elderly are more prone to develop adverse drug reactions (ADRs). Important causes of ADRs in elderly patients are multimorbidity and polypharmacy resulting in increased risk for drug-drug interactions.

In this chapter we will discuss the alterations in pharmacokinetic processes in elderly patients and the increased potential for ADRs in this population. Changes in pharmacodynamics, including changes in the number, affinity and responsiveness of drug receptors, and changes in physiological reserve and in response to injury also affect the risk of drug toxicity in elderly patients. However, in this chapter we will focus on age-related pharmacokinetic changes.

7.1 Introduction

Due to increasing life expectancy both the proportion and absolute number of older people are increasing dramatically worldwide. At the global level in 2019, approximately 9% of people are aged 65 or older. The proportion of persons ≥65 years old in the world is expected to reach ~16% in 2050 and could reach ~23% by 2100 [1] (see also ▶ Chap. 1 for a more elaborate discussion on the epidemiology of ageing). With increasing age, various anatomical and physiological changes take place, which may impact drug pharmacokinetics and pharmacodynamics [2]. Elderly patients might have alterations in several pharmacokinetic processes (i.e. absorption, distribution, metabolism and excretion (ADME)). Moreover, the higher prevalence of multimorbidity and polypharmacy in the elderly population results in an increased risk for drug-drug interactions [3].

7.2 Adverse Drug Reactions

Older adults are more prone to develop adverse drug reactions (ADRs) since they exhibit numerous risk factors, like multimorbidity which is often associated with polypharmacy (see also ▶ Chaps. 8 and 9 on Multimorbidity and Multipharmacy on the Older Adult) [3]. The prevalence of multimorbidity in the elderly population varies between 55% and 98%, with increasing prevalence in very old persons [4]. In a cross-sectional study of 1.75 million people registered in primary care in Scotland, the prevalence of multimorbidity was ~82% in people ≥85 years old [5]. Common conditions in these patients (≥ 75 years old) were hypertension (62%), coronary heart disease (31%), chronic kidney disease (19%), depression (17%) and diabetes (17%) [6].

Polypharmacy has been consistently identified as a risk factor for ADRs. The risk of ADRs increases from 13% in a person taking two medicines to 38% when taking five and 82% when taking seven or more [7]. In an Irish retrospective cohort study of community-dwelling people over 70 years old, almost 80% reported at least one ADR during the previous 6 months [8]. A meta-analysis demonstrated that approximately 9% of all hospitalisations of older patients are directly related to ADRs [9]. Non-steroidal anti-inflammatory drugs (NSAIDs) were most frequently related to hospital admissions, followed by other common medications used in patients of older age, such as β-blockers, antibiotics, oral anticoagulants, digoxin, ACE inhibitors, anticancer drugs, calcium-channel blockers, opioids and oral antidiabetics [9]. In most of the cases, ADRs are probably preventable, for example, by adequate dosing considering the renal function (e.g. in the case of digoxin) or by identification of particular groups at risk of bleeding (e.g. in the case of NSAIDs or oral anticoagulants) [9]. Unfortunately, ADRs do not only account for morbidity but are also related to deaths in elderly patients [10, 11]. Wu et al. showed that age was an independent risk factor for severe ADRs, defined as requiring hospitalisation or resulting in death. The odds of experiencing severe ADRs increased by 3% per 1-year increase in age. Furthermore, severe ADRs occurred more frequently in patients who had many coexisting conditions [11].

7.3 Frailty

Older age is frequently accompanied by frailty, which increases in prevalence with advancing age. Frailty is defined as "a clinically recognizable state of increased vulnerability resulting from ageing-associated decline in reserve and function across multiple physiologic systems such that the ability to cope with everyday or acute stressors is compromised" (see also ▶ Chap. 11). A systematic review showed that approximately one in ten independently living adults aged 65 and older is frail [12]. In a prospective multicentre study in Europe, frailty (defined as a clinical frailty scale (CFS) ≥5) was found to be present in 43% of very old critically ill patients admitted to the ICU (≥80 years old) [13]. Polypharmacy is associated with frailty [14, 15]. Patients concomitantly using five of more drugs (polypharmacy) or ten or more drugs (hyperpolypharmacy) had a 1.5- and two-fold higher risk, respectively, for developing frailty within 3 years [15].

7.4 Changes in Pharmacokinetics in the Elderly

Many anatomical and physiological changes that occur with ageing potentially impact the pharmacokinetics and pharmacodynamics of drugs [2, 16]. Older people, and especially frail patients, have a marked decline in skeletal muscle mass (sarcopenia; see also ▶ Chap. 10) [17, 18], which may be accompanied by increased adiposity [19], resulting in an increase in volume of distribution of lipid-soluble drugs. Other important pharmacokinetic changes include a reduction in renal and hepatic clearance [20]. When frailty and physical decline progress, this will have implications for pharmacokinetics and drug dosing [21].

7.5 Absorption After Oral Drug Administration

It has been proposed that advancing age results in a decline in gastric acid secretion. However, data are conflicting as it was shown that in the absence of gastric mucosal atrophy, there was no relationship between ageing and reduced acid secretion [22, 23]. Drugs that require an acidic environment for absorption, such as ketoconazole and iron, may have a reduced extent of absorption in elderly patients with hypochlorhydria secondary to gastric pathology and in those taking medications that increase gastric pH, such as proton pump inhibitors and H2 antagonists, potentially leading to subtherapeutical plasma levels [16, 24, 25].

Healthy ageing seems associated with modest slowing of gastric emptying, but emptying generally remains within the normal range for young subjects [26, 27]. However, several diseases that increase in prevalence with advancing age, such as Parkinson's disease and diabetes, frequently have an impact on gut function, including gastric emptying [27].

Beyond the stomach, the small intestine retains much of its normal motility [28, 29]. Passive intestinal transport of most substrates is not affected by ageing [30–32]. The permeability of drugs appears unchanged in older adults when medication is absorbed by passive diffusion (e.g. penicillins, diazepam, metronidazole) [33]. However, in laboratory animals (old-age rats), there is increased permeability of the intestines to higher molecular mass compounds [34]. This may indicate that the intestinal protective barrier function to some harmful substances is less efficient in old animals. Furthermore, the active transport of glucose [32], calcium [35] and vitamin B12 [36] is impaired in the small intestines of aged rats.

A transporter that has recently received attention is P-glycoprotein (P-gp), an efflux transporter that is found in the luminal surface of the intestine in addition to other places in the body including the blood-brain barrier, kidneys and lymphocytes. P-gp actively transports drugs and xenobiotics back into the gut lumen, decreasing absorption [37]. A large number of drugs appear to be P-gp substrates including antibiotics, anticancer drugs and calcium-channel blockers. Studies on the impact of advancing age on P-gp activity and expression have provided conflicting results. Some studies have demonstrated an increase in P-gp activity and/or expression with age, whereas others showed a significant reduction or minor effects, also depending on the type of tissue studied [38].

The colonic transit time of radio-nuclear labelled material appears to be slower in elderly patients [39, 40]. This might result in slower gastrointestinal absorption of drugs, in such a way that the maximal plasma concentration is achieved later (longer T_{max}) and is lower (lower C_{max}). In general, for most drugs, the absorption is unchanged in older patients and the area under the concentration-time curve (AUC, bioavailability) is not much affected [16].

7.6 Absorption After Non-oral Drug Administration

While medication is most commonly administered via the oral route, administration via alternative routes such as the skin or lungs is also possible for specific drugs. The advantages of transdermal drug administration compared to oral administration include bypassing of the gastrointestinal route and hepatic first-pass metabolism (see also paragraph on bioavailability), improved patient compliance and less fluctuation in plasma drug concentrations, minimising the risk of adverse effects [41, 42]. Changes in skin barrier function in the elderly may impact the percutaneous absorption. With increasing age, the skin undergoes many structural and functional changes. For example, aged skin shows a thinner epidermis and is often dry [43]. Moreover, increased age may be associated with decreased cutaneous perfusion [43]. However, in general no clinically relevant changes in absorption of transdermal drugs have been demonstrated between young and old individuals [41], although more research on age-related changes in skin barrier function in the very old patient is required. Additional studies may elucidate if different transdermal dosing regimens should be applied for elderly patients to ensure effective treatment, while minimising the risk of adverse effects. This is especially important for medication with a narrow therapeutic window, such as fentanyl [44].

The ageing process also alters the intrinsic structure of the lung as well as the supportive extrapulmonary structures, i.e. chest wall, spine and respiratory muscles. These changes lead to unfavourable mechanisms associated with decreased expiratory flows, increased air trapping and decreased gas exchange [45]. Age-related reductions in chest wall compliance, total alveolar surface area and ventilation-perfusion matching may decrease the absorption of drugs via inhalation [46]. Furthermore, decrements in cognition and fine manual dexterity can lead to suboptimal inhaler technique. For example, inhaled bronchodilators for the treatment of asthma and chronic obstructive pulmonary disease (COPD) need to reach the small- and medium-sized airways in sufficient quantities to be effective [46].

7.7 Bioavailability

The bioavailability of a drug is the fraction of an administered dose that reaches the systemic circulation. Oral bioavailability of some drugs is reduced due to first-pass metabolism which mainly occurs in the liver but also in the gut. Ageing may be associated with a reduction in first-pass metabolism, most likely due to reduced liver blood flow and liver volume (as discussed further below, see paragraph metabolism). Oral bioavailability and plasma levels of certain drugs with extensive first-pass metabolism are substantially higher in elderly individuals compared to younger subjects. Typical examples include beta-blockers, such as labetalol, and the calcium-channel blocker verapamil [47]. As a consequence, drugs with an extensive first-pass metabolism, and especially those with a narrow therapeutic window, should be initiated at a low dose. On the other hand, first-pass activation of several prodrugs (e.g. codeine [48], simvastatin [49], and the angiotensin-converting enzyme (ACE) inhibitors enalapril [50] and perindopril [51]) might be slowed or reduced with advancing age, but the clinical significance of this is unclear. Higher doses of prodrugs may be required in an elderly patient to achieve the same AUC for the active drug (metabolite) compared a younger patient [16].

7.8 Distribution

7.8.1 Body Composition

Significant changes in body composition occur with advancing age. There is a progressive reduction in total body water and lean body mass, resulting in a relative increase in body fat [52, 53]. This means that water-soluble drugs tend to have a smaller volume of distribution resulting in higher serum levels in older people. Typical examples of medication that need a lower loading dose in elderly people are gentamicin, digoxin, theophylline and cimetidine [20, 54–57]. The smaller volume of distribution most likely also explains the higher peak ethanol levels found in the blood after ethanol administration in the old compared with younger subjects [58]. Lipid-soluble drugs, in contrast, generally have a higher volume of distribution in elderly patients and subsequently a prolonged half-life ($t_{1/2}$) (e.g. diazepam) [55, 59]. Consequently, after cessation of treatment, adverse effects may continue for a longer period of time [55]. The reduction in volume of distribution of water-soluble compounds should result in a decreased $t_{1/2}$ but often renal clearance is diminished as well [20]. The net effect on $t_{1/2}$ of these alterations is often small but basically unpredictable.

Another reason for a change in the volume of distribution might be a difference of permeability of body compartments. This is illustrated by a study in healthy volunteers that showed that the volume of distribution of verapamil (a substrate of P-gp) in the brain increases in old age, consistent with dysfunction of the blood-brain barrier [60]. This could also indicate that the ageing brain could be at higher risk for increased brain penetration of drugs that are actively pumped out of the brain by P-gp, such as digoxin, loperamide and cyclosporin A [61].

7.8.2 Protein Binding

The main factor determining drug effect is the free (unbound) concentration of the drug. Drugs that bind to plasma proteins have a smaller apparent volume of distribution and a lower free fraction. The two main drug-binding proteins in the plasma are albumin and alpha-1-acid glycoprotein. Acidic compounds (e.g. diazepam, phenytoin, warfarin, acetylsalicylic acid) mainly bind to albumin, whereas basic drugs (e.g. lidocaine, propranolol) bind to alpha-1-acid glycoprotein [56, 62]. Blood albumin concentrations decrease with age and are approximately 10% reduced in older people [63, 64]. Albumin is commonly reduced in malnutrition, cachexia or acute illness [20, 56]. Especially in critically ill patients rapid reductions in serum albumin may lead to toxicity because serum concentrations of unbound (free) drug may increase. Phenytoin and warfarin are examples of drugs with a higher risk of toxic effects when the serum albumin level decreases. In contrast, alpha-1-glycoprotein concentrations can be increased in older people, although this is usually attributed to acute illness or chronic inflammatory diseases, rather than age per se [20, 53, 65]. While alpha-1-glycoprotein represents a relatively small portion (~1–3%) of the total plasma proteins, compared to albumin (~60%), it can play a prominent role in drug binding and pharmacokinetics [65].

The clinical implication of a rise in alpha-1-glycoprotein depends on the degree of binding of a drug to the protein and may cause a reduction in the unbound fraction of certain drugs (such as propranolol) [66, 67].

7.9 Metabolism

Hepatic drug clearance depends on portal and arterial hepatic blood flow and elimination by metabolism and/or secretion into the bile. Hepatic clearance of highly extracted substrates is determined mostly by hepatic blood flow and is known as "flow-limited metabolism". Liver blood flow declines linearly with age, beginning in the third decade of life, showing a reduction of approximately 20–40% in 80–90-year-old individuals [47]. There is a consistent effect of age on the clearance of flow-limited drugs (such as morphine, propranolol, verapamil and amitriptyline), most of which are reduced by about 30% to 40%, correlating well with the age-related reduction in blood flow [16, 68, 69]. On the other hand, hepatic clearance of poorly extracted chemicals is described as "capacity-limited metabolism" because the intrinsic clearance (metabolising capacity) is the rate-limiting step. In elderly patients there is a decrease in liver mass of approximately 20–30% [70]. Compared to "flow-limited" drugs, there is a less consistent reduction in metabolism of "capacity-limited" drugs, such as theophylline, diazepam and phenytoin [69].

The metabolic system transforms lipophilic, water-insoluble drugs into more polar and water-soluble metabolites, which are more easily excreted from the body. Although almost every organ like the intestinal wall, skin, lung and kidney has some ability to metabolise drugs, the liver represents the principal organ of drug metabolism [71]. Xenobiotic metabolism has been traditionally classified into two phases. Phase I reactions involve oxidation, reduction or hydrolysis of the parent drug. The most important enzyme system of phase I metabolism is cytochrome P-450 (CYP450), a superfamily of isoezymes that catalyse the oxidation of many drugs. Phase II reactions involve conjugation with an endogenous substance (e.g. sulphate, glucuronic acid, glutathione) to increase its water solubility.

Whether increasing age results in decreased metabolisation capacity of enzymes is controversial [62, 72]. Although few studies have shown decreased CYP450 content in liver biopsies of elderly individuals [73, 74] (specifically CYP2E1 and CYP3A [73]), most studies show that enzymatic capacity of various CYP450 isoenzymes seems to be quite well preserved in advanced age, at least in the fit elderly [53, 70]. The content and activities of various CYP450 enzymes in liver biopsy samples did not decline with age (in the range of 10–85 years) [75–78]. In frailty, phase I metabolism seems to be somewhat impaired, but data are conflicting [79]. For example, frailty was associated with higher inflammatory markers and lower plasma esterase activity [80]. However, frail older people did not have reduced CYP3A and P-glycoprotein metabolism [81]. Inflammation has the potential to down-regulate the expression of CYP450 [82]. This is especially relevant for critically ill patients, as inflammatory responses can result in a reduction of the clearance of some drugs (e.g. drugs with a narrow therapeutic window).

Phase II pathways, such as glucuronidation or sulphation, seem to be quite normal in the elderly [53, 76]. For example, human in vitro glucuronidation and sulphation of paracetamol are not impaired significantly with normal ageing [83]. Furthermore, no difference was found in the clearance of temazepam (metabolised predominantly by glucuronidation) between healthy young and old individuals [84, 85]. However, phase II metabolism may be impaired in frail older people [79]. For example, the clearance of metoclopramide via sulphation is reduced in frail older people [86]. Moreover, the glucuronidation of paracetamol was significantly more reduced in frail older individuals compared to their healthy counterparts [87]. A reduction in phase II glucuronidation of paracetamol will lead to a greater metabolism via the alternative (phase I CYP-mediated) pathway. This leads to production of a toxic metabolite, which is usually neutralised via conjugation with glutathione. However, as frailty is associated with malnutrition, glutathione stores may be depleted. Therefore, the frail have a greater risk of paracetamol-induced liver toxicity [53, 88].

In conclusion, there is much debate whether an individual's drug-metabolising capacity declines with advancing age. Currently, there is only minimal evidence that drug metabolism itself is less efficient in healthy elderly patients than in younger patients. However, frailty more than age per se contributes to impairments in drug metabolism. In addition, various diseases, especially liver dysfunction, will reduce the metabolic rate for many drugs in the elderly. In addition, polypharmacy in elderly patients is a significant risk factor for ADRs through drug-drug interactions. As the hepatic function of elderly patients varies greatly from person to person, dose adjustments should be individualised and the efficacy and safety of administered drugs should be monitored carefully.

7.9.1 The Impact of Genetic Polymorphisms on Drug Metabolism in the Elderly

Important genetic polymorphisms exist for CYP450 enzymes, accounting for a substantial interindividual variability in drug metabolism, with potential severe clinical consequences including therapeutic failure or ADRs [89]. Commonly implicated drugs include NSAIDs metabolised by CYP2C9, proton pump inhibitors metabolised by CYP2C19 and beta-blockers and several antipsychotics and antidepressants metabolised by CYP2D6 [90]. Pharmacogenetic testing of genes coding for drug-metabolising enzymes could optimise medication prescribing. Older patients may especially benefit from pharmacogenetic testing as they are at increased risk for ADRs due to polypharmacy, e.g. by inhibition or induction of CYP450. Indeed, pharmacogenetic testing of polypharmacy patients aged 50 years and older considerably reduced the number of re-hospitalisations and ED visits [91].

Ducker et al. studied the combined effects of age and metabolic genotype on pharmacokinetics. In drugs with pharmacokinetics significantly modulated by genetic polymorphisms, old age caused on average a moderate 1.5-fold increase in systemic exposure, but in a few drugs, systemic exposure in the elderly was twofold or more, including zolpidem, clomipramine, paroxetine and fluvoxamine [92].

Especially in critically ill patients, many factors contribute to the wide variability in drug response. In addition to genetic variation, impaired organ function, co-morbidities, polypharmacy and drug interactions should be considered when administering drugs [93]. Many of these factors are more prominent in elderly patients than in their younger counterparts. Limited data is available on the impact of genetic polymorphisms on ADR risk in the (old) critically ill patient. Future studies may determine the relative contribution of genetics to drug response in critically ill patients, potentially decreasing ADRs by improvements in drug selection or dosage modification [93].

7.10 Excretion

Excretion is the process of removing a drug and its metabolites from the body, e.g. via the lungs, urine, faeces and sweat. The kidneys are the main organs of excretion. This involves glomerular filtration, tubular secretion and tubular reabsorption (see also ▶ Chap. 5 on 5.3 Renal Function/Functional Alterations). At the glomerulus, unbound drugs are passively filtered through the glomerular membrane. The glomerular filtration rate (GFR) is the total volume of glomerular filtrate produced per unit time by all nephrons and is approximately 120 ml/min in a young and healthy adult. In normal ageing, the GFR is reduced by roughly 15–40% [69]. It has been estimated that after the age of 30 there is a mean decrease in GFR of approximately 8 ml/min/decade [94, 95]. The decrease in renal weight, reduced renal blood flow, decreased number of functioning glomeruli and reduced permeability were thought to be the cause of the reduced GFR in the elderly [95]. However, the age-related decrease in GFR varies substantially from person to person [96]. Moreover, many age-related diseases (e.g. hypertension, heart failure and diabetes) as well as chronic exposure to nephrotoxic drugs (e.g. non-steroidal anti-inflammatory drugs (NSAIDs)) can directly influence GFR and may confound the actual effect of ageing on renal function [53, 97].

Drugs may also enter the renal tubules through active secretion. The unfiltered fraction of plasma and the particles too large to enter the glomerular filtrate (including drugs bound to proteins) pass through the efferent arterioles to the vessels supplying the renal tubules. The majority of tubular secretion occurs in the proximal tubule and depends on active transport by specific saturable transporters, such as P-gp. These transporters can be blocked by other drugs. For example, serum concentrations of digoxin, a drug that relies both on passive glomerular filtration and active tubular secretion, increased in a stepwise fashion with an increasing number of co-administered P-gp inhibitors [98]. The number of tubules, tubular length and tubular volume decrease with age [99]. The reduction in tubular secretion in old age is potentially greater than the decrease in GFR [16].

Drugs that have been filtered at the glomerulus or secreted in the proximal tubule may be passively reabsorbed from the tubular fluid in the proximal and distal tubules. Only non-ionised drugs are reabsorbed. Proximal tubule functions are generally preserved in healthy ageing, with near-normal production of erythropoietin and normal sodium reabsorption in the proximal tubules [16]. However, in old age, the clearance of some ions (like lithium) is reduced [100] and the overall tubular function is decreased, which results in an impairment to concentrate or dilute urine maximally [95, 99].

The clinical importance of decreased renal excretion is dependent on the potential toxicity of the drug. Toxicity may develop slowly because concentrations of chronically used drugs increase for 5 to 6 half-lives, until a steady state is achieved. For example, certain benzodiazepines or their active metabolites have a prolonged $t_{1/2}$ in older patients and, therefore, signs of toxicity may not appear until days or weeks after therapy is started. Moreover, drugs with a narrow therapeutic window, such as digoxin [101], lithium [102], gentamicin [103] and dabigatran [104], might cause serious adverse effects if they accumulate only slightly more than intended. Maintenance doses of drugs that are renally excreted must be adjusted for the individual patient's renal function. When possible, therapeutic drug monitoring (TDM) should be engaged to guide dosing (in combination with assessment of drug response) to prevent toxicity. Unfortunately, GFR is particularly difficult to assess in elderly patients. Usually we assume that the serum creatinine concentration is a good approximation of creatinine clearance. However, in older people, endogenous creatinine production is reduced as a result of muscle wasting, which leads to a lower serum creatinine concentration and hence an overestimation of the GFR [69]. This is definitely exacerbated in critical illness. Muscle wasting is excessive in the first days of critical illness [105]. Another problem with using GFR to guide dosing is that not all drugs are handled by the kidney in exactly the same way as creatinine is. For example, reduced renal function might also mean reduced reabsorption of medication (e.g. fluconazole) in the distal tubules of the nephron.

Fliser et al. have questioned the importance of age-related reduction in renal functioning in affecting pharmacokinetics. Although clearance of drugs with different mechanisms of renal excretion (such as atenolol and hydrochlorothiazide) was slightly reduced in the healthy elderly, pharmacokinetics (i.e. AUC and Cmax) were similar to younger subjects [106]. However, a pharmacokinetic study of gentamicin, as a marker of renal drug clearance by glomerular filtration, showed that frail patients had an approximately 12% lower gentamicin clearance than non-frail patients [107].

ADME	Possible changes in older adults	Clinical significance	Example drugs
Absorption	Reduced gastric acid production [a]	In case of increased gastric pH: Potential reduced absorption of drugs that require an acidic environment for absorption	Ketoconazole, iron
	Transit time: [b] Stomach: Modest decrease in gastric emptying Small intestines: Mostly unchanged motility Colon: Colonic transit time might be slower	Unlikely to have clinical significance	–
	Reduced active intestinal transport[c]	Reduced absorption of certain nutrients	Glucose, calcium, Vitamin B12
	Decreased or increased P-glycoprotein activity	Unclear	–
	Reduced first-pass metabolism (due to reduced liver blood flow and liver volume)	Increased oral bioavailability of drugs with extensive first-pass metabolism First-pass activation of pro-drugs might be reduced	Labetalol, verapamil Codeine, simvastatin, enalapril, perindopril

ADME	Possible changes in older adults	Clinical significance	Example drugs
Distribution	Body composition: Reduction in total body water Reduction in muscle mass Relative increase in body fat	Water-soluble drugs tend to have a smaller volume of distribution (resulting in increased plasma concentrations) Lipid-soluble drugs generally have a higher volume of distribution (prolonged half-life)	Digoxin, gentamicin, cimetidine Diazepam
	Plasma protein binding: Reduction in plasma albumin (commonly reduced in malnutrition or acute illness) Increased α1-acid glycoprotein (usually due to acute illness or chronic inflammatory diseases)	A reduction in plasma albumin leads to increased unbound (free) concentration of specific acidic drugs A rise in α1-acid glycoprotein may cause a reduction in the unbound (free) concentration of specific basic drugs	Phenytoin, warfarin Propranolol
	Decreased P-glycoprotein activity in blood-brain barrier	Potential increase in brain penetration of drugs that are actively pumped out of the brain by P-glycoprotein	Digoxin, loperamide, cyclosporine A
Metabolism	Reduced hepatic blood flow	Reduced hepatic clearance of "flow-limited" drugs	Morphine, propranolol, verapamil, amitriptyline
	Reduced hepatic mass	Less consistent reduction in hepatic clearance of "capacity-limited" drugs	Diazepam, phenytoin
	Metabolising capacity: Phase I: Both reduced and unaltered CYP450 content/ activity are reported Phase II: In general no change with normal ageing. May be impaired in frail older people	Reduced CYP450 activity results in reduction in metabolism of drugs that undergo phase I metabolism In frail older people, impaired phase II reactions (e.g. glucuronidation, sulphation) have been reported	Paracetamol, metoclopramide
Elimination	Reduced renal blood flow Reduced renal mass Decreased GFR Reduced tubular function	Decreased drug removal. Accumulation of drug in plasma	Digoxin, lithium, gentamicin, dabigatran

CYP450: cytochrome P-450; GFR: glomerular filtration rate

[a]Hypochlorhydria due to gastric mucosal atrophy is more common in the elderly. Reduced gastric acid production (increased gastric pH) may also be caused by medication use, e.g. proton pump inhibitors and H2 antagonists

[b]Transit time may also be reduced by certain comorbidities (e.g. diabetes, Parkinson's disease) and certain drugs (e.g. anticholinergics and opioids)

[c]Passive intestinal transport of most substrates is not affected by ageing

7.11   Knowledge Gap: Under-Representation of Older Patients in Clinical Trials

As discussed previously, the elderly have a significant higher disease burden than younger individuals. Despite the higher incidence of diseases in the elderly, geriatric patients are often excluded from clinical trials. Under-representation of older patients in clinical trials may occur for several reasons. For example, older patients are excluded, in addition to the advanced age per se, due to comorbidities, polypharmacy, cognitive impairment and frailty [108]. Ageing is a heterogeneous process which could introduce higher variability in response to treatment, which makes it more difficult to achieve statistically significant clinical trial end points. Currently, there are limited data available on the use of many drugs in the elderly population, and doses prescribed in older patients are often reduced, generally for safety reasons. Evidence of the efficacy and safety of a drug should result from clinical trials conducted in a representative patient population. Therefore, a sufficient number of elderly patients should be included in clinical trials. When elderly patients are excluded, the efficacy and safety concerns unique to this population will not be detected making it difficult to establish the risks versus the benefits of a specific treatment [108]. To improve our knowledge on the impact of ageing on pharmacokinetics and pharmacodynamics, future geriatric studies should provide a more detailed characterisation of the included subjects, in order to differentiate the fit from the frail elderly. Dividing the elderly in different age groups (such as 65–75, 76–85 and > 85 years) might help to elucidate the various ageing processes.

> **Conclusions**
>
> Older patients and particularly old critically ill patients handle their medications differently than their younger counterparts. Clinicians are often unaware of the anatomical and physiological changes that occur with ageing and the impact of these alterations on pharmacokinetics in the elderly. It is difficult to establish what changes are purely caused by ageing. For example, comorbidities such as liver and kidney disease, affecting drug metabolism and elimination, are more common in elderly patients. Moreover, the increased prevalence of polypharmacy and therefore increased risk for ADRs make it also difficult to determine the actual effect of ageing on pharmacokinetics. When possible, TDM, metabolic geno- or phenotyping and appropriate measurements of renal clearance should be performed to prevent either sub- or supra-therapeutic plasma concentrations. Old (critically ill) patients are often excluded from clinical trials, making it difficult to assess the benefits and risks of a specific drug used in the elderly population This basically means that we are blindfoldedly treating our geriatric patients. Future research should focus on these issues if we want to prevent ADRs in this growing proportion of ICU patients.

> **Take-Home Messages**
>
> - With advancing age, several anatomical and physiological changes can occur that potentially affect pharmacokinetics (i.e. absorption, distribution, metabolism and excretion (ADME)).
> - Interindividual variability in drug disposition is particularly prominent in the elderly population due to comorbidities and polypharmacy.
> - Drug dosing in the elderly should be adjusted to alterations in pharmacokinetics, but changes in pharmacodynamics should also be considered.
> - Older adults should be treated according to clinical response. Dose adjustments should be individualised and the efficacy and safety of administered drugs should be monitored carefully.
> - Although the elderly use a disproportionate share of prescription drugs, few of these drugs are adequately tested in older adults. Therefore, there is an urgent need to generate more clinical data for the growing elderly population.

References

1. United Nations, Department of economic and social affairs, population Division (2019). World population prospects 2019: highlights (ST/ESA/SER.A/423); 2019.
2. Waring RH, Harris RM, Mitchell SC. Drug metabolism in the elderly: a multifactorial problem? Maturitas. 2017;100:27–32.
3. Davies EA, O'Mahony MS. Adverse drug reactions in special populations - the elderly. Br J Clin Pharmacol. 2015;80(4):796–807.
4. Marengoni A, Angleman S, Melis R, Mangialasche F, Karp A, Garmen A, et al. Aging with multimorbidity: a systematic review of the literature. Ageing Res Rev. 2011;10(4):430–9.
5. Barnett K, Mercer SW, Norbury M, Watt G, Wyke S, Guthrie B. Epidemiology of multimorbidity and implications for health care, research, and medical education: a cross-sectional study. Lancet. 2012;380(9836):37–43.
6. McLean G, Gunn J, Wyke S, Guthrie B, Watt GC, Blane DN, et al. The influence of socioeconomic deprivation on multimorbidity at different ages: a cross-sectional study. Br J Gen Pract. 2014;64(624):e440–7.
7. Goldberg RM, Mabee J, Chan L, Wong S. Drug-drug and drug-disease interactions in the ED: analysis of a high-risk population. Am J Emerg Med. 1996;14(5):447–50.
8. Cahir C, Bennett K, Teljeur C, Fahey T. Potentially inappropriate prescribing and adverse health outcomes in community dwelling older patients. Br J Clin Pharmacol. 2014;77(1):201–10.
9. Oscanoa TJ, Lizaraso F, Carvajal A. Hospital admissions due to adverse drug reactions in the elderly. A meta-analysis. Eur J Clin Pharmacol. 2017;73(6):759–70.
10. Wester K, Jonsson A, Spigset O, Hagg S. Spontaneously reported fatal suspected adverse drug reactions: a 10-year survey from Sweden. Pharmacoepidemiol Drug Saf. 2007;16(2):173–80.
11. Wu C, Bell CM, Wodchis WP. Incidence and economic burden of adverse drug reactions among elderly patients in Ontario emergency departments: a retrospective study. Drug Saf. 2012;35(9):769–81.
12. Collard RM, Boter H, Schoevers RA, Oude Voshaar RC. Prevalence of frailty in community-dwelling older persons: a systematic review. J Am Geriatr Soc. 2012;60(8):1487–92.
13. Flaatten H, de Lange DW, Morandi A, Andersen FH, Artigas A, Bertolini G, et al. The impact of frailty on ICU and 30-day mortality and the level of care in very elderly patients (≥ 80 years). Intensive Care Med. 2017;43(12):1820–8.
14. Herr M, Robine JM, Pinot J, Arvieu JJ, Ankri J. Polypharmacy and frailty: prevalence, relationship, and impact on mortality in a French sample of 2350 old people. Pharmacoepidemiol Drug Saf. 2015;24(6):637–46.

15. Saum KU, Schottker B, Meid AD, Holleczek B, Haefeli WE, Hauer K, et al. Is polypharmacy associated with frailty in older people? Results from the ESTHER cohort study. J Am Geriatr Soc. 2017;65(2):e27–32.
16. Hilmer SN. ADME-tox issues for the elderly. Expert Opin Drug Metab Toxicol. 2008;4(10):1321–31.
17. Buch A, Carmeli E, Boker LK, Marcus Y, Shefer G, Kis O, et al. Muscle function and fat content in relation to sarcopenia, obesity and frailty of old age--An overview. Exp Gerontol. 2016;76:25–32.
18. Marzetti E, Calvani R, Tosato M, Cesari M, Di Bari M, Cherubini A, et al. Sarcopenia: an overview. Aging Clin Exp Res. 2017;29(1):11–7.
19. Cesari M, Leeuwenburgh C, Lauretani F, Onder G, Bandinelli S, Maraldi C, et al. Frailty syndrome and skeletal muscle: results from the Invecchiare in chianti study. Am J Clin Nutr. 2006;83(5):1142–8.
20. Mangoni AA, Jackson SHD. Age-related changes in pharmacokinetics and pharmacodynamics: basic principles and practical applications. Br J Clin Pharmacol. 2004;57(1):6–14.
21. Johnston C, Kirkpatrick CM, McLachlan AJ, Hilmer SN. Physiologically based pharmacokinetic modeling at the extremes of age. Clin Pharmacol Ther. 2013;93(2):148.
22. Hurwitz A, Brady DA, Schaal SE, Samloff IM, Dedon J, Ruhl CE. Gastric acidity in older adults. JAMA. 1997;278(8):659–62.
23. Nakamura K, Ogoshi K, Makuuchi H. Influence of aging, gastric mucosal atrophy and dietary habits on gastric secretion. Hepato-Gastroenterology. 2006;53(70):624–8.
24. Hurwitz A, Ruhl CE, Kimler BF, Topp EM, Mayo MS. Gastric function in the elderly: effects on absorption of ketoconazole. J Clin Pharmacol. 2003;43(9):996–1002.
25. Tay HS, Soiza RL. Systematic review and meta-analysis: what is the evidence for oral iron supplementation in treating anaemia in elderly people? Drugs Aging. 2015;32(2):149–58.
26. Gainsborough N, Maskrey VL, Nelson ML, Keating J, Sherwood RA, Jackson SH, et al. The association of age with gastric emptying. Age Ageing. 1993;22(1):37–40.
27. Soenen S, Rayner CK, Horowitz M, Jones KL. Gastric emptying in the elderly. Clin Geriatr Med. 2015;31(3):339–53.
28. Husebye E, Engedal K. The patterns of motility are maintained in the human small intestine throughout the process of aging. Scand J Gastroenterol. 1992;27(5):397–404.
29. O'Mahony D, O'Leary P, Quigley EM. Aging and intestinal motility: a review of factors that affect intestinal motility in the aged. Drugs Aging. 2002;19(7):515–27.
30. Saltzman JR, Kowdley KV, Perrone G, Russell RM. Changes in small-intestine permeability with aging. J Am Geriatr Soc. 1995;43(2):160–4.
31. Valentini L, Ramminger S, Haas V, Postrach E, Werich M, Fischer A, et al. Small intestinal permeability in older adults. Physiol Rep. 2014;2(4):e00281.
32. Yuasa H, Soga N, Kimura Y, Watanabe J. Effect of aging on the intestinal transport of hydrophilic drugs in the rat small intestine. Biol Pharm Bull. 1997;20(11):1188–92.
33. Schmucker DL. Aging and drug disposition: an update. Pharmacol Rev. 1985;37(2):133–48.
34. Hollander D, Tarnawski H. Aging-associated increase in intestinal absorption of macromolecules. Gerontology. 1985;31(3):133–7.
35. Armbrecht HJ, Boltz MA, Kumar VB. Intestinal plasma membrane calcium pump protein and its induction by 1,25(OH)(2)D(3) decrease with age. Am J Phys. 1999;277(1):G41–7.
36. Toyoshima M, Inada M, Kameyama M. Effects of aging on intracellular transport of vitamin B12 (B12) in rat enterocytes. J Nutr Sci Vitaminol (Tokyo). 1983;29(1):1–10.
37. Doherty MM, Charman WN. The mucosa of the small intestine: how clinically relevant as an organ of drug metabolism? Clin Pharmacokinet. 2002;41(4):235–53.
38. Mangoni AA. The impact of advancing age on P-glycoprotein expression and activity: current knowledge and future directions. Expert Opin Drug Metab Toxicol. 2007;3(3):315–20.
39. Madsen JL. Effects of gender, age, and body mass index on gastrointestinal transit times. Dig Dis Sci. 1992;37(10):1548–53.
40. Madsen JL, Graff J. Effects of ageing on gastrointestinal motor function. Age Ageing. 2004;33(2):154–9.
41. Konda S, Meier-Davis SR, Cayme B, Shudo J, Maibach HI. Age-related percutaneous penetration part 2: effect of age on dermatopharmacokinetics and overview of transdermal products. Skin Therapy Lett. 2012;17(6):5–7.

42. Tanner T, Marks R. Delivering drugs by the transdermal route: review and comment. Skin Res Technol. 2008;14(3):249–60.
43. Kaestli LZ, Wasilewski-Rasca AF, Bonnabry P, Vogt-Ferrier N. Use of transdermal drug formulations in the elderly. Drugs Aging. 2008;25(4):269–80.
44. Nelson L, Schwaner R. Transdermal fentanyl: pharmacology and toxicology. J Med Toxicol. 2009;5(4):230–41.
45. Skloot GS. The effects of aging on lung structure and function. Clin Geriatr Med. 2017;33(4):447–57.
46. Allen S. Are inhaled systemic therapies a viable option for the treatment of the elderly patient? Drugs Aging. 2008;25(2):89–94.
47. Wilkinson GR. The effects of diet, aging and disease-states on presystemic elimination and oral drug bioavailability in humans. Adv Drug Deliv Rev. 1997;27:129–59.
48. Prommer E. Role of codeine in palliative care. J Opioid Manag. 2011;7(5):401–6.
49. Schachter M. Chemical, pharmacokinetic and pharmacodynamic properties of statins: an update. Fundam Clin Pharmacol. 2004;19(1):117–25.
50. Davies RO, Gomez HJ, Irvin JD, Walker JF. An overview of the clinical pharmacology of enalapril. Br J Clin Pharmacol. 1984;18(Suppl 2):215S–29S.
51. Todd PA, Perindopril FA. A review of its pharmacological properties and therapeutic use in cardiovascular disorders. Drugs. 1991;42(1):90–114.
52. Fulop T Jr, Worum I, Csongor J, Foris G, Leovey A. Body composition in elderly people. I. Determination of body composition by multiisotope method and the elimination kinetics of these isotopes in healthy elderly subjects. Gerontology. 1985;31(1):6–14.
53. Reeve E, Wiese MD, Mangoni AA. Alterations in drug disposition in older adults. Expert Opin Drug Metab Toxicol. 2015;11(4):491–508.
54. Cusack B, Kelly J, O'Malley K, Noel J, Lavan J, Horgan J. Digoxin in the elderly: pharmacokinetic consequences of old age. Clin Pharmacol Ther. 1979;25(6):772–6.
55. Drenth-van Maanen AC, Wilting I, Jansen PAF. Prescribing medicines to older people-how to consider the impact of ageing on human organ and body functions. Br J Clin Pharmacol. 2020;86(10):1921–30.
56. Jansen PA, Brouwers JR. Clinical pharmacology in old persons. Scientifica (Cairo). 2012;2012:723678.
57. Redolfi A, Borgogelli E, Lodola E. Blood level of cimetidine in relation to age. Eur J Clin Pharmacol. 1979;15(4):257–61.
58. Vestal RE, McGuire EA, Tobin JD, Andres R, Norris AH, Mezey E. Aging and ethanol metabolism. Clin Pharmacol Ther. 1977;21(3):343–54.
59. Herman RJ, Wilkinson GR. Disposition of diazepam in young and elderly subjects after acute and chronic dosing. Br J Clin Pharmacol. 1996;42(2):147–55.
60. Toornvliet R, van Berckel BN, Luurtsema G, Lubberink M, Geldof AA, Bosch TM, et al. Effect of age on functional P-glycoprotein in the blood-brain barrier measured by use of (R)-[(11)C] verapamil and positron emission tomography. Clin Pharmacol Ther. 2006;79(6):540–8.
61. Schinkel AH. P-glycoprotein, a gatekeeper in the blood-brain barrier. Adv Drug Deliv Rev. 1999;36(2–3):179–94.
62. Butler JM, Begg EJ. Free drug metabolic clearance in elderly people. Clin Pharmacokinet. 2008;47(5):297–321.
63. Greenblatt DJ. Reduced serum albumin concentration in the elderly: a report from the Boston collaborative drug surveillance program. J Am Geriatr Soc. 1979;27(1):20–2.
64. Weaving G, Batstone GF, Jones RG. Age and sex variation in serum albumin concentration: an observational study. Ann Clin Biochem. 2016;53(1):106–11.
65. Smith SA, Waters NJ. Pharmacokinetic and Pharmacodynamic considerations for drugs binding to Alpha-1-acid glycoprotein. Pharm Res. 2019;36(2):30.
66. Tenero DM, Bottorff MB, Burlew BS, Williams JB, Lalonde RL. Altered beta-adrenergic sensitivity and protein binding to 1-propranolol in the elderly. J Cardiovasc Pharmacol. 1990;16(5):702–7.
67. Woo J, Chan HS, Or KH, Arumanayagam M. Effect of age and disease on two drug binding proteins: albumin and alpha-1- acid glycoprotein. Clin Biochem. 1994;27(4):289–92.
68. Le Couteur DG, McLean AJ. The aging liver. Drug clearance and an oxygen diffusion barrier hypothesis. Clin Pharmacokinet. 1998;34(5):359–73.

69. McLean AJ, Le Couteur DG. Aging biology and geriatric clinical pharmacology. Pharmacol Rev. 2004;56(2):163–84.
70. Herrlinger C, Klotz U. Drug metabolism and drug interactions in the elderly. Best Pract Res Clin Gastroenterol. 2001;15(6):897–918.
71. Shi S, Klotz U. Age-related changes in pharmacokinetics. Curr Drug Metab. 2011;12(7):601–10.
72. Schmucker DL. Liver function and phase I drug metabolism in the elderly: a paradox. Drugs Aging. 2001;18(11):837–51.
73. George J, Byth K, Farrell GC. Age but not gender selectively affects expression of individual cytochrome P450 proteins in human liver. Biochem Pharmacol. 1995;50(5):727–30.
74. Sotaniemi EA, Arranto AJ, Pelkonen O, Pasanen M. Age and cytochrome P450-linked drug metabolism in humans: an analysis of 226 subjects with equal histopathologic conditions. Clin Pharmacol Ther. 1997;61(3):331–9.
75. Hunt CM, Westerkam WR, Stave GM. Effect of age and gender on the activity of human hepatic CYP3A. Biochem Pharmacol. 1992;44(2):275–83.
76. Klotz U. Pharmacokinetics and drug metabolism in the elderly. Drug Metab Rev. 2009;41(2):67–76.
77. Schmucker DL, Woodhouse KW, Wang RK, Wynne H, James OF, McManus M, et al. Effects of age and gender on in vitro properties of human liver microsomal monooxygenases. Clin Pharmacol Ther. 1990;48(4):365–74.
78. Shimada T, Yamazaki H, Mimura M, Inui Y, Guengerich FP. Interindividual variations in human liver cytochrome P-450 enzymes involved in the oxidation of drugs, carcinogens and toxic chemicals: studies with liver microsomes of 30 Japanese and 30 Caucasians. J Pharmacol Exp Ther. 1994;270(1):414–23.
79. Hilmer SN, Wu H, Zhang M. Biology of frailty: implications for clinical pharmacology and drug therapy in frail older people. Mech Ageing Dev. 2019;181:22–8.
80. Hubbard RE, O'Mahony MS, Calver BL, Woodhouse KW. Plasma esterases and inflammation in ageing and frailty. Eur J Clin Pharmacol. 2008;64(9):895–900.
81. Schwartz JB. Erythromycin breath test results in elderly, very elderly, and frail elderly persons. Clin Pharmacol Ther. 2006;79(5):440–8.
82. Renton KW. Regulation of drug metabolism and disposition during inflammation and infection. Expert Opin Drug Metab Toxicol. 2005;1(4):629–40.
83. Herd B, Wynne H, Wright P, James O, Woodhouse K. The effect of age on glucuronidation and sulphation of paracetamol by human liver fractions. Br J Clin Pharmacol. 1991;32(6):768–70.
84. Divoll M, Greenblatt DJ, Harmatz JS, Shader RI. Effect of age and gender on disposition of temazepam. J Pharm Sci. 1981;70(10):1104–7.
85. Ghabrial H, Desmond PV, Watson KJ, Gijsbers AJ, Harman PJ, Breen KJ, et al. The effects of age and chronic liver disease on the elimination of temazepam. Eur J Clin Pharmacol. 1986;30(1):93–7.
86. Wynne HA, Yelland C, Cope LH, Boddy A, Woodhouse KW, Bateman DN. The association of age and frailty with the pharmacokinetics and pharmacodynamics of metoclopramide. Age Ageing. 1993;22(5):354–9.
87. Wynne HA, Cope LH, Herd B, Rawlins MD, James OF, Woodhouse KW. The association of age and frailty with paracetamol conjugation in man. Age Ageing. 1990;19(6):419–24.
88. Mitchell SJ, Kane AE, Hilmer SN. Age-related changes in the hepatic pharmacology and toxicology of paracetamol. Curr Gerontol Geriatr Res. 2011;2011:624156.
89. Seripa D, Pilotto A, Panza F, Matera MG, Pilotto A. Pharmacogenetics of cytochrome P450 (CYP) in the elderly. Ageing Res Rev. 2010;9(4):457–74.
90. Tannenbaum C, Sheehan NL. Understanding and preventing drug-drug and drug-gene interactions. Expert Rev Clin Pharmacol. 2014;7(4):533–44.
91. Elliott LS, Henderson JC, Neradilek MB, Moyer NA, Ashcraft KC, Thirumaran RK. Clinical impact of pharmacogenetic profiling with a clinical decision support tool in polypharmacy home health patients: a prospective pilot randomized controlled trial. PLoS One. 2017;12(2):e0170905.
92. Ducker CM, Brockmoller J. Genomic variation and pharmacokinetics in old age: a quantitative review of age- vs. Genotype-related differences. Clin Pharmacol Ther. 2019;105(3):625–40.
93. Empey PE. Genetic predisposition to adverse drug reactions in the intensive care unit. Crit Care Med. 2010;38(6 Suppl):S106–16.

94. Lindeman RD, Tobin J, Shock NW. Longitudinal studies on the rate of decline in renal function with age. J Am Geriatr Soc. 1985;33(4):278–85.

95. Muhlberg W, Platt D. Age-dependent changes of the kidneys: pharmacological implications. Gerontology. 1999;45(5):243–53.

96. Fliser D. Ren sanus in corpore Sano: the myth of the inexorable decline of renal function with senescence. Nephrol Dial Transplant. 2005;20(3):482–5.

97. Sesso R, Prado F, Vicioso B, Ramos LR. Prospective study of progression of kidney dysfunction in community-dwelling older adults. Nephrology (Carlton). 2008;13(2):99–103.

98. Englund G, Hallberg P, Artursson P, Michaelsson K, Melhus H. Association between the number of coadministered P-glycoprotein inhibitors and serum digoxin levels in patients on therapeutic drug monitoring. BMC Med. 2004;2:8.

99. Bolignano D, Mattace-Raso F, Sijbrands EJ, Zoccali C. The aging kidney revisited: a systematic review. Ageing Res Rev. 2014;14:65–80.

100. Sproule BA, Hardy BG, Shulman KI. Differential pharmacokinetics of lithium in elderly patients. Drugs Aging. 2000;16(3):165–77.

101. Currie GM, Wheat JM, Kiat H. Pharmacokinetic considerations for digoxin in older people. Open Cardiovasc Med J. 2011;5:130–5.

102. Tueth MJ, Murphy TK, Evans DL. Special considerations: use of lithium in children, adolescents, and elderly populations. J Clin Psychiatry. 1998;59(Suppl 6):66–73.

103. Triggs E, Charles B. Pharmacokinetics and therapeutic drug monitoring of gentamicin in the elderly. Clin Pharmacokinet. 1999;37(4):331–41.

104. Harper P, Young L, Merriman E. Bleeding risk with dabigatran in the frail elderly. N Engl J Med. 2012;366(9):864–6.

105. Puthucheary ZA, Rawal J, McPhail M, Connolly B, Ratnayake G, Chan P, et al. Acute skeletal muscle wasting in critical illness. JAMA. 2013;310(15):1591–600.

106. Fliser D, Bischoff I, Hanses A, Block S, Joest M, Ritz E, et al. Renal handling of drugs in the healthy elderly. Creatinine clearance underestimates renal function and pharmacokinetics remain virtually unchanged. Eur J Clin Pharmacol. 1999;55(3):205–11.

107. Johnston C, Hilmer SN, McLachlan AJ, Matthews ST, Carroll PR, Kirkpatrick CM. The impact of frailty on pharmacokinetics in older people: using gentamicin population pharmacokinetic modeling to investigate changes in renal drug clearance by glomerular filtration. Eur J Clin Pharmacol. 2014;70(5):549–55.

108. van Marum RJ. Underrepresentation of the elderly in clinical trials, time for action. Br J Clin Pharmacol. 2020;86(10):2014–6.

Geriatric Syndroms

Contents

Multimorbidity

Claire Roubaud-Baudron and Florent Guerville

Contents

> **Learning Objectives**
> - To understand the concept and operational definitions of multimorbidity.
> - To understand the consequences of multimorbidity on survival, functional status and quality of life.
> - To understand that multimorbidity assessment is one element of the comprehensive geriatric assessment and is necessary for clinical decision making and management in ICU.

8.1 Introduction

Multimorbidity, defined by the co-occurrence of multiple chronic diseases, increases with age and represents several challenges for care, in health systems designed with a 'single-disease approach'. Especially, multimorbidity is one of the geriatric conditions which needs to be assessed and managed in intensive care units (ICU). The assessment of chronic medical conditions is a one of the steps helping to decide an ICU admission and the intensity of ICU treatments and will also be helpful to manage the patient once admitted in the ICU. Apart from the treatment of the acute event resulting in ICU admission, management of chronic underlying diseases is crucial to avoid a cascade of exacerbations. Old patients with multimorbidity admitted to the ICU are more prone, in addition to the acute illness, to develop other subsequent organ failures and finally have an increased related mortality. In the first part of the present chapter, we summarize current knowledge on multimorbidity in older persons: definitions, epidemiology, consequences and models of care. The second part of this chapter is dedicated to provide tools to assess multimorbidity at the bedside of the patient at triage and to anticipate and prevent future failures of chronic health conditions during the ICU stay.

8.2 Multimorbidity in the Older Population: What Do We Know?

8.2.1 History and Conceptual Definition

The term 'multimorbidity' was introduced in Germany in 1976 [1] as an addition to the concept of 'comorbidity' introduced in 1970 [2, 3]. The latter one prevailed until the concept of multimorbidity gained an international attraction through research in 1990 [4, 5]. Comorbidity refers to additional diseases beyond an index condition, with an influence on the prognosis of the index disease. This implies care focused on a main condition. Conversely, multimorbidity refers to multiple diseases co-occurring in the same patient [6]. This new term implies a shift of interest towards a holistic view of medical problems, which are considered according to their impact in a given patient. Instead of being focused on an index disease, care is oriented towards outcomes that matter to the patient [3, 7]. This comprehensive, functional (versus disease centred) view seems particularly useful for long-term care and family medicine. Indeed, clinical care and research are still too much focused on a single disease paradigm, inappropriate for older patients with complex multimorbidity [5].

Based on a systematic review of literature, Le Reste et al. [5] proposed an integrative definition: Multimorbidity is defined as 'any combination of chronic disease with at least one other disease (acute or chronic) or biopsychosocial factor (associated or not) or somatic risk factor. Any biopsychosocial factor, any somatic risk factor, the social network, the burden of diseases, the health care consumption, and the patient's coping strategies may function as modifiers of the effects of multimorbidity on health. Multimorbidity may modify the health outcomes and lead to an increased disability or a decreased quality of life or frailty.'

There is an epidemiological overlap between multimorbidity and frailty, which is conceptualized as a reduction in physiological reserve in multiple systems, increasing vulnerability to stressors [8]. Frailty and multimorbidity can thus be conceptually viewed as diverse expressions of the same phenomenon: age-related loss of resilience and inability to cope with external stressors. The main difference is that metrics of frailty should aim at identifying a preclinical condition of vulnerability to stressors, whereas metrics of multimorbidity provide a measure of the clinical expression of such vulnerability [9]. In the NHATS study, it has been shown that both multimorbidity patterns and frailty phenotype are independently associated with mortality, suggesting that assessing both frailty and multimorbidity and their interplay could improve risk prediction and facilitate individualized care of older people [10].

8.2.2 Operational Definitions

Several operational definitions of multimorbidity have been proposed so far [3], with three main different approaches:

- **Number**: commonly ≥ 2 or 3 co-occurrent diseases in the same patient. This definition is easy to use in epidemiological studies, but includes patients with diseases controlled by lifestyle or drugs with few symptoms, as well as patients with severe functional loss consequently to diseases.
- **Number and severity:** this approach is useful to identify patients at high risk of poor health outcome in clinical studies. One of the most popular examples is the Charlson Comorbidity Index [7, 11] developed in a sample of patients hospitalized in a medical centre and predictive of 1-year mortality. A specific version of the Cumulative Illness Rating Scale was validated for Geriatrics [12].
- **Number and functional implications**: this approach considers diseases/symptoms as well as physical/cognitive functional implication of diseases. It is thus suitable to identify patients with complex health problems, who need multi-professional care. This is considered the most relevant approach for clinical care of older patients.

Despite a lack of a standardized operational approach, it is admitted that indices of multimorbidity should include highly prevalent conditions and strong risk factors for disability [9], and that disease severity, duration and interaction between acute and chronic conditions are more important than diseases count [3].

8.2.3 Epidemiology

Multimorbidity is clearly associated with older age. According to a meta-analysis of 41 studies [3] defining multimorbidity as ≥ 2 co-occurrent diseases, the prevalence of multimorbidity was estimated between 20% and 30% (all ages) but rose to 55–98% in older persons (60+ to 80+ years old). In the same work, risk factors for multimorbidity incidence (four studies, all ages) were older age, female sex, number of previous diseases, lower education and thinner social network.

One could ask whether the accumulation of multiple chronic diseases in some individuals is random or not. In a landmark study using data from general practice, Van Den Akker et al. [13] found that statistical clustering was stronger than expected: compared to pure chance, more people had no disease and more people had ≥4 diseases. These findings opened a research field about clustering of chronic diseases.

Nevertheless, studies of patterns of associative multimorbidity found inconsistent results, notably because of a lack of standardization of multimorbidity measurements [9]. But could this kind of research have clinical implications, beyond describing common pathophysiological pathways among diseases from the same pattern? One hypothesis would be that the rate of accumulation of multiple diseases in the same individual would serve as a proxy measure of the speed of ageing, indicating loss of resilience and homeostasis [9]. Therefore, we need longitudinal analyses of chronic disease incidence in order to better understand their dynamic and prognosis. Such a 12-year longitudinal study in older persons described changes over time from one multimorbidity cluster to another and differences in mortality rate between clusters [14].

Studies showing statistical clustering of chronic diseases also raise the question of the causes of multimorbidity. Co-occurrence of chronic diseases in an individual may theoretically be due to random chance, common risk factors and/or biological mechanisms, or iatrogenic cascades. To date, very little is known about genetic, lifestyle, biological or environmental contributors to multimorbidity. Over the last decade, a research field called *Geroscience* gained attraction. This field is built on the following hypothesis: the accumulation of diseases and functional loss during ageing is driven by common biological mechanisms [15]. Several hallmarks or pillars of biological ageing were described [15, 16], including (but not limited to) cell senescence, chronic low-grade inflammation, stem cell exhaustion and metabolic dysfunction. This research could lead to biomarker and therapeutic intervention discoveries but has not yet been translated in clinical practice.

8.2.4 Consequences and Prognosis

According to two meta-analyses [3, 9], multimorbidity predicts functional decline/disability and is associated with low quality of life (especially its physical component) and healthcare utilization (including number of drugs, hospitalization, physician referrals and costs). Unexpectedly, the association with mortality is more controversial, but an increase in multimorbidity indexes over time could be a better predictor of death than a transversal measure [17]. Interestingly, in older community-dwelling adults, the association of multimorbidity with death may be mediated by disability [18]. In a clinical perspective, this underlines the importance of assessing functional consequences of chronic diseases in daily life and implementing personalized healthcare plan to reduce disability and other adverse outcomes.

8.2.5 Models and Quality of Care

Actual medicine, inherited from the twentieth century, is designed to treat single diseases. Multimorbid, frail older patients (i.e. most patients hospitalized in 'superspecialized' departments) find this medicine confusing, impersonal and challenging [19]. Their complex medical problems are managed with many specialist referrals, often inefficient and ineffective. In many cases, 'the patient fails by not fitting the service'. We thus need a 'XXIth century care model that count past one' [20], shifting to the era of multimorbidity medicine. To this aim, we need to promote a holistic patient-centred approach with continuous collaboration across specialties, including both medical care and social services.

Several challenges should be emphasized. We lack specific guidelines because multimorbid older patients are mostly excluded from randomized controlled trials. Most trials focus on survival or specific disease measures or events and do not include function, symptom relief, quality of life or other outcomes important to older persons [21].

Clinicians struggle for applying single disease-specific guidelines in patients with multimorbidity [22]. It is often unclear which condition(s) contributes to an individual's function, symptoms, quality of life or survival, and consequently, which conditions should be the main treatment targets. Following disease-specific clinical guidelines in multimorbid older patients may lead to adverse interaction between drugs and diseases [23]. In the same line, following several disease-specific guidelines concomitantly may lead to deleterious treatment burden, with uncertain benefit [24]. Healthcare in which each clinician focuses only on his/her own domain and condition-specific outcomes leads to fragmentation, conflicting recommendations, treatment burden and care that is not always focused on what matters most to patients [21]. More than 40% of older adults acknowledge some degree of treatment burden that represents an underappreciated yet modifiable source of nonadherence [25, 26].

In this challenging context, which principles should guide clinical decision making? In 2019, an *American Geriatrics Society* working group proposed the following principles [21]:

- Elicit and incorporate patient (and family/caregiver) preferences into medical decision making.
- Recognize the limitations of the evidence base and interpret and apply the medical literature specifically for this population.
- Frame clinical management decisions within the context of harms, burdens, benefits and prognosis (e.g. remaining life expectancy, functional status and quality of life).
- Consider treatment complexity and feasibility when making clinical management decisions.
- Use strategies for choosing therapies that optimize benefit, minimize harm and enhance quality of life.

From these principles, the following recommended actions were inferred:

1. **Identify and communicate** patients' health priorities and health trajectory (i.e. prognosis, likely patterns of change in function, health status and quality of life, over a defined period).
2. **Decide**: stop, start or continue care based on health priorities and trajectory and potential benefit vs harm/burden. *For example,* stop medications deemed inap-

propriate in older adults, avoid medication cascades and discontinue treatment no longer indicated or needed. Consider health trajectory and time to benefit for preventive interventions. Explain cessation of screening and prevention as a shift in priorities, using positive messaging.

3. **Align** decisions and care among patients, caregivers and clinicians with patients' health priorities and trajectory. Such approach lessens the likelihood of conflicting recommendations and treatment burden if all clinicians focus on the same priorities. *For example,* affirm shared understanding of patients' health priorities. Link decisions to something meaningful for the patient. Accept patients' decisions. Acknowledge absence of one 'right answer'. Use collaborative negotiation to arrive at shared recommendations.

8.3 Multimorbidity and Critical Care

8.3.1 Multimorbidity and Decision of ICU Admission

Multimorbidity per se but also its consequences on functional independence and frailty should be considered when deciding or not an ICU admission. Because older patients and patients with multimorbidity are excluded from clinical trials, no recommendation have been established in decision making and management of older adults with multimorbidity eligible to an admission to ICU. As described above (see 'Models and Quality of Care' section), some guiding principles have been established by panel experts to improve the management of older patients with multimorbidity [21] but not specifically those with theoretical indication to an ICU transfer.

Multimorbidity is associated with an increased mortality in ICU whatever the diagnosis at admission (acute myocardial infarction [27], sepsis [28], emergency general surgery [29], etc.). Prediction of mortality in ICU is based on acute physiology scores like the Simplified Acute Physiology Score (SAPS) [30] or the Acute Physiology and Chronic Health Evaluation (APACHE) [31]. Most recent versions of these scores incorporate a limited number of health chronic conditions like cancer, chemotherapy-induced immunosuppression or chronic heart failure. Because studies establishing such scores included a small proportion of very old patients, some frequent comorbidities are lacking like neurocognitive disorders or diabetes. Hence, these scores are less efficient to evaluate the illness severity with increasing age [32].

In a systematic review of the literature selecting 129 studies, different factors associated with in-hospital mortality were reported in older population admitted to ICU. Apart from well-known factors at admission like diagnosis and severity score, comorbidities, functional status and frailty were also reported as risk factors for mortality. Noteworthy, these items were occasionally reported and this review of the literature underlined a great heterogeneity of the data collected. For instance, comorbidities were reported as a selection of chronic diseases and the performance of a standardized comorbidity score was most of the time lacking [33].

As stated above, multimorbidity and frailty are both indirect markers of decreased organ reserve capacities and have some overlap. Studies reporting prevalence of frailty and multimorbidity in participants older than 80 years found that frailty was present in multimorbid people in 27% of cases, whereas multimorbidity concerned

63% of the frail individuals [34], signifying that they can both be complementary criteria to describe an old patient. As a prognostic factor, frailty assessment predicted more accurately COVID-19 survival compared to multimorbidity or age [35].

The impact of multimorbidity on survival may be an addition of the impacts of separate chronic health conditions, but possibly specific combination of comorbidities may have a synergic effect on survival. Although most of the studies reported the impact of a sum of comorbidities considering the weight of the comorbidity or its severity (for instance using Charlson Comorbidity Index [11] or the Cumulative Illness Rating Scale (CIRS-G [12], some authors tried to study the impact of combinations of comorbidities (clusters) and identify high-risk patient groups with an increased risk of organ failure, sepsis and mortality [14, 28]. While this latter reported several different clusters associated to specific trajectories (for instance the cluster of patients combining severe hepatic disease and drug abuse was composed of younger patients who were more prone to develop sepsis liver disease), more studies are needed to precisely define these specific clusters in order to define their needs and to personalize care. Interestingly, several studies reported that change in comorbidities over time (multimorbidity trajectories) was more predictive on mortality than multimorbidity at a given moment, including long-term history disease before ICU admission [17].

In real life, at the bedside of the patients, assessing an older patient with multimorbidity may be very complex and challenging; multimorbidity assessment includes the number of chronic diseases, their severity, their interactions, their impact on functional status, the adverse effects of multimorbidity-induced polypharmacy and finally their prognosis (see ▶ Box 8.1). In fact, one trap would be to overestimate or underestimate the severity of a chronic condition.

For instance, a history of major neurocognitive disorder does not mean that the illness is severe; the term major means that the cognitive impairment interferes with independence in everyday activities including elaborate activities like paying bills or managing medication. In that case, it is important to evaluate the impact of the disease in daily living. Example of traps would be to refuse an ICU admission because of a false label of 'severely cognitive impaired' for a patient with a low impact of her/his cognitive impairment on daily living, but to accept admission of another patient, ignoring that she/he is bedridden all day and needs help for all the daily activities. ▶ Box 8.1 is a toolbox that may help to evaluate promptly the severity of a disease.

Box 8.1 Tools to Evaluate the Severity of Chronic Health Conditions at Bedside of the Patient

- **Healthcare utilization**: how many episodes of exacerbation (how many episodes of acute heart failure? delirium? aspiration pneumonia in the last 6 months? Number of hospitalizations in the last 6 months? How many hospital-free days in the last 3 months?)?
- **Usual markers** (although not perfect) evaluating the severity/control of a chronic disease like left ventricular ejection fraction for chronic heart failure, level of glycosylated haemoglobin in the case of type 2 diabetes mellitus, Mini-Mental Status score in the case of neurocognitive disorders and glomerular filtration rate for chronic renal disease.

> — **Impact on functional independence** may be assessed by activities of daily living (ADL) and instrumental-ADL score or by asking questions about intervention of caregiver. Be careful, a nurse can intervene for basic ADL like toileting but also for IADL (like medication).
> — **The number of medications** may be a good indicator of multimorbidity and severity (but is not always appropriate to patient's actual needs).

8.3.2 Management of Multimorbidity in the ICU

Multimorbidity is one of the factors increasing the complexity of the management of older adults in the ICU. Patients with multimorbidity admitted to the ICU are at higher risk of multiorgan dysfunction and death.

With ageing, organ functions decline over time without reaching the threshold of insufficiency (■ Fig. 8.1, line 1); the decline is increased with the occurrence of a chronic disease (line 2, note that the slope of the line is steeper) and may reach the insufficiency threshold after several years of chronic disease progression. The area under line 1 or line 2 also decreases over time and represents the organ capacity or reserve. When an acute disease occurs, the organ function collapses and failure appears.

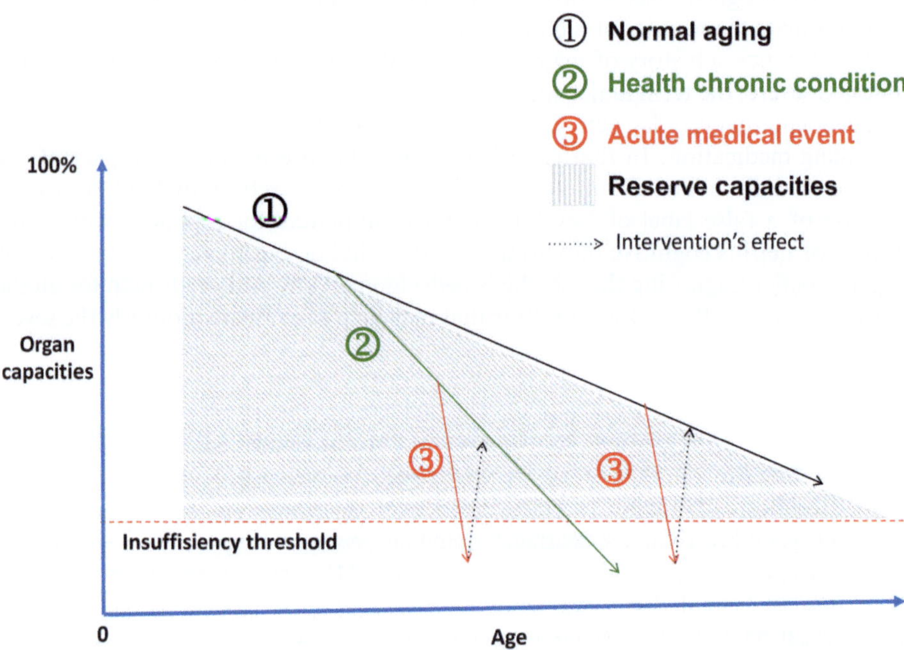

■ **Fig. 8.1** 1 + 3 or how to try to be efficient in geriatrics (Professor Jean Pierre Bouchon). This figure explains the concept of organ capacity (shaded area) decreasing with ageing (line 1) and decreasing faster with the occurrence of a chronic medical condition (line 2). The occurrence of an acute organ failure requires an investigation of the cause (line 3). Note that the acute exacerbation is reversible and transient

☑ Figure 8.1 illustrates the organ function across life and helps physician to understand how an acute event, even minor, may jeopardize a medical stability in an older patient. For instance, an acute anaemia from a gut ulcer may induce congestive heart failure, especially if the patient has a chronic heart disease. In the case of multimorbidity, it is important to understand that an acute medical event may induce several other medical events (by exacerbating several chronic diseases), a phenomenon also named 'geriatric cascade'. For instance, a fever and fatigue induced by an infection result in dehydration with an acute renal failure, responsible for an increased plasmatic level of drugs (antibiotics) leading to the occurrence of delirium and falls [36]. One challenge in the ICU is to prevent organ decompensations and adverse drugs events.

8.3.2.1 Avoiding a Cascade of Organ Failures

Multimorbidity is one of the geriatric conditions which may be destabilized in the ICU. As illustrated in ☑ Fig. 8.1, an acute medical event may induce chronic disease(s) exacerbation(s). Causative factors may be i. the acute illness leading to ICU admission (a sepsis may induce a delirium or an acute heart failure), ii. the treatment of the acute disease (antibiotics prescribed for a sepsis may be responsible for an acute renal failure and/or delirium) and iii. The ICU environment by itself: noise, sleep deprivation, sensory deprivation, new medications and invasive procedures.

8.3.2.2 Avoiding Adverse Drug Events

Multimorbidity is associated with polypharmacy and older patients admitted to hospital take around seven drugs daily. The first most important step to avoid adverse drug events is to determine which drugs the patient is actually taking (current medication list). One patient may have several medication orders from different physicians (general practitioner, cardiologist, dermatologist, ophthalmologist, etc.). To establish a comprehensive list of current medication, asking several sources is necessary: patient, caregivers, nurses, general practitioner, pharmacist, etc. This first effective step is time consuming but may save time in the long run and be very helpful for diagnosis (one in five patients older than 75 is addressed to the emergency department for an adverse drug event [37]). Such a comprehensive assessment of actual drug list may also avoid medication errors (omission, dose error, wrong time, etc.) at each transition step of care trajectory (admission, transfer and discharge) [38]. Moreover, older patients are more prone to develop adverse events compared to youngers. For each acute medical event or exacerbation, questioning about the implication of medication should become a habit. Tools are available to help appropriate prescription in older population (see dedicated chapter).

Limiting medication during an acute medical event is sometimes necessary, for instance, stopping psychotropic drugs in case of altered level of consciousness, switching oral antidiabetics to insulin, stopping diuretics in case of dehydration or anti-thrombotics in case of haemorrhage or in case of risk of overdosage to due unstable kidney function. Some drugs may also be evaluated as temporarily futile like a cholinesterase inhibitor, vitamins or statins. On the contrary, some drug withdrawal must be deleterious and should be frequently re-evaluated (benzodiazepines, antithrombotic treatments, diuretics, etc.). Traps and tips of the management of multimorbidity in older patients are presented in ☑ Fig. 8.2.

Frequent traps to avoid and useful tips !

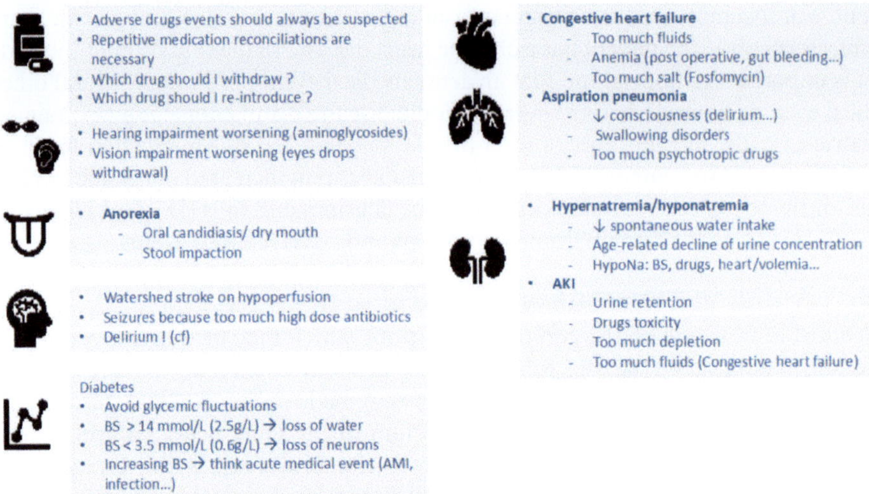

Fig. 8.2 Practical implications. Proposition of frequent traps encountered in geriatrics regarding multimorbidity and tips to avoid a geriatric cascade. AKI: acute kidney injury. BS: blood sugar

Conclusions and Perspectives

Multimorbidity is frequent in older patients, and because this population is under-represented in clinical trials, mortality risk prediction is less efficient with ageing. Assessment of multimorbidity is based on the number and the severity (healthcare utilization, number of medication and impact on daily independence) of distinct chronic medical conditions so far, but the analysis of their combinations and trajectories will probably be more useful in the future to predict their impact on survival.

Intensivists are experts in managing complex acute medical illnesses. Incorporating some geriatric principles about multimorbidity in their daily practice would improve management of older patients in the ICU. Such an approach is based on screening and preventing adverse drug events, evaluating organ reserves/capacities and anticipating/detecting possible chronic disease exacerbations, thereby avoiding geriatric cascades.

Take-Home Messages/Practical Implications

- Contrarily to 'comorbidity', which implies care focused on a main condition, 'multimorbidity' refers to multiple diseases co-occurring in the same patient. This implies a shift of interest towards a holistic view of medical problems.
- There are multiple scales to assess multimorbidity. The most relevant approach is to consider a number of diseases as well as their functional implications.
- We lack evidence-based guidelines to take care of older multimorbid patients, and the crude addition of single disease-specific guidelines in the same patient leads to inappropriate care.

- Patients' health priorities should be recognized and should guide clinical decisions.
- Multimorbidity is associated with an increased risk of mortality in ICU.
- Multimorbidity assessment (number of chronic health conditions, their severity and impact on daily living) is helpful to determine whether an older patient is eligible to an admission to ICU.
- Once admitted to ICU, management of multimorbidity is based on screening and preventing adverse drug events, evaluating organ reserves/capacities and anticipating possible chronic disease exacerbations, thereby avoiding geriatric cascades.

References

1. Brandlmeier P. Multimorbidity among elderly patients in an urban general practice. ZFA (Stuttgart). 1976;52(25):1269–75.
2. Feinstein AR. The pre-therapeutic classification of co-morbidity in chronic disease. J Chronic Dis. 1970;23(7):455–68.
3. Marengoni A, Angleman S, Melis R, Mangialasche F, Karp A, Garmen A, et al. Aging with multimorbidity: a systematic review of the literature. Ageing Res Rev. 2011;10(4):430–9.
4. Heuft G. Future research perspectives of a psychoanalytical gerontopsychophysiology--personality and the aging process. Z Gerontol. 1990;23(5):262–6.
5. Le Reste JY, Nabbe P, Lygidakis C, Doerr C, Lingner H, Czachowski S, et al. A research group from the European general practice research network (EGPRN) explores the concept of multimorbidity for further research into long term care. J Am Med Dir Assoc. 2013;14(2):132–3.
6. Batstra L, Bos EH, Neeleman J. Quantifying psychiatric comorbidity--lessions from chronic disease epidemiology. Soc Psychiatry Psychiatr Epidemiol. 2002;37(3):105–11.
7. Nicholson K, Almirall J, Fortin M. The measurement of multimorbidity. Health Psychol. 2019;38(9):783–90.
8. Clegg A, Young J, Iliffe S, Rikkert MO, Rockwood K. Frailty in elderly people. Lancet. 2013;381(9868):752–62.
9. Fabbri E, Zoli M, Gonzalez-Freire M, Salive ME, Studenski SA, Ferrucci L. Aging and multimorbidity: new tasks, priorities, and Frontiers for integrated Gerontological and clinical research. J Am Med Dir Assoc. 2015;16(8):640–7.
10. Nguyen QD, Wu C, Odden MC, Kim DH. Multimorbidity patterns, frailty, and survival in community-dwelling older adults. J Gerontol A Biol Sci Med Sci. 2019;74(8):1265–70.
11. Charlson ME, Pompei P, Ales KL, MacKenzie CR. A new method of classifying prognostic comorbidity in longitudinal studies: development and validation. J Chronic Dis. 1987;40(5):373–83.
12. Miller MD, Paradis CF, Houck PR, Mazumdar S, Stack JA, Rifai AH, et al. Rating chronic medical illness burden in geropsychiatric practice and research: application of the cumulative illness rating scale. Psychiatry Res. 1992;41(3):237–48.
13. van den Akker M, Buntinx F, Metsemakers JF, Roos S, Knottnerus JA. Multimorbidity in general practice: prevalence, incidence, and determinants of co-occurring chronic and recurrent diseases. J Clin Epidemiol. 1998;51(5):367–75.
14. Vetrano DL, Roso-Llorach A, Fernandez S, Guisado-Clavero M, Violan C, Onder G, et al. Twelve-year clinical trajectories of multimorbidity in a population of older adults. Nat Commun. 2020;11(1):3223.
15. Kennedy BK, Berger SL, Brunet A, Campisi J, Cuervo AM, Epel ES, et al. Geroscience: linking aging to chronic disease. Cell. 2014;159(4):709–13.
16. Lopez-Otin C, Blasco MA, Partridge L, Serrano M, Kroemer G. The hallmarks of aging. Cell. 2013;153(6):1194–217.

17. Fraccaro P, Kontopantelis E, Sperrin M, Peek N, Mallen C, Urban P, et al. Predicting mortality from change-over-time in the Charlson comorbidity index: a retrospective cohort study in a data-intensive UK health system. Medicine (Baltimore). 2016;95(43):e4973.
18. St John PD, Tyas SL, Menec V, Tate R. Multimorbidity, disability, and mortality in community-dwelling older adults. Can Fam Physician. 2014;60(5):e272–80.
19. Mason B, Nanton V, Epiphaniou E, Murray SA, Donaldson A, Shipman C, et al. 'My body's falling apart'. Understanding the experiences of patients with advanced multimorbidity to improve care: serial interviews with patients and carers. BMJ Support Palliat Care. 2016;6(1):60–5.
20. Banerjee S. Multimorbidity--older adults need health care that can count past one. Lancet. 2015;385(9968):587–9.
21. Boyd C, Smith CD, Masoudi FA, Blaum CS, Dodson JA, Green AR, et al. Decision making for older adults with multiple chronic conditions: executive summary for the American Geriatrics Society guiding principles on the Care of Older Adults with Multimorbidity. J Am Geriatr Soc. 2019;67(4):665–73.
22. Fried TR, Tinetti ME, Iannone L. Primary care clinicians' experiences with treatment decision making for older persons with multiple conditions. Arch Intern Med. 2011;171(1):75–80.
23. Boyd CM, Darer J, Boult C, Fried LP, Boult L, Wu AW. Clinical practice guidelines and quality of care for older patients with multiple comorbid diseases: implications for pay for performance. JAMA. 2005;294(6):716–24.
24. Tinetti ME, Fried TR, Boyd CM. Designing health care for the most common chronic condition--multimorbidity. JAMA. 2012;307(23):2493–4.
25. Naik AD, Dyer CB, Kunik ME, McCullough LB. Patient autonomy for the management of chronic conditions: a two-component re-conceptualization. Am J Bioeth. 2009;9(2):23–30.
26. Wolff JL, Boyd CM. A look at person- and family-centered care among older adults: results from a National Survey [corrected]. J Gen Intern Med. 2015;30(10):1497–504.
27. Hall M, Dondo TB, Yan AT, Mamas MA, Timmis AD, Deanfield JE, et al. Multimorbidity and survival for patients with acute myocardial infarction in England and Wales: latent class analysis of a nationwide population-based cohort. PLoS Med. 2018;15(3):e1002501.
28. Zador Z, Landry A, Cusimano MD, Geifman N. Multimorbidity states associated with higher mortality rates in organ dysfunction and sepsis: a data-driven analysis in critical care. Crit Care. 2019;23(1):247.
29. Ho VP, Schiltz NK, Reimer AP, Madigan EA, Koroukian SM. High-risk comorbidity combinations in older patients undergoing emergency general surgery. J Am Geriatr Soc. 2019;67(3):503–10.
30. Le Gall JR, Lemeshow S, Saulnier F. A new simplified acute physiology score (SAPS II) based on a European/north American multicenter study. JAMA. 1993;270(24):2957–63.
31. Zimmerman JE, Kramer AA, McNair DS, Malila FM. Acute physiology and chronic health evaluation (APACHE) IV: hospital mortality assessment for today's critically ill patients. Crit Care Med. 2006;34(5):1297–310.
32. Flaatten H, de Lange DW, Artigas A, Bin D, Moreno R, Christensen S, et al. The status of intensive care medicine research and a future agenda for very old patients in the ICU. Intensive Care Med. 2017;43(9):1319–28.
33. Vallet H, Schwarz GL, Flaatten H, de Lange DW, Guidet B, Dechartres A. Mortality of older patients admitted to an ICU: a systematic review. Crit Care Med. 2021;49(2):324–34.
34. Vetrano DL, Palmer K, Marengoni A, Marzetti E, Lattanzio F, Roller-Wirnsberger R, et al. Frailty and multimorbidity: a systematic review and meta-analysis. J Gerontol A Biol Sci Med Sci. 2019;74(5):659–66.
35. Hewitt J, Carter B, Vilches-Moraga A, Quinn TJ, Braude P, Verduri A, et al. The effect of frailty on survival in patients with COVID-19 (COPE): a multicentre, European, observational cohort study. Lancet Public Health. 2020;5(8):e444–e51.
36. Bouchon J. 1 + 3 ou comment tenter d'être efficace en gériatrie. Rev Prat Méd Gén. 1984;34:888.
37. Shehab N, Lovegrove MC, Geller AI, Rose KO, Weidle NJ, Budnitz DS. US emergency department visits for outpatient adverse drug events, 2013-2014. JAMA. 2016;316(20):2115–25.
38. Dautzenberg L. Bretagne L. Tsokani S, Zevgiti S, Rodondi N, et al. Medication review interventions to reduce hospital readmissions in older people. J Am Geriatr Soc: Koek HL; 2021.

Multipharmacy on the Older Adult

Lozano Vicario Lucía, Gutiérrez-Valencia Marta, and Martínez-Velilla Nicolas

Contents

> **Learning Objectives**
> - To understand the main concepts of polypharmacy, hyperpolypharmacy, PIM, and prescribing cascade.
> - To know the epidemiology of drug therapy.
> - To understand the impact of pharmacokinetics and pharmacodynamics in the older adult and their consequences.
> - To define different consequences of polypharmacy.
> - To know the risk factors involved in polypharmacy.
> - To know the drugs with anticholinergic effects: the importance of anticholinergic burden.
> - To understand the relationship between polypharmacy and other geriatric syndromes: frailty and cognitive impairment.
> - To understand that medications in older patients should be individually adapted according to therapeutic goals.
> - To describe practical approaches to prescribe medications to older patients.

9.1 Introduction

The use of medications in the elderly is a complex issue influenced by many health- and non-health-related factors. Drug therapy is one of the most important tools available for preserving and improving health. However, polypharmacy and the inappropriate use of medications can imply adverse effects and situations of vulnerability that trigger many negative health outcomes: reduced adherence, increased risk of hospitalization, nursing home admissions, adverse drug events (ADEs), emergency department (ED) visits, poor quality of life, and mortality.

Polypharmacy is also a geriatric syndrome that is closely related to falls, delirium, cognitive impairment, malnutrition, and frailty, among others.

In this chapter, we will analyze the concept of polypharmacy, hyperpolypharmacy, and potentially inappropriate medications (PIMs) as well as their impact on the older adult, and the practical implications that those factors may play in the management of appropriate drug prescription (and deprescription).

9.1.1 Concepts

9.1.1.1 Polypharmacy

There is not a universal consensus about the definition of polypharmacy, although the use of five or more medications is the most common threshold [1]. Hyperpolypharmacy is often considered the use of ten or more medications. An increased number of medications have been associated with a higher cost, an increase in drug-drug and drug-disease interactions, poorer medication adherence, or prescription cascades [2, 3]. Therefore, polypharmacy goes beyond the high number of drugs used in quantitative terms but is related to taking more drugs than clinically appropriate in qualitative terms. Although polypharmacy could be appropriate and necessary in some cases, it is very unlikely to happen if the treatment is comprehensively reviewed and monitored. For this reason, there is an additional concept to polypharmacy: the potentially inappropriate medications (PIMs).

9.1.1.2 PIM

It is the use of medicines that introduce a significant risk of an adverse drug-related event where there is evidence for an equally or more effective but lower-risk alternative therapy available for treating the same condition. It also includes the use of medicines at a higher frequency and for longer than clinically indicated, the use of multiple medicines that have recognized drug-drug interactions and drug-disease interactions, and the under-use of beneficial medicines that are clinically indicated but not prescribed for ageist or irrational reasons [4].

Consequently, PIMs may offer an opportunity to improve care through deprescription or, if required, may be replaced by a safer alternative.

9.1.1.3 Prescribing Cascade

The prescribing cascade concept was first proposed by Rochon and Gurwitz in 1997 [5] and it is the prescription of new drugs to treat an adverse drug reaction associated with another medicine. For example, the drug-induced parkinsonism: antidopaminergic-related adverse effects associated with antipsychotic agents have long been recognized, including the development of extrapyramidal signs and symptoms. This drug-related symptom may be potentially misdiagnosed as a new medical condition (i.e., Parkinson's disease) and treated with a new drug (dopamine agonist) producing another medical condition (◘ Table 9.1).

9.2 Epidemiology of Drug Therapy

Polypharmacy is directly associated with aging, and as a result of the aging population, the prevalence of polypharmacy is increasing all over the world. Some population studies performed in patients over 65 years in primary care estimated that the

◘ **Table 9.1** Examples of prescribing cascades

Initial drug therapy	New medical condition	New drug treatment
Antipsychotic or metoclopramide	Parkinsonism	Anti-Parkinson therapy
Cholinesterase inhibitor	Urinary incontinence	Anticholinergic bladder therapy
Tricyclic antidepressant	Delirium	Antipsychotic
Nonsteroidal anti-inflammatory drug (NSAID)	Gout	Antigout therapy
Nonsteroidal anti-inflammatory drug (NSAID)	Hypertension	Antihypertensive therapy

prevalence of polypharmacy reached 44% in Sweden [6], 39% in the United States [7], and 41.2% in Switzerland [8]. A recent study carried out across Europe estimates a prevalence of polypharmacy between 26.3 and 39.9%, being the highest prevalence of medication use among women [9]. A recent cross-sectional analysis of 100% US Medicare claims data showed that the patient-level mean concurrent medication rate was 5.6 in people older than 65 years old [10]. Polypharmacy is most often chronic, although a substantial number of older adults experience short, recurring episodes of polypharmacy and are thus exposed to its potential harms in a transient rather than persistent pattern. A longitudinal cohort study using register data of all 711,432 older adults living in Sweden with 5 or more prescription drugs assessed the chronicity of polypharmacy and identified factors associated with chronic polypharmacy [11]. Overall, 82% were continuously exposed to polypharmacy for 6 months or longer and 74% for 12 months or longer. The proportion of individuals who remained exposed until the end of the study was 55%. Factors associated with chronic polypharmacy included higher age, female sex, living in an institution, chronic multimorbidity, and multidose prescriptions.

The **prevalence** of PIMs in older adults ranges between 20% and 60%, depending on the healthcare setting (e.g., community vs. hospital or nursing homes) or criteria used to define inappropriate prescribing (American Geriatrics Society Beers Criteria vs. STOPP/START criteria). According to Gallagher, the prevalence of PIM across European hospitals was 51.3% using STOPP criteria, varying from 34.7% in Prague to 77.3% in Geneva, and 30.4% using Beer's criteria, varying from 22.7% in Prague to 43.3% in Geneva. Using START criteria, the overall potentially inappropriate prescribing omissions (PPOs) prevalence rate was 59.4%, ranging from 51.3% in Cork to 72.7% in Perugia [12]. According to the World Health Organization (OMS), more than 50% of the medicines that are prescribed, dispensed, or sold are PIMs, and half of the patients do not take them properly. It seems clear that polypharmacy can be a particularly relevant problem in people with certain characteristics, and therefore in specific settings such as nursing homes or some areas of hospitalization, due to the high prevalence of polypharmacy and associated factors in these settings and the complexity and vulnerability of this type of patients.

The prevalence of polypharmacy in **long-term care settings** (LTCS) is very high. A systematic review of 44 studies assessing medication use in long-term care facilities reported a 38.1–91.2% prevalence of polypharmacy, where polypharmacy was defined as ≥5 medications. When defined as ≥9 medications, the prevalence ranged from 12.8–74.4% and 10.6–65.0% when considered as ≥10 medications [13]. Residents often have multiple comorbidities with resulting complex medication regimens; multimorbidity often leads to the use of multiple inappropriate or unnecessary medications and it's a strong risk factor of iatrogenia. Associations with polypharmacy were reported for comorbidity, recent hospital discharge, and the number of prescribers. Older age, cognitive impairment, disability, and length of stay in the LTCS were inversely associated with polypharmacy as well [13]. The older adults living in nursing homes have many peculiarities in relation to the use of medicines. Some studies have suggested that polypharmacy rates in nursing homes are the highest in older populations, as well as the use of potentially inappropriate medications. This is likely due to the profile of older adults admitted to nursing homes: very old age, multimorbidity, and high prevalence of cognitive impairment and advanced disability [14]. However, a recent study has shown that although the prevalence of polypharmacy is higher in nursing homes than in the community, when adjusting for confounders, living in nursing homes is associated with a lower risk of the prevalence and incidence of polypharmacy [6]. It's very important at this point to keep in mind the big heterogeneity in the type of LTCS. Due to the particularities in this population, the same rules cannot be applied as those to the rest of the elderly population. Health and polypharmacy determinants in older nursing home residents emerge from those usually accounted for in the general population. In another recent study done in nursing homes in Spain, frail participants generally took fewer medications than non-frail participants [15], in contrast with other settings. This may be related to the short life expectancy of this population. In nursing homes, advanced disability, severe cognitive impairment, and frailty may be perceived as the end-of-life features, which may influence decision-making regarding medications.

More than half of **hospitalized** older patients present PIMs [16]. The most commonly prescribed PIMs at discharge included benzodiazepines and proton pump inhibitors. For example, the administration of benzodiazepines for sleep during hospitalization is, unfortunately, standard practice in many institutions, as is the administration of proton pump inhibitors within intensive care units for gastroprotection or the use of antipsychotics for delirium or sleep. However, these medications may be inadvertently continued once patients leave the hospital.

On the other hand, herbal medicines are frequently used by older adults, and physicians often do not inquire about their use. More than one-third of the US adult population is estimated to take herbal medicine or supplement such as ginseng, ginkgo biloba extract, and glucosamine that may interact with prescribed drug therapies leading to adverse events [17].

The damaging effects of PIMs, by excess, default, or misuse, cause an economic loss of 7.2 billion dollars per year in community-dwelling older adults in the United States [18].

9.3 Pharmacokinetics and Pharmacodynamics

When prescribing medications to older adults, it is very important to consider pharmacokinetics and pharmacodynamics changes that occur with normal aging.

Pharmacokinetics relates to the way that the body handles a drug and involves the drug absorption, distribution across the body compartments, metabolism in the liver, and elimination by the kidneys.

There are few changes in the drug absorption with aging; however, changes in drug distribution, metabolism, and excretion can impact the clearance of medication from the body in older adults [19].

Age-related changes in body composition can affect the volume of distribution of a drug. Older people have less body mass and greater fat stores than younger people. An example is a therapy with benzodiazepines (BZDs). BZDs are lipid-soluble and their use in the older adults can cause ADEs because they have an increased volume of distribution and consequently prolonged clearance rates.

Older people have a reduced oxidative metabolism by cytochrome P450 (CYP) enzymes in the liver, and renal function often declines with aging as well. Therefore, it is very important to take special care prescribing drug dosing for older patients, particularly in the case of highly lipid-soluble drugs, medications metabolized via reactions catalyzed by CYP enzymes, and drugs excreted by the kidneys.

On the other hand, **pharmacodynamics** relates to the effect that a drug has on the body. Aging is associated with a greater sensitivity to a number of drug therapies. For example, older people are more sensitive to the effects of benzodiazepines, opioids, and warfarin, regardless of whether pharmacokinetic changes might exist.

9.4 Consequences of Polypharmacy

(a) **Consequences on therapeutic adherence**:

The lack of adherence to treatment increases with the complexity of the therapeutic regimen and with the number of drugs to be consumed. Thus, in patients with chronic diseases such as diabetes or congestive heart failure, non-compliance was 15% when taking only one medication, 25% when taking 2–3 drugs, and 35% when taking four or more medicines [20]. As a result, the patient no longer benefits from the drugs, which can trigger decompensations or lack of achievement of the proposed therapeutic objectives.

(b) **Consequences on ADEs**:

The incidence of ADEs increases exponentially with the number of drugs consumed. Most ADEs are due to unnecessary or even contraindicated drugs and drug interactions. It has been reported that up to 35% of outpatients and 40% of hospitalized elderly experience an ADE. Furthermore, approximately 10% of emergency room visits may be attributed to an ADE. In a population-based study, outpatients taking five or more medications had an 88% increased risk of experiencing an ADE compared to those who were taking fewer medications [21].

(c) **Consequences of drug interactions**:

A higher number of medications are associated with a higher probability of producing drug interactions with each other. It has also been found that a factor associated with drug interactions is the fact that there are several prescribing physicians. Interactions that lead to a reduction in the effectiveness of the medication may be overlooked more often than those that result in a synergistic effect, because other reasons may be found to explain the ineffectiveness (e.g., therapeutic failure, disease resistance to medication, etc.). These hasty and erroneous conclusions can lead to an increase in dose or the introduction of a new drug, putting the patient at greater risk of a drug interaction.

(d) **Consequences on the risk of hospitalization, morbidity, and mortality**:

It is estimated that between 10% and 20% of the hospital admissions in older people would be related to adverse drug effects, polypharmacy being one of the associated factors [22].

PIM use by community-dwelling patients has been associated with a 10% to 30% increased risk of hospitalization, as well as increased risk of ADEs, ED visits, and poor quality of life [23–25].

Different studies have shown an association between polypharmacy and mortality, using both discrete and categorical definitions, and a dose-response relationship was observed across escalating thresholds for defining polypharmacy [26].

(e) **Consequences on the economy**:
The geriatric patients, for several reasons, are the main group involved, with 17% of the population being responsible for 70% of pharmaceutical expenditure [27]. The economic consequences of polypharmacy are manifold. The increase in adverse effects, interactions, duplication, etc. leads to an increase in the use of health resources. The magnitude of hospital admissions due to drug incidents is very high and about half of them are preventable. It is estimated that mismanaged polypharmacy contributed to 4% of the world's total avoidable costs due to sub-optimal medicine use. A total of US$ 18 billion, 0.3% of the global total health expenditure, could be avoided by appropriate polypharmacy management [28].

9.5 Risk Factors Involved in Polypharmacy

— Factors related to patients:

The development of chronic diseases is one of the factors mainly involved in poly-pharmacy. The diseases most closely associated with polypharmacy are cardiovascular diseases, diabetes, high blood pressure, and digestive symptoms.

Aging, the number of medications, female sex, and poor perception of health are also risk factors involved in polypharmacy [29].

— Social factors:

Polypharmacy and the use of potentially inappropriate medicines have been linked to various social factors, such as living alone, having a low educational, and socioeconomic level and living in rural areas. These findings illustrate the need to influence the comprehensive approach of patients with polypharmacy, and especially the older adults, on social factors with resources that go beyond aspects of the healthcare system.

— Factors related to the health system:

One of the factors identified is the fact that usually there are several physicians and pharmacists involved in the drug prescription and dispensing of the same patient, which favors the lack of coordination. Therefore, poor control and review of the medication result in duplication and interaction between drugs. Health systems are socially linked to prescription: 75% of medical consultations end with a prescription. On the other hand, many older adults self-medicate, which can cause important consequences. At a physician level, less experience time since medical school graduation and bigger practice size have been associated with higher rates of polypharmacy [10]. The application of clinical practice guidelines focused on a particular pathology, without considering multimorbidity, and the application of therapeutic objectives set for the general population is also a frequent cause of polypharmacy in this population. Older adults are often under-represented both in clinical practice guidelines and in the studies on which these guidelines are based.

Overtreatment, which occurs in all types of populations and healthcare settings, especially affects older people and is another cause of polypharmacy. Some of the reasons are defensive medicine, therapeutic inertia, abuse of preventive medicine, and the medicalization of life (◘ Fig. 9.1).

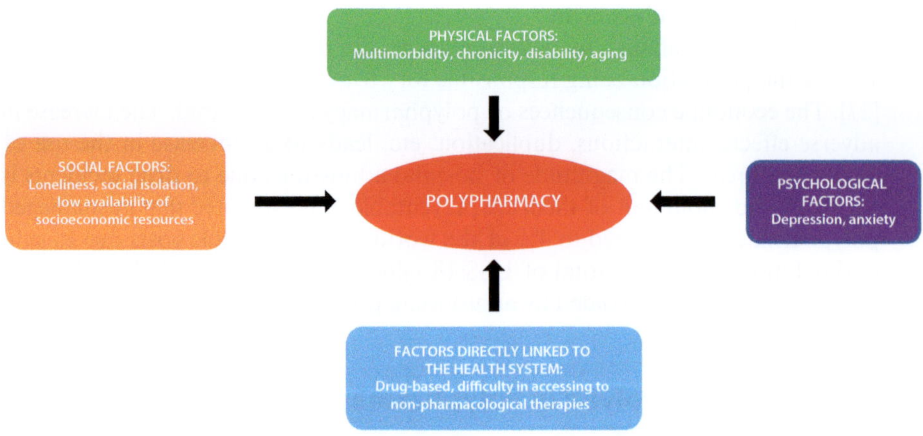

Fig. 9.1 Risk factors involved in polypharmacy

9.6 Drugs with Anticholinergic Effects (DACEs) and Anticholinergic Burden

Older people are commonly exposed to drugs that have anticholinergic properties. DACEs are commonly prescribed for the management of different conditions such as depression, psychosis, Parkinson's disease, muscle spasms, allergy, excessive gastric acid, nausea and vomiting, intestinal motility disorders, overactive bladder, and chronic obstructive pulmonary disease. Older adults have a relatively high probability of being exposed to DACEs due to their high medical comorbidity and the number of prescribed medications.

It has been found that the use of drugs with anticholinergic properties is more frequent in frail patients and that the risk of developing frailty increases proportionally with anticholinergic load [30–32].

The wide distribution of muscarinic acetylcholine receptor subtypes (M1–M5) in the central nervous system (CNS) and in the rest of the body leads to a great variety of peripheral and CNS adverse effects with DACEs. Peripheral effects include constipation, dry mouth, dry eyes, tachycardia, and urinary retention. CNS effects include agitation, confusion, delirium, falls, hallucinations, and cognitive dysfunction.

The neurotransmitter acetylcholine (Ach) is critical for communication between neurons and muscle at the neuromuscular junction for modulating posture and movement, direct neurotransmission in autonomic ganglia, and pathways in the brain that are involved in memory and cognitive function. In the nucleus basalis, identified basal forebrain cholinergic neurons innervate the cerebral cortex, amygdaloid complex, or hippocampus and are necessary for learning and memory formation. It has been observed that the use of an anticholinergic drug administered to healthy volunteers resulted in impairment of memory function, similar to that seen in Alzheimer's disease.

Recent evidence has also demonstrated that DACEs may impair cognitive performance as well as physical function in older adults. For instance, normal age-related decline in memory could increase with DACEs. In addition, comorbid conditions in older adults, like Parkinson's disease and type 2 diabetes, can also predispose to a decline in cognition and amplify the effects of DACEs on cognitive function.

The cumulative exposure to multiple medicines with anticholinergic properties is known as **anticholinergic burden**. A systematic review and meta-analysis done by Ruxton et al. found that higher anticholinergic burden in older people is associated with greater risk of morbidity and mortality, longer hospital length of stay (LOS), institutionalization, and functional and cognitive decline [33].

Cognitive impairment, falls, and a decline in the ability to ambulate are associated with a reduction in performing daily activities, high care needs, social isolation, increased hospitalizations, long-term institutionalization, and death in older adults.

Traditional methods for assessing exposure to DACEs were previously based on a dichotomous yes/no approach or the total number of DACEs taken by the patient. However, other characteristics such as the daily dose, binding affinity to the muscarinic receptor(s), the permeability of the blood-brain barrier, and serum and tissue concentrations all influence the risk of anticholinergic effects. These characteristics, and the identification of an increasing number of DACEs, have led to the development of several DACE scoring systems. Currently, there are nine tools to measure anticholinergic burden. The most used scales are the Anticholinergic Risk Scale (ARS), the Anticholinergic Cognitive Burden (ACB) Scale, the Anticholinergic Drug Scale (ADS), and the anticholinergic component of the drug burden index (DBIAC). These scales may provide a more useful way to examine the association between the overall exposure to DACEs and adverse outcomes than looking at individual medications or classes of medications separately.

Salahudeen et al. found that there were substantial differences in the estimation of anticholinergic burden exposure between the scales so there is not one standardized scale to measure anticholinergic burden [34]. However, this situation provides an opportunity for updating and refining such instruments.

9.7 Polypharmacy and Geriatric Syndromes: Frailty and Cognitive Impairment

Frailty is a geriatric syndrome characterized by age-related decreases in physiologic reserves, resulting in vulnerability to health declines following even minor stressor events [35]. It is often associated with multiple chronic medical conditions and polypharmacy and is linked with multiple adverse outcomes including functional decline, hospitalization, nursing home admission, and death.

While frailty and polypharmacy often coexist and have been studied extensively and individually, little is known about their relationship which is likely complex and bidirectional. Systematic reviews have demonstrated a significant association between an increased number of medications and frailty [36, 37]. It can be hypothesized that drug therapies are being prescribed to manage the chronic medical conditions that accompany frailty and that drug therapies are the stress events that trigger a series of declines that eventually meet the criteria for frailty. The risk of developing frailty was 40% greater among individuals with polypharmacy compared to individuals without polypharmacy; however, 75% of those with polypharmacy were prefrail or frail.

Potentially inappropriate medications have also shown a relationship with frailty. A significant correlation between the frailty index and the number of STOPP criteria was found in a study with older hospital inpatients [38]. Patients above a frailty index score threshold were more likely to experience a STOPP criterion and to develop an ADR. A longitudinal study including community-dwelling older adults showed that patients with frailty had increased odds of both taking a PIM and getting PIM prescriptions in the future, according to Beers Criteria [39]. Frail patients could also be more exposed to underprescribing, according to the START criteria [40]. On the other hand, it has been suggested that the presence of PIMs increases the risk of becoming frail in a 3-year follow-up period [41].

Although estimates of frailty prevalence vary substantially by the definition chosen, it is clear that frailty is common among older adults, with approximately 15% and 45% of US community-dwelling older adults meeting the definitions of frail and prefrail, respectively [42]. As such, developing strategies to delay or prevent the onset of frailty have the potential to improve health outcomes for older adults internationally. Proposed interventions to reduce the burden of frailty on individuals and society include exercise, nutrition, and pharmacologic interventions. This is very important because polypharmacy is a potentially modifiable risk factor for mortality among older adults. Reducing polypharmacy has been suggested as a recommended measure for both the prevention and management of frailty.

It seems clear that frailty is an important issue that must be taken into account for decision-making in drug prescribing to older patients, and that polypharmacy should be assessed with special caution in frail older adults. Incorporating frailty assessment into primary care is increasingly encouraged to identify individuals at greater risk of mortality, hospitalization, and susceptibility to adverse health outcomes.

Polypharmacy is also common among older adults with dementia. Around 70% of people with dementia live with comorbidity and are prescribed multiple medications, and 64% are prescribed at least one PIM [43]. These patients may be exposed to central nervous system-acting medications, including antipsychotics, antidepressants, benzodiazepines (BZDs), and medications with anticholinergic effects in order to treat comorbidities and manage behavioral and psychological symptoms. However, these medications are associated with adverse cardiovascular side effects, hypotension, falls, delirium, detrimental effects on cognition, and mortality. People with dementia may be more susceptible to adverse effects of central nervous system-acting medications due to age-related and disease-related pharmacokinetic and pharmacodynamic changes, including alterations in the blood-brain barrier permeability associated with Alzheimer's disease.

9.8 Medications and Therapeutic Goals

The development of some diseases leads to an advanced and chronic status with limited life expectancy and a need for palliative care, including patients with advanced oncological or hematological disease, patients with advanced organic disease, and patients with advanced dementia. For all these patients and situations, therapeutic objectives must be in line with their life goals. For chronic patients with good baseline health and a long life expectancy, the use of preventive strategies is important. For complex chronic patients, where life expectancy is more limited, preserving functionality may be a priority objective. Meanwhile, for patients with advanced disease in a situation of limited life prognosis, symptomatic management should be a priority. A differentiation between preventive, etiological, or symptomatic objectives can help in the decision-making.

Holmes et al. proposed a model for appropriate prescribing for patients late in life [44]. The model finds four steps in the medication decision-making: remaining life expectancy, time until benefit, goals of care, and treatment targets. This model is visually represented in a pyramid, showing the appropriate medications at any level. At the top are represented patients with limited life expectancy, whose drugs should have a short time until benefit, goals of care are palliative, and treatment targets should be focused on symptom management. Moving toward the bottom, the patient's life expectancy is longer, time until benefit may be longer, goals of care are more aggressive, and treatment targets also include preventive strategies. The bottom of the pyramid therefore contains all medications that are otherwise appropriate according to evidence-based existing criteria for patients 65 years and older.

In the last period of life, polypharmacy is accentuated, and it also has specific features. A recent study carried out in Sweden with more than half a million people over 65 years analyzed the drug consumption during the last year of life of the participants [45].

The results showed that drug consumption increased progressively until death and that people who had taken at least 10 drugs increased from 30.3 to 47.2% during this period. Furthermore, they pointed out that this high pharmacological load in the last month of life was not only attributable to symptomatic treatments but also to medicines with a clear long-term preventive objective. As an example, in that last month of life, more than 50% of the participants consumed antithrombotics, more than 40% beta-blockers, more than 20% ACE inhibitors, and more than 15% statins. These data suggest the use of treatments with little potential benefit, or even inappropriate treatments (considering the clinical and functional situation of the patient, their life expectancy, and therapeutic goals). In these circumstances, the balance between harm and the real benefit is certainly unstable and often unpredictable.

9.9 Management of Polypharmacy in the Elderly

Selecting the right medication and the right dose for an older patient is difficult because so little evidence is available to guide choices. Decision-making often has to be drawn on information obtained from clinical trials of patients that are very different from those that we see in our clinical practice. Therefore, the findings of clinical trials for conditions commonly affecting older people cannot directly be extrapolated to that age group, as older patients, particularly frail patients and those with multiple chronic illnesses, have often been excluded from participation in such studies. This poses the challenge to the adoption of clinical practice guidelines developed to improve the quality of healthcare for many chronic conditions.

Appropriateness of prescribing can be assessed by process or outcome measures that are **explicit** (criterion-based) or **implicit** (judgment-based) [46]. Explicit methods are usually developed from expert opinions through literature reviews and consensus techniques. Evidence-based information about drug treatments in older people is frequently absent, so expert opinion is often needed in geriatric medicine. These measures are usually drug- or disease-oriented, need little or no clinical judgment to be applied, and can be applied on large prescribing databases when valid clinical details are registered.

However, explicit criteria don't take into account individual factors like comorbidities, life expectancy, or patients' preferences. Moreover, consensus approaches have little evidence of validity and reliability.

The American Geriatrics Society (AGS) **Beers** Criteria for Potentially Inappropriate Medication (PIM) Use in Older Adults [47] and **STOPP** (Screening Tool of Older Persons' Prescriptions) and **START** (Screening Tool to Alert to Right Treatment) [48] are the most widely used explicit list of PIM for assessing medication appropriateness.

Beers Criteria have been developed by the American Geriatrics Society (AGS) to assist clinicians with identifying and avoiding potentially inappropriate medications for older adults. These criteria were last updated in 2019 and are intended for use in adults 65 years and older in all ambulatory, acute, and institutionalized settings of care, except for the hospice and palliative care settings. Consumers, researchers, pharmacy benefit managers, regulators, and policymakers also widely use them. The intention of the AGS Beers Criteria is to improve medication selection, educate clinicians and patients, reduce adverse drug events, and serve as a tool for evaluating the quality of care, cost, and patterns of drug use of older adults.

The STOPP and START are the European criteria that facilitate medication review in multimorbid older people in most clinical settings. They were last updated in 2015. These criteria are designed to detect common and/or important potentially inappropriate medications (PIMs – STOPP criteria) and potential prescribing omissions (PPOs – START criteria). Several clinical trials show that the use of STOPP/START criteria significantly improves medication appropriateness, reduces medication cost, reduces falls, and diminishes ADEs.

Explicit tools have also been developed for more specific older population groups. The STOPP-Frail, developed in 2017, comprises 27 criteria relating to medications that are potentially inappropriate in frail older patients with limited life expectancy and may assist physicians in deprescribing medications in these patients [49]. It has been recently updated to make the tool more practical, patient-centered, and complete [50].

In implicit approaches, a clinician uses information from the patient and drug published evidence to make judgments about appropriateness. The focus is usually on the patient rather than on drugs or diseases. So it is more sensitive and can account for patients' preferences. However, this model is time-consuming, depends on the user's knowledge and attitudes, and can have low reliability [46]. The Medication Appropriateness Index (MAI) is one of the most widespread implicit tools [51]. It is a measure of prescribing appropriateness that assesses ten elements of prescribing: indication, effectiveness, dose, correct directions, practical directions, drug-drug interactions, drug-disease interactions, duplication, duration, and cost. Clinical judgment is needed, but the index has operational definitions and explicit instructions to standardize the rating process. The ratings generate a weighted score that can be used as a summary measure of prescribing appropriateness.

MEDICATION APPROPRIATENESS INDEX	
1.	Is there an indication for the drug?
2.	Is the medication effective for the condition?
3.	Is the dosage correct?
4.	Are the directions correct?
5.	Are the directions practical?
6.	Are there clinically significant drug-drug interactions?
7.	Are there clinically significant drug-disease/condition interactions?
8.	Is there unnecessary duplication with other drug(s)?
9.	Is the duration of therapy acceptable?
10.	Is this drug the least expensive alternative compared with others of equal utility?

Fig. 9.2 Medication Appropriateness Index (MAI)

There is no ideal measure, but the strengths and weaknesses of both approaches should be considered (Fig. 9.2).

Prescribing medicines taking into account all the particularities of geriatric patients is a complex task, but the consequences of polypharmacy and the frequency of inappropriate medication make it increasingly necessary to accompany it with deprescription.

Deprescribing can be referred to as a process of withdrawing inappropriate medications, supervised by a healthcare professional with the goal of managing polypharmacy and improving patient outcomes [52].

While there is growing evidence to support the deprescribing process, withdrawing medications is often found to be difficult by health professionals. An algorithm to guide the deprescribing process to reduce inappropriate polypharmacy in clinical practice has been proposed by the Australian Deprescribing Network, which includes five steps [53]: (1) ascertain all drugs the patient is currently taking and the reasons for each one, (2) consider the overall risk of drug-induced harm in individual patients in determining the required intensity of deprescribing intervention, (3) assess each drug in regard to its current or future benefit potential compared with current or future harm or burden potential, (4) prioritize drugs for discontinuation that have the lowest benefit-harm ratio and lowest likelihood of adverse withdrawal reactions or disease rebound syndromes, and (5) implement a discontinuation regimen and monitor patients closely for improvement in outcomes or onset of adverse effects. The Canadian Deprescribing Network is focusing efforts on developing deprescribing guidelines for specific medications (▶ https://www.deprescribingnetwork.ca/).

Many different interventions for deprescribing have been proposed. A structured, multidisciplinary approach including medication reconciliation, medication review conducted by a pharmacist, or use of assessment tools to detect medications known to increase the risk of adverse events may improve medication appropriateness. Moreover, an integrated approach taking into account patient perspectives may result in more successful deprescribing interventions. The importance of shared decision-making and patient preferences in guiding the deprescribing process has been highlighted, although implementation in the clinical practice may be challenging [54]. Computerized decision support tools consistently reduced the number of potentially inappropriate prescriptions started and the mean number of potentially inappropriate prescriptions per patient, and also increased potentially inappropriate prescription discontinuation and drug appropriateness [55] (► http://www.medbase.fi/en/professionals/renbase; ► http://www.medbase.fi/en/professionals/inxbase; ► https://www.ema.europa.eu/ema; ► http://www.medbase.fi/en/professionals/riskbase; ► https://deprescribing.org/). More randomized controlled trials assessing the impact of computerized decision support tools are needed to evaluate the use of medication targets defined by explicit criteria, adverse drug reactions, quality of life measurements, patient satisfaction, or professional satisfaction with a reasonable follow-up, which could clarify the clinical usefulness of these tools.

The outcomes of deprescribing are inconsistent and vary by setting and on the intervention being evaluated. Evidence on interventions to address polypharmacy summarized in six systematic reviews, mostly focused on older adults, shows that, despite the low quality of evidence in the underlying primary studies, they improved medication appropriateness [56]. However, there was no consistent evidence of any impact on downstream patient-centered outcomes such as healthcare utilization, morbidity, or mortality. A more recent meta-analysis shows that medication deprescribing interventions may provide reductions in mortality and the use of potentially inappropriate medications in community-dwelling older adults [57].

There is emerging evidence regarding deprescribing strategies targeting specific populations and medication classes in older adults. For example, a systematic review assessing outcomes of deprescribing interventions in older patients with life-limiting illness and limited life expectancy found that these interventions can improve medication appropriateness and have the potential for enhancement of several clinical outcomes and cost savings, but the evidence needs to be better established [58]. A Cochrane systematic review concluded that there is no evidence of an effect of discontinuing compared with continuing antihypertensives used for hypertension or primary prevention of cardiovascular disease in older adults on all-cause mortality and myocardial infarction. Limitations such as small studies and low event rates prevent from having firm conclusions about the effect of deprescribing antihypertensives on these outcomes [52].

Different barriers and facilitators of deprescribing have been found [59]. Cultural and organizational barriers include a culture of diagnosing and prescribing, evidence-based guidance focused on single diseases, a lack of evidence-based guidelines for the care of older people with multimorbidities, and a lack of shared communication, decision-making systems, tools, and resources. Interpersonal and individual-level barriers include professional etiquette, fragmented care, prescribers' and patients' uncertainties, and gaps in tailored support. Facilitators include prudent prescribing, greater availability and acceptability of nonpharmacological alternatives, resources, improved communication, collaboration, knowledge, and understanding, patient-centered care, and shared decision-making.

Hospitalization is an especially key event for the elderly and is associated with higher morbidity and mortality and cognitive and functional impairment. The incorporation of new prescribers and the increase in the number of drugs during hospitalization contribute to the risk of iatrogenesis and the complexity of administering drugs. In contrast, hospitalization enables strict follow- up, access to different specialists, and specific resources, so it could be an appropriate setting for the deprescribing process. It has been found that the therapeutic appropriateness of elderly hospitalized patients can be improved by interventions with various approaches (medication reviews, computerized decision support tools, and detection of explicit criteria of the inappropriate prescription), implemented by various healthcare professionals (clinical pharmacists, geriatricians, multidisciplinary teams, etc.). The best results in improving important health outcomes, such as readmissions or emergency room visits, have been shown in multifaceted multidisciplinary interventions [60, 61].

Medicine optimization strategies in geriatric populations should be multidimensional and interdisciplinary to meet the needs of older adults with chronic diseases and complexity. The medication history, the clinical interview by the pharmacist, and a comprehensive geriatric assessment (CGA) have been proven as the building blocks of deprescribing strategies in hospitalized older adults.

Attention must be paid to the problems of medication reconciliation derived from the transitions of care, like hospital admission and discharge, or nursing home admission, and the presence of different prescribers. Medication reconciliation is the process of obtaining and documenting a complete and accurate list of current patient medications and comparing this list with medication orders at each point of care transition to identify and rectify any discrepancies before patient harm occurs, and should be implemented in transitions of care, especially in patients with polypharmacy [62]. Patients and responsible physicians, nurses, and pharmacists should be involved in the medication reconciliation process. This reconciliation is done in order to avoid medication errors such as omissions, duplications, dosing errors, or drug interactions. Changes in medication like different doses, discontinued therapies, additional therapies, etc. are common during transitions between hospital and nursing homes and home and are a frequent source of medication errors and confusion. ADEs attributed to medication changes occurred in 20% of patients on transfer from hospital to a nursing home, happening most commonly for patients on readmission to the nursing home. Due to the very low-quality evidence, it is not clear if medication reconciliation alone may have a measurable impact on medication discrepancies or clinical outcomes [63].

9.9.1 Practical Approach to Prescribing Medications to Older Adults

Older people often receive care from multiple providers, and they may fill prescriptions at several pharmacies. That's why patients should be instructed to bring in all current medications (both prescription and nonprescription medications) to each visit, for thorough medication reconciliation and to check for potential drug-drug interactions. In order to do a proper review, the physician should ask the patient to bring to the visit all the bottles of pills that they are using. For example, many patients do not consider vitamins, ophthalmic preparations, or herbal medicines to be drug therapies, but they may have ADEs or drug interactions as a result.

It is important to promote communication and integration between the different professionals (hospital and primary care) who care for the patient. Creating an appropriate relationship between the healthcare professional and the patient facilitates the development of a therapeutic plan. Periodic evaluation of the drug regimen that a patient is taking is an essential component of the medical care of older adults in order to do changes. These changes may include discontinuation of a therapy prescribed for an indication that no longer exists, the substitution of a required therapy with a potentially safer agent, reduction in dosage of a drug that the patient still needs to take, or an increase in dose or even addition of a new medication.

Physicians are often reluctant to stop medications, especially if they did not initiate the treatment and the patient seems to be tolerating the therapy. However, drugs with limited or no therapeutic benefit can expose the patient to the risks for an adverse event, so that stopping potentially unnecessary therapy is a must.

The value of an individual drug therapy needs to be considered in the context of and individual's life course. Consideration also needs to be given to the lag time to benefit as well as the recipient's expected life expectancy when determining if a drug is beneficial.

Physicians should limit prescribing a new drug therapy to situations in which benefits clearly outweigh risks and always after safer alternatives have been attempted. In this regard, nonpharmacological approaches have to be considered. An illustrative example is the use of nonpharmacological approaches to managing behavioral symptoms such as wandering and agitation in older adults with dementia. These symptoms frequently result in prescriptions for psychotropic medications such as antipsychotic drugs, but these drugs are on average only modestly effective and can provoke serious adverse effects. Nonpharmacological strategies could be recommended as first-line treatments also with the implementation of exercise and nutrition programs to manage cardiovascular risk factors, diabetes, hypertension, etc. Some interventions consist of encouraging caregivers to describe to the clinician the presenting behavior in detail, then the provider investigates possible underlying causes of the behavior problem like medication side effects, pain, sleeplessness, etc. and works with the caregiver to treat them (changing medications, controlling the pain, treating insomnia, music therapy, exercising, giving the patients busy tasks to do, etc.). After nonpharmacological measures have been tried, consideration may be given to the use of pharmacologic interventions, taking into account potential risks associated with them. For example, selective serotonin reuptake inhibitors (SSRIs) can reduce anxiety and agitation but may increase the risk of falls, gait disorders, and hyponatremia.

Many ADEs are dose-related, so it is important to reduce the dose as much as possible. A classic example is the association between the use of long elimination half-life hypnotic-anxiolytics, antipsychotics, and tricyclic antidepressants and the development of hip fracture as a result of increasing falls. Another example involves the intensity of diabetes treatment. A very tight glycemic control has little evidence of benefit but it has been consistently found that it produces higher rates of hypoglycemia which leads to increased risk of falls, cognitive impairment, and confusion.

Clinicians should also beware of the "prescribing cascade" in order to avoid an additional medication therapy instead of prompting a medication review and discontinuation of the offending drug.

The interventions to be implemented must be individualized taking into account the specific circumstances and characteristics of each patient. It is important to balance guidelines for chronic disease management with the individual patient's goals of care, as well as risk factors for adverse drug events such as cognitive impairment, frailty, and renal impairment.

> **Clinical Protocol**
>
> Medication reconciliation systems and processes have successfully reduced medication errors in many healthcare organizations. The **practical steps to optimize drug regimens** for older patients are:
> 1. Review current drug therapy: develop a list of current medications.
> 2. Discontinue unnecessary therapy.
> 3. Consider ADEs as a potential cause for any new symptom.
> 4. Consider nonpharmacologic approaches.
> 5. Substitute with safer alternatives.
> 6. Reduce the dose.

Conclusions

Polypharmacy is a potentially modifiable risk factor for mortality and other adverse outcomes among older adults as hospitalization, disability, nursing home admissions, ADEs, ED visits, and poor quality of life.

There is a need to implement medication optimization strategies in very old and complex patients in order to avoid polypharmacy and its consequences. Reducing polypharmacy and improving therapeutic appropriateness could therefore help minimize the problem.

Enhancing the inclusion of frail older people in drug trials would help in decision-making because data could be extrapolated to standard clinical practice. Moreover, further research is required to explore the role of a reduction in polypharmacy in the development, reversion, or delay of frailty and the possible benefits of screening frailty in older people to lead interventions on excessive polypharmacy.

We must also advance in the optimization of medications in elderly people living in nursing homes through specific strategies, given the particularities of this population.

Take-Home Messages

- Prescribing for older adults is an important challenge because they take more medications than younger people and their particular conditions (frailty, cognitive impairment, falls, malnutrition, etc.) present an increased risk of drug interactions and ADEs.
- Many complex factors are likely to be involved in making the best prescribing decisions for an individual patient, and it is essential that the risks are balanced against the benefits of each medication. Important stress exists between avoiding inappropriate medications and the underuse of potentially beneficial drugs.
- Prescribing cascades are common and important to consider in older adults with multiple chronic diseases who are likely to be prescribed multiple drug therapies.
- Anticholinergic drugs lead to many ADEs. We can do an estimation of anticholinergic burden exposure, using scales.
- The relationship between polypharmacy and frailty is complex and bidirectional. Reducing polypharmacy has been suggested for both prevention and management of frailty.

- People with dementia may be more susceptible to polypharmacy. Polypharmacy should be assessed with special caution in older adults with cognitive impairment.
- AGS Beers Criteria, STOPP/START criteria, and STOPP-Frail criteria have been developed by experts internationally to assess the quality of medication use in older adults that can be applied in clinical practice.
- Practical steps can be taken to optimize prescribing for older adults that include reviewing current drug therapies, discontinuing potentially unnecessary drug therapies when no longer indicated, reducing the dose, and considering nonpharmacologic treatment approaches.
- Hospitalization can provide an opportunity to review and optimize a patient's medication regimen in order to reduce ED visits and readmissions by preventing drug interactions and adverse effects. Engaging providers and teams or expert consultation can facilitate medication rationalization and deprescribing for an individual old patient. A multidisciplinary team can improve the care of elderly patients.

References

1. Masnoon N, Shakib S, Kalisch-Ellett L, Caughey GE. What is polypharmacy? A systematic review of definitions. BMC Geriatr. 2017; https://doi.org/10.1186/s12877-017-0621-2.
2. Hajjar ER, Cafiero AC, Hanlon JT. Polypharmacy in elderly patients. Am J Geriatr Pharmacother. 2007;5:345–51.
3. Rochon PA, Gurwitz JH. The prescribing cascade revisited. Lancet. 2017;389:1778–80.
4. Gallagher P, Barry P, O'Mahony D. Inappropriate prescribing in the elderly. J Clin Pharm Ther. 2007;32:113–21.
5. Rochon PA, Gurwitz JH. Optimising drug treatment for elderly people: the prescribing cascade. Br Med J. 1997;315:1096–9.
6. Morin L, Johnell K, Laroche ML, Fastbom J, Wastesson JW. The epidemiology of polypharmacy in older adults: register-based prospective cohort study. Clin Epidemiol. 2018;10:289–98.
7. Kantor ED, Rehm CD, Haas JS, Chan AT, Giovannucci EL. Trends in prescription drug use among adults in the United States from 1999-2012. JAMA - J Am Med Assoc. 2015;314:1818–31.
8. Blozik E, Rapold R, Von Overbeck J, Reich O. Polypharmacy and potentially inappropriate medication in the adult, community-dwelling population in Switzerland. Drugs Aging. 2013;30:561–8.
9. Midão L, Giardini A, Menditto E, Kardas P, Costa E. Polypharmacy prevalence among older adults based on the survey of health, ageing and retirement in Europe. Arch Gerontol Geriatr. 2018;78:213–20.
10. Ellenbogen MI, Wang P, Overton HN, Fahim C, Park A, Bruhn WE, Carnahan JL, Linsky AM, Balogun SA, Makary MA. Frequency and predictors of polypharmacy in US Medicare patients: a cross-sectional analysis at the patient and physician levels. Drugs Aging. 2020;37:57–65.
11. Wastesson JW, Morin L, Laroche ML, Johnell K. How chronic is polypharmacy in old age? A longitudinal Nationwide cohort study. J Am Geriatr Soc. 2019;67:455–62.
12. Gallagher P, Lang PO, Cherubini A, et al. Prevalence of potentially inappropriate prescribing in an acutely ill population of older patients admitted to six European hospitals. Eur J Clin Pharmacol. 2011;67:1175–88.
13. Jokanovic N, Tan ECK, Dooley MJ, Kirkpatrick CM, Bell JS. Prevalence and factors associated with polypharmacy in Long-term care facilities: a systematic review. J Am Med Dir Assoc. 2015;16:535.e1–12.
14. Rolland Y, Abellan Van Kan G, Hermabessiere S, Gerard S, Guyonnet-Gillette S, Vellas B. Descriptive study of nursing home residents from the REHPA network. J Nutr Heal Aging. 2009;13:679–83.

15. Gutiérrez-Valencia M, Izquierdo M, Lacalle-Fabo E, Marín-Epelde I, Ramón-Espinoza MF, Domene-Domene T, Casas-Herrero Á, Galbete A, Martínez-Velilla N. Relationship between frailty, polypharmacy, and underprescription in older adults living in nursing homes. Eur J Clin Pharmacol. 2018;74:961–70.
16. Tosato M, Landi F, Martone AM, Cherubini A, Corsonello A, Volpato S, Bernabei R, Onder G. Potentially inappropriate drug use among hospitalised older adults: results from the CRIME study. Age Ageing. 2014;43:767–73.
17. Rashrash M, Schommer JC, Brown LM. Prevalence and predictors of herbal medicine use among adults in the United States. J Patient Exp. 2017;4:108–13.
18. Fu AZ, Jiang JZ, Reeves JH, Fincham JE, Liu GG, Perri M. Potentially inappropriate medication use and healthcare expenditures in the US community-dwelling elderly. Med Care. 2007;45:472–6.
19. Corsonello A, Pedone C, Incalzi R. Age-related pharmacokinetic and Pharmacodynamic changes and related risk of adverse drug reactions. Curr Med Chem. 2010;17:571–84.
20. Hulka BS, Kupper LL, Cassel JC, Efird RL, Burdette JA. Medication use and misuse: physician-patient discrepancies. J Chronic Dis. 1975;28:7–21.
21. Maher RL, Hanlon J, Hajjar ER. Clinical consequences of polypharmacy in elderly. Expert Opin Drug Saf. 2014;13:57–65.
22. Cabré M, Elias L, Garcia M, Palomera E, Serra-Prat M. Avoidable hospitalizations due to adverse drug reactions in an acute geriatric unit. Analysis of 3,292 patients. Med Clin (Barc). 2018;150:209–14.
23. Hill-Taylor B, Sketris I, Hayden J, Byrne S, O'Sullivan D, Christie R. Application of the STOPP/START criteria: a systematic review of the prevalence of potentially inappropriate prescribing in older adults, and evidence of clinical, humanistic and economic impact. J Clin Pharm Ther. 2013;38:360–72.
24. Pérez T, Moriarty F, Wallace E, McDowell R, Redmond P, Fahey T. Prevalence of potentially inappropriate prescribing in older people in primary care and its association with hospital admission: longitudinal study. BMJ. 2018; https://doi.org/10.1136/bmj.k4524.
25. Hamilton H, Gallagher P, Ryan C, Byrne S, O'Mahony D. Potentially inappropriate medications defined by STOPP criteria and the risk of adverse drug events in older hospitalized patients. Arch Intern Med. 2011;171:1013–9.
26. Leelakanok N, Holcombe AL, Lund BC, Gu X, Schweizer ML. Association between polypharmacy and death: a systematic review and meta-analysis. J Am Pharm Assoc. 2017;57:729–38.e10.
27. Campins L, Serra-Prat M, Palomera E, Bolibar I, Martínez MÀ, Gallo P. Reduction of pharmaceutical expenditure by a drug appropriateness intervention in polymedicated elderly subjects in Catalonia (Spain). Gac Sanit. 2019;33:106–11.
28. Medication Safety in Polypharmacy. Geneva: World Health Organization; 2019 (WHO/UHC/SDS/2019.11). Licence: CC BY-NC-SA 3.0 IG.
29. Hovstadius B, Petersson G. Factors leading to excessive polypharmacy. Clin Geriatr Med. 2012;28:159–72.
30. Herr M, Sirven N, Grondin H, Pichetti S, Sermet C. Frailty, polypharmacy, and potentially inappropriate medications in old people: findings in a representative sample of the French population. Eur J Clin Pharmacol. 2017;73:1165–72.
31. Moulis F, Moulis G, Balardy L, et al. Exposure to atropinic drugs and frailty status. J Am Med Dir Assoc. 2015;16:253–7.
32. Jamsen KM, Bell JS, Hilmer SN, et al. Effects of changes in number of medications and drug burden index exposure on transitions between frailty states and death: the Concord health and ageing in men project cohort study. J Am Geriatr Soc. 2016;64:89–95.
33. Ruxton K, Woodman RJ, Mangoni AA. Drugs with anticholinergic effects and cognitive impairment, falls and all-cause mortality in older adults: a systematic review and meta-analysis. Br J Clin Pharmacol. 2015;80:209–20.
34. Salahudeen MS, Hilmer SN, Nishtala PS. Comparison of anticholinergic risk scales and associations with adverse health outcomes in older people. J Am Geriatr Soc. 2015;63:85–90.
35. Clegg A, Young J, Iliffe S, Rikkert MO, Rockwood K. Frailty in elderly people. In: Lancet. Lancet Publishing Group; 2013. p. 752–62.
36. Gutiérrez-Valencia M, Izquierdo M, Cesari M, Casas-Herrero IM, Martínez-Velilla N. The relationship between frailty and polypharmacy in older people: a systematic review. Br J Clin Pharmacol. 2018;84:1432–44.

37. Palmer K, Villani ER, Vetrano DL, et al. Association of polypharmacy and hyperpolypharmacy with frailty states: a systematic review and meta-analysis. Eur Geriatr Med. 2019;10:9–36.
38. Cullinan S, O'Mahony D, O'Sullivan D, Byrne S. Use of a frailty index to identify potentially inappropriate prescribing and adverse drug reaction risks in older patients. Age Ageing. 2016;45:115–20.
39. Muhlack DC, Hoppe LK, Stock C, Haefeli WE, Brenner H, Schöttker B. The associations of geriatric syndromes and other patient characteristics with the current and future use of potentially inappropriate medications in a large cohort study. Eur J Clin Pharmacol. 2018;74:1633–44.
40. Meid AD, Quinzler R, Freigofas J, Saum KU, Schöttker B, Holleczek B, Heider D, König HH, Brenner H, Haefeli WE. Medication underuse in aging outpatients with cardiovascular disease: prevalence, determinants, and outcomes in a prospective cohort study. PLoS One. 2015; https://doi.org/10.1371/journal.pone.0136339.
41. Martinot P, Landré B, Zins M, Goldberg M, Ankri J, Herr M. Association between potentially inappropriate medications and frailty in the early old age: a longitudinal study in the GAZEL cohort. J Am Med Dir Assoc. 2018;19:967–73.e3.
42. Bandeen-Roche K, Seplaki CL, Huang J, Buta B, Kalyani RR, Varadhan R, Xue QL, Walston JD, Kasper JD. Frailty in older adults: a nationally representative profile in the United States. Journals Gerontol - Ser A Biol Sci Med Sci. 2015;70:1427–34.
43. Porter B, Arthur A, Savva GM. How do potentially inappropriate medications and polypharmacy affect mortality in frail and non-frail cognitively impaired older adults? A cohort study. BMJ Open. 2019; https://doi.org/10.1136/bmjopen-2018-026171.
44. Holmes HM, Hayley DC, Alexander GC, Sachs GA. Reconsidering medication appropriateness for patients late in life. Arch Intern Med. 2006;166:605–9.
45. Morin L, Vetrano DL, Rizzuto D, Calderón-Larrañaga A, Fastbom J, Johnell K. Choosing wisely? Measuring the burden of medications in older adults near the end of life: Nationwide, longitudinal cohort study. Am J Med. 2017;130:927–36.e9.
46. Spinewine A, Schmader KE, Barber N, Hughes C, Lapane KL, Swine C, Hanlon JT. Appropriate prescribing in elderly people: how well can it be measured and optimised? Lancet. 2007;370:173–84.
47. Fick DM, Semla TP, Steinman M, et al. American Geriatrics Society 2019 updated AGS beers criteria® for potentially inappropriate medication use in older adults. J Am Geriatr Soc. 2019;67:674–94.
48. O'Mahony D, O'Sullivan D, Byrne S, O'Connor MN, Ryan C, Gallagher P. STOPP/START criteria for potentially inappropriate prescribing in older people: version 2. Age Ageing. 2015;44:213–8.
49. Lavan AH, Gallagher P, Parsons C, O'Mahony D. STOPPFrail (screening tool of older persons prescriptions in frail adults with limited life expectancy): consensus validation. Age Ageing. 2017;46:600–7.
50. Curtin D, Gallagher P, O'Mahony D. Deprescribing in older people approaching end-of-life: development and validation of STOPPFrail version 2. Age Ageing. 2020; https://doi.org/10.1093/ageing/afaa159.
51. Hanlon JT, Schmader KE, Samsa GP, Weinberger M, Uttech KM, Lewis IK, Cohen HJ, Feussner JR. A method for assessing drug therapy appropriateness. J Clin Epidemiol. 1992;45:1045–51.
52. Reeve E, Gnjidic D, Long J, Hilmer S. A systematic review of the emerging definition of "deprescribing" with network analysis: implications for future research and clinical practice. Br J Clin Pharmacol. 2015;80:1254–68.
53. Scott IA, Hilmer SN, Reeve E, et al. Reducing inappropriate polypharmacy: the process of deprescribing. JAMA Intern Med. 2015;175:827–34.
54. Jansen J, Naganathan V, Carter SM, et al. Too much medicine in older people? Deprescribing through shared decision making. BMJ. 2016; https://doi.org/10.1136/bmj.i2893.
55. Monteiro L, Maricoto T, Solha I, Ribeiro-Vaz I, Martins C, Monteiro-Soares M. Reducing potentially inappropriate prescriptions for older patients using computerized decision support tools: systematic review. J Med Internet Res. 2019; https://doi.org/10.2196/15385.
56. Anderson LJ, Schnipper JL, Nuckols TK, Shane R, Sarkisian C, Le MM, Pevnick JM, Hughes CM, Jackevicius CA, O'Mahony D. A systematic overview of systematic reviews evaluating interventions addressing polypharmacy. Am J Heal Pharm. 2019;76:1777–87.
57. Bloomfield HE, Greer N, Linsky AM, Bolduc J, Naidl T, Vardeny O, MacDonald R, McKenzie L, Wilt TJ. Deprescribing for community-dwelling older adults: a systematic review and meta-analysis. J Gen Intern Med. 2020; https://doi.org/10.1007/s11606-020-06089-2.

58. Shrestha S, Poudel A, Steadman K, Nissen L. Outcomes of deprescribing interventions in older patients with life-limiting illness and limited life expectancy: a systematic review. Br J Clin Pharmacol. 2020;86:1931–45.
59. Doherty AJ, Boland P, Reed J, Clegg AJ, Stephani AM, Williams NH, Shaw B, Hedgecoe L, Hill R, Walker L. Barriers and facilitators to deprescribing in primary care: a systematic review. BJGP Open. 2020; https://doi.org/10.3399/bjgpopen20X101096.
60. Van Der Linden L, Hias J, Dreessen L, Milisen K, Flamaing J, Spriet I, Tournoy J. Medication review versus usual care to improve drug therapies in older inpatients not admitted to geriatric wards: a quasi-experimental study (RASP-IGCT). BMC Geriatr. 2018; https://doi.org/10.1186/s12877-018-0843-y.
61. Gillespie U, Alassaad A, Henrohn D, Garmo H, Hammarlund-Udenaes M, Toss H, Kettis-Lindblad Å, Melhus H, Mörlin C. A comprehensive pharmacist intervention to reduce morbidity in patients 80 years or older: a randomized controlled trial. Arch Intern Med. 2009;169:894–900.
62. Lehnbom EC, Stewart MJ, Manias E, Westbrook JI. Impact of medication reconciliation and review on clinical outcomes. Ann Pharmacother. 2014;48:1298–312.
63. Anderson LJ, Schnipper JL, Nuckols TK, et al. Effect of medication reconciliation interventions on outcomes: a systematic overview of systematic reviews. Am J Heal Pharm. 2019;76:2028–40.

Sarcopenia: An Overview

Laura Orlandini, Tiziano Nestola, and Matteo Cesari

Contents

> **Learning Objectives**
>
> Sarcopenia is a highly prevalent condition in older patients across clinical settings. Even if its role is traditionally overshadowed, muscle health is central for the global homeostasis of the individual, especially in critically ill patients. After the reading of this chapter, the reader should be able to:
> - Define and classify sarcopenia, including the novel concept of acute sarcopenia.
> - Differentiate and see the overlappings of sarcopenia with related constructs like cachexia and frailty.
> - Identify the available clinical tools for the screening and assessment of muscle mass, strength, and function.
> - Familiarize with the strategies and recommendations for the management of sarcopenia.

Practical Implications

Sarcopenia is multifactorial in its etiology and heterogeneous in its diagnosis. Despite its heterogeneity, the clinician must be familiar with the condition and ready to detect it. In fact, sarcopenia has a significant impact in prognostic terms across clinical settings. As detailed in the chapter:
- Sarcopenia is associated with adverse outcomes both at the individual (i.e., reduced quality of life, increased risk of disability and mortality) and healthcare system (i.e., prolonged hospitalization, institutionalization, and increased healthcare costs) level.
- Multiple tools are available for clinicians to assess muscle health during the routine practice.
- Tailored interventions to increase muscle strength and function should follow the identification of sarcopenia to promote healthy aging.

10.1 Introduction

The skeletal muscle mass and strength tend to decrease after the age of 40. To define the pathological reduction and promote the necessary clinical visibility of it, the term sarcopenia was coined. Sarcopenia is today considered one of the major geriatric syndromes. Its origin is multifactorial, including unhealthy lifestyle and diseases. It is strongly related to the concept of frailty.

A growing body of the literature today differentiates sarcopenia from cachexia, a highly prevalent condition in patients with wasting diseases (e.g., cancer, chronic respiratory failure). Both sarcopenia and cachexia are predictive of adverse outcomes [1]. In particular, cachexia is associated with increased chemotherapy toxicity, postoperative complications, and mortality [2]; it occurs independently of the cancer stage [3].

Interestingly, it has been recently proposed to consider a novel form of muscle decline, known as acute sarcopenia. It refers to that kind of sarcopenia occurring as a consequence of acute illnesses since the very first days of immobility due to the acuteness. It represents a risk factor for the development of chronic sarcopenia and implies similar negative effects over the long term.

10.2 **Sarcopenia**

In 1988, Dr. Irwin Rosenberg noted that "no decline with age is as dramatic as or potentially more significant than the decline in lean body mass." To describe the phenomenon, he coined the term "sarcopenia," from the two Greek words *"sarx"* (for flesh) and *"penia"* (for loss) [4]. Rosenberg intended to draw the attention of the scientific community to the process of muscle decline that accompanies aging as a critical factor in the development of many disabling (and potentially reversible) conditions of older persons.

Over the subsequent years, researchers have been trying to provide an operational definition of sarcopenia suitable for the translation of the theoretical construct of sarcopenia in the clinical setting. In the initial works, sarcopenia was primarily defined on the basis of the low muscle mass alone. Consistently with what was previously done in the field of osteoporosis, Baumgartner and colleagues [5] defined sarcopenia as an appendicular skeletal muscle mass lower than two standard deviations below the mean observed in a reference group of young individuals.

Further evidence, however, exposed the limits of a definition of sarcopenia solely determined by the quantification of muscle mass. Low muscle mass alone, in fact, is not or only partially associated with adverse outcomes such as mortality and disability [6, 7]. On the contrary, muscle strength and physical performance (i.e., the overt expressions of the muscle quality) represent strong predictors of negative health-related events [8, 9], thus better serving for providing the needed clinical relevance to the construct of sarcopenia. In other words, a bidimensional sarcopenia considering both the muscle quality (expressed by muscle strength/performance) and quantity (i.e., muscle mass) was felt to better mirror the health status of the individual. Such evolution of the sarcopenia condition was supported in several consensus articles published by different panels of international experts in the field [10–13]. Among these, the document produced by the European Working Group on Sarcopenia in Older People (EWGSOP) [10] received a particularly large diffusion. According to this model, sarcopenia was defined by (1) the presence of low appendicular lean mass (assessed by dual-energy X-ray absorptiometry [DXA]) combined with (2) muscle weakness (measured with a handheld dynamometer and expressed by poor handgrip strength) and/or impaired mobility (measured as slow gait speed).

The major weakness of the EWSGOP algorithm was indicated in being the result of consensus/arbitrary decision and not sufficiently data driven. Furthermore, many argued about the similar weight given to the two dimensions in the definition of sarcopenia.

To overcome these limitations, the Foundation for the National Institutes of Health-Sarcopenia Project (FNIH) [11] published in 2014 a series of articles on the topic. The FNIH investigators conducted ad hoc statistical analyses on multiple cohorts to obtain clear thresholds for the key sarcopenia components. Moreover, the choice of the instruments that could best capture each sarcopenia dimension was not based on the experts' consensus, but left to the statistical models. As a result, sex-specific cut-points for both muscle weakness and low appendicular mass were generated for the variables that were best predicting muscle-related adverse outcomes.

The recognition of a specific ICD-10 code for sarcopenia in 2016 has represented another significant step towards the recognition of sarcopenia as a clinically relevant condition [12]. In fact, it has legitimated its presence in the clinical field, raised awareness about the importance of physical function in older persons, and opened the venue to more research targeting the muscle decline.

More recently, the EWGSOP document was updated (i.e., EWGSOP2) [13], given the large body of new evidence produced in the last years. In the EWGSOP2 definition, a new algorithm is proposed. Screening tools (as the SARC-F) are proposed to initiate the process. Sarcopenia is now considered as *probable* as soon as muscle weakness (assessed through handgrip strength or poor results at the chair stand test) is detected. The diagnosis is then confirmed by the presence of low muscle quantity (measured via a DXA scan). *Poor physical performance* is finally used to measure the severity of the sarcopenia condition (using the gait speed, short physical performance battery [SPPB], Timed Up-and-Go test [TUG], and/or the 400-meter walk test). The rationale behind the evolution of the algorithm is that assessing muscle strength is more feasible and clinically relevant than assessing the muscle quantity. This may raise awareness among clinicians and better answer to the unmet clinical need raised by patients.

Important innovations on the sarcopenia classification can also be found in the EWGSOP2 document. Sarcopenia is here classified as "primary," or age-related, and "secondary," when single or multiple causes other than or in addition to aging can be identified. Systemic diseases (i.e., cancer or organ failure), physical inactivity, and inadequate energy intake (i.e., anorexia, malabsorption, limited ability to eat, limited access to healthy foods) are possible causal factors for secondary sarcopenia. More importantly, sarcopenia is more clearly framed as a muscle disease (rather than a syndrome as before) that can acutely and/or progressively occur. Sarcopenia is acute when it relates to an acute illness or injury, and its duration is inferior to 6 months. On the other hand, it is chronic when it is associated with chronic or progressive conditions and lasts more than 6 months.

Differences in definitions and cut-points of sarcopenia are exemplified in
◘ Table 10.1.

10.3   Assessment of Muscle Mass, Strength, and Performance

A wide variety of tests and tools are available for the assessment of sarcopenia. However, first of all, the patient's characteristics (i.e., mobility, clinical conditions), the access and availability of healthcare resources (i.e., community versus hospital setting), and the purpose of the testing (i.e., screening versus diagnosis) should guide the clinician in the selection of the best instruments to use in the diagnostic process [14, 15].

■ Screening Tests

The SARC-F questionnaire is a five-item test that asks the patient about perceived limitation in strength, walking ability, rising from a chair, stair climbing, and recent experience with falls [16]. It is a validated, inexpensive, and convenient method for identifying patients at risk for sarcopenia in clinical practice. However, given its moderate sensitivity and high specificity for low muscle strength, it is particularly suitable for detecting the most severe cases of sarcopenia [17].

Table 10.1 Proposed operational definitions and cut-points for sarcopenia. Modified from Beaudart and colleagues (*Archives of Public Health* 2014)

Criteria	Muscle mass	Muscle function	
		Muscle strength	Physical performance
Baumgartner et al.	ASM/height^2 >2 SD below young healthy mean	No	No
European working group on Sarcopenia in older people (EWGSOP)	ALM/height^2 Men ≤7.23 kg/m^2 Women ≤5.67 kg/m^2	Yes/no[a] Grip strength Men <30 kg Women <20 kg	Yes/no[a] Gait speed <0.8 m/s
Foundation of NIH Sarcopenia project (FNIH)	ALM$_{BMI}$ Men <0.789 Women <0.512	Grip strength Men <30 kg Women <20 kg	Gait speed <0.8 m/s
European working group on Sarcopenia in older people (EWGSOP2)	ASM Men <20 kg Women <15 kgOr ALM/height [2] Men ≤7 kg/m^2 Women ≤5.5 kg/m^2	Grip strength Men <27 kg Women <16 kgOr Chair stand test >15 sec	Yes/no[b] Gait speed ≤0.8 m/s *Or* SPPB ≤8 *Or* TUG ≥20 sec *Or* 400 m walk test ≥6 minutes/ non-completion

ASM appendicular skeletal muscle mass; ASM/height^2 ratio of appendicular skeletal muscle mass over height squared; ALM/height^2 ratio between appendicular lean mass and squared height; ALM$_{BMI}$ ratio between appendicular lean mass and body mass index; SPPB short physical performance battery; TUG Timed Up-and-Go test; SD standard deviation
[a]The authors suggest using muscle strength and/or muscle performance to confirm sarcopenia
[b]The authors suggest the use of physical performance to assess the degree of severity of sarcopenia

Members of the European Society for Clinical and Economic Aspects of Osteoporosis and Osteoarthritis (ESCEO) working group recently recommended the application of the so-called "red flag" method [15]. "Red flags" are clinical presentations that can be easily and quickly assessed during a standard medical consultation that are closely associated with the high likelihood of sarcopenia. The proposed signs/symptoms/conditions stem from the assessment of physical function (i.e., general weakness, loss of muscle mass and/or strength, fatigue, weight loss, falls), nutrition status, and lifestyle. The presence of one or more "red flags" should immediately alert the clinician about the risk of sarcopenia and prompt to further evaluation.

◼ Muscle Quantity

The DXA is a well-established and safe technique that provides reproducible muscle mass measurements (in particular, total body lean tissue mass and appendicular skeletal muscle mass) [18]. It is acknowledged that the accuracy of DXA results varies across age groups, and some conditions may alter its findings. Moreover, some body composition parameters of growing interest in the field (i.e., intramuscular fat) are not measurable with DXA. However, bearing these limitations in mind, given its convenience and availability in clinical settings, the DXA remains, to date, the favored method for assessing muscle mass in sarcopenia [13].

Despite potentially representing the gold standard for muscle mass measurement [15], the cost, lack of portability, need of qualified personnel, and the absence of specific defining cut-points limit the use of magnetic resonance imaging (MRI) and computerized tomography (CT) to the research setting in sarcopenia.

The bioelectrical impedance analysis (BIA) provides an indirect measurement of muscle mass. For its affordability and portability, the BIA measurements may be easier to access than DXA. However, among the limitation of the procedure, it is important to consider that validated, population-specific reference cut-points for the raw measurement are lacking [19, 20].

Although operational definitions of sarcopenia generally agree on the use of DXA or BIA, many heterogeneous methodologies have been proposed or under study to assess body composition and skeletal muscle. Among these, the ultrasound is probably the one with the broadest diffusion. Ultrasound has shown good reliability in estimating muscle mass in older subjects compared to DXA, MRI, and CT scan [21]. The technique has the clear advantage of assessing muscle quantity (i.e., pennate muscle thickness and cross-sectional area) and muscle quality (i.e., echogenicity). Initially used in the research setting, the wide ultrasound availability and bed-side utilization have raised the interest in its potential for detecting sarcopenia in routine clinical practice [22].

Finally, the urinary excretion of creatine provides a direct measure of the organism's muscle mass.

The administration per os of deuterium-marked creatine and its subsequent assessment in a urine sample are today attracting a growing interest.

For a more detailed description of the pros and cons associated with available methodologies for muscle quantity determinations, refer to ◘ Table 10.2.

■ Muscle Strength

Being simple, inexpensive, and highly predictive of poor outcomes [23], the handgrip strength is frequently used for measuring muscle strength in clinical settings [15, 24]. The standardized assessment of the handgrip strength via a calibrated dynamometer is guaranteed by specific protocols demonstrating the correct way for measuring it [25] and the availability of population-specific thresholds of risk [26]. In the EWGSOP2 document [13], the chair stand test is indicated as an alternative measure of strength. The test, providing a proxy of lower extremity muscle strength, is designed to time how long is needed for a patient to rise five times from a seated position as quickly as possible [8, 27].

■ Physical Performance

In terms of reliability and ability to predict adverse outcomes [26, 28], gait speed is perhaps the most recommended instrument to measure the individual's physical performance. Gait speed can be measured alone or as part of a test battery, in particular the short physical performance battery (SPPB). Despite being highly predictive of negative outcomes [29], the time needed to assess the SPPB (approximately 10 minutes) makes it less suitable for clinical practice and of more interest for the research

▣ Table 10.2 Characteristics of the most frequently used methods for the assessment of skeletal muscle

Method	Strengths	Limitations
MRI	High resolution Assessment of muscle quality Quantification of lean and fat mass	Expensive equipment and need of qualified personnel Time-consuming Space requirements Cross-sectional results specific of a body district
CT	Assessment of muscle quality quantification of lean and fat mass	Expensive equipment and need of qualified personnel Time-consuming Exposure to radiations Space requirements Cross-sectional results specific of a body district
DXA	Quantification of lean and fat mass Commonly available and frequently used in the clinical setting Relatively inexpensive exam No special training Whole-body and specific body district quantification of body composition components	No muscle quality assessment Space requirements Low-dose radiations No difference between water and bone-free lean tissue Expensive equipment
BIA	Relatively cheap and portable device Inexpensive exam	No muscle quality assessment Low accuracy
Anthropometry	Easy and inexpensive to assess	Minimal accuracy
Ultrasound	Unexpensive Qualitative assessment of (specific) muscle structure	Relatively high costs for the equipment and need of qualified personnel Evaluation of a specific body district Operator-dependent Limited evidence coming from this technique
Creatine dilution method	Accurate estimate of whole-body muscle mass	Use limited to the research setting Limited number of studies adopting the technique No possibility of exploring specific body districts Need of a lab (with qualified personnel) and time-consuming

MRI magnetic resonance imaging; CT computerized tomography; DXA dual-energy X-ray absorptiometry; BIA bioelectrical impedance analysis

Modified from Pahor and colleagues (*The Journal of Nutrition, Health and Ageing*, 2009) [81]

setting. In the EWGSOP2 document [13], the Timed Up-and-Go test (TUG) and the 400-meter walk test are also listed as valid alternatives for capturing the physical performance. In the TUG [30], the individual is asked to rise from a chair, walk for 3 meters along a track, turn, walk back, and sit down again. Instead, the 400-meter walk test represents a valid indicator for defining mobility disability. The 400-meter distance is considered as a surrogate of the distance a person should be able to cover in daily life for remaining mobility independent. For this test, the person is asked to complete 20 laps of a 20-meter long track at the usual pace.

10.4 The Etiology of Sarcopenia

Sarcopenia and cachexia (i.e., a wasting disorder that causes extreme weight loss and muscle wasting and can include loss of body fat; see also below) have a multifactorial etiology that only apparently overlaps. Lifestyle, diseases, malnutrition, and age-related biological conditions (e.g., *inflamm-aging*, mitochondrial changes, reduction of neuro-muscular junctions and muscular regenerative potential, endocrinal disorders, vascular dysfunction) are crucial for the onset and development of sarcopenia [31]. Instead, the major determinant of cachexia is represented by the late stage of a serious/terminal disease (e.g., cancer, chronic obstructive pulmonary disease, congestive heart failure) and related conditions (e.g., chemotherapy toxicity, postoperative complications). Both sarcopenia and cachexia are predictive of negative health-related outcomes.

Sarcopenia is associated with falls, disability, institutionalization, and mortality [32]. After the age of 35–40 years, the muscle mass declines at a rate of 1–2% per year and strength of 1.5%, increasing to 3% per year after the age of 60 [33]. Alongside the loss of muscle mass and strength, fat increases 0.45 kg per year after the age of 30 [34], potentially masking the loss of lean mass in the extreme condition of sarcopenic obesity [32]. Regarding lifestyle factors, sedentary behavior and malnutrition are undoubtedly among the most influential determinants of sarcopenia [35]. Thus, physical activity and healthy nutrition assume a crucial role in preventing and treating muscle loss. The endocrine role in sarcopenia etiology results in decreased anabolic hormones (i.e., testosterone, estrogen, growth hormone, and insulin-like growth factor-1) [36], modifications in the renin-angiotensin system [37], and vitamin D deficiency [38]. *Inflamm-aging* acts on sarcopenia through (1) mediators such as interleukin (IL) 6 and tumor-necrosis factor α (TNF-α), (2) mitochondrial dysfunction, and (3) oxidative stress [39]. At a biological level, an imbalance between anabolic and catabolic processes leads to protein and loss of myocytes, then to loss of muscle mass (predominantly in the type II fibers), and finally to muscle function [40].

10.5 Prevalence and Outcomes of Sarcopenia

Despite the heterogeneity of available operational definitions and cut-points, sarcopenia consistently remains a highly prevalent and detrimental condition in older subjects [41]. Its prevalence tends to vary across clinical settings, with the lowest prevalence reported in the community (about 10%) [42, 43] and the highest in nursing homes (about 40%) [42, 44].

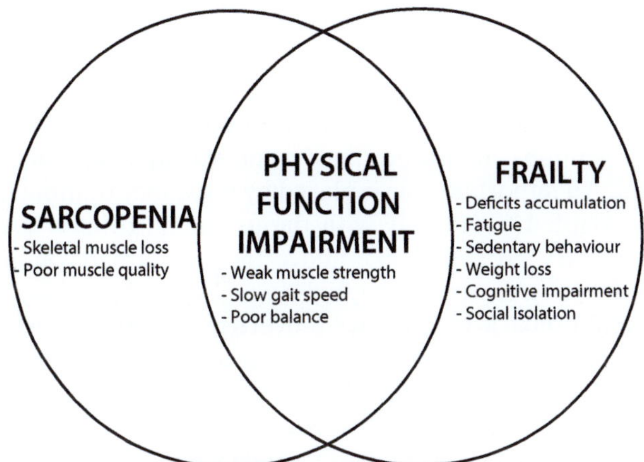

■ Fig. 10.1 The relationship among sarcopenia, physical function impairment, and frailty. Published by Cesari and colleagues (*Front Aging Neuroscience* 2014) in an open-access article, distributed under the terms of the Creative Commons Attribution License (CC BY)

Sarcopenia has a significant impact on the person and the public health. Sarcopenia increases the risk of fracture by direct (i.e., negative interaction between muscle and bone) [45, 46] and indirect (i.e., increased risk of falling) [47] effects. As mentioned, it predicts functional decline and physical disability [48], as well as short- and long-term mortality in both hospitalized [49] and nursing home patients [50]. Persons with sarcopenia have shown a reduced quality of life [51]. Furthermore, sarcopenia represents a relevant burden for the healthcare systems as it increases the risk of prolonged hospitalization [52], institutionalization [53], and increased healthcare costs [54, 55].

Under this perspective, sarcopenia does not seem to fit into the classical age-related, standalone disease profile. Taking into account the fact that (1) it has a multifactorial etiology and is associated with multiple risk factors, (2) it is closely associated with aging, and (3) its presence induces poor health outcomes, sarcopenia has long been included as one of the major geriatric syndromes [56]. Sarcopenia is also associated with other geriatric syndromes, particularly frailty (a multidimensional medical condition characterized by reduced homeostatic reserves and increased vulnerability to stressors) [57]. It has been discussed that sarcopenia and frailty may overlap, sharing that physical impairment represents the first step of the disabling cascade (■ Fig. 10.1) [58]. As soon as sarcopenia is considered as a geriatric syndrome, the clinical approach for its management requires a comprehensive assessment aimed to personalize care, as documented in the literature for every multidimensional geriatric condition [59].

10.6 The Management of Sarcopenia

Since sarcopenia has gained an ICD-10-CM code and officially recognized as a nosological condition, specific recommendations for its clinical management have been proposed by a task force of the Society on Sarcopenia, Cachexia and Wasting

Disorders. It has been solicited that physicians screen for sarcopenia using validated tools, as the SARC-F questionnaire. Subsequently, the diagnosis should be confirmed, measuring both the muscle strength (e.g., handgrip, chair stand test) and muscle mass (via DXA, CT scan, ultrasound). Once the diagnosis has been confirmed, interventions should be aimed at increasing muscle mass and, in particular, function. An important role is played by resistance training [60]. Moreover, diet should be adapted (eventually with the use of nutritional supplements) for increasing the dietary protein intake above the standard recommended dietary allowances (for 0.9 g/kg/day to 1–1.5 g/kg/day and up to 2 g/kg/day in the presence of catabolic conditions) [61, 62]. The β-hydroxy β-methylbutyrate (HMB) has shown to be beneficial in increasing muscle mass and function in frail patients with sarcopenia [63]. Positive effects have also been documented for vitamin D supplementation in deficient persons [64]. Testosterone is not currently recommended in the absence of hypogonadism as no strong evidence supports its safe use in sarcopenic persons although it surely has an anabolic action on the muscle [65]. Similarly, anti-myostatin inhibitors and molecules acting on the growth hormone axis might be promising but still lack sufficient evidence supporting their clinical use [66, 67]. Anti-cytokine/myokine treatments include antibody agents against pro-inflammatory factors (e.g., anti-TNF-α, anti-IL-1, anti-IL-6) that limit the loss of skeletal muscle mass. For example, positive findings have been reported for the anti-TNF agent infliximab in treating sarcopenia in patients with Crohn's disease [68]. Agents against IL-6 (influencing energy homeostasis and muscle substrate utilization) have demonstrated benefits in some specific forms of cachexia (e.g., siltuximab reduced anorexia and cachexia in ovarian, prostate, and lung cancer patients) [69].

10.7 Cachexia

Cachexia, derived from the Greek terms *kakos* (i.e., bad) and *hexis* (i.e., condition), is a complex multifactorial syndrome characterized by severe body weight loss (greater than 5% of body weight in 12 months or less) due to an underlying severe illness [70]. Cancer, chronic heart failure, chronic renal failure, and chronic obstructive pulmonary disease are the most frequent underlying conditions responsible for specific phenotypes of cachexia. Cases of cachexia secondary to rheumatoid arthritis and HIV are also observed.

Weight loss secondary to loss of muscle mass (associated or not with loss of fat mass) represents the primary clinical and diagnostic criterion of cachexia. Five secondary criteria have been indicated, three of which need to be present to confirm the diagnosis (❏ Table 10.3). The secondary criteria refer to decreased muscle mass (i.e., fatigue, low fat-free mass index, decreased muscle strength) and inflammation (i.e., anorexia and biochemical abnormalities) and were defined according to the main pathophysiological mechanisms involved. In 2010, the European Society for Clinical Nutrition and Metabolism (ESPEN) [71] completed the existing definition by including different stages of cachexia (❏ Table 10.4) to facilitate an earlier identification (and hopefully treatment) of the condition.

◘ Table 10.3 Proposed definitions of cachexia in adults proposed by Evans and colleagues (*Clinical Nutrition*, 2008)

Main criterion	*Essential for diagnosis*
Weight loss	At least 5% reduction of weight occurred within 12 months in the presence of underlying illness, or BMI <20 kg/m2 if weight loss cannot be documented
Secondary criteria	*At least three criteria present for diagnosis*
Decreased muscle strength	Poor handgrip strength
Fatigue	Physical and/or mental weariness resulting from exertion. Inability to continue exercise at the same intensity with consequent deterioration of performance
Anorexia	Limited food intake (i.e., total caloric intake less than 20 kcal/kg of body weight/day; less than 70% of usual food intake) or poor appetite
Low fat-free mass index	Lean tissue depletion (i.e., low mid-upper arm muscle circumference, low appendicular skeletal muscle index)
Abnormal biochemistry	Increased inflammatory status (CRP >5.0 mg/L; IL-6 > 4.0 pg/mL)

BMI body mass index; CRP C-reactive protein; IL-6: interleukin 6

◘ Table 10.4 Proposed staging of cachexia in adults

ESPEN-SIG (2010)	Precachexia	All the following criteria have to be present: Unintentional weight loss $\leq$5% of the usual body weight during the last 6 months Underlying chronic disease Chronic or recurrent systemic inflammatory response[a] Anorexia or anorexia-related symptoms
Evans et al. 2008	Mild cachexia	Unintentional weight > 5% of usual body weight loss within the previous 12 months
	Moderate cachexia	Unintentional weight loss >10% of usual body weight within the previous 12 months
	Severe cachexia	Unintentional weight loss >15% of usual body weight within the previous 12 months

[a]Cancer, chronic heart failure, chronic respiratory disease, liver failure, chronic kidney disease, rheumatoid arthritis, and HIV

Modified by Muscaritoli et al. (*Clinical Nutrition, 2010*)

10.8   The Etiology of Cachexia

Muscle mass loss is the most relevant feature of cachexia, irrespective of the causative disease. It is mainly secondary to the accelerated proteolysis of skeletal muscle cells [72]. Different proteolytic mechanisms are involved in the accelerated muscle wasting process, the ubiquitin-dependent pathway being the most important.

Systemic inflammation is the driving force behind the muscle protein breakdown in cachexia [73]. Systemic inflammation is caused by the imbalance between pro- and anti-inflammatory cytokines, produced by the acute disease, immunological abnormalities, and the growing adipose tissue [74].

Anorexia contributes to cachexia by causing reduced food intake and favoring weight loss. It is defined as the reduction (or loss) in the desire to eat [75]. The cachexia-related anorexia is different from the anorexia nervosa, because it is defined by the presence of a primary catabolic condition. Its genesis is complex and multifactorial; the underlying hypothesized mechanism resides in the inappropriate response of the hypothalamic axis to the appetite and satiety stimuli, although other factors (i.e., depression, pain, dysphagia) may play a role in its etiology as well [76].

Malnutrition (i.e., a state of nutrition in which a deficiency, imbalance, or excess of nutrients causes measurable adverse effects on body form and function and produces negative clinical outcomes) is also another major component of cachexia [77]. However, it is noteworthy that not all malnourished patients have cachexia, but all cachectic patients are malnourished.

10.9   The Overlap Between Cachexia and Sarcopenia

Comparing cachexia and sarcopenia, it becomes clear how close the two constructs are. Both conditions share a similar biological substratum in which several factors interplay (i.e., age, comorbidity, metabolic abnormalities). Moreover, as one condition may lead to the other and vice versa, sarcopenia and cachexia could be considered as part of the same continuum of muscle decline, which leads to negative health outcomes. However, in clinical practice, it may be challenging or even impossible to assess and disentangle the specific contribution of each of the two in the loss of the individual's muscle mass and function.

Differences between the two conditions can be mentioned (◘ Table 10.5). Although muscle mass loss is featured in both conditions, the process is usually rapid and acute in cachexia, whereas it is more gradual and progressive in sarcopenia. Although low-grade inflammation has been identified as a contributor for the development of sarcopenia, inflammation is more prominent in cachexia, for which it represents a core feature.

The partial overlap between cachexia and sarcopenia has important implications in terms of therapeutic strategies. Ongoing research is exploring pharmacological and non-pharmacological options that aim at reducing muscle loss in both by acting as the shared biological mechanisms.

Table 10.5 Comparison between sarcopenia and cachexia, modified from Argilès and colleagues (*Current Opinion in Pharmacology* 2015)

	Sarcopenia	Cachexia
Weight loss	Might be present	Might be present
Muscle mass	Decreased	Decreased
Fat mass	Increased	Decreased
Underlying catabolic disease	Yes/no	Yes
Inflammation (systemic)	+	+++
Anorexia	+	++
Resting energy expenditure	Decreased	Increased
Muscle protein degradation	+++	+
Impaired muscle protein synthesis	Yes	Yes/no
Insulin resistance	Yes	Yes

10.10 Management of Cachexia

Just like sarcopenia, the ultimate goal of treating cachexia remains the attenuation of losing muscle mass and function. Given the complex pathogenesis for both conditions, the approach must always consider different factors, including age, comorbidities, medications, inflammatory status, metabolism, nutritional status, and lifestyle.

Several therapies designed for sarcopenia have shown some potential also in cachexia, given the common biological background. For example, anamorelin can increase body weight and lean body mass while reducing some cachexia symptoms; unfortunately, no effect has been demonstrated on muscle strength [78]. Enobosarm has a similar impact on body composition in both sarcopenia and cachexia, but (again) no effect on muscle function [79–81]. Biological agents against inflammation targeting MABp1 have shown benefits in preventing muscle loss due to cancer, but no gain in function has emerged [82]. Recent research focuses on the potential role of anti-microRNAs (miRs) agents to counteract muscle loss [83, 84].

The absence of benefits on muscular function of biological treatments in cachexia can be explained by the fact that chronic diseases and systemic inflammation alter the direct relationship between muscle mass and muscle strength [79]. Thus, the potential benefits of the biological treatments can be fully achieved only if nutritional and metabolic interventions and physical exercise act against muscle wasting in a multimodal approach. Moreover, the severity of the underlying catabolic condition (the primary cause of cachexia) cannot be neglected.

10.11 Acute Sarcopenia

Inactivity and periods of bed rest secondary to acute illnesses and hospitalization have a dramatic impact on muscle mass and function. A study demonstrated a significant decrease in muscle protein synthesis (−0.027% per hour), muscle mass (−1.5 kg in whole-body lean mass), and strength (−19 Newton-meters per second) in a cohort of healthy older patients after 10 days of bedrest [85]. The effect of bedrest on muscle mass is particularly accentuated in older people compared to their younger counterparts [86]. The inactivity-induced loss of muscle mass is more rapid during the initial phases of immobility and predominantly affects the lower body musculature [86, 87]. Unlike cachexia, prolonged bedrest induces muscle mass loss through the inhibition of protein synthesis [88].

Endocrine deregulation and systemic inflammatory play a role in acute illnesses and lead to a rapid decline in muscle mass and function. Sepsis, for example, is associated with endocrine alterations, rise in inflammatory cytokines, and a decrease in muscle function [89]. Surgery, trauma, and burns have a similar effect on the muscles [90].

In a recent review, Welsh and colleagues [91] state that the combined effect of inactivity, systemic inflammation, and endocrine alterations witnessed during significant events (i.e., acute illnesses, surgery, trauma, burns) may precipitate the development of secondary sarcopenia [92]. This condition, defined acute sarcopenia, is defined as "a change in muscle mass and function within 28 days of a significant stressor event sufficient to meet criteria for sarcopenia using previously defined cut-off points." During the recovery process, the individual may or may not return to his/her pre-illness level of muscle function and mass. In other words, acute sarcopenia can lead to the "usual" chronic sarcopenia.

Further research is needed to establish the risk factors and the long-term outcomes associated with acute sarcopenia. Interventional studies that target acute sarcopenia are needed. The prevention and treatment of acute sarcopenia are likely to be beneficial for the individual patients (reducing the risk of developing chronic sarcopenia) and the health system (limiting the length of hospital stay and rehabilitation costs).

> **Conclusions**
>
> Sarcopenia has evolved in its meaning since its origin more than 20 years ago, encompassing not only the condition of reduction in muscular appendicular mass, but also the loss of muscular function. Multiple instruments have been developed and validated over the past years for screening and diagnosing sarcopenia. Decisional algorithms have been proposed. Sarcopenia is now dissected in different forms (primary vs. secondary; disease vs. syndrome; acute vs. chronic), implicitly demonstrating the interest in this condition because it has impacts on the person and public health systems. The growing body of literature focused on cachexia further shows how the skeletal muscle quantity and quality become more relevant in the clinical and research field.
>
> Aging and frailty are connected with all these forms of muscle loss that seem to share common pathways in their physiopathology, potentially favoring the development of therapeutic solutions. It is crucial for clinicians to familiarize with these new conditions and adapt their routines to accommodate the assessment of the patient's muscle health. This is feasible in every setting, given the broad spectrum of instruments that are today available. Overlooking the individual's muscle quality and quantity should be considered malpractice.

> **Take-Home Messages**
> - Sarcopenia is a multifactorial condition highly prevalent in older subjects, characterized by a decline in muscle mass and quality.
> - Cachexia, defined by severe body weight loss due to an underlying severe illness, only partially overlaps with sarcopenia.
> - An acute form of sarcopenia exists and has important clinical implications in critically ill old patients.
> - Tailored interventions that increase muscle strength and function can limit the negative outcomes that this condition has on the individual and on the healthcare system.
> - Screening and assessment of sarcopenia should become part of routine clinical practice.

References

1. M. Pahor M. Sarcopenia: clinical evaluation, biological markers and other evaluation tools. J Nutr Health Aging. 2009;13(8):724. https://doi.org/10.1007/s12603-009-0204-9
2. Sm K-B, Vc M. V B. computed tomography-defined muscle and fat wasting are associated with cancer clinical outcomes. Semin Cell Dev Biol. https://doi.org/10.1016/j.semcdb.2015.09.001.
3. van Vledder MG, Levolger S, Ayez N, Verhoef C, Tran TCK, IJzermans JNM. Body composition and outcome in patients undergoing resection of colorectal liver metastases. BJS Br J Surg. 2012;99(4):550–7. https://doi.org/10.1002/bjs.7823.
4. Rosenberg IH. Sarcopenia: origins and clinical relevance. J Nutr. 1997;127(5 Suppl):990S–1S. https://doi.org/10.1093/jn/127.5.990S.
5. Baumgartner RN, Koehler KM, Gallagher D, et al. Epidemiology of sarcopenia among the elderly in New Mexico. Am J Epidemiol. 1998;147(8):755–63. https://doi.org/10.1093/oxfordjournals.aje.a009520.
6. Newman AB, Kupelian V, Visser M, et al. Strength, but not muscle mass, is associated with mortality in the health, aging and body composition study cohort. J Gerontol A Biol Sci Med Sci. 2006;61(1):72–7. https://doi.org/10.1093/gerona/61.1.72.
7. Visser M, Kritchevsky SB, Goodpaster BH, et al. Leg muscle mass and composition in relation to lower extremity performance in men and women aged 70 to 79: the health, aging and body composition study. J Am Geriatr Soc. 2002;50(5):897–904. https://doi.org/10.1046/j.1532-5415.2002.50217.x.
8. Cesari M, Kritchevsky SB, Newman AB, et al. Added value of physical performance measures in predicting adverse health-related events: results from the health, aging, and body composition study. J Am Geriatr Soc. 2009;57(2):251–9. https://doi.org/10.1111/j.1532-5415.2008.02126.x.
9. Lauretani F, Russo CR, Bandinelli S, et al. Age-associated changes in skeletal muscles and their effect on mobility: an operational diagnosis of sarcopenia. J Appl Physiol. 2003;95(5):1851–60. https://doi.org/10.1152/japplphysiol.00246.2003.
10. Cruz-Jentoft AJ, Baeyens JP, Bauer JM, et al. Sarcopenia: European consensus on definition and diagnosis. Age Ageing. 2010;39(4):412–23. https://doi.org/10.1093/ageing/afq034.
11. Studenski SA, Peters KW, Alley DE, et al. The FNIH Sarcopenia project: rationale, study description, conference recommendations, and final estimates. J Gerontol A Biol Sci Med Sci. 2014;69(5):547–58. https://doi.org/10.1093/gerona/glu010.
12. Anker SD, Morley JE, von Haehling S. Welcome to the ICD-10 code for sarcopenia. J Cachexia Sarcopenia Muscle. 2016;7(5):512–4. https://doi.org/10.1002/jcsm.12147.
13. Cruz-Jentoft AJ, Bahat G, Bauer J, et al. Sarcopenia: revised European consensus on definition and diagnosis. Age Ageing. 2019;48(1):16–31. https://doi.org/10.1093/ageing/afy169.
14. Cesari M, Vellas B. Sarcopenia: a novel clinical condition or still a matter for research? J Am Med Dir Assoc. 2012;13(9):766–7. https://doi.org/10.1016/j.jamda.2012.07.020.

15. Beaudart C, McCloskey E, Bruyère O, et al. Sarcopenia in daily practice: assessment and management. BMC Geriatr. 2016;16 https://doi.org/10.1186/s12877-016-0349-4.

16. Malmstrom TK, Miller DK, Simonsick EM, Ferrucci L, Morley JE. SARC-F: a symptom score to predict persons with sarcopenia at risk for poor functional outcomes. J Cachexia Sarcopenia Muscle. 2016;7(1):28–36. https://doi.org/10.1002/jcsm.12048.

17. Bahat G, Yilmaz O, Kılıç C, Oren MM, Karan MA. Performance of SARC-F in regard to Sarcopenia definitions, muscle mass and functional measures. J Nutr Health Aging. 2018;22(8):898–903. https://doi.org/10.1007/s12603-018-1067-8.

18. Validity of fan-beam dual-energy X-ray absorptiometry for measuring fat-free mass and leg muscle mass. Health, Aging, and Body Composition Study--Dual-Energy X-ray Absorptiometry and Body Composition Working Group - PubMed. Accessed 1 Sep, 2020. https://pubmed.ncbi.nlm.nih.gov/10517786/

19. Reiss J, Iglseder B, Kreutzer M, et al. Case finding for sarcopenia in geriatric inpatients: performance of bioimpedance analysis in comparison to dual X-ray absorptiometry. BMC Geriatr. 2016;16 https://doi.org/10.1186/s12877-016-0228-z.

20. Gonzalez MC, Heymsfield SB. Bioelectrical impedance analysis for diagnosing sarcopenia and cachexia: what are we really estimating? J Cachexia Sarcopenia Muscle. 2017;8(2):187–9. https://doi.org/10.1002/jcsm.12159.

21. Nijholt W, Scafoglieri A, Jager-Wittenaar H, Hobbelen JSM, van der Schans CP. The reliability and validity of ultrasound to quantify muscles in older adults: a systematic review. J Cachexia Sarcopenia Muscle. 2017;8(5):702–12. https://doi.org/10.1002/jcsm.12210.

22. Ticinesi A, Narici MV, Lauretani F, et al. Assessing sarcopenia with vastus lateralis muscle ultrasound: an operative protocol. Aging Clin Exp Res. 2018;30(12):1437–43. https://doi.org/10.1007/s40520-018-0958-1.

23. Leong DP, Teo KK, Rangarajan S, et al. Prognostic value of grip strength: findings from the prospective urban rural epidemiology (PURE) study. Lancet Lond Engl. 2015;386(9990):266–73. https://doi.org/10.1016/S0140-6736(14)62000-6.

24. Rossi AP, Fantin F, Micciolo R, et al. Identifying sarcopenia in acute care setting patients. J Am Med Dir Assoc. 2014;15(4):303.e7–12. https://doi.org/10.1016/j.jamda.2013.11.018

25. Patrizio E, Calvani R, Marzetti E, Cesari M. Physical functional assessment in older adults. J Frailty Aging. 2021;10(2):141–9. https://doi.org/10.14283/jfa.2020.61

26. Roberts HC, Denison HJ, Martin HJ, et al. A review of the measurement of grip strength in clinical and epidemiological studies: towards a standardised approach. Age Ageing. 2011;40(4):423–9. https://doi.org/10.1093/ageing/afr051.

27. Jones CJ, Rikli RE, Beam WC. A 30-s chair-stand test as a measure of lower body strength in community-residing older adults. Res Q Exerc Sport. 1999;70(2):113–9. https://doi.org/10.1080/02701367.1999.10608028.

28. Studenski S, Perera S, Patel K, et al. Gait speed and survival in older adults. JAMA. 2011;305(1):50–8. https://doi.org/10.1001/jama.2010.1923.

29. Pavasini R, Guralnik J, Brown JC, et al. Short physical performance battery and all-cause mortality: systematic review and meta-analysis. BMC Med. 2016;14(1):215. https://doi.org/10.1186/s12916-016-0763-7.

30. Podsiadlo D, Richardson S. The timed "up & go": a test of basic functional mobility for frail elderly persons. J Am Geriatr Soc. 1991;39(2):142–8. https://doi.org/10.1111/j.1532-5415.1991.tb01616.x.

31. Sarcopenia: an undiagnosed condition in older adults. current consensus definition: prevalence, etiology, and consequences. J Am Med Dir Assoc. 2011;12(4):249–56. https://doi.org/10.1016/j.jamda.2011.01.003

32. Rolland Y, Czerwinski S, van Kan GA, et al. Sarcopenia: its assessment, etiology, pathogenesis, consequences and future perspectives. J Nutr Health Aging. 2008;12(7):433–50. https://doi.org/10.1007/BF02982704.

33. Landi F, Calvani R, Tosato M, et al. Age-related variations of muscle mass, strength, and physical performance in community-dwellers: results from the milan EXPO survey. J Am Med Dir Assoc. 2017;18(1):88.e17–24. https://doi.org/10.1016/j.jamda.2016.10.007

34. Forbes GB. Longitudinal changes in adult fat-free mass: influence of body weight. Am J Clin Nutr. 1999;70(6):1025–31. https://doi.org/10.1093/ajcn/70.6.1025.

35. Skeletal muscle loss: cachexia, sarcopenia, and inactivity | The American Journal of Clinical Nutrition | Oxford Academic. Accessed 29 Sep, 2020. https://academic-oup-com.pros.lib.unimi.it/ajcn/article/91/4/1123S/4597225

36. Sakuma K, Yamaguchi A. Sarcopenia and cachexia: the adaptations of negative regulators of skeletal muscle mass. J Cachexia Sarcopenia Muscle. 2012;3(2):77–94. https://doi.org/10.1007/s13539-011-0052-4.

37. Carter CS, Onder G, Kritchevsky SB, Pahor M. Angiotensin-converting enzyme inhibition intervention in elderly persons: effects on body composition and physical performance. J Gerontol Ser A. 2005;60(11):1437–46. https://doi.org/10.1093/gerona/60.11.1437.

38. Cesari M, Incalzi RA, Zamboni V, Pahor M. Vitamin D hormone: a multitude of actions potentially influencing the physical function decline in older persons. Geriatr Gerontol Int. 2011;11(2):133–42. https://doi.org/10.1111/j.1447-0594.2010.00668.x.

39. Marzetti E, Calvani R, Cesari M, et al. Mitochondrial dysfunction and sarcopenia of aging: from signaling pathways to clinical trials. Int J Biochem Cell Biol. 2013;45(10):2288–301. https://doi.org/10.1016/j.biocel.2013.06.024.

40. Marzetti E, Lees HA, Wohlgemuth SE, Leeuwenburgh C. Sarcopenia of aging: underlying cellular mechanisms and protection by calorie restriction. BioFactors Oxf Engl. 2009;35(1):28–35. https://doi.org/10.1002/biof.5.

41. Iannuzzi-Sucich M, Prestwood KM, Kenny AM. Prevalence of sarcopenia and predictors of skeletal muscle mass in healthy, older men and women. J Gerontol A Biol Sci Med Sci. 2002;57(12):M772–7. https://doi.org/10.1093/gerona/57.12.m772.

42. Papadopoulou SK, Tsintavis P, Potsaki G, Papandreou D. Differences in the prevalence of Sarcopenia in community-dwelling, nursing home and hospitalized individuals. A systematic review and meta-analysis. J Nutr Health Aging. 2020;24(1):83–90. https://doi.org/10.1007/s12603-019-1267-x.

43. Shafiee G, Keshtkar A, Soltani A, Ahadi Z, Larijani B, Heshmat R. Prevalence of sarcopenia in the world: a systematic review and meta- analysis of general population studies. J Diabetes Metab Disord. 2017;16 https://doi.org/10.1186/s40200-017-0302-x.

44. Shen Y, Chen J, Chen X, Hou L, Lin X, Yang M. Prevalence and associated factors of Sarcopenia in nursing home residents: a systematic review and meta-analysis. J Am Med Dir Assoc. 2019;20(1):5–13. https://doi.org/10.1016/j.jamda.2018.09.012.

45. Cianferotti L, Brandi ML. Muscle-bone interactions: basic and clinical aspects. Endocrine. 2014;45(2):165–77. https://doi.org/10.1007/s12020-013-0026-8.

46. Brotto M, Johnson ML. Endocrine crosstalk between muscle and bone. Curr Osteoporos Rep. 2014;12(2):135–41. https://doi.org/10.1007/s11914-014-0209-0.

47. Bischoff-Ferrari HA, Orav JE, Kanis JA, et al. Comparative performance of current definitions of sarcopenia against the prospective incidence of falls among community-dwelling seniors age 65 and older. Osteoporos Int J Establ Result Coop Eur Found Osteoporos Natl Osteoporos Found USA. 2015;26(12):2793–802. https://doi.org/10.1007/s00198-015-3194-y.

48. Tanimoto Y, Watanabe M, Sun W, et al. Association of sarcopenia with functional decline in community-dwelling elderly subjects in Japan. Geriatr Gerontol Int. 2013;13(4):958–63. https://doi.org/10.1111/ggi.12037.

49. Vetrano DL, Landi F, Volpato S, et al. Association of sarcopenia with short- and long-term mortality in older adults admitted to acute care wards: results from the CRIME study. J Gerontol A Biol Sci Med Sci. 2014;69(9):1154–61. https://doi.org/10.1093/gerona/glu034.

50. Landi F, Liperoti R, Fusco D, et al. Prevalence and risk factors of sarcopenia among nursing home older residents. J Gerontol A Biol Sci Med Sci. 2012;67(1):48–55. https://doi.org/10.1093/gerona/glr035.

51. Rizzoli R, Reginster J-Y, Arnal J-F, et al. Quality of life in sarcopenia and frailty. Calcif Tissue Int. 2013;93(2):101–20. https://doi.org/10.1007/s00223-013-9758-y.

52. Sousa AS, Guerra RS, Fonseca I, Pichel F, Amaral TF. Sarcopenia and length of hospital stay. Eur J Clin Nutr. 2016;70(5):595–601. https://doi.org/10.1038/ejcn.2015.207.

53. Hirani V, Blyth F, Naganathan V, et al. Sarcopenia is associated with incident disability, institutionalization, and mortality in community-dwelling older men: the Concord health and ageing in men project. J Am Med Dir Assoc. 2015;16(7):607–13. https://doi.org/10.1016/j.jamda.2015.02.006.

54. Sheetz KH, Waits SA, Terjimanian MN, et al. Cost of major surgery in the sarcopenic patient. J Am Coll Surg. 2013;217(5):813–8. https://doi.org/10.1016/j.jamcollsurg.2013.04.042.

55. Janssen I, Shepard DS, Katzmarzyk PT, Roubenoff R. The healthcare costs of sarcopenia in the United States. J Am Geriatr Soc. 2004;52(1):80–5. https://doi.org/10.1111/j.1532-5415.2004.52014.x.

56. Cruz-Jentoft AJ, Landi F, Topinková E. Michel J-P. Understanding sarcopenia as a geriatric syndrome: Curr Opin Clin Nutr Metab Care. 2010;13(1):1–7. https://doi.org/10.1097/MCO.0b013e328333c1c1.

57. Clegg A, Young J, Iliffe S, Rikkert MO, Rockwood K. Frailty in elderly people. Lancet. 2013;381(9868):752–62. https://doi.org/10.1016/S0140-6736(12)62167-9.

58. Cesari M, Landi F, Vellas B, Bernabei R, Marzetti E. Sarcopenia and physical frailty: two sides of the same coin. Front Aging Neurosci. 2014;6 https://doi.org/10.3389/fnagi.2014.00192.

59. Pitkälä KH, Laurila JV, Strandberg TE, Tilvis RS. Multicomponent geriatric intervention for elderly inpatients with delirium: a randomized, controlled trial. J Gerontol A Biol Sci Med Sci. 2006;61(2):176–81. https://doi.org/10.1093/gerona/61.2.176.

60. Vlietstra L, Hendrickx W, Waters DL. Exercise interventions in healthy older adults with sarcopenia: a systematic review and meta-analysis. Australas J Ageing. 2018;37(3):169–83. https://doi.org/10.1111/ajag.12521.

61. Bauer J, Biolo G, Cederholm T, et al. Evidence-based recommendations for optimal dietary protein intake in older people: a position paper from the PROT-AGE study group. J Am Med Dir Assoc. 2013;14(8):542–59. https://doi.org/10.1016/j.jamda.2013.05.021.

62. Bauer JM, Verlaan S, Bautmans I, et al. Effects of a vitamin D and leucine-enriched whey protein nutritional supplement on measures of Sarcopenia in older adults, the PROVIDE study: a randomized, double-blind, placebo-controlled trial. J Am Med Dir Assoc. 2015;16(9):740–7. https://doi.org/10.1016/j.jamda.2015.05.021.

63. Bear DE, Langan A, Dimidi E, et al. β-Hydroxy-β-methylbutyrate and its impact on skeletal muscle mass and physical function in clinical practice: a systematic review and meta-analysis. Am J Clin Nutr. 2019;109(4):1119–32. https://doi.org/10.1093/ajcn/nqy373.

64. Beaudart C, Buckinx F, Rabenda V, et al. The effects of vitamin D on skeletal muscle strength, muscle mass and muscle power: a systematic review and meta-analysis of randomized controlled trials. J Clin Endocrinol Metab;11.

65. Skinner JW, Otzel DM, Bowser A, et al. Muscular responses to testosterone replacement vary by administration route: a systematic review and meta-analysis. J Cachexia Sarcopenia Muscle. 2018;9(3):465–81. https://doi.org/10.1002/jcsm.12291.

66. Anker SD, Coats AJS, Morley JE. Evidence for partial pharmaceutical reversal of the cancer anorexia–cachexia syndrome: the case of anamorelin. J Cachexia Sarcopenia Muscle. 2015;6(4):275–7. https://doi.org/10.1002/jcsm.12063.

67. Kouw IWK, Groen BBL, Smeets JSJ, et al. One week of hospitalization following elective hip surgery induces substantial muscle atrophy in older patients. J Am Med Dir Assoc. 2019;20(1):35–42. https://doi.org/10.1016/j.jamda.2018.06.018.

68. Ticinesi A, Meschi T, Narici MV, Lauretani F, Maggio M. Muscle ultrasound and Sarcopenia in older individuals: a clinical perspective. J Am Med Dir Assoc. 2017;18(4):290–300. https://doi.org/10.1016/j.jamda.2016.11.013.

69. Shankaran M, Czerwieniec G, Fessler C, et al. Dilution of oral D3-Creatine to measure creatine pool size and estimate skeletal muscle mass: development of a correction algorithm. J Cachexia Sarcopenia Muscle. 2018;9(3):540–6. https://doi.org/10.1002/jcsm.12278.

70. Evans WJ, Morley JE, Argilés J, et al. Cachexia: a new definition. Clin Nutr Edinb Scotl. 2008;27(6):793–9. https://doi.org/10.1016/j.clnu.2008.06.013.

71. Muscaritoli M, Anker SD, Argilés J, et al. Consensus definition of sarcopenia, cachexia and pre-cachexia: joint document elaborated by Special Interest Groups (SIG) "cachexia-anorexia in chronic wasting diseases" and "nutrition in geriatrics". Clin Nutr Edinb Scotl. 2010;29(2):154–9. https://doi.org/10.1016/j.clnu.2009.12.004.

72. Biolo G, Cederholm T, Muscaritoli M. Muscle contractile and metabolic dysfunction is a common feature of sarcopenia of aging and chronic diseases: from sarcopenic obesity to cachexia. Clin Nutr. 2014;33(5):737–48. https://doi.org/10.1016/j.clnu.2014.03.007.

73. Deans C, Wigmore SJ. Systemic inflammation, cachexia and prognosis in patients with cancer. Curr Opin Clin Nutr Metab Care. 2005;8(3):265–9. https://doi.org/10.1097/01.mco.0000165004.93707.88.

74. Prins JB. Adipose tissue as an endocrine organ. Best Pract Res Clin Endocrinol Metab. 2002;16(4):639–51. https://doi.org/10.1053/beem.2002.0222.

75. Chapman IM, MacIntosh CG, Morley JE, Horowitz M. The anorexia of ageing. Biogerontology. 2002;3(1):67–71. https://doi.org/10.1023/A:1015211530695.

76. Cancer anorexia: clinical implications, pathogenesis, and therapeutic strategies. - Abstract - Europe PMC. Accessed 2 Sep, 2020. https://europepmc.org/article/med/14602249

77. Lochs H, Allison SP, Meier R, et al. Introductory to the ESPEN guidelines on enteral nutrition: terminology, Definitions and General Topics. Clin Nutr. 2006;25(2):180–6. https://doi.org/10.1016/j.clnu.2006.02.007.

78. Garcia JM, Boccia RV, Graham CD, et al. Anamorelin for patients with cancer cachexia: an integrated analysis of two phase 2, randomised, placebo-controlled, double-blind trials. Lancet Oncol. 2015;16(1):108–16. https://doi.org/10.1016/S1470-2045(14)71154-4.

79. Dobs AS, Boccia RV, Croot CC, et al. Effects of enobosarm on muscle wasting and physical function in patients with cancer: a double-blind, randomised controlled phase 2 trial. Lancet Oncol. 2013;14(4):335–45. https://doi.org/10.1016/S1470-2045(13)70055-X.

80. Dubois V, Simitsidellis I, Laurent MR, et al. Enobosarm (GTx-024) modulates adult skeletal muscle mass independently of the androgen receptor in the satellite cell lineage. Endocrinology. 2015;156(12):4522–33. https://doi.org/10.1210/en.2015-1479.

81. Enobosarm (GTx-024) Modulates Adult Skeletal Muscle Mass Independently of the Androgen Receptor in the Satellite Cell Lineage | Endocrinology | Oxford Academic. Accessed 29 Sep, 2020. https://academic-oup-com.pros.lib.unimi.it/endo/article/156/12/4522/2422756

82. Hong DS, Hui D, Bruera E, et al. MABp1, a first-in-class true human antibody targeting interleukin-1α in refractory cancers: an open-label, phase 1 dose-escalation and expansion study. Lancet Oncol. 2014;15(6):656–66. https://doi.org/10.1016/S1470-2045(14)70155-X.

83. McCarthy JJ. The role of microRNAs in skeletal muscle health and disease. Front Biosci. 2015;20(1):37–77. https://doi.org/10.2741/4298.

84. He WA, Calore F, Londhe P, Canella A, Guttridge DC, Croce CM. Microvesicles containing miR-NAs promote muscle cell death in cancer cachexia via TLR7. Proc Natl Acad Sci U S A. 2014;111(12):4525–9. https://doi.org/10.1073/pnas.1402714111.

85. Kortebein P, Ferrando A, Lombeida J, Wolfe R, Evans WJ. Effect of 10 days of bed rest on skeletal muscle in healthy older adults. JAMA. 2007;297(16):1772–4. https://doi.org/10.1001/jama.297.16.1772-b.

86. Ferrando AA, Tipton KD, Bamman MM, Wolfe RR. Resistance exercise maintains skeletal muscle protein synthesis during bed rest. J Appl Physiol Bethesda Md 1985. 1997;82(3):807–10. https://doi.org/10.1152/jappl.1997.82.3.807

87. LeBlanc AD, Schneider VS, Evans HJ, Pientok C, Rowe R, Spector E. Regional changes in muscle mass following 17 weeks of bed rest. J Appl Physiol Bethesda Md 1985. 1992;73(5):2172–8. https://doi.org/10.1152/jappl.1992.73.5.2172

88. Symons TB, Sheffield-Moore M, Chinkes DL, Ferrando AA, Paddon-Jones D. Artificial gravity maintains skeletal muscle protein synthesis during 21 days of simulated microgravity. J Appl Physiol. 2009;107(1):34–8. https://doi.org/10.1152/japplphysiol.91137.2008.

89. Brough W, Horne G, Blount A, Irving MH, Jeejeebhoy KN. Effects of nutrient intake, surgery, sepsis, and long term administration of steroids on muscle function. Br Med J Clin Res Ed. 1986;293(6553):983–8.

90. Finnerty CC, Mabvuure NT, Ali A, Kozar RA, Herndon DN. The surgically induced stress response. JPEN J Parenter Enteral Nutr. 2013;37(5 0):21S–9S. https://doi.org/10.1177/0148607113496117

91. Welch CK, Hassan-Smith ZA, Greig CM, Lord JA, Jackson T. Acute Sarcopenia Secondary to Hospitalisation - An Emerging Condition Affecting Older Adults. Aging Dis. 2018;9(1):151–64. https://doi.org/10.14336/AD.2017.0315

92. English KL, Paddon-Jones D. Protecting muscle mass and function in older adults during bed rest. Curr Opin Clin Nutr Metab Care. 2010;13(1):34–9. https://doi.org/10.1097/MCO.0b013e328333aa66.

Geriatric Syndromes: Frailty

R. Walford, T. Lawton, and A. Clegg

Contents

> **⌂ Learning Objectives**
>
> Having read this chapter, you will be able to:
> - Define frailty and explain its pathophysiology.
> - Understand the two reference standard models of frailty: the phenotype model and cumulative deficit model.
> - Appreciate the limitations of these two models for clinical practice and have an understanding of alternative simple instruments for assessing frailty in critically unwell older people.
> - Understand the implications of our ageing population and the epidemiology of frailty in critical care units.
> - Appreciate the clinical utility of frailty in critical care, including its role in triage decisions, predicting prognosis and identifying people for therapeutic interventions, as well as its potential future role as a therapeutic target.

11.1 Introduction

Population ageing worldwide is accelerating rapidly, with major implications for the planning and delivery of healthcare services. The ageing global demographic has been accompanied by a notable increase in the proportion of older people admitted to critical care facilities [1]. However, chronological age is not a universal predictor of inferior outcomes, and the concept of frailty more accurately identifies older people at increased risk of adverse outcomes, compared to people of the same chronological age. Frailty encapsulates the variable vulnerability to stressor events observed in older age, helping to explain why some older individuals are more resilient and are able to withstand stressors, whilst others only need a minor insult, such as a simple infection to trigger a sudden, disproportionate change in their health [2].

Globally, the prevalence of frailty in older adults is estimated to range from 7 to 26% [3], and this population with frailty is at increased risks of falls, disability and death. Older people with frailty are recognised as core users of health and social care services internationally, accounting for a considerable proportion of healthcare expenditure [4]. Over the past 20 years, there has been a considerable expansion in research to improve our understanding of the pathophysiology of frailty and its implications for healthcare services, which have historically mainly been designed to meet the needs of younger people with single long-term conditions. In this chapter, we discuss the definition, pathophysiology and epidemiology of frailty as well as present instruments to assess frailty in critically unwell older adults alongside an overall focus on the clinical importance of recognising frailty in critical care.

11.2 Frailty Definition and Pathophysiology

Frailty is a condition characterised by loss of biological reserves, failure of physiological mechanisms and increased vulnerability to a range of adverse outcomes. It develops as the result of accelerated ageing-associated decline across multiple physiological systems. This cumulative physiological decline diminishes homeostatic reserve, until stressor events trigger disproportionate and dramatic changes in health status [5]. For

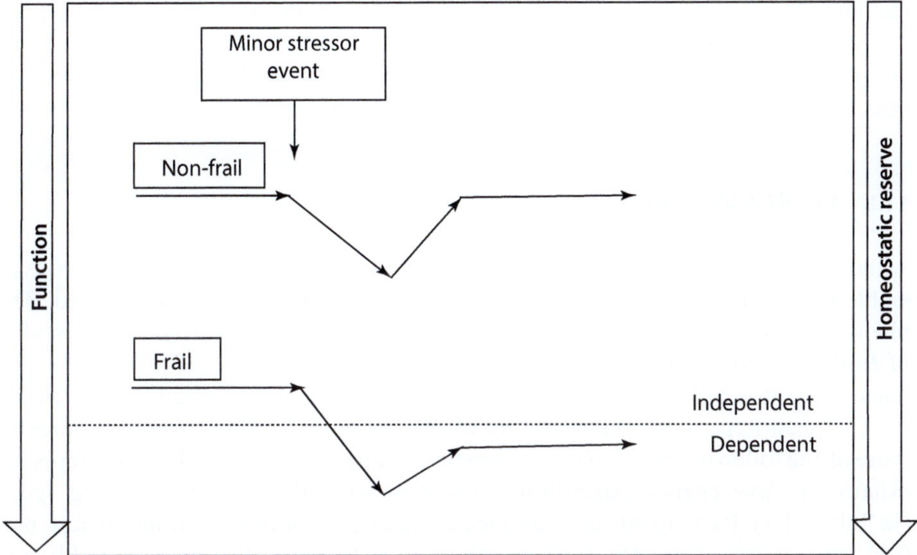

Fig. 11.1 Schematic epresentation of the typical clinical presentation of frailty [6]

example, a new medication, a 'minor' surgical procedure or an infection can translate into marked deteriorations in function and a transition from being independent to dependent, mobile to immobile and lucid to delirious (■ Fig. 11.1) [6]. The sudden, disproportionate change in health observed in frailty is typically followed by a prolonged period of recovery, frequently requiring an extended hospital stay, including a period of rehabilitation.

The brain, endocrine system, immune system and skeletal muscle are the physiological systems which have been most extensively investigated in frailty, [6] and cumulative decline in these systems has particular importance in the context of critical illness. In general, the cumulative decline across multiple systems in frailty identifies an individual whose homeostatic mechanisms are on the verge of a tipping point from which it may be impossible to recover, with an additional stressor of a critical illness leading to complete homeostatic failure and death. Considering specific organ systems, the gradual loss of skeletal muscle strength and function (sarcopenia) that is commonly observed in frailty can be particularly problematic with the addition of an acute severe illness, such as sepsis, or major surgical procedure. This is because the breakdown of muscle protein to produce amino acids for energy and antigenic peptides for the immune response to an inflammatory stimulus can further diminish already depleted skeletal muscle. When this is combined with additional muscle atrophy through immobility in hospital, the result can potentially be a major loss of independence that might not be recoverable, even with a prolonged period of rehabilitation. Furthermore, the changes to the brain that are observed with frailty can increase the risk of delirium, which is commonly encountered in the critical care setting, and an extremely unpleasant and upsetting experience for patients, families and staff.

Although the brain, endocrine system, immune system and skeletal muscle have been best studied, it is recognised that cumulative decline across other key systems including the cardiovascular, respiratory and renal systems contributes to the overall development of frailty. Indeed, research has indicated that it is the total amount of decline across multiple organ systems that drives the development of frailty, as opposed to impairment in one particular system alone [7].

11.3 Frailty Models

Although the concept of frailty has been established in geriatric medicine for considerable time, it is only more recently that frailty models have been developed. The phenotype model and the cumulative deficit model are the two international models of frailty that are best established as reference standards. Both are extensively validated and, although conceptually different, have overlap in identification of frailty.

The phenotype model identifies frailty on the basis of the presence of three or more of the following physical characteristics: unintentional weight loss, self-reported exhaustion, low energy expenditure, low grip strength and slow walking speed (■ Table 11.1). Participants are classified as frail (three or more characteristics), pre-frail (one or two characteristics) or robust (no characteristics present). Although widely recognised as a reference standard, the main limitations of the phenotype model have been that the time required for assessment of the five characteristics means that it more suited as a research tool, rather than for routine clinical practice. An additional limitation is that the components can potentially conflate acute illness with frailty.

The cumulative deficit model identifies frailty on the basis of the accumulation of a range of health deficits (clinical signs, symptoms, diseases, disabilities, impairments), on the simple principle that the more small things an individual has wrong with them, the more likely they are to have frailty. The model is flexible in terms of the number and type of deficit variables that are required – a minimum number of 30 deficit variables is required for a valid model [9]. The deficit variables can be combined to calculate a frailty index (FI) score as the total number present in an individual as an equally weighted proportion of the total possible. A higher frailty index score is typically associated with worse outcomes [10]. With a theoretical range of

■ **Table 11.1** The five phenotype model indicators of frailty and their associated measures [8]

Frailty indicator	Measure
Unintentional weight loss	Self-reported weight loss of more than 10 pounds or recorded weight loss of ≥5% per annum
Self-reported exhaustion	Self-reported exhaustion on CES-D score (3–4 days per week or most of the time)
Low energy expenditure	Energy expenditure <383 kcal/week (males) or <270 kcal/week (females)
Slow gait speed	Standardised cut-off times to walk 15 feet, stratified for sex and height
Weak grip strength	Grip strength, stratified by sex and BMI

between 0 and 1, a value of 0.70 represents a level of frailty beyond which further deficit accumulation is not sustainable [10]. Similar to the phenotype model, a key historical limitation of the cumulative deficit model is that it has been mainly suited to the research setting, although more recent research has extended the model to critical care.

11.4 Instruments for Assessing Frailty in Critically Unwell Older People

The limitations of the original phenotype and cumulative deficit models for routine assessment of critically unwell older people have led to interest in instruments that are feasible to complete in the time-pressured environment of an acute hospital but retain good reliability. Although there is a very extensive range of instruments for identifying frailty in community settings, many of these include performance-based items, such as measures of mobility (e.g. gait speed, timed-up-and-go test), which can conflate frailty with acute illness. Furthermore, frailty assessment in critically ill older people presents additional challenges, including the frequent presence of acute delirium, underlying dementia or reduced level of consciousness that can accompany critical illness. Useful instruments also need to take into account both the possibility of proxy completion and the challenges presented when there is no proxy available in the setting of an acute hospitalisation.

A 2018 systematic review of the feasibility and reliability of frailty assessment instruments in critically unwell older people identified six studies that assessed different frailty instruments in the critical care setting [11].

11.4.1 Modified Phenotype Model

A modified frailty phenotype model has been used in research studies investigating frailty in critical care. One version operationalised the five phenotype model domains for use in critical care, and a second version extended the modified domains to include cognitive impairment and sensory impairment (◘ Table 11.2) [11].

In studies that have used the modified phenotype model, limitations in terms of difficulties completing some components, even with adaptations for critical care, were reported. Although the modified frailty phenotype has been used by both research and clinical staff, the time required for completion has not been reported, which means that resource required for routine implementation is currently uncertain.

11.4.2 Cumulative Deficit Model

A 43-item proxy-reported questionnaire based on the cumulative deficit model of frailty has been developed and tested in 610 critical care patients (◘ Table 11.3) [13]. The questionnaire is completed using variables drawn from the health record, supplemented by proxy completion of variables collected from family members, based on the condition of the patient 2 weeks prior to hospital admission. Each deficit

Table 11.2   Assessment of frailty according to modified frailty phenotype model [12]

Frailty domain	Measure
Shrinking	Reported weight loss and BMI <24 or ≥5% weight loss
Weakness	Unable to rise from a chair without using arms
Slowness	Falls or need for assistance with mobility inside or outside the home in the past year
Low physical activity	Unable to climb flight of stairs or undertake moderate activity, e.g. pushing a vacuum cleaner or bowling
Exhaustion	Feeling that everything the patient does is an effort and/or the feeling that he could not get going, in past 4 weeks; number of times he/she had a lot of energy in past 4 weeks
Cognitive impairment	Memory impairment screen, or modified version of the short-form informant questionnaire on cognitive decline in the elderly
Sensory impairment	Problems in daily life because of poor vision or impaired hearing in last year

variable is coded as 0 (absent), 1 (present) or 0.5 (where intermediate values are possible).

The frailty index was a better predictor of adverse outcomes after critical care admission than age, illness severity or comorbidity. Higher baseline physical function and lower frailty index scores were robust predictors of survival and long-term physical function. In the validation study, the questionnaire was completed by trained researchers, and feasibility of use in routine clinical care requires further evaluation. A 52-item frailty index has also been operationalised for critical care, and validated in a sample of 155 patients, demonstrating good prediction of survival [14].

11.4.3   Clinical Frailty Scale

The Clinical Frailty Scale (CFS) is a method of summarising the overall level of fitness or frailty of an older individual after a clinical evaluation. The original CFS was a seven-item pictorial scale, ranging from level 1 (very fit) to level 7 (severely frail). More recently, a nine-item version has been developed, including two additional categories – very severe frailty (level 8) and terminally ill (level 9) (Fig. 11.2). The CFS has been used by a broad range of clinical and research staff, with high rates of completion in studies that evaluated reliability in critical care, reflecting its relative simplicity and ease of use. Furthermore, good inter-rater reliability has been reported for the CFS when used by different clinical staff, providing further support for its use [15]. It is gaining popularity in critical care as a frailty assessment instrument that is aligned with implementation in time-pressured clinical environments. One limitation of the CFS is that it mainly assesses function of an individual, so it may not account for the cumulative decline across multiple physiological systems that is characteristic of frailty. Despite this, the CFS correlates well with the research standard cumulative

■ Table 11.3 43 items included in a cumulative deficit frailty index developed for use in critical care, including items completed using information from the health record and proxy completion

#	Items contributed to the FI
1	Overall health of the patient?
2	Do you think the patient was depressed?
3	Do you think the patient worried a lot or got anxious?
4	Do you think the patient felt exhausted or tired all the time?
5	Did the patient have sleep problems?
6	Did the patient have problems with memory or thinking?
7	Did the patient have any problems speaking to make him–/herself understood?
8	Did the patient have difficulty hearing?
9	Did the patient have problems with eyesight (even when wearing glasses)?
10	Did the patient have problems with balance?
11	Did the patient complain of feeling dizzy or lightheaded?
12	Did the patient need assistance of a person or aid to prevent falling?
13	Did the patient hold on to furniture to keep from failing?
14	Was the patient able to walk alone?
15	Was the patient able to get out of a bed or chair alone?
16	Did the patient have problems with bowel control?
17	Did the patient have problems with bladder control?
18	Did the patient experience any unplanned weight loss in the last 6 months?
19	What was the patient's food intake in the week prior to ICU admission?
20	Was the patient able to carry out some day-to-day tasks?
21	Feed himself/herself?
22	Take a bath or shower?
23	Dress himself/herself?
24	Drive?
25	Look after his/her own medications?
26	Do day-to-day shopping?
27	Do day-to-day household cleaning?
28	Cook well enough to maintain his/her nutrition?
29	Look after his/her own banking and financial affairs?
30	Overall health of the patient?
31	Myocardial infarct

(continued)

◩ Table 11.3 (continued)

#	Items contributed to the FI
32	Congestive heart failure
33	Peripheral vascular disease
34	Cerebrovascular disease +/− hemiplegia
35	Dementia
36	Chronic pulmonary disease
37	Connective tissue disease
38	Ulcer disease
39	Any liver disease
40	Diabetes
41	Moderate or several renal diseases
42	Diabetes with end organ damage
43	Any tumour

Clinical Frailty Scale*

1   Very Fit – People who are robust, active, energetic and motivated. These people commonly exercise regularly. They are among the fittest for their age.

2   Well – People who have **no active disease symptoms** but are less fit than category 1. Often, they exercise or are very **active occasionally**, e.g. seasonally.

3   Managing Well – People whose **medical problems are well controlled**, but are **not regularly active** beyond routine walking.

4   Vulnerable – While **not dependent** on others for daily help, often **symptoms limit activities**. A common complaint is being "slowed up", and/or being tired during the day.

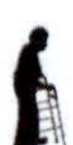

5   Mildly Frail – These people often have **more evident slowing**, and need help in **high order IADLs** (finances, transportation, heavy housework, medications). Typically, mild frailty progressively impairs shopping and walking outside alone, meal preparation and housework.

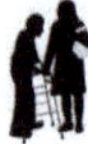

6   Moderately Frail – People need help with **all outside activities** and with **keeping house**. Inside, they often have problems with stairs and need **help with bathing** and might need minimal assistance (cuing, standby) with dressing.

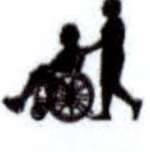

7   Severely Frail – **Completely dependent for personal care**, from whatever cause (physical or cognitive). Even so, they seem stable and not at high risk of dying (within ~ 6 months).

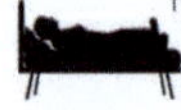

8   Very Severely Frail – Completely dependent, approaching the end of life. Typically, they could not recover even from a minor illness.

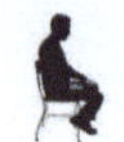

9. Terminally Ill - Approaching the end of life. This category applies to people with **a life expectancy <6 months**, who are **not otherwise evidently frail**.

Scoring frailty in people with dementia

The degree of frailty corresponds to the degree of dementia. Common **symptoms in mild dementia** include forgetting the details of a recent event, though still remembering the event itself, repeating the same question/story and social withdrawal.

In **moderate dementia**, recent memory is very impaired, even though they seemingly can remember their past life events well. They can do personal care with prompting.

In **severe dementia**, they cannot do personal care without help.

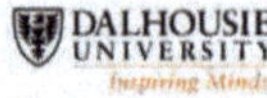

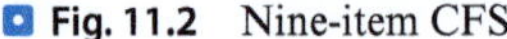

◩ Fig. 11.2   Nine-item CFS

deficit model, which includes variables that span the range of systems that are typically impaired in frailty.

11.4.4 Identifying Frailty Using Routine Electronic Health Record Data

The use of routine electronic health record data to identify frailty in critically unwell older people is an attractive option but has a range of considerations. In the UK, an electronic frailty index (eFI) has been developed using routinely available primary care electronic health record data, and implemented nationally, but is not currently available in secondary care health record systems [16] and requires validation in a critical care context. A Hospital Frailty Risk Score (HFRS) has also been developed and validated using International Classification of Diseases version 10 (ICD-10) coding, [17] but has not yet been validated in critical care or been widely implemented. A modified frailty index (mFI), constructed using 11 and 19 items, has been developed and tested using critical care registry data from 129,680 patients in Brazil, with higher scores demonstrating good prediction of in-hospital mortality and lower likelihood of returning home [18]. However, the index included fewer items than the recommended minimum of 30 variables required for a valid frailty index, and only 1 item assessing physical function was included in the shorter version, meaning that the index mainly includes comorbidities, rather than aligning with the wider multidimensional construct of frailty [19]. The use of routine electronic health record data to identify frailty in critically unwell older adults is an attractive area of ongoing work.

11.5 Epidemiology of Frailty

A notable consequence of the increased global life expectancy observed across the twentieth century is the demographic shift towards an ageing population, which has been most marked in higher-income countries [20]. By 2070, it is predicted that 18.9% of the global population will be older than 65 years and 28.7% in high-income countries [20].

Globally the prevalence of frailty amongst community-dwelling older adults (≥ 50) ranges from 7 to 26%, depending on the definition used and population examined [21]. Prevalence is associated with social and economic factors and has consistently been demonstrated to be greater in women independent of age [8, 21]. Frailty is a dynamic process whereby people transition between different frailty states over time. The most common trajectory is for individuals to progress to a worse frailty state, although frailty has been observed to improve to some degree in almost a quarter of people. However, transitioning from established frailty to a non-frail state is typically very rare [22]. Older people typically comprise up to two-thirds of the acute inpatient population, and estimates indicate that around half of these patients have frailty [23].

11.5.1 Epidemiology of Frailty in Critical Care Units

One of the consequences of population ageing is that older critically ill patients are a rapidly expanding group in critical care units. A growing older population with frailty at risk of sudden, dramatic changes in health with acute illness has major implications for the design and operational delivery of critical care, and robust information on epidemiology of frailty in critical care is required for planning services. A landmark 2017 systematic review of the prevalence of frailty in critical care facilities and its impact on outcomes of critically ill patients identified 10 studies, with a total of 3050 patients [22]. These ten studies along with additional key studies that were conducted following this review are summarised in ◘ Table 11.4. The frailty rates in patients admitted to critical care units differ considerably between studies, with rates ranging between 12 and 60%. This likely represents different eligibility criteria and frailty scores used across studies, alongside differences in service model delivery in different countries globally. A large, transnational study spanning 21 European countries investigating the impact of frailty in 5021 intensive care unit patients used a standardised assessment of frailty – the Clinical Frailty Scale – and reported notable differences in frailty prevalence [24]. Rates of frailty in older intensive care unit patients were lowest in Western Europe (35.1%) compared to Eastern Europe (55.3%), with intermediate rates in Central Europe (48.9%), Northern Europe (48.4%) and Southern Europe (38.6%). As the frailty assessment measure was standardised across settings, these differences most likely reflect how service models have been established in these geographical regions, with a greater emphasis on triage of critically unwell older patients prior to transfer to intensive care units in Western and Southern Europe.

11.6 Clinical Utility of Frailty in Critical Care

Interest in identifying frailty in critical care has grown in recent years, particularly in view of triage decisions potentially required in the COVID-19 pandemic [41]. The most common scale used clinically is the Clinical Frailty Scale, aligned with the evidence for its feasibility and reliability in critical care settings as it is considered easy to estimate with minimal training and even without the involvement of a patient's family [11]. A major concern with the use of frailty scores on ICU is that patients may be far from their baseline and this could cloud judgement. Although the CFS appears to have a high inter-rater reliability, a 2019 study reported a difference of one category or more in 47% of cases [15].

11.6.1 Prognosis

There are many scoring systems which predict outcomes in critical care, but in the main these are only recommended for use in aggregate and not for individuals [42]. Frailty as measured by CFS and frailty index predicts mortality independent of age and acute scoring systems such as APACHE II and SOFA [24, 36]. In the Muscedere et al. meta-analysis, [43] frailty was a predictor of hospital (risk ratio (RR), 1.71; 95%

⬡ Table 11.4 Major studies exploring frailty prevalence in the critically ill

Reference	Year	Country	Cohort size (N)	Age criteria (years)	Prevalence (%)	Frailty criteria
Bagshaw [25]	2014	Canada	421	$\geq$50	33	9-point CFS ($\geq$5 points)
Brummell [26]	2020	USA	567	$\geq$18	24	7-point CFS ($\geq$5 points)
Brummel [27]	2017	USA	1040	$\geq$18	30	7-point CFS ($\geq$3 points)
Darvall [28]	2019	New Zealand, Australia	15,613	$\geq$80	40	8-point CFS ($\geq$5 points)
Ferrante [29]	2016	USA	391	$\geq$70	55	FP ($\geq$3 points)
Fisher [30]	2015	Australia	205	$\geq$18	28	9-point CFS ($\geq$5 points)
Flaatten [24]	2017	21 European countries	5021	$\geq$80	43	9-point CFS ($\geq$5 points)
Geense [31]	2020	The Netherlands	1300	$\geq$18	12	9-point CFS ($\geq$5 points)
Hessey [32]	2020	Canada	11,816	$\geq$18	29	9-point CFS ($\geq$5 points)
Heyland [13, 33]	2015	Canada	610	$\geq$80	32 (CFS) 59 (FI)	7-point CFS ($\geq$5 points) 43-item FI (>0.2)
Hope [34, 35]	2015	USA	84	$\geq$18	35 (CFS) 27 (FAT-ICU)	9-point CFS ($\geq$5 points) FAT-ICU (>3 points)
Hope [12]	2017	USA	95	$\geq$18	36	9-point CFS ($\geq$5 points)
Kizilarslanoglu [36]	2017	Turkey	122	>60	21	55-item FI (>0.4)
Le Maguet [3]	2014	France	196	>65	41 (FP) 24 (CFS)	FP ($\geq$3 points) 9-point CFS ($\geq$5 points)
Lopez [37]	2019	Spain	132	$\geq$65	35	FRAIL scale ($\geq$3 points)
Montgomery [38]	2019	Canada	15,238	$\geq$18	28	9-point CFS ($\geq$5 points)

(continued)

■ Table 11.4 (continued)

Reference	Year	Country	Cohort size (N)	Age criteria (years)	Prevalence (%)	Frailty criteria
Mueller [39]	2016	USA	102	>18	38	50-item FI FI (>0.25)
Takaoka [40]	2020	Canada	66	≥18	26	9-point CFS (≥5 points)
Zampieri [18]	2018	Brazil	129,680	≥18	19	11-point modified FI (≥3 points)
Zeng [14]	2015	China	155	>65	60	52-item FI (>0.22)

CFS, clinical frailty scale; FI, frailty index; FP, frailty phenotype; FAT-ICU, frailty assessment tool for intensive care unit

confidence interval (CI), 1.43 to 2.05) and long-term (RR, 1.53; 95% CI, 1.40 to 1.68) mortality independent of age, illness severity and comorbidity. Additionally, frail patients were less likely to be discharged home (RR 0.59; 95% CI 0.49 to 0.71) and reported a reduced quality of life at 1 year.

Even as a strong prognostic factor, it is not clear that frailty can be used on its own to identify futility in critical care decision making. Survival is possible even for patients considered 'very severely frail', [24] and acceptable outcomes will vary by patient, so frailty must for now remain as one factor in a comprehensive assessment and discussion which incorporates patient wishes and acute illness severity [44].

11.6.2   Identifying People for Therapeutic Interventions

Admission to critical care is itself a therapeutic intervention, and many scoring systems are validated on patients already admitted to critical care, making it problematic to use them to guide admission [42]. It has therefore not historically been recommended that any scoring system be used to guide critical care admission, [45] though during the COVID-19 pandemic, UK guidance from the National Institute for Health and Care Excellence (NICE) suggested critical care treatment may be inappropriate for patients with a CFS score of 5 or more [41, 44]. The use of prognostic indicators in general to guide decisions to intervene with admission to critical care or an escalation of treatment, when failing to intervene, may result in death, risks becoming a self-fulfilling prophecy even when based on reliable evidence [46].

Recognising that it is not usually possible to accurately determine which patients may respond best to the initiation of critical care treatment, there is interest in 'ICU trials' where a patient is admitted to critical care but treatment is withdrawn early if they are not responsive in the first 24–48 hours [47, 48]. However, whilst medical and bioethical literature frequently combines withdrawal and withholding of life-sustaining treatment by invoking the 'Equivalence Thesis', it appears that most doctors feel on safer ground withholding rather than withdrawing treatment [49]. This may risk patients missing out on treatments who may have benefitted, or subjecting patients to the indignity and discomfort of futile treatment, and work to reduce the disparity between ethical theory and medical practice could produce real patient benefit.

Despite these ethical concerns, it is clear that both treatment withdrawal and treatment withholding are used in critical care when limiting life-sustaining treatments (LSTs) [47]. As might be expected, frailty, age and acute organ failure all predict LST limitation in older adults in critical care. However, this varies across Europe, where LST limitation appears to be more common in countries where there are greater levels of religious atheism, or higher GDP per capita, and highest in Northern Europe.

11.6.3 The Future: Frailty as a Therapeutic Target?

As we improve our understanding of frailty as a syndrome distinct from ageing, there is interest in identifying treatments which can target underlying elements [50].

Box 11.1

Inflammation	Inflammatory cytokines may perpetuate frailty, but no therapy has yet proven helpful; monoclonal antibodies can reduce inflammation but may worsen infection. Statin therapy has been studied without outcome improvement. Omega-3 fatty acid supplementation shows some promising signs but needs further study in this population
Myopathy	Early mobilisation may improve later function, but interventions on the ward or later after ICU have not been shown to be beneficial. Electrical stimulation and in-bed cycling in ICU also seem to have limited effect on critical illness myopathy. Medications targeting muscle atrophy are of interest, but not yet in human trials
Neuro-endo-crine	Frailty and prolonged ICU stay can be associated with hormone suppression, and this may potentiate muscle loss, weakness and fatigue. Therapeutics targeting the somatotrophic and gonadal axes have not been tested. Targeting the adrenal axis is more problematic because of cortisol's role as an immunosuppressant along with evidence it may increase mortality, but vitamin D supplementation may affect cortisol regulation, and trials are ongoing, though so far without improvement being demonstrated

Conclusion

Frailty is a common condition in older age that has clinical utility in guiding complex clinical decisions in the context of critical care admission and life-sustaining treatment decisions. A range of frailty instruments are available for use in critical care, with the CFS being one example of a tool that is simple to use, with evidence for predictive validity, feasibility and reliability that is gaining adoption in routine practice. Although useful as a prognostic factor, decisions about admission to critical care and life-sustaining treatments should not ordinarily be made on the basis of frailty alone, but as part of a holistic assessment of the patient and the context of the critical illness, as part of shared decision making in full partnership with patients and their families.

> **Take-Home Messages**
> - Frailty is a condition characterised by loss of biological reserve, failure of homeostatic mechanisms and resultant increased vulnerability to stressors.
> - Across Europe, the prevalence of frailty in critical care is lower in Western and Southern Europe. This likely reflects the differences in service models and emphasis on triage.
> - The two most extensively validated models of frailty are the phenotype model (based on five physical characteristics) and the cumulative deficit model (based on the accumulation of a range of health deficits spanning clinical signs, symptoms, diseases, disabilities and impairments).
> - Alternative simple instruments have been developed which are more feasible to complete in the time-pressured acute hospital environment and have fewer performance-based measures which may be confounded by acute illness. The Clinical Frailty Scale (CFS), a nine-item pictorial scale, has gained popularity given it is relatively simple to use and has shown good inter-rater reliability.
> - Frailty is a strong prognostic factor regarding hospital and long-term mortality, severity of illness and morbidity after critical care admission. Frailty serves as a valuable component to the comprehensive assessment required for critical care decision making.

References

1. Ihra GC, Lehberger J, Hochrieser H, Bauer P, Schmutz R, Metnitz B, et al. Development of demographics and outcome of very old critically ill patients admitted to intensive care units. Intensive Care Med. 2012;38(4):620–6.
2. De Biasio JC, Mittel AM, Mueller AL, Ferrante LE, Kim DH, Shaefi S. Frailty in critical care medicine: a review. Anesth Analg. 2020;130(6):1462–73.
3. Le Maguet P, Roquilly A, Lasocki S, Asehnoune K, Carise E, Saint Martin M, et al. Prevalence and impact of frailty on mortality in elderly ICU patients: a prospective, multicenter, observational study. Intensive Care Med. 2014;40(5):674–82.
4. Han L, Clegg A, Doran T, Fraser L. The impact of frailty on healthcare resource use: a longitudinal analysis using the clinical practice research datalink in England. Age Ageing. 2019;48(5):665–71.
5. Xue QL. The frailty syndrome: definition and natural history. Clin Geriatr Med. 2011;27(1):1–15.
6. Clegg A, Young J, Iliffe S, Rikkert MO, Rockwood K. Frailty in elderly people. Lancet. 2013;381(9868):752–62.
7. Fried LP, Xue QL, Cappola AR, Ferrucci L, Chaves P, Varadhan R, et al. Nonlinear multisystem physiological dysregulation associated with frailty in older women: implications for etiology and treatment. J Gerontol A Biol Sci Med Sci. 2009;64(10):1049–57.
8. Fried LP, Tangen CM, Walston J, Newman AB, Hirsch C, Gottdiener J, et al. Frailty in older adults: evidence for a phenotype. J Gerontol A Biol Sci Med Sci. 2001;56(3):M146–56.
9. Searle SD, Mitnitski A, Gahbauer EA, Gill TM, Rockwood K. A standard procedure for creating a frailty index. BMC Geriatr. 2008;8:24.
10. Rockwood K, Mitnitski A. Limits to deficit accumulation in elderly people. Mech Ageing Dev. 2006;127(5):494–6.
11. Pugh RJ, Ellison A, Pye K, Subbe CP, Thorpe CM, Lone NI, et al. Feasibility and reliability of frailty assessment in the critically ill: a systematic review. Crit Care. 2018;22(1):49.
12. Hope AA, Hsieh SJ, Petti A, Hurtado-Sbordoni M, Verghese J, Gong MN. Assessing the usefulness and validity of frailty markers in critically ill adults. Ann Am Thorac Soc. 2017;14(6):952–9.
13. Heyland DK, Garland A, Bagshaw SM, Cook D, Rockwood K, Stelfox HT, et al. Recovery after critical illness in patients aged 80 years or older: a multi-center prospective observational cohort study. Intensive Care Med. 2015;41(11):1911–20.

14. Zeng A, Song X, Dong J, Mitnitski A, Liu J, Guo Z, et al. Mortality in relation to frailty in patients admitted to a specialized geriatric intensive care unit. J Gerontol A Biol Sci Med Sci. 2015;70(12):1586–94.
15. Pugh RJ, Battle CE, Thorpe C, Lynch C, Williams JP, Campbell A, et al. Reliability of frailty assessment in the critically ill: a multicentre prospective observational study. Anaesthesia. 2019;74(6):758–64.
16. Clegg A, Bates C, Young J, Ryan R, Nichols L, Ann Teale E, et al. Development and validation of an electronic frailty index using routine primary care electronic health record data. Age Ageing. 2016;45(3):353–60.
17. Gilbert T, Neuburger J, Kraindler J, Keeble E, Smith P, Ariti C, et al. Development and validation of a hospital frailty risk score focusing on older people in acute care settings using electronic hospital records: an observational study. Lancet. 2018;391(10132):1775–82.
18. Zampieri FG, Iwashyna TJ, Viglianti EM, Taniguchi LU, Viana WN, Costa R, et al. Association of frailty with short-term outcomes, organ support and resource use in critically ill patients. Intensive Care Med. 2018;44(9):1512–20.
19. Flaatten H, Clegg A. Frailty: we need valid and reliable tools in critical care. Intensive Care Med. 2018;44(11):1973–5.
20. World Populat Prospects. 2019. United Nations Department of economic and social affairs (DESA)/population division.
21. O'Caoimh R, Sezgin D, O'Donovan MR, Molloy DW, Clegg A, Rockwood K, et al. Prevalence of frailty in 62 countries across the world: a systematic review and meta-analysis of population-level studies. Age Ageing. 2020;
22. Gill TM, Gahbauer EA, Allore HG, Han L. Transitions between frailty states among community-living older persons. Arch Intern Med. 2006;166(4):418–23.
23. Hilmer SN, Perera V, Mitchell S, Murnion BP, Dent J, Bajorek B, et al. The assessment of frailty in older people in acute care. Australas J Ageing. 2009;28(4):182–8.
24. Flaatten H, De Lange DW, Morandi A, Andersen FH, Artigas A, Bertolini G, et al. The impact of frailty on ICU and 30-day mortality and the level of care in very elderly patients (≥80 years). Intensive Care Med. 2017;43(12):1820–8.
25. Bagshaw SM, Stelfox HT, McDermid RC, Rolfson DB, Tsuyuki RT, Baig N, et al. Association between frailty and short- and long-term outcomes among critically ill patients: a multicentre prospective cohort study. CMAJ. 2014;186(2):E95–102.
26. Brummel NE, Girard TD, Pandharipande PP, Thompson JL, Jarrett RT, Raman R, et al. Prevalence and course of frailty in survivors of critical illness. Crit Care Med. 2020;48(10):1419–26.
27. Brummel NE, Bell SP, Girard TD, Pandharipande PP, Jackson JC, Morandi A, et al. Frailty and subsequent disability and mortality among patients with critical illness. Am J Respir Crit Care Med. 2017;196(1):64–72.
28. Darvall JN, Bellomo R, Paul E, Subramaniam A, Santamaria JD, Bagshaw SM, et al. Frailty in very old critically ill patients in Australia and New Zealand: a population-based cohort study. Med J Aust. 2019;211(7):318–23.
29. Ferrante LE, Pisani MA, Murphy TE, Gahbauer EA, Leo-Summers LS, Gill TM. The Association of Frailty with Post-ICU disability, nursing home admission, and mortality: a longitudinal study. Chest. 2018;153(6):1378–86.
30. Fisher C, Karalapillai DK, Bailey M, Glassford NG, Bellomo R, Jones D. Predicting intensive care and hospital outcome with the Dalhousie clinical frailty scale: a pilot assessment. Anaesth Intensive Care. 2015;43(3):361–8.
31. Geense W, Zegers M, Dieperink P, Vermeulen H, van der Hoeven J, van den Boogaard M. Changes in frailty among ICU survivors and associated factors: results of a one-year prospective cohort study using the Dutch clinical frailty scale. J Crit Care. 2020;55:184–93.
32. Hessey E, Montgomery C, Zuege DJ, Rolfson D, Stelfox HT, Fiest KM, et al. Sex-specific prevalence and outcomes of frailty in critically ill patients. J Intensive Care. 2020;8:75.
33. Heyland D, Cook D, Bagshaw SM, Garland A, Stelfox HT, Mehta S, et al. The very elderly admitted to ICU: a quality finish? Crit Care Med. 2015;43(7):1352–60.
34. Hope A, Hsieh S, Hurtado-Sbordoni M, Petti A, Gong N. Frailty assessment and hospital outcomes in critically ill patients. Am J Respir Crit Care Med. 2015:A2285.
35. Hope A, Petti A, Hurtado-Sbordoni M, Gong M. Bedside frailty assessment and hospital outcomes in critically ill patients. J Am Geriatr Soc. 2015:S180.

36. Kizilarslanoglu MC, Civelek R, Kilic MK, Sumer F, Varan HD, Kara O, et al. Is frailty a prognostic factor for critically ill elderly patients? Aging Clin Exp Res. 2017;29(2):247–55.
37. López Cuenca S, Oteiza López L, Lázaro Martín N, Irazabal Jaimes MM, Ibarz Villamayor M, Artigas A, et al. Frailty in patients over 65 years of age admitted to intensive care units (FRAIL-ICU). Med Intensiva. 2019;43(7):395–401.
38. Montgomery CL, Zuege DJ, Rolfson DB, Opgenorth D, Hudson D, Stelfox HT, et al. Implementation of population-level screening for frailty among patients admitted to adult intensive care in Alberta. Canada Can J Anaesth. 2019;66(11):1310–9.
39. Mueller N, Murthy S, Tainter CR, Lee J, Riddell K, Fintelmann FJ, et al. Can sarcopenia quantified by ultrasound of the rectus Femoris muscle predict adverse outcome of surgical intensive care unit patients as well as frailty? A prospective. Observat Cohort Study Ann Surg. 2016;264(6):1116–24.
40. Takaoka A, Heels-Andsdell D, Cook DJ, Kho M. The association between frailty and short-term outcomes in an intensive care unit rehabilitation trial: an exploratory analysis. J Frailty Aging. 2020;
41. COVID-19 rapid guideline: critical care in adults. National Institute for Health and Care Excellence. 2020. p. 14. Report No.: NG159.
42. Hyzy RC. ICU scoring and clinical decision making. Chest. 1995;107(6):1482–3.
43. Muscedere J, Waters B, Varambally A, Bagshaw SM, Boyd JG, Maslove D, et al. The impact of frailty on intensive care unit outcomes: a systematic review and meta-analysis. Intensive Care Med. 2017;43(8):1105–22.
44. Wilkinson DJC. Frailty triage: is rationing intensive medical treatment on the grounds of frailty ethical? Am J Bioeth. 2020;1-22
45. Desai N, Gross J. Scoring systems in the critically ill: uses, cautions, and future directions. BJA Educ. 2019;19(7):212–8.
46. Wilkinson D. The self-fulfilling prophecy in intensive care. Theor Med Bioeth. 2009;30(6):401–10.
47. Guidet B, Flaatten H, Boumendil A, Morandi A, Andersen FH, Artigas A, et al. Withholding or withdrawing of life-sustaining therapy in older adults (≥80 years) admitted to the intensive care unit. Intensive Care Med. 2018;44(7):1027–38.
48. Guidet B, Hodgson E, Feldman C, Paruk F, Lipman J, Koh Y, et al. The Durban world congress ethics round table conference report: II. Withholding or withdrawing of treatment in elderly patients admitted to the intensive care unit. J Crit Care. 2014;29(6):896–901.
49. Wilkinson D, Savulescu J. A costly separation between withdrawing and withholding treatment in intensive care. Bioethics. 2014;28(3):127–37.
50. Paul JA, Whittington RA, Baldwin MR. Critical illness and the frailty syndrome: mechanisms and potential therapeutic targets. Anesth Analg. 2020;130(6):1545–55.

Malnutrition

Lahaye Clement

Contents

> **Learning Objectives**
> - Understand the concept of malnutrition and metabolic disturbances at the origin of a particular nutritional risk in the elderly.
> - Discuss the interest and the limits of the nutritional assessment methods concerning the elderly in critical care.
> - Know the impact of malnutrition on morbidity and mortality in ICU.
> - Discover the particularities of nutritional support for the elderly in intensive care.

12.1 Introduction

Malnutrition is one of the most common geriatric syndromes, and patients in the intensive care unit (ICU) are particularly exposed to a degradation of their nutritional status.

Non-detection of malnutrition deprives the clinician of a central prognostic factor, which compromises the relevance of certain treatments.

Insufficient nutritional support exposes the occurrence of complications that will prolong the length of stay and reduce the functional recovery capacities and survival.

In the elderly, nutritional support is one of the cornerstones of maintaining and optimizing functional status and quality of life during and after critical care.

In this chapter, we will present the definition and risk factors of malnutrition in the elderly, the different nutritional assessment methods, the impact of malnutrition on prognosis, and finally the major aspects of nutritional support.

12.2 Definition and Risk Factors of Malnutrition in the Elderly

Malnutrition consists of a combination of reduced food intake or assimilation and varying degrees of acute or chronic inflammation, leading to altered body composition and diminished biological function [1].

Altered body composition manifests as a decrease in any marker of muscle mass (fat-free mass, muscle mass index, or body cell mass). Malnutrition is associated with adverse functional and clinical outcomes.

The prevalence of malnutrition in elderly ICU patients on admission is high but varies from 20 to 60% depending on the assessment methods used [2, 3] similar to the prevalence observed in other hospital wards [4, 5].

In an effort of consensus between the major global clinical nutrition societies, the GLIM (Global Leadership Initiative on Malnutrition) recently proposed diagnostic criteria based on the combination of a phenotypic criterion and an etiological criterion [1] (> Fig. 12.1).

Patients in critical care therefore naturally meet the etiological criterion. However, the phenotypic criterion must be sought. We will see below the physiological and pathophysiological modifications that may favour the occurrence of this phenotypic criterion.

Aging is associated with a reduction in the ability to respond to acute stress. Nutritional reserves are one of the major factors limiting the body's adaptation to an acute illness.

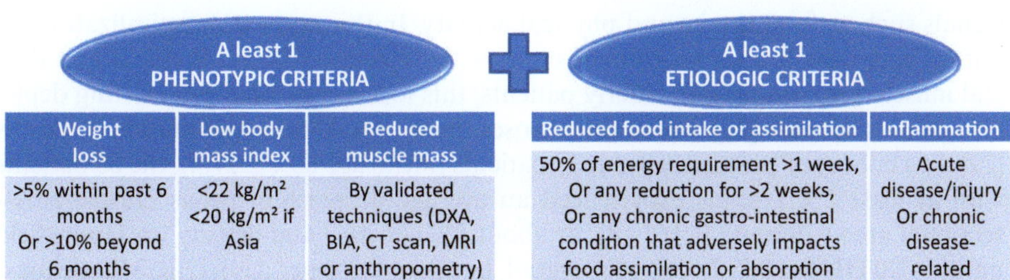

Weight loss	Low body mass index	Reduced muscle mass	Reduced food intake or assimilation	Inflammation
>5% within past 6 months Or >10% beyond 6 months	<22 kg/m² <20 kg/m² if Asia	By validated techniques (DXA, BIA, CT scan, MRI or anthropometry)	50% of energy requirement >1 week, Or any reduction for >2 weeks, Or any chronic gastro-intestinal condition that adversely impacts food assimilation or absorption	Acute disease/injury Or chronic disease-related

Fig. 12.1 Phenotypic and etiological criteria for the diagnosis of malnutrition for patients over 70 years, according to the 2018 GLIM consensus. (*DXA* dual-energy X-ray absorptiometry, *BIA* bioelectrical impedance analysis, *CT* computerized tomography, *MRI* magnetic resonance imaging)

The nutritional aspect of aging is characterized by a progressive modification of body composition linked to alterations in the control of homeostasis and metabolic adaptations (Traité de nutrition Clinique SFNCM 2016 ▶ Chap. 33).

At the macroscopic scale, fat mass increases steadily between 20 and 70 years, going from 18–25 to 35–40% in women and from 13–18% to 30–35% in men [6]. This increase mainly concerns perivisceral and intermuscular adipose tissue and this is at the expense of lean mass. Thus, muscle mass decreases by 3 to 8% per decade from age 30 and with a faster decline beyond age 60 [7], without significant change in the overall mass of other organs. The functional loss is even more marked than the loss of muscle mass and reflects a decrease in the number of type II fibres (with rapid contraction and glycolytic metabolism), a reduction in the number of active motor units, or myosteatosis [8–10].

Aging is accompanied by an alteration of the mechanisms regulating food intake [11].

Moreover, the frequency of chronic organ pathologies, chronic pain, depression, and cognitive disorders contribute to a decrease in appetite and premature satiation [12, 13]. These elements contribute to a chronic deficit in the protein-energy balance in the elderly, in particular in the case of multiple pathologies.

There are many changes at the metabolic and cellular levels. A tendency towards metabolic acidosis, especially after the age of 50, contributes to the loss of muscle and bone mass [14]. Insulin resistance promoted by the decrease in physical activity and low-grade inflammation is accompanied by a decrease in the muscular capacities to oxidize fatty acids and to use glucose [15].

These changes were associated with fat accumulation in muscle and liver tissue, and mitochondrial dysfunction [16]. Post-prandial protein anabolism is reduced, while there is a lack of catabolism inhibition, contributing to a gradual reduction in muscle mass [17]. This loss of response to anabolic stimuli has several origins such as insulin resistance [18], low-grade inflammation [19], increased splanchnic extraction [20], or vitamin D deficiency [21].

This anabolic resistance justifies a higher daily protein intake requirements for older healthy subjects, i.e. 1 to 1.2 g of protein/kg/d versus 0.8 g/kg/d in the adult population [22, 23]. Interestingly, physical activity, in particular resistance training, can improve muscle anabolic effect of protein intake, even in elderly subjects [24–26].

Any acute illness is accompanied by hypermetabolism and increased protein catabolism (in particular in inflammatory events) [27, 28] and a decrease in anabolic signals such as food intake and physical activity. In this context, hospitalizations in critical care rapidly alter nutritional status with depletion of both body fat and skeletal muscle proteins [27]. In elderly patients, this loss occurs on a pre-existing depletion of muscle mass [22], which predisposes them to ICU-acquired muscle weakness [29]. In a cohort of postoperative ICU patients (mean age 60.1 ± 17.4), the 65 patients with at least 2 CT scans experienced an average decrease in psoas muscle cross-sectional area (−9 mm2 [−16, −4], or about 1% per day) and density (in Hounsfield units (−1.0 HU [−10.2, 7.0] (2.3%) overall, or about 0.3% per day)) [30]. Muscle mass loss assessed by ultrasound occurs early in ICU patients (age 55+/−17 years), and the extent of the loss is typically between 14% and 21% within the first week of admittance [31]. In addition to the loss of muscle mass, forced immobilization in the event of acute illness as in ICU is accompanied by further alterations in muscle metabolism and quality such as a decrease in the ability of muscles to oxidize lipids with a shift in muscle fuel utilization from lipids towards glucose, causing accumulation of lipids in the muscle [32, 33]. These metabolic effects of short-term physical are less reversible on resumption of habitual physical activity in older adults than in younger people [34].

12.3 Nutritional Assessment in ICU and Prognosis

Malnutrition in critically ill patients is associated with increased risk for infections and extended lengths of stay and may lead to poor quality of life, disability, and morbidities long after ICU discharge [35, 36]. An early assessment of nutritional status, although essential to refine the patient's prognosis and identify patients who will benefit most from an intensive nutrition strategy, is not always based on consensual criteria or threshold value. Until a specific tool has been validated, the European Society for Clinical Nutrition and Metabolism recommends the use of anamnesis (weight loss or recent decrease in physical performance), physical examination, and general assessment of body composition and muscle mass and strength [35]. In addition, since screening and diagnostic tools have often not been specifically evaluated in the elderly population, these recommendations apply regardless of age [37].

Weight loss and reduced energy intake are major criteria for identifying malnutrition in hospitalized patients [38]. However, these criteria aren't always assessable in the event of critical care (vigilance or cognitive disorders, rapid change in hydration status, etc.). In the same way, anthropometric measurements are often unreliable due to inter-operator variability and especially in critical care due to the presence of oedema [39].

Among conventional methods for nutritional assessment, BMI seems the most accessible. A J-shaped association between body mass index (BMI) and all-cause mortality has been identified in populations [40]. In the healthy older population, BMI range from 25 to 30 is associated with the best prognosis in terms of disability-free years and life expectancy [41–43]. In nutritionDay, a worldwide inpatient survey, BMI range of 25–29.9 or ≥30 was associated with lower risks of in-hospital mortality, compared to normal (18.5–24.9) or low (<18.5) BMI, even among 75+ [44]. Both severe obesity (BMI >35) and underweight (BMI <20) have been reported as independent risk factors for postoperative complications in cardiac surgical ICU patients (median age, 70 y) [45]. In a Japanese nationwide database of ICU patients (median age, 70; IQR, 60–78), Sasabuchi et al. found an inverse J-shaped association between BMI and in-hospital mortality. The lowest mortality was observed in subjects with a BMI of approximately 24 kg/m^2 in the non-ventilated group and of 23 kg/m^2 in the mechanically ventilated group [46].

However, BMI is a very rough estimate of nutritional status and only imperfectly reflects body composition. Thus, the use of imaging techniques is developing in particular to assess lean mass. The use of computed tomography (CT) scan, frequently performed in ICU, is a promising method to improve nutritional assessment although not yet available in current practice. In particular, skeletal muscle and adipose tissue cross-sectional area (quantified by single-slice CT scans at the third lumbar vertebra) are strongly correlated to whole-body muscle and adipose tissue mass [47, 48]. A CT-measured skeletal muscle cross-sectional area at L3, divided by height in meters squared (defining muscle index), was measured in a cohort of 149 injured elderly ICU patients (median age 79 y) [49]. Among the 71% of patients with low muscle index (less than 38.9 cm2/m2 for females and less than 55.4 cm2/m2 for males [48]), 9% were underweight, 44% normal weight, and 47% overweight/obese (based on BMI). In multivariate analysis, low muscle index was associated with increased mortality and decreased ventilator-free and ICU-free days. Neither BMI, serum albumin, nor total adipose tissue on admission was indicative of survival or ventilator-free or ICU-free days [49]. In addition to quantity, muscle quality, assessed on CT scans by analysing skeletal muscle density (SMD) or the amount of intermuscular adipose tissue (IMAT), may be an important prognostic factor. In a retrospective study including 491 mechanically ventilated critically ill adult patients (mean age 58 ± 18 years), low SMD but not IMAT was independently associated with higher 6-month mortality [50].

Muscular ultrasonography allows visualization and classification of both muscle quantity (cross-sectional area, muscle layer thickness) and quality (echo intensity by grayscale and pennation angle) [51]. Although this technique offers a non-invasive and easily repeatable method during hospitalization, it still suffers from problems of standardization of measurements and a lack of consensus standards according to age [52, 53].

Bioelectrical impedance analysis (BIA) can be used to assess body composition (fat mass or fat-free mass), but these measures are often unsuitable in ICU unstable patients with fluid compartment shifts [54]. Most of the studies in ICU focus on the use of a more reliable BIA parameter, phase angle, as a good marker of nutritional status and prognosis of critically ill patients [55–57]. As ultrasonography, BIA is not yet used in common practice.

Many malnutrition screening tools based on clinical diagnosis, biological results, physical examination, anthropometric measurements, food/nutrient intake, and functional assessment were created during the last 30 years and aim to identify patients who would most benefit from nutritional support. Some tools, such as Nutritional Risk Screening 2002 or Mini Nutritional Assessment, are commonly used in the elderly population (in- or outpatients) but are often unsuitable for patients in the ICU. Other such tests have been used in ICU. Thus, moderate or severe malnourishment according to the subjective global assessment (SGA ranking B or C) is associated with higher intra-hospital mortality [58] even after 65 years [59]. In a prospective cohort of 76 surgical patients admitted to ICU (mean age, 60.36 ± 16.24 years), malnourished patients according to SGA (ranking B or C) had lower body mass index, mid-arm circumference, calf circumference, and serum albumin but higher hospital mortality compared to well-nourished patients (SGA A) [2]. Some studies do not find a link between these tests and the prognosis. In another cohort, the SGA at ICU admission (73.1 +/− 5.4 years) isn't associated with serum albumin value, length of stay, or mortality [60]. In a prospective cohort of 109 ICU patients (mean age, 76.5 ± 9.6 y) in India, 1-year mortality was associated with APACHE II score ($P < 0.001$; OR, 1.2; 95% CI, 1.1–1.3), severe risk of malnutrition (Malnutrition Universal Screening Tool score $\geq$2) (P = 0.006; OR, 0.08; 95% CI, 0.01–0.48), and delirium (P = 0.03; OR, 0.32; 95% CI, 0.11–0.9) [61].

Heyland et al. have developed the Nutrition Risk in the Critically Ill (NUTRIC) score as the first nutritional risk assessment tool for ICU patients. It is based on age, Acute Physiology and Chronic Health Evaluation (APACHE) II score, Sequential Organ Failure Assessment (SOFA) score, number of comorbidities, days from hospital admission to ICU admission, and serum interleukin 6 (IL-6) level [62]. In a recent review, NUTRIC score successfully predicts length of stay and mortality in ICU [63]. A modified NUTRIC score, composed of all variables except for IL-6 level, has showed similar performance to predict 28-day mortality (AUC, 0.757; 95% CI, 0.713–0.801) to the initial NUTRIC score [64]. In a retrospective cohort of 136 critically ill COVID-19 patients (median age, 69 y; IQR, 57–77), NUTRIC score predicted complications in the ICU such as acute respiratory distress syndrome (ARDS), shock, acute myocardial injury, secondary infection, and death in the ICU after 28 days of hospitalization [65]. However, there is no consensus on the best tool to identify malnutrition in ICU and the rates of malnutrition are very variable according to the tests [66]. None of these studies have compared the performance of these tools according to age groups.

Vitamin D insufficiency is the most common nutritional deficiency concerning 40% to 60% in the healthy general adult population and is also common in ICU patients (60–95% of deficiency or insufficiency) at any age (40–75 y) [67]. Vitamin D-deficient patients at ICU admission exhibit higher severity scores such as APACHE II or SOFA [68–70]; more complications such as acute respiratory insufficiency, acute liver failure, or infections [71]; and longer length of stay [72]. In another prospective study, vitamin D insufficiency (cut-off, 11 ng/ml) at ICU admission is associated with mortality at 28 days and with acute kidney injury [73]. Serum 25(OH)D levels below 20 ng/ml at ICU admission are associated with 28-day mortality in septic patients [69]. In a retrospective cohort of 655 surgical and nonsurgical critically ill patients (median age, 65 y; IQR, 23), adjusted hospital mortality is multiplied by 2 in case of low 25(OH)D status (overall less than 20 ng/ml with seasonal variations) [70]. Beyond its well-known role in bone metabolism, vitamin D deficiency in the general population has been associated with a decrease in muscular performance, increased all-cause and cardiovascular mortality, and cardiovascular events [74, 75]. Besides, vitamin D appears to be actively involved in the immune system, both innate and adaptive [76]. More than just a marker of overall health or acute disease severity, vitamin D deficiency (various cut-off between 11 and 25 ng/ml) could be a factor of complication especially infectious and length of stay [67]. Under these conditions, the fragile elderly population is particularly exposed to a deterioration of its prognostic. However, there is still a lack of interventional studies to validate this hypothesis.

Albumin and transthyretin (TTR also known as prealbumin) levels are widely used in clinical practice to assess, respectively, nutritional status and recent nutritional intake for hospital patients and outpatients [77]. However, the use of albumin level has evolved in recent years from a nutritional marker to an overall prognostic marker [35]. In particular, its level is inversely proportional to the intensity of inflammation, the presence of proteinuria, or liver failure. Albumin level on admission to ICU (for sepsis or surgery) is an independent risk factor for mortality [78, 79] or intensive respiratory or vasopressor support [80], with variable thresholds between 24 and 30 g/L [79–81]. Low TTR levels at ICU admission are also independently associated with higher in-hospital mortality, more infectious complications, longer total hospital length of stay (LOS), and ICU LOS [82]. Thanks to their prognostic performance, albumin and prealbumin levels remain the most widely used "nutritional" biological markers [83]. However, calorie and/or protein delivery in the ICU is not associated with changes in serum albumin [84]. TTR and retinol-binding protein (RBP), as rapid turnover proteins, have an interest in monitoring nutritional therapy lasting more than a week and are correlated with energy intake and nitrogen balance in ICU [85, 86]. Higher TTR levels over time were independently associated with lower in-hospital mortality, fewer infectious complications, shorter total hospital and ICU LOS, and fewer ventilator days [82]. Nevertheless, the normal values of the TTR decrease after 50 years in connection with the evolution of the lean mass [87]. Moreover, these studies included only a few elderly subjects. Efficient and accessible biomarkers of the nutritional risk or the efficacy of a nutritional intervention in elderly ICU patients still have to be identified [88].

As ICUs take care of populations with increasing age and BMI, the coexistence of obesity and malnutrition tends to be more frequent [89]. Determining nutritional status is even more difficult in the obese population (BMI ≥30), leading to missed or delayed detection of malnutrition and therefore to inadequate care.

12.4 Nutritional Intervention in Critically Ill Older Adults

Nutritional support is one of the cornerstones of maintaining and optimizing functional status and quality of life in critically ill older adults.

Oral diet and oral nutrition supplements remain the first-line intervention for the non-ventilated patient when permitted by the clinical condition and level of vigilance [35]. However, energy intake is likely to be suboptimal in elderly ICU patients [90], due to decreased appetite, alterations in taste and smell, gastrointestinal symptoms, weakness, delirium, or abulia [91, 92]. Dietary monitoring is essential to assess inadequate oral intakes and decide without delay when to implement artificial nutrition. Particular attention should be paid to screening for swallowing disorders that are particularly present in the elderly population during an acute phase, and texture-adapted food must then be proposed.

If oral intake is not possible or insufficient, ESPEN guideline on clinical nutrition in ICU recommends a nutritional support within 48 hours for enteral nutrition (EN) or within 3–7 days for parenteral nutrition (PN) in case enteral nutrition is not possible [35]. The use of EN over PN in elderly patients with an intact gastrointestinal tract is recommended in particular to reduce complications particularly frequent in the elderly such as infection, or thrombosis [23]. In a meta-analysis comparing enteral vs. parenteral feeding strategy in ICU, enteral was not associated with significantly reduced overall mortality but reduces rates of ICU-induced infection and length of stay [93].

While a calorie target of 70 to 100% of REE is usually recommended with a gradual increase during the acute phase (first week), the optimal amount of calories and timing is also controversial. Indirect calorimetry is the recommended tool to assess REE but remains rarely available in practice. Calculation by the respirators of REE from the measurement of the carbon dioxide production (VCO2) or oxygen consumption (VO2) seems to be a reliable method for ventilated patients. Some equations have been determined to estimate REE with basic clinical information such as weight, height, and age. The Harris and Benedict equation, which has been validated on a cohort of healthy elderly subjects aged 70 to 98 years, is the most widely used in practice [94, 95]. However, these predictions are difficult to extrapolate to heterogeneous hospitalized elderly population and are often inaccurate in ICU [96–98]. In the absence of indirect calorimetry or VCO2 measurements, simple weight-based equations (such as 20–25 kcal/kg/d during the acute phase and 30–35 kcal/kg/d thereafter) can also be used to prevent under- or overfeeding [35, 99].

Recent observations suggest that the risk for hyperglycaemia and overfeeding warrants a reduced caloric load of 15 kcal/kg/d for hypercatabolic patients during their first week in ICU [100]. In a retrospective cohort of 1171 ICU patients (median age 60 years), Zusman et al. [101] found that a calorie intake equivalent to 70% of the REE is associated with the lowest mortality, length of stay, and ventilation in ICU patients. Normocaloric enteral nutrition (100% of REE, 19.7 ± 5.7 kcal/k) was associated with less frequent nosocomial infection compared to hypocaloric (50% of REE 11.3 ± 3.1 kcal/kg) nutrition (11.1% vs. 26.1%, respectively) without effect on ICU mortality in a cohort of 100 ICU patients (mean age 65.8 ± 11.6 years) [102]. In a meta-analysis including 2517 patients (mean age 53 ± 5 years), there was no difference in the risk of acquired infections, hospital mortality, ICU length of stay, or ventilator-free days between patients receiving intentional hypocaloric as compared to normocaloric feeding [103]. However, no studies have been specifically conducted in an elderly population. Thus, hypocaloric diet, aiming to achieve 70–80% of REE during the acute phase, with progression to isocaloric when appropriate/feasible has been recently proposed for the older critically ill adult to avoid complications of overfeeding [104].

Most of the studies highlighting the deleterious effects of high-calorie intake (above 100–110% of REE) implicate a possible refeeding syndrome. Refeeding syndrome is a potentially fatal condition, characterized by hydroelectrolyte disturbances (hypophosphatemia, hypokalaemia, etc.), fluid retention, and metabolic and clinical complications (dysglycemia, dyspnoea, etc.). Elderly malnourished patients are particularly at risk of this syndrome caused by rapid initiation of refeeding after a period of undernutrition [70]. This is explained by the decrease of physiological reserves with aging, by the frequency of certain comorbidities (diabetes, cancer) and of certain treatments (diuretics, antacids), and by the severity of the acute illness. In a prospective cohort of 109 Malaysian ICU patients (mean age 51 ± 16 y), the 44 (42.6%) patients that experienced refeeding hypophosphataemia had similar age, higher SOFA score, and lower serum albumin [71]. Prevention is based on daily clinical and biological monitoring, initially limited caloric intake (10 kcal/kg/j), the correction of hydroelectrolytic imbalance, and a polysupplementation in vitamins and trace elements.

Protein intake seems to be a crucial prognostic factor, especially in the acute phase. Recommendations for adult dietary protein intake are based on nitrogen balance, i.e. the difference between nitrogen intake (food or artificial nutrition) and loss (urinary urea nitrogen excretion plus a constant of 4 g/day) [22, 105]. Thus, a negative nitrogen balance reflects a loss of total body protein and a catabolic state. Healthy elderly people tend to need higher protein intakes to balance their nitrogen balance [106]. Even under nutritional support, the majority of critically ill patients are affected by a negative nitrogen balance with an average loss of 11 g/d [107]. The protein deficit during the first 7 days impacts muscle quality with a decrease in muscle density on CT scan [30] and is associated with longer ICU stay and fewer ventilator-free days [108].

Moreover, most of the studies suggest that high protein intake (1.2–2 g/kg/d) could improve nitrogen balance and prognosis in critically ill patients [109, 110]. In a prospective cohort of 113 ICU patients (mean age 59 ± 17.2 y), a higher mean protein intake (1.5 g/kg/d vs. 1.1 g/kg/d or 0.8/kg/d) was associated with a lower nitrogen imbalance (−2.6 g/day vs. − 4.6 g/day vs. − 6.6 g/day) and a lower ICU mortality (16% vs. 24% vs. 27%) [110]. However, the provision of energy was not related to survival. In a cohort of 54 ICU older patients (>65 y), Dickerson et al. found that protein intakes of 1.5 to 2.5/kg/d are necessary to significantly improve nitrogen balance, with a considerable variability in nitrogen balance response to incremental increases in protein intake [105]. In the Critically Ill International Nutrition Surveys, a large cohort on 4040 ICU patients (mean age 60 ± 17 y) achieving ≥80% of prescribed protein intake was associated with reduced 60-day mortality and time to discharge alive, but ≥80% of prescribed energy intake has no significant impact on these factors [111].

These elements are at the origin of recent recommendations of ESPEN proposing 1.3 g protein/kg/d during critical illness [35], while the American Society for Parenteral and Enteral Nutrition (ASPEN) and the Society of Critical Care Medicine nutrition guidelines recommend 1.2–2.0 g protein/kg/d [99].

Some articles also underline the important gap between prescription and effective protein-energy intake, which represents 60 to 70% of the prescribed dose [111]. This difference may be even more marked in the elderly population due to physiologically slowed gastric emptying. In order to decrease gastric feeding intolerance, intravenous erythromycin (preferable to metoclopramide) may be used transitorily as prokinetic therapy while monitoring the risk of QT prolongation and cardiac arrhythmias.

Classical enteral isocaloric (1 kcal/kg/d) and normoprotidic (15% of total energy intake related to proteins) formula are not suitable to achieve reduced energy but high protein goals and could lead to insufficient protein intake [112]. New commercial formulas have therefore been developed over the past 5 years to maximize protein intake while limiting excessive caloric intake [113].

Physical activity is recommended to improve the beneficial effects of nutritional therapy [35].

Early exercise training (passive or active cycling) in ICU survivors enhanced recovery of functional exercise capacity, and muscle force at hospital discharge [114]. In a cohort of 200 surgical ICU patients (mean age 65 years), early mobilization shortened patient length of stay in the ICU and improved patients' functional mobility at hospital discharge [115]. However, a physical rehabilitation programme started in ICU fails to prove a benefit on quality of life at 12 months [116]. A Cochrane review, analysing early intervention (mobilization or active exercise) commenced in the ICU, concluded on poor evidence of benefit on physical function or performance, muscle strength, or health-related quality of life [117].

Micronutrient intakes (vitamins and trace elements) at least equal to the daily requirements are recommended in critical care [35, 118]. This is the case with at least 1500 kcal of enteral nutrition administered per day, but this requires a specific contribution in case of parenteral nutrition. Furthermore, deficiencies in certain micronutrients (iron, copper, selenium, vitamins D, B1, B6, and C) are common in cases of malnutrition and may be further aggravated by the increased needs during acute illness or by refeeding. Questioning for risk factors (alcoholism, previous bariatric surgery, restrictive diet, etc.) and targeted biological dosages must determine which vitamins or trace elements will require specific supplementation beyond the recommended daily allowance. As in general elderly population, ICU patients with measured low plasma levels (25-hydroxy-vitamin D <12.5 ng/ml, or 50 nmol/l) could benefit from supplementation. Randomized supplementation trials in ICU have shown mortality reduction when compared to placebo even with a 6-month follow-up [119, 120]. No particular side effects have been observed with doses between 200,000 and 540,000 units administered by the enteral, intramuscular, or intravenous routes. ESPEN recommends a high dose of vitamin D3 (500,000 UI) as a single dose within a week after admission [35].

As in other areas, caregivers can be auxiliary to nutritional care in addition to healthcare professionals. Family-centred intervention based on nutrition education sessions and nutrition diary may also improve nutrition in the recovery phase after a critical illness [121] (see ▶ Chap. 7) (◘ Fig. 12.2).

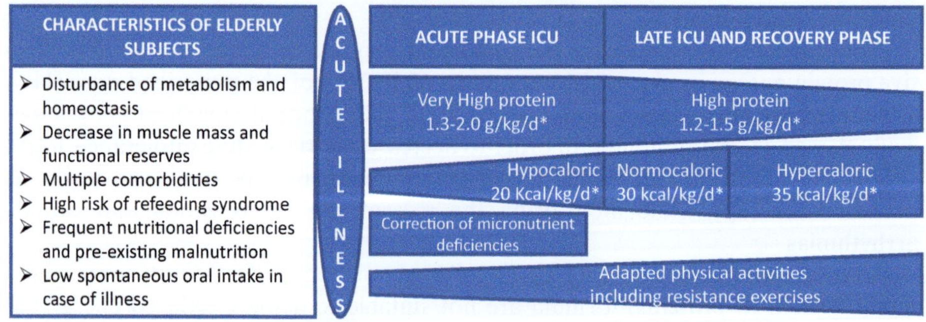

◘ **Fig. 12.2** Main characteristics of the elderly population and principles of nutritional support according to the ICU phase. (*Indicative values that need to be modulated according to the level of hypercatabolism and previous nutritional status)

Conclusion

Malnutrition is common in critically ill patients, especially in the elderly population which cumulates many risk factors.

Severe illness and intensive care constitute major metabolic challenges for elderly organisms and contribute to degrading their nutritional status.

Malnutrition is accompanied by more frequent hospital complications, an increase in the length of stay, a prolonged impairment of functional capacities, and a decrease in survival.

Usual methods of investigating nutritional status have serious limitations in critical care.

Nutritional interventions based on a standard protein-energy intake have evolved to adapt to very heterogeneous needs, particularly in elderly subjects.

Associated therapies such as physical activity and correction of vitamin D deficiency have significant synergistic effects.

The need for new studies is important to better take into account the specificities of the elderly population which is increasingly represented in ICU.

Take-Home Messages

- Malnutrition is accompanied by a deterioration of survival but also functional prognosis, in particular in the elderly population.
- An early nutritional assessment (by any available means) is mandatory for defining an individualized scope of care.
- High protein but normocaloric nutrition, resistance training, and vitamin deficiency supplementation are the main elements of nutritional care.

References

1. Cederholm T, Jensen GL, Correia MITD, Gonzalez MC, Fukushima R, Higashiguchi T, et al. GLIM criteria for the diagnosis of malnutrition - a consensus report from the global clinical nutrition community. J Cachexia Sarcopenia Muscle. 2019;10(1):207–17.
2. Gattermann Pereira T, da Silva FJ, Tosatti JAG, Silva FM. Subjective global assessment can be performed in critically ill surgical patients as a predictor of poor clinical outcomes. Nutr Clin Pract. 2019;34(1):131–6.
3. Sheean PM, Peterson SJ, Chen Y, Liu D, Lateef O, Braunschweig CA. Utilizing multiple methods to classify malnutrition among elderly patients admitted to the medical and surgical intensive care units (ICU). Clin Nutr. 2013;32(5):752–7.
4. Barker LA, Gout BS, Crowe TC. Hospital malnutrition: prevalence, identification and impact on patients and the healthcare system. Int J Environ Res Public Health. 2011;8(2):514–27.
5. Elia M, Zellipour L, Stratton RJ. To screen or not to screen for adult malnutrition? Clin Nutr. 2005;24(6):867–84.
6. Cohn SH, Vartsky D, Yasumura S, Sawitsky A, Zanzi I, Vaswani A, et al. Compartmental body composition based on total-body nitrogen, potassium, and calcium. Am J Phys. 1980;239(6):E524–30.
7. Fleg JL, Lakatta EG. Role of muscle loss in the age-associated reduction in VO2 max. J Appl Physiol (1985). 1988;65(3):1147–51.
8. Brooks SV, Faulkner JA. Skeletal muscle weakness in old age: underlying mechanisms. Med Sci Sports Exerc. 1994;26(4):432–9.
9. Lexell J. Evidence for nervous system degeneration with advancing age. J Nutr. 1997;127(5 Suppl):1011S–3S.

10. Delmonico MJ, Harris TB, Visser M, Park SW, Conroy MB, Velasquez-Mieyer P, et al. Longitudinal study of muscle strength, quality, and adipose tissue infiltration. Am J Clin Nutr. 2009;90(6):1579–85.

11. Hetherington MM. Taste and appetite regulation in the elderly. Proc Nutr Soc. 1998;57(4):625–31.

12. Donini LM, Savina C, Cannella C. Eating habits and appetite control in the elderly: the anorexia of aging. Int Psychogeriatr. 2003;15(1):73–87.

13. MacIntosh C, Morley JE, Chapman IM. The anorexia of aging. Nutrition. 2000;16(10):983–95.

14. Frassetto L, Sebastian A. Age and systemic acid-base equilibrium: analysis of published data. J Gerontol A Biol Sci Med Sci. 1996;51(1):B91–9.

15. Rimbert V, Boirie Y, Bedu M, Hocquette J-F, Ritz P, Morio B. Muscle fat oxidative capacity is not impaired by age but by physical inactivity: association with insulin sensitivity. FASEB J. 2004;18(6):737–9.

16. Petersen KF, Befroy D, Dufour S, Dziura J, Ariyan C, Rothman DL, et al. Mitochondrial dysfunction in the elderly: possible role in insulin resistance. Science. 2003;300(5622):1140–2.

17. Rolland Y, Czerwinski S. Abellan Van Kan G, Morley JE, Cesari M, Onder G, et al. sarcopenia: its assessment, etiology, pathogenesis, consequences and future perspectives. J Nutr Health Aging. 2008;12(7):433–50.

18. Guillet C, Prod'homme M, Balage M, Gachon P, Giraudet C, Morin L, et al. Impaired anabolic response of muscle protein synthesis is associated with S6K1 dysregulation in elderly humans. FASEB J. 2004;18(13):1586–7.

19. Balage M, Averous J, Rémond D, Bos C, Pujos-Guillot E, Papet I, et al. Presence of low-grade inflammation impaired postprandial stimulation of muscle protein synthesis in old rats. J Nutr Biochem. 2010;21(4):325–31.

20. Volpi E, Mittendorfer B, Wolf SE, Wolfe RR. Oral amino acids stimulate muscle protein anabolism in the elderly despite higher first-pass splanchnic extraction. Am J Phys. 1999;277(3):E513–20.

21. Salles J, Chanet A, Giraudet C, Patrac V, Pierre P, Jourdan M, et al. 1,25(OH)2-vitamin D3 enhances the stimulating effect of leucine and insulin on protein synthesis rate through Akt/PKB and mTOR mediated pathways in murine C2C12 skeletal myotubes. Mol Nutr Food Res. 2013;57(12):2137–46.

22. Bauer J, Biolo G, Cederholm T, Cesari M, Cruz-Jentoft AJ, Morley JE, et al. Evidence-based recommendations for optimal dietary protein intake in older people: a position paper from the PROT-AGE study group. J Am Med Dir Assoc. 2013;14(8):542–59.

23. Volkert D, Beck AM, Cederholm T, Cruz-Jentoft A, Goisser S, Hooper L, et al. ESPEN guideline on clinical nutrition and hydration in geriatrics. Clin Nutr. 2018.

24. Biolo G, Tipton KD, Klein S, Wolfe RR. An abundant supply of amino acids enhances the metabolic effect of exercise on muscle protein. Am J Phys. 1997;273(1 Pt 1):E122–9.

25. Endo Y, Nourmahnad A, Sinha I. Optimizing skeletal muscle anabolic response to resistance training in aging. Front Physiol [Internet]. 2020 Jul 23 [cited 2021 Apr 17];11. Available from: https://www.ncbi.nlm.nih.gov/pmc/articles/PMC7390896/

26. Yang Y, Breen L, Burd NA, Hector AJ, Churchward-Venne TA, Josse AR, et al. Resistance exercise enhances myofibrillar protein synthesis with graded intakes of whey protein in older men. Br J Nutr. 2012;108(10):1780–8.

27. Monk DN, Plank LD, Franch-Arcas G, Finn PJ, Streat SJ, Hill GL. Sequential changes in the metabolic response in critically injured patients during the first 25 days after blunt trauma. Ann Surg. 1996;223(4):395–405.

28. Biolo G. Protein metabolism and requirements. World Rev Nutr Diet. 2013;105:12–20.

29. Phillips SM, Dickerson RN, Moore FA, Paddon-Jones D, Weijs PJM. Protein turnover and metabolism in the elderly intensive care unit patient. Nutr Clin Pract. 2017;32(1_suppl):112S–20S.

30. Yeh DD, Ortiz-Reyes LA, Quraishi SA, Chokengarmwong N, Avery L, Kaafarani HMA, et al. Early nutritional inadequacy is associated with psoas muscle deterioration and worse clinical outcomes in critically ill surgical patients. J Crit Care. 2018;45:7–13.

31. Gruther W, Benesch T, Zorn C, Paternostro-Sluga T, Quittan M, Fialka-Moser V, et al. Muscle wasting in intensive care patients: ultrasound observation of the M. quadriceps femoris muscle layer. J Rehabil Med. 2008;40(3):185–9.

32. Stein TP, Wade CE. Metabolic consequences of muscle disuse atrophy. J Nutr. 2005;135(7):1824S–8S.

33. Casaer MP, Langouche L, Coudyzer W, Vanbeckevoort D, De Dobbelaer B, Güiza FG, et al. Impact of early parenteral nutrition on muscle and adipose tissue compartments during critical illness. Crit Care Med. 2013;41(10):2298–309.

34. Bowden Davies KA, Pickles S, Sprung VS, Kemp GJ, Alam U, Moore DR, et al. Reduced physical activity in young and older adults: metabolic and musculoskeletal implications. Therapeut Adv Endocrinol. 2019;10:2042018819888824.

35. Singer P, Blaser AR, Berger MM, Alhazzani W, Calder PC, Casaer MP, et al. ESPEN guideline on clinical nutrition in the intensive care unit. Clin Nutr. 2019;38(1):48–79.

36. Wieske L, Dettling-Ihnenfeldt DS, Verhamme C, Nollet F, van Schaik IN, Schultz MJ, et al. Impact of ICU-acquired weakness on post-ICU physical functioning: a follow-up study. Crit Care. 2015;19:196.

37. Tatucu O, Lambell K, Ridley E. Nutritional Management of the Critically Ill Older Adult. 2020 [cited 2021 Apr 18]; Available from: https://research.monash.edu/en/publications/nutritional-management-of-the-critically-ill-older-adult

38. Vest MT, Papas MA, Shapero M, McGraw P, Capizzi A, Jurkovitz C. Characteristics and outcomes of adult inpatients with malnutrition. JPEN J Parenter Enteral Nutr. 2018;42(6):1009–16.

39. Cheng AT, Plank LD, Hill GL. Prolonged overexpansion of extracellular water in elderly patients with sepsis. Arch Surg. 1998;133(7):745–51.

40. Bhaskaran K. dos-Santos-Silva I, Leon DA, Douglas IJ, Smeeth L. association of BMI with overall and cause-specific mortality: a population-based cohort study of 3·6 million adults in the UK. Lancet Diabetes Endocrinol. 2018;6(12):944–53.

41. Al Snih S, Ottenbacher KJ, Markides KS, Kuo Y-F, Eschbach K, Goodwin JS. The effect of obesity on disability vs mortality in older Americans. Arch Intern Med. 2007;167(8):774–80.

42. Flegal KM, Kit BK, Orpana H, Graubard BI. Association of all-cause mortality with overweight and obesity using standard body mass index categories: a systematic review and meta-analysis. JAMA. 2013;309(1):71–82.

43. Oreopoulos A, Kalantar-Zadeh K, Sharma AM, Fonarow GC. The obesity paradox in the elderly: potential mechanisms and clinical implications. Clin Geriatr Med. 2009;25(4):643–59.

44. Cereda E, Klersy C, Hiesmayr M, Schindler K, Singer P, Laviano A, et al. Body mass index, age and in-hospital mortality: the NutritionDay multinational survey. Clin Nutr. 2017;36(3):839–47.

45. Zittermann A, Becker T, Gummert JF, Börgermann J. Body mass index, cardiac surgery and clinical outcome. A single-center experience with 9125 patients. Nutr Metab Cardiovasc Dis. 2014;24(2):168–75.

46. Sasabuchi Y, Yasunaga H, Matsui H, Lefor AT, Horiguchi H, Fushimi K, et al. The dose-response relationship between body mass index and mortality in subjects admitted to the ICU with and without mechanical ventilation. Respir Care. 2015;60(7):983–91.

47. Shen W, Punyanitya M, Wang Z, Gallagher D, St-Onge M-P, Albu J, et al. Total body skeletal muscle and adipose tissue volumes: estimation from a single abdominal cross-sectional image. J Appl Physiol. 2004;97(6):2333–8.

48. Mourtzakis M, Prado CMM, Lieffers JR, Reiman T, McCargar LJ, Baracos VE. A practical and precise approach to quantification of body composition in cancer patients using computed tomography images acquired during routine care. Appl Physiol Nutr Metab. 2008;33(5):997–1006.

49. Moisey LL, Mourtzakis M, Cotton BA, Premji T, Heyland DK, Wade CE, et al. Skeletal muscle predicts ventilator-free days, ICU-free days, and mortality in elderly ICU patients. Crit Care. 2013;17(5):R206.

50. Looijaard WGPM, Dekker IM, Stapel SN, Girbes ARJ, Twisk JWR, Oudemans-van Straaten HM, et al. Skeletal muscle quality as assessed by CT-derived skeletal muscle density is associated with 6-month mortality in mechanically ventilated critically ill patients. Crit Care. 2016;20(1):386.

51. Formenti P, Umbrello M, Coppola S, Froio S, Chiumello D. Clinical review: peripheral muscular ultrasound in the ICU. Ann Intensive Care [Internet]. 2019 17 [cited 2021 Apr 17];9. Available from: https://www.ncbi.nlm.nih.gov/pmc/articles/PMC6525229/

52. Mourtzakis M, Parry S, Connolly B, Puthucheary Z. Skeletal muscle ultrasound in critical care: a tool in need of translation. Ann Am Thorac Soc. 2017;14(10):1495–503.

53. Nakanishi N, Tsutsumi R, Okayama Y, Takashima T, Ueno Y, Itagaki T, et al. Monitoring of muscle mass in critically ill patients: comparison of ultrasound and two bioelectrical impedance analysis devices. J Intensive Care. 2019;7(1):61.

54. Savalle M, Gillaizeau F, Maruani G, Puymirat E, Bellenfant F, Houillier P, et al. Assessment of body cell mass at bedside in critically ill patients. Am J Physiol Endocrinol Metabolism. 2012;303(3):E389–96.
55. Kuchnia A, Earthman C, Teigen L, Cole A, Mourtzakis M, Paris M, et al. Evaluation of bioelectrical impedance analysis in critically ill patients: results of a multicenter prospective study. J Parenter Enter Nutr. 2017;41(7):1131–8.
56. Lee Y, Kwon O, Shin CS, Lee SM. Use of bioelectrical impedance analysis for the assessment of nutritional status in critically ill patients. Clini Nutr Res. 2015;4(1):32–40.
57. Reis de Lima e Silva R, Porto Sabino Pinho C, Galvão Rodrigues I, Gildo de Moura Monteiro Júnior J. [Phase angle as an indicator of nutritional status and prognosis in critically ill patients]. Nutr Hosp. 2014;31(3):1278–85.
58. Bector S, Vagianos K, Suh M, Duerksen DR. Does the subjective global assessment predict outcome in critically ill medical patients? J Intensive Care Med. 2016;31(7):485–9.
59. Giannasi SE, Venuti MS, Midley AD, Roux N, Kecskes C, San RE. Mortality risk factors in elderly patients in intensive care without limitation of therapeutic effort. Med Intensiva. 2018;42(8):482–9.
60. Atalay BG, Yagmur C, Nursal TZ, Atalay H, Noyan T. Use of subjective global assessment and clinical outcomes in critically ill geriatric patients receiving nutrition support. JPEN J Parenter Enteral Nutr. 2008;32(4):454–9.
61. Tripathy S, Mishra JC, Dash SC. Critically ill elderly patients in a developing world—mortality and functional outcome at 1 year: A prospective single-center study. Journal of Critical Care. 2014;29(3):474.e7–13.
62. Heyland DK, Dhaliwal R, Jiang X, Day AG. Identifying critically ill patients who benefit the most from nutrition therapy: the development and initial validation of a novel risk assessment tool. Crit Care. 2011;15(6):R268.
63. Reis AMD, Fructhenicht AVG, Moreira LF. NUTRIC score use around the world: a systematic review. Rev Bras Ter Intensiva. 2019;31(3):379–85.
64. Jeong DH, Hong S-B, Lim C-M, Koh Y, Seo J, Kim Y, et al. Comparison of accuracy of NUTRIC and modified NUTRIC scores in predicting 28-Day mortality in patients with sepsis: a single center retrospective study. Nutrients. 2018;17:10(7).
65. Zhang P, He Z, Yu G, Peng D, Feng Y, Ling J, et al. The modified NUTRIC score can be used for nutritional risk assessment as well as prognosis prediction in critically ill COVID-19 patients. Clin Nutr. 2021;40(2):534–41.
66. Coltman A, Peterson S, Roehl K, Roosevelt H, Sowa D. Use of 3 tools to assess nutrition risk in the intensive care unit. JPEN J Parenter Enteral Nutr. 2015;39(1):28–33.
67. de Haan K, Groeneveld ABJ, de Geus HRH, Egal M, Struijs A. Vitamin D deficiency as a risk factor for infection, sepsis and mortality in the critically ill: systematic review and meta-analysis. Crit Care. 2014;18(6):660.
68. Anwar E, Hamdy G, Taher E, Fawzy E, Abdulattif S, Attia MH. Burden and outcome of vitamin D deficiency among critically ill patients: a prospective study. Nutr Clin Pract. 2017;32(3):378–84.
69. Chen Z, Luo Z, Zhao X, Chen Q, Hu J, Qin H, et al. Association of vitamin D status of septic patients in intensive care units with altered procalcitonin levels and mortality. J Clin Endocrinol Metab. 2015;100(2):516–23.
70. Amrein K, Zajic P, Schnedl C, Waltensdorfer A, Fruhwald S, Holl A, et al. Vitamin D status and its association with season, hospital and sepsis mortality in critical illness. Crit Care. 2014;18(2):R47.
71. Gomes TL, Fernandes RC, Vieira LL, Schincaglia RM, Mota JF, Nóbrega MS, et al. Low vitamin D at ICU admission is associated with cancer, infections, acute respiratory insufficiency, and liver failure. Nutrition. 2019;60:235–40.
72. Lr M, Y A, Kl W, Dd G, Ok D. Worsening severity of vitamin D deficiency is associated with increased length of stay, surgical intensive care unit cost, and mortality rate in surgical intensive care unit patients. American journal of surgery [Internet]. 2012 Jul [cited 2021 Apr 3];204(1). Available from: https://pubmed.ncbi.nlm.nih.gov/22325335/
73. Zapatero A, Dot I, Diaz Y, Gracia MP, Pérez-Terán P, Climent C, et al. Severe vitamin D deficiency upon admission in critically ill patients is related to acute kidney injury and a poor prognosis. Med Intensiva. 2018;42(4):216–24.
74. Holick MF. Vitamin D deficiency. N Engl J Med. 2007;357(3):266–81.

75. Dobnig H, Pilz S, Scharnagl H, Renner W, Seelhorst U, Wellnitz B, et al. Independent association of low serum 25-hydroxyvitamin d and 1,25-dihydroxyvitamin d levels with all-cause and cardiovascular mortality. Arch Intern Med. 2008;168(12):1340–9.

76. Hewison M. Vitamin D and innate and adaptive immunity. Vitam Horm. 2011;86:23–62.

77. Dellière S, Cynober L. Is transthyretin a good marker of nutritional status? Clin Nutr. 2017;36(2):364–70.

78. Basile-Filho A, Lago AF, Menegueti MG, Nicolini EA, De Rodrigues LAB, Nunes RS, et al. The use of APACHE II, SOFA, SAPS 3, C-reactive protein/albumin ratio, and lactate to predict mortality of surgical critically ill patients: a retrospective cohort study. Medicine (Baltimore). 2019;98(26):e16204.

79. Kendall H, Abreu E, Cheng A-L. Serum albumin trend is a predictor of mortality in ICU patients with sepsis. Biol Res Nurs. 2019;21(3):237–44.

80. Wi YM, Kim JM, Peck KR. Serum albumin level as a predictor of intensive respiratory or vasopressor support in influenza a (H1N1) virus infection. Int J Clin Pract. 2014;68(2):222–9.

81. Yin M, Si L, Qin W, Li C, Zhang J, Yang H, et al. Predictive value of serum albumin level for the prognosis of severe sepsis without exogenous human albumin administration: a prospective cohort study. J Intensive Care Med. 2018;33(12):687–94.

82. Haltmeier T, Inaba K, Durso J, Khan M, Siboni S, Cheng V, et al. Transthyretin at admission and over time as a marker for clinical outcomes in critically ill trauma patients: a prospective single-center study. World J Surg. 2020;44(1):115–23.

83. Ferrie S, Tsang E. Monitoring nutrition in critical illness: what can we use? Nutr Clin Pract. 2018;33(1):133–46.

84. Yeh DD, Johnson E, Harrison T, Kaafarani HMA, Lee J, Fagenholz P, et al. Serum levels of albumin and Prealbumin do not correlate with nutrient delivery in surgical intensive care unit patients. Nutr Clin Pract. 2018;33(3):419–25.

85. Parent B, Seaton M, O'Keefe GE. Biochemical markers of nutrition support in critically ill trauma victims. JPEN J Parenter Enteral Nutr. 2018;42(2):335–42.

86. Casati A, Muttini S, Leggieri C, Colombo S, Giorgi E, Torri G. Rapid turnover proteins in critically ill ICU patients. Negative acute phase proteins or nutritional indicators? Minerva Anestesiol. 1998;64(7–8):345–50.

87. Ingenbleek Y. Plasma transthyretin as a biomarker of sarcopenia in elderly subjects. Nutrients. 2019;21:11(4).

88. Stoppe C, Wendt S, Mehta NM, Compher C, Preiser J-C, Heyland DK, et al. Biomarkers in critical care nutrition. Crit Care. 2020;24(1):499.

89. Mauldin K, O'Leary-Kelley C. New guidelines for assessment of malnutrition in adults: obese critically ill patients. Crit Care Nurse. 2015;35(4):24–30.

90. Chapple L, Gan M, Louis R, Yaxley A, Murphy A, Yandell R. Nutrition-related outcomes and dietary intake in non–mechanically ventilated critically ill adult patients: a pilot observational descriptive study. Aust Crit Care. 2020;33(3):300–8.

91. Bryczkowski SB, Lopreiato MC, Yonclas PP, Sacca JJ, Mosenthal AC. Risk factors for delirium in older trauma patients admitted to the surgical intensive care unit. J Trauma Acute Care Surg. 2014;77(6):944–51.

92. Reid MB, Allard-Gould P. Malnutrition and the critically ill elderly patient. Crit Care Nurs Clin North Am. 2004;16(4):531–6.

93. Elke G, van Zanten ARH, Lemieux M, McCall M, Jeejeebhoy KN, Kott M, et al. Enteral versus parenteral nutrition in critically ill patients: an updated systematic review and meta-analysis of randomized controlled trials. Crit Care. 2016;20(1):117.

94. Harris JA, Benedict FG. A biometric study of human basal metabolism. Proc Natl Acad Sci U S A. 1918;4(12):370–3.

95. Melzer K, Laurie Karsegard V, Genton L, Kossovsky MP, Kayser B, Pichard C. Comparison of equations for estimating resting metabolic rate in healthy subjects over 70 years of age. Clin Nutr. 2007;26(4):498–505.

96. Neelemaat F, van Bokhorst-de van der Schueren MAE, Thijs A, Seidell JC, Weijs PJM. Resting energy expenditure in malnourished older patients at hospital admission and three months after discharge: predictive equations versus measurements. Clin Nutr. 2012;31(6):958–66.

97. Zusman O, Kagan I, Bendavid I, Theilla M, Cohen J, Singer P. Predictive equations versus measured energy expenditure by indirect calorimetry: a retrospective validation. Clin Nutr. 2019;38(3):1206–10.
98. Segadilha NLAL, Rocha EEM, Tanaka LMS, Gomes KLP, Espinoza REA, Peres WAF. Energy expenditure in critically ill elderly patients: indirect calorimetry vs predictive equations. JPEN J Parenter Enteral Nutr. 2017;41(5):776–84.
99. McClave SA, Taylor BE, Martindale RG, Warren MM, Johnson DR, Braunschweig C, et al. Guidelines for the provision and assessment of nutrition support therapy in the adult critically ill patient: Society of Critical Care Medicine (SCCM) and American Society for Parenteral and Enteral Nutrition (a.S.P.E.N.). JPEN J Parenter Enteral Nutr. 2016;40(2):159–211.
100. Rugeles SJ, Ochoa Gautier JB, Dickerson RN, Coss-Bu JA, Wernerman J, Paddon-Jones D. How many nonprotein calories does a critically ill patient require? a case for hypocaloric nutrition in the critically ill patient. Nutr Clin Pract. 2017;32(1_suppl):72S–6S.
101. Zusman O, Theilla M, Cohen J, Kagan I, Bendavid I, Singer P. Resting energy expenditure, calorie and protein consumption in critically ill patients: a retrospective cohort study. Crit Care. 2016;20(1):367.
102. Petros S, Horbach M, Seidel F, Weidhase L. Hypocaloric vs Normocaloric nutrition in critically ill patients: a prospective randomized pilot trial. JPEN J Parenter Enteral Nutr. 2016;40(2):242–9.
103. Marik PE, Hooper MH. Normocaloric versus hypocaloric feeding on the outcomes of ICU patients: a systematic review and meta-analysis. Intensive Care Med. 2016;42(3):316–23.
104. McKendry J, Thomas ACQ, Phillips SM. Muscle mass loss in the older critically ill population: potential therapeutic strategies. Nutr Clin Pract. 2020;35(4):607–16.
105. Dickerson RN. Nitrogen balance and protein requirements for critically ill older patients. Nutrients. 2016;8(4):226.
106. Morse MH, Haub MD, Evans WJ, Campbell WW. Protein requirement of elderly women: nitrogen balance responses to three levels of protein intake. J Gerontol A Biol Sci Med Sci. 2001;56(11):M724–30.
107. Dickerson RN, Pitts SL, Maish GO, Schroeppel TJ, Magnotti LJ, Croce MA, et al. A reappraisal of nitrogen requirements for patients with critical illness and trauma. J Trauma Acute Care Surg. 2012;73(3):549–57.
108. Yeh DD, Fuentes E, Quraishi SA, Lee J, Kaafarani HMA, Fagenholz P, et al. Early protein inadequacy is associated with longer intensive care unit stay and fewer ventilator-free days: a retrospective analysis of patients with prolonged surgical intensive care unit stay. JPEN J Parenter Enteral Nutr. 2018;42(1):212–8.
109. Scheinkestel CD, Kar L, Marshall K, Bailey M, Davies A, Nyulasi I, et al. Prospective randomized trial to assess caloric and protein needs of critically ill, anuric, ventilated patients requiring continuous renal replacement therapy. Nutrition. 2003;19(11–12):909–16.
110. Allingstrup MJ, Esmailzadeh N, Wilkens Knudsen A, Espersen K, Hartvig Jensen T, Wiis J, et al. Provision of protein and energy in relation to measured requirements in intensive care patients. Clin Nutr. 2012;31(4):462–8.
111. Nicolo M, Heyland DK, Chittams J, Sammarco T, Compher C. Clinical outcomes related to protein delivery in a critically ill population: a multicenter, multinational observation study. JPEN J Parenter Enteral Nutr. 2016;40(1):45–51.
112. Berger MM, Soguel L, Charrière M, Thériault B, Pralong F, Schaller MD. Impact of the reduction of the recommended energy target in the ICU on protein delivery and clinical outcomes. Clin Nutr. 2017;36(1):281–7.
113. ApSimon M, Johnston C, Winder B, Cohen SS, Hopkins B. Narrowing the protein deficit gap in critically ill patients using a very high-protein enteral formula. Nutr Clin Pract. 2020;35(3):533–9.
114. Burtin C, Clerckx B, Robbeets C, Ferdinande P, Langer D, Troosters T, et al. Early exercise in critically ill patients enhances short-term functional recovery. Crit Care Med. 2009;37(9):2499–505.
115. Schaller SJ, Anstey M, Blobner M, Edrich T, Grabitz SD, Gradwohl-Matis I, et al. Early, goal-directed mobilisation in the surgical intensive care unit: a randomised controlled trial. Lancet. 2016;388(10052):1377–88.
116. Cuthbertson BH, Rattray J, Campbell MK, Gager M, Roughton S, Smith A, et al. The PRaCTICaL study of nurse led, intensive care follow-up programmes for improving long term outcomes from critical illness: a pragmatic randomised controlled trial. BMJ. 2009;339:b3723.

12

117. Doiron KA, Hoffmann TC, Beller EM. Early intervention (mobilization or active exercise) for critically ill adults in the intensive care unit. Cochrane Database of Systematic Reviews [Internet]. 2018 [cited 2021 Apr 17];(3). Available from: https://doi.org/10.1002/14651858.CD010754.pub2/full

118. Lefrant J-Y, Hurel D, Cano NJ, Ichai C, Preiser J-C, Tamion F, et al. Guidelines for nutrition support in critically ill patient. Ann Fr Anesth Reanim. 2014;33(3):202–18.

119. Zajic P, Amrein K. Vitamin D deficiency in the ICU: a systematic review. Minerva Endocrinol. 2014;39(4):275–87.

120. Putzu A, Belletti A, Cassina T, Clivio S, Monti G, Zangrillo A, et al. Vitamin D and outcomes in adult critically ill patients. A systematic review and meta-analysis of randomized trials. J Crit Care. 2017;38:109–14.

121. Marshall AP, Lemieux M, Dhaliwal R, Seyler H, MacEachern KN, Heyland DK. Novel, family-centered intervention to improve nutrition in patients recovering from critical illness: a feasibility study. Nutr Clin Pract. 2017;32(3):392–9.

Functional Status and Older Age

Nazir I. Lone, Lisa Salisbury, and Atul Anand

Contents

© The Author(s), under exclusive license to Springer Nature Switzerland AG 2022
H. Flaatten et al. (eds.), *The Very Old Critically Ill Patients*, Lessons from the ICU,
https://doi.org/10.1007/978-3-030-94133-8_13

> **🎓 Learning Objectives**
> 1. To understand the changes in functional status associated with normal ageing, and risk factors of change in functional status.
> 2. To compare instruments used to measure functional status in older people, and their specific application in the ICU setting.
> 3. To evaluate the literature relating to functional status and its impact on ICU triage and outcomes for older adults admitted to intensive care.

13.1 Introduction

Functional status is an important component of clinical assessment when considering older adults for ICU admission, and their ability to survive and recover from an episode of critical illness. In those who survive, many older adults will experience a decline in physical function. Functional status is intrinsically linked to other features associated with ageing, including frailty, disability and comorbidity. For this reason, intensive care clinicians will benefit from an understanding of functional status in the context of normal ageing, and how an individual's pre-illness function impacts on ICU outcomes.

In this chapter, we will evaluate the interaction between chronological ageing and changes in functional status, as well as risk factors for decline in functional status in the older general population. We will then critically evaluate current instruments used to measure functional status in older people, with a particular focus on assessment in the critical care unit. We conclude the chapter with an analysis of the evidence base relating to premorbid functional status and its relationship with outcomes for critically ill older people.

13.2 Normal Ageing and Predictors for Change in Functional Status

13.2.1 Changes in Functional Status in Normal Ageing

The World Health Organization (WHO) places the maintenance of functional ability at the core of healthy ageing and wellbeing [1]. Sufficient functional ability is described as the capability of people 'to be and do what they have reason to value'. [2] This person-centred definition has replaced previous benchmarking against expectations for the age of an individual [3]. Evaluating 'normal' ageing is therefore more nuanced, although some common changes in functional status are observable across populations. The degree to which these processes are influenced or even confounded by factors independent of ageing, most notably comorbidity and socioeconomic deprivation, is still a matter of debate. Until midlife, disability is most commonly related to the profound effect of trauma or a single disease process [4]. However, across older populations, such simple causal links are usually missing; multifactorial disability is often seen without a simple disease focus. The interplay between normal ageing and the compounded effect of multiple simultaneous chronic diseases (multimorbidity) is particularly complicated. This is important given the dramatic increase in the age-specific prevalence of chronic degenerative diseases in older populations across high-income countries [5], although the rate of this growth may be falling [6].

Longitudinal observational cohort studies with decades of follow-up have provided much of the evidence around normal ageing. These have revealed the influence of early and midlife factors on an individual's trajectory of functional change and have attempted to separate age-related declines from other causes. There is now consensus around a hierarchical loss of function with age. For example, in the Newcastle 85+ UK cohort, 'cutting toenails' was identified as the most difficult measured function in older age and the earliest where independence is lost. In contrast, 'self-feeding' was observed to be the simplest and therefore last function compromised [7]. The American Longitudinal Study of Aging (LSOA) noted independent walking at the top of the hierarchy as an early functional loss but also reported loss of self-feeding as the most advanced stage of decline [8]. In younger participants (60–64 years old), difficulty walking up a flight of stairs may be an earlier marker of functional decline [9]. Variation in the functional activities included within these hierarchical scales does not necessarily imply disagreement; direct comparison between cohorts is difficult because of the different tools used to measure function [10]. This methodological challenge is likely to explain some of the variation in reported estimates for population prevalence of any disability, such as between 6% and 35% across broadly similar European nations [11].

Some aspects of functional decline may differ between women and men. Tasks related to strength appear more difficult at an earlier age for women, while older men may be quicker to report difficulty walking [7]. Some of these findings may reflect sex differences in traditional societal roles, such as housework and shopping. However, loss of muscle strength and impaired lower limb balance appear common precipitants of early functional decline in older age, across multiple longitudinal studies [4, 7, 9, 12]. Muscle strength is easily measurable in a clinical setting using a handgrip dynamometer and may be considered a pre-frailty marker [13]. Age-related loss of muscle strength must be distinguished from sarcopenia, a condition in which both muscle strength and muscle mass and/or function are diminished. Sarcopenia is a clear risk factor for functional decline and death but is not an inevitable state of older age [14, 15].

The rate of decline in function varies between individuals, but longitudinal observational data from Europe has suggested it is possible to assign one of the three common trajectories over 10 years of follow-up in people aged 60–70 years old: rapid, intermediate or low/no decline in function [16]. However, as individuals approach the end of life, patterns of functional loss become much less predictable. In the Precipitating Events Project (PEP), progression of disability was recorded on a monthly basis for participants in their final year of life. Over this much shorter period, five distinct trajectories of functional decline were noted. These groups had similar numbers but limited common predictors: persistent severe, steadily progressive, early accelerated, late catastrophic and no disability [17]. In the absence of a single common pathway of normal ageing, it is more straightforward to classify changes in functional status in terms of observable domains like muscle strength, balance and manual dexterity. Task-based approaches within disability models, such as those measuring activities of daily living, often fail to account for the heterogeneity of older adults, particularly towards the end of life.

13.2.2 Risk Factors and Predictors of Change in Functional Status

Studies that have helped to define the concept of normal ageing through observation of older adults over time have also accumulated evidence for associations with change in functional status. The evidence level for many of these factors varies widely. In this section, the most commonly reported features observed across multiple studies are discussed. These may be broadly divided into groups (see 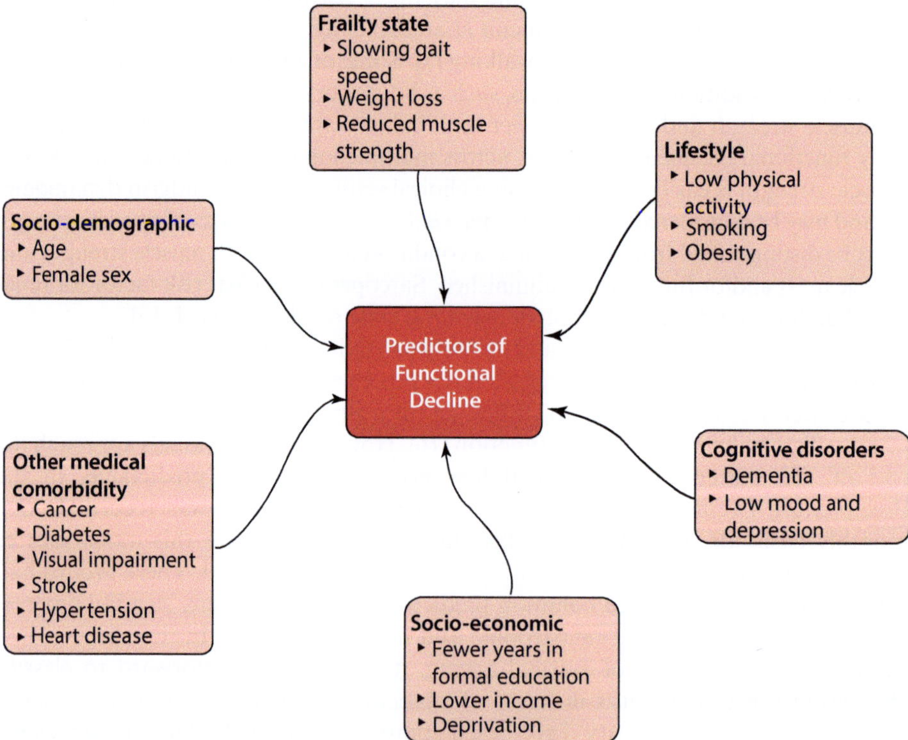 Fig. 13.1).

Some of these predictors are non-modifiable, such as socio-demographic risk factors like increasing age. Numerous studies have reported females to be at greater risk than males for functional decline [18–20]. This relationship is only partly explained by longer life expectancy in women. Other risk factors are arguably modifiable at a societal level. On average more rapid declines in functional status are observed in individuals with lower formal educational attainment, lower household income and other forms of socioeconomic deprivation [21].

Frailty is a commonly used term to describe vulnerability to dependency or death when faced with an acute stressor [22]. However, even without such a stressor event, frail individuals experience a decline in functional status at a faster rate than non-frail counterparts. Conceptually, frailty is seen as a process independent of age, but ultimately the term can be used to describe the variation in ageing patterns between individuals [23]. The physical frailty phenotype was first described in 2001 as comprising five traits: slowness, weakness, weight loss, exhaustion and low physical activ-

Fig. 13.1   Summary of major predictors of functional decline

ity [13]. For an individual to be considered frail, they must display at least three of these features, with cut-off thresholds broadly based on the lowest 20% from population normal values. In the original description from the Cardiovascular Health Study of over 5000 community-dwelling older adults, frailty by this definition was associated with a doubling of the risk of functional decline over 3 years, compared to non-frail individuals. This was after adjustment for important potential confounders such as age, sex, medical comorbidity and baseline functional status. Frailty, multimorbidity and disability are closely linked states but affect individuals in different ways [24]. Overall however, frailty appears to be a strong and independent predictor of future disability.

In a systematic review assessing the impact of individual frailty traits, slowness and low physical activity were shown to be the most important predictors for future functional decline, but all except self-reported exhaustion appear important [25]. This shows the potential importance of a 'pre-frail' state with single frailty markers as early indicators of the risk of developing dependency. It is easy to imagine how a 'frailty cycle' can develop, such as an individual with declining muscle strength (weakness) leading to slower gait speed (slowness) and reduced participation (low physical activity). This can become a vicious cycle that results in a full frailty state and ultimately disability [13].

Executive cognitive function is critical to successful completion of activities of daily living. It is unsurprising that disorders of cognitive function are powerful predictors of functional decline. Of the dementias, there is some evidence that the Alzheimer's subtype, particularly when features of behavioural disturbance are present, is a particularly significant risk factor [26, 27]. Functioning eyesight is another foundational component for independence in older age; longitudinal data suggests a threefold increase in unadjusted risk of dependence with activities of daily living in those with impaired vision compared to those without [28]. Mood disorders are an important differential diagnosis for dementia states, but depression by itself has been reported as a risk for declining functional status in older adults [29, 30]. In consideration of broader chronic health conditions, the number of self-reported comorbidities has also been associated with poorer function. Specific conditions merit particular attention, such as stroke, diabetes, hypertension and chronic lung and ischaemic heart disease, but the additive effect of multimorbidity is also important [19, 31]. Extremes of both low and high body weight, which may be strongly related to advanced progression of these other health conditions, are also risk factors for functional decline [21, 30].

Individual lifestyle choices are potentially attractive targets for healthcare interventions, but it is worth acknowledging the powerful role of social determinants that arguably require wider societal-level change [32]. Active smoking is one such risk factor for functional decline, although this association is less clear amongst those who have stopped smoking [18, 19]. A sedentary lifestyle contributes to the risk of disability, but as noted previously, such low physical activity may represent the development of a wider frailty state. While there is some evidence that married couples gain protection against functional decline, observational studies are inconsistent on the effect of single living, isolation or poorer social networks, with generally weak associations with functional status [20, 21].

13.2.3 Successful Ageing

There is increased research and policy focus on compression of functional decline, attempting to shift individuals onto a trajectory that shortens their years lived with disability and promotes functional independence for as long as possible [10]. Based on our understanding of the predictors of functional decline, successful ageing cannot simply be considered as a process of old age. This is an issue for the whole life course, with some non-modifiable risks embedded from birth, influenced by health behaviours and activity in early and middle age. These concepts have been crystallised in the concept of *intrinsic capacity* – the composite of all physical and mental capacities of an individual. This may be seen as a reserve against future disability [33]. If age-related declines in function were constant, individuals who have accrued the greatest intrinsic capacity in midlife are likely to be protected for longer against disability in later life.

Successful ageing is about more than just the absence of disease and disability. Varied definitions have included engagement with active family life, development of new skills in a 'third age' of learning and preservation of cognitive and physical function. This makes direct comparisons between studies challenging, although common themes do emerge [34]. As may be expected from the predictors of functional decline, sustained physical activity is by far the most powerful and consistently reported predictor of successful ageing. In 1 meta-analysis of 9 longitudinal studies including over 17,000 participants, medium to high physical activity such as daily recreational walking was associated with a 49% reduction in the risk of new impairment in activities of daily living over 10 years of follow-up [35]. A similar risk reduction was noted for progression of existing disability. Other cohorts have focused on a wider concept of successful ageing, such as the English Longitudinal Study of Ageing. In over 3000 participants, a dose-dependent relationship was observed between the amount of physical activity undertaken and the probability of surviving free of major chronic disease, depression or physical or cognitive impairment over 8 years of follow-up [36]. Research in this important area has largely been conducted in richer Western countries, and there remains limited evidence from low- and middle-income nations [37].

It is important to not completely exclude the importance of disease management to successful ageing. Careful control of multimorbid conditions is essential to provide the foundations for successful ageing and to enable participation in protective physical activities [38]. Cognitive decline and dementia lack effective medical treatments and these conditions are powerful risk factors for functional decline. Targeted cognitive training in older adults without dementia has been shown to reduce decline in instrumental activities of daily living in one randomised trial, [39] although there is arguably a much stronger evidence base for the protective effects of physical activity on the development of future cognitive decline [40]. Ultimately physical activity is likely to be the single most effective intervention to promote successful ageing.

13.3 Measurement of Functional Status

The measurement of functional status is not standardised across practice with a plethora of measures used to capture functional status in older populations [41–43]. This variation reflects the complexity of functional status as a concept [44]. For example, an ability to walk and sit to stand may not automatically result in the ability to use a toilet, and environmental differences such as different toilet heights or availability of rails can affect the ability to independently use a toilet. This complexity is mirrored in the measurement of functional status as a concept, and different approaches to measuring functional status exist.

The World Health Organization International Classification of Functioning, Disability and Health [45] (WHO-ICF) is a conceptual framework identifying the components of health and the complex interactions between them required to function. The WHO-ICF framework comprises three distinct domains of body functions and structure (e.g. strength), activities (execution of a task or action undertaken by an individual) and participation (involvement in a life situation) with consideration of environmental and personal contextual factors considered across all domains. The WHO-ICF domains of activity and participation fit most closely with functional status with further sub-division of the domains into Learning and Applying Knowledge; General Tasks and Demands; Communication; Mobility; Self-Care; Domestic Life; Interpersonal Interactions and Relationships; Major Life Areas; and Community and Social and Civic Life. The WHO-ICF framework illuminates the complex interactions between domains and is a useful framework to consider when measuring functional status, for example, What aspects of functional status are an instrument assessing? It may be that one measure is not sufficient to reflect functional status and that a battery of measures needs to be considered. The following section will consider some of the instruments used to measure functional status in the older person.

13.3.1 Instruments Used to Measure Functional Status in the Older Person

There are a range of instruments in existence that measure functional status in the older person with most reflecting the mobility and self-care domains of the WHO-ICF. Measures range from simple self-rating, for example, independent versus not in a single functional activity, to ordinal scales containing multiple functional activities. ■ Table 13.1 provides a summary of validated measurement instruments commonly used to reflect functional status in older populations. This list is not exhaustive but includes outcome measures frequently reported in the literature and used in clinical practice.

13.3.1.1 Mobility

Some instruments measure mobility to reflect functional status and range from reflecting one construct to the evaluation of multiple functional activities. The Functional Reach [46] assesses dynamic postural control through a forward lean. This is a simple and quick test of balance requiring little equipment but only assesses

Table 13.1 Summary of validated measurement instruments of functional status in older populations

Measurement instrument	WHO-ICF activity and participation subcategories
Functional reach	Mobility/body functions and structures
180-degree turn	Mobility/body functions and structures
The five times sit-to-stand	Mobility
Timed up and go	Mobility
6 minute walk test	Mobility
Tinetti	Mobility
Elderly mobility scale	Mobility
Katz activities of daily living	Self-care
Lawton activities of daily living	Self-care
Barthel index	Self-care
FIM	Self-care

in one direction and may be limited by reduced flexibility and strength and fear. The 180-degree turn [47] assesses dynamic postural stability by assessing an individual as they independently step through 180 degrees with the number of steps taken counted. While both these measures conceptually assess a component of normal movement required for mobility, it could be argued the underlying construct being measured is balance and should therefore be categorised as body functions and structures on the WHO-ICF. In isolation, these instruments are limited in their ability to measure functional status.

Other mobility measures use duration of time needed to achieve a functional goal to assess functional activities. The Five Times Sit-to-Stand Test (FTSST) was first reported as a simple measure of lower extremity muscle strength, assessed by the time required to sit to stand ten consecutive times [48] with variations over the years resulting in the commonly used timed FTSST [49]. The FTSST was evaluated in older intensive care patients [50] and found to be both safe and reliable but limited to high-functioning older adults. Timed walking tests include the 10-metre walk test, which measures gait velocity over 10 metres using any aid and at the individuals preferred speed [51], and the 6-Minute Walk Test, which measures the distance walked in 6 minutes as a submaximal test of aerobic capacity and endurance [52]. These timed measures only assess one functional activity and can have a floor effect as individuals need to be independent in the functional activity before measurement can be carried out.

Further measures combine more than one functional activity within a measurement instrument. The Timed Up and Go records the time taken to stand up from a chair, walk 3 m, turn around, walk back and sit back down [53]. The Performance-Oriented Mobility Assessment (POMA) was described by Tinetti [54] and includes nine balance and eight gait activities each allocated scores of 0 to 2. Amended versions of the POMA are available including the Problem-Oriented Assessment of Mobility and the Tinetti Scales of Gait or Balance each reflecting slight variations in the aspect of functional status being measured. The Elderly Mobility Scale assesses seven activities including transfers, standing, gait and the functional reach [55] all graded on an ordinal scale with a total maximum score of 20. Scores under 10 generally mean an individual is dependent in functional activities and 10–13 borderline for safety and independence in functional activities, and scores over 14 indicate an individual would be safe and independent. It could be argued the measures containing multiple mobility activities provide a more comprehensive measurement of functional status although they are still only focused on mobility activities and do not consider self-care activities.

13.3.1.2 Self-Care

Activities undertaken as part of normal daily living are termed activities of daily living (ADL) including bathing, dressing, eating, using the toilet, transferring and continence. Instrumental activities of daily living (IADL) are more complex activities such as using the telephone, shopping, preparing food, housekeeping, doing laundry, using transport and managing medicines and finance. ADL and IADL would be categorised under self-care in the WHO-ICF framework.

Measurement of individual ADL can be undertaken by broad categorisation of an activity, for example, independent, needing some assistance, mostly dependent and completely dependent. This approach could lead to bias and be open to interpretation if the categories are not well-defined. However, this bias can be overcome with the use of a validated scale. The Katz Index of Independence in Activities of Daily Living (Katz ADL) was designed to measure the function of older adults with chronic conditions and assesses six ADL. Each ADL is rated as 0 (dependence) or 1 (independence) with clear definitions for each category [56, 57]. The Lawton Instrumental Activities of Daily Living Scale [58] evaluates eight IADL that rely on both physical and cognitive function. Despite the development of both the Katz and Lawton measures taking place decades ago, they are still frequently used to measure ADL in older populations [59]. Other measures of ADL available, although not specifically developed for an elderly population, are the Barthel Index, a measure of 10 ADL [60], and the Functional Independence Measure which has 18 separate components, some of which reflect the construct of self-care [61].

13.3.2 Instruments Used to Measure Functional Status in the ICU Setting

In the ICU the functional status of an individual can be impacted by both critical illness and ICU-acquired weakness [62]. Several measurement tools have been designed to capture functional status in the ICU. These instruments have not been exclusively designed to assess the older person, but the content of many of the measures reflects the instruments used to assess functional status in older persons.

The Physical Function in Intensive Care Test (PFIT) was originally designed as a five-component score [63] and subsequently validated as an ordinal scale (PFIT-s) with four components measuring upper and lower limb strength and the functional activities of standing up from a chair and marching on the spot [64]. The Functional Status Score for the Intensive Care Unit (FSS-ICU) uses the 0 (total assistance) to 7 (complete independence) scoring from the Functional Independence Measure (FIM). However, the FSS-ICU only adopts the walking component from the FIM and added four further activities (rolling, supine to sit, sit to stand and sitting edge of bed) and uses the FIM scoring system to assess each activity resulting in a total score ranging from 0 to 35 [65]. The PFIT-s and FSS-ICU only contain four or five categories, while other measures have included a wider range of functional activities. The Manchester Mobility Score [66] is an ordinal scale containing seven functional activities ranging from bed interventions to moving/walking with a score of 0 to 7 used to describe the level of mobility. The Critical Care Functional Rehabilitation Outcome Measure [67] evaluates nine functional activities from a straight leg raise to walking a minimum of ten steps using the same scoring system of 0 to 7 used by the FIM and FSS-ICU. The Chelsea Critical Care Physical Assessment Tool [68] measures seven functional activities as well as grip strength, respiratory function and cough. All activities are measured on an ordinal level of 0 to 5 resulting in an overall score of between 0 and 50. The Perme score [69] contains 15 scored items to reflect mobility status ranging from the ability to follow commands to the distance walked in 2 minutes, while the de Morton Mobility Index [70] also contains 15 hierarchical activities from bridging to jumping scored as 0 or 1 and for some activities 2 providing an overall score. The ICU Mobility Scale (IMS) [71] was developed in response to the variability of instruments available to measure functional status in the ICU which can make comparison of datasets challenging. The IMS was developed by an international team and includes 10 mobility milestones with an 11-point ordinal scale ranging from 0 (able to do nothing) to walking independently without a gait aid with each of the 11 classifications scored 0 or 1 using well-defined criteria.

It is evident there is a range of instruments available to measure functional status in the ICU setting but with differing numbers of activities and scoring approaches. Core outcome sets (COS) are an agreed standardised set of outcome measures that would be reported as a minimum in clinical trials [72] and are helpful to identify an agreed common measure. A COS to evaluate physical rehabilitation in critical care is currently being identified and will be helpful to guide choice of functional status measures in the future [73].

13.4 Functional Status and Its Impact on ICU Triage and Outcomes

An individual's pre-illness functional status influences their likely outcome after ICU admission. For this reason, an evaluation of functional status has a role when weighing the benefits and burdens of treatment in ICU at the time of admission. Clinicians can draw on a growing literature that quantifies the relationship between functional status and both mortality and physical function outcomes. Pre-illness functional status, at its simplest, can be measured at a single time point pre-admission through patient or family recall. However, studies have progressed to explore the impact of a change in function during a defined period before admission on outcomes. Similarly, physical function as an outcome can be measured at a single time point after ICU discharge or can incorporate a change in function from baseline to the time point of measurement of post-ICU outcomes. The range of instruments used to define pre-illness physical function, or more often the ability to perform activities of daily living, varies. This section reviews the literature relating to how pre-illness functional status impacts on ICU outcomes for older patients, as well as on admission triage.

13.4.1 Functional Status and Outcomes

13.4.1.1 Mortality Outcomes

Mortality is the primary outcome used in risk prediction models that are frequently used to benchmark care in ICUs globally. However, commonly used models, such as APACHE II, do not include a measure of pre-admission functional status. The ICNARC model, derived from the Case Mix Programme database comprising admissions to ICUs in England, Wales and Northern Ireland, was updated in 2015 to evaluate whether inclusion of additional variables would improve model performance [74]. One of these variables was a measure of pre-admission functional status. This variable contained three levels relating to the assistance required with activities of daily living: none, some and total. Despite the model demonstrating excellent discrimination in predicting in-hospital mortality in ICU patients, addition of this variable to the model improved model performance as was independently associated with mortality (some assistance with daily activities vs none, OR 1.61; total assistance vs no assistance, OR 2.43). In a single-centre study undertaken in the USA, a similar three-category variable measuring pre-admission performance of activities of daily living was independently associated with hospital mortality, even with inclusion of APACHE IV predicted mortality in multivariable models [75]. These studies demonstrate that functional status is an independent predictor of mortality and improves model performance, even when added to high performing risk prediction models.

13.4.1.2 Physical Function Outcomes

Studies often do not include a clearly validated measure of physical function at baseline. However, simplified objective measures such as 'living independently at home' are often recorded. Such measures, which combine impairments, and restrictions in function, activities and participation, with environmental and personal factors, are often used due to ease of collection and fewer issues with patient or proxy recall. One such study which identified risk factors for physical impairment 6 months after acute lung injury reported both an objectively assessed measure of physical function, the 6-Minute Walk Test, and a self-reported measure of physical function, SF-36 Physical Function [76]. Those living independently at home before their critical illness had significantly higher 6-Minute Walk Test and SF-36 Physical Function scores as a proportion of predicted. These associations remained significant in multivariable models. Importantly, multivariable models adjusted for comorbidity using an index of conditions specifically validated for physical function outcomes, the Functional Comorbidity Index, [77] in addition to the more commonly used Charlson Comorbidity Index [78]. The Functional Comorbidity Index was developed and validated using the SF-36 Physical Function score as the outcome, rather than using mortality, which is by far the most commonly used outcome in development and validation of comorbidity indices.

In contrast, Heyland and colleagues used a validated measure of pre-illness functional status in a cohort study of patients aged 80 years and older admitted to ICU study [79]. The study aimed to identify characteristics associated with return to baseline physical function. Importantly, the researchers included measures of comorbidity, frailty and baseline physical function in the multivariable predictor model. Baseline physical function was defined using the physical functioning domain of the 36-Item Short Form Survey. This is a validated 36-item instrument which is a self-reported survey of general health status, ranging between 0 and 100, in which a higher score represents better function. The baseline physical function (PF) score in the 610 participants in the cohort was 40, indicating significant impairment. The study identified that a higher baseline PF score was associated with a higher likelihood of 12-month survival and a better physical function at 12-month follow-up in survivors. However, the primary outcome of the study, a return to baseline physical function, was defined as being alive at 12 months and reporting a PF score within 10 points of baseline score and a minimum PF score of 10 to avoid floor effects. This outcome combined mortality with functional status in a binary format. In multivariable models using this outcome as the dependent variable, good pre-admission physical function (defined as a higher baseline PF score) was associated with lower likelihood of being alive and returning to baseline function. The authors explained this somewhat counterintuitive finding as being due to their chosen outcome: returning to within 10 points of baseline PF score was more difficult to achieve for patients who started with a higher baseline score than those who started with a lower baseline score. This is evident in stratified unadjusted analyses of outcomes stratified by baseline PF <40 compared with ≥40 (◘ Fig. 13.2).

This study by Heyland and colleagues is important as it extends outcome measurement so that we can better distinguish between pre-existing functional impairment and new impairment after ICU admission, which can be causally attributed to critical illness. However, once a non-mortality outcome is chosen in a study, the analysis needs to explicitly state how to handle those who die during follow-up [80]. The disadvantage of combining non-recovery and death is that this effectively equates these two outcomes as having equal value. While some may argue that patients may place more value on being alive rather than functional impairment, this is not what was reported in a community-based survey [81].

A further study conducted in 754 people aged 70 years or older investigated pre-ICU admission factors associated with functional recovery within 6 months of ICU admission [82]. Functional recovery was defined as the return to a total disability count less than or equal to pre-ICU admission disability count. Physical function was measured by the Short Physical Performance Battery, which is an objective assessment of physical function, in contrast to the self-reported SF-36 PF score used in the study by Heyland and colleagues. In univariable analyses, low physical capacity (SPPB score 0–3) pre-ICU admission was associated with a lower likelihood of functional recovery relative to high physical function (SPPB score 8–12) (HR 0.46, 95% CI 0.28–0.77, $p = 0.003$).

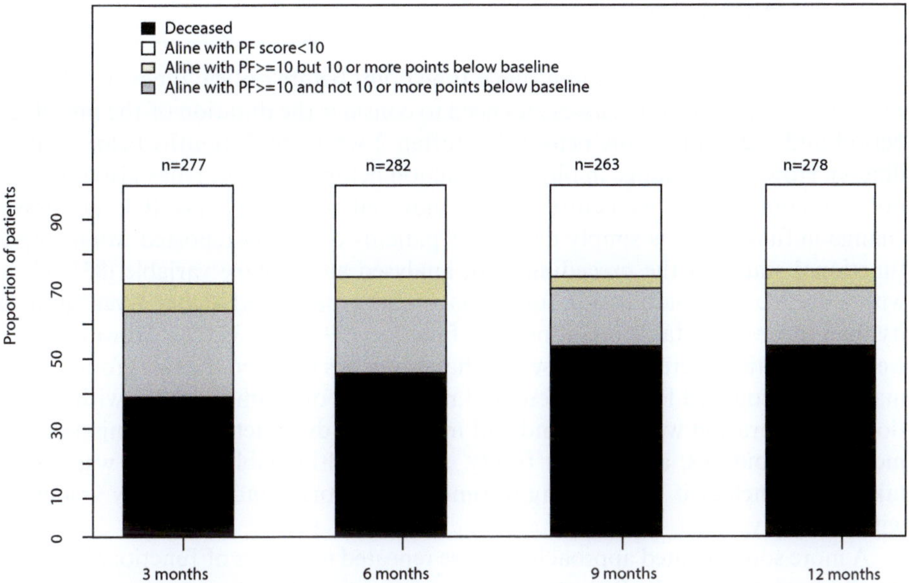

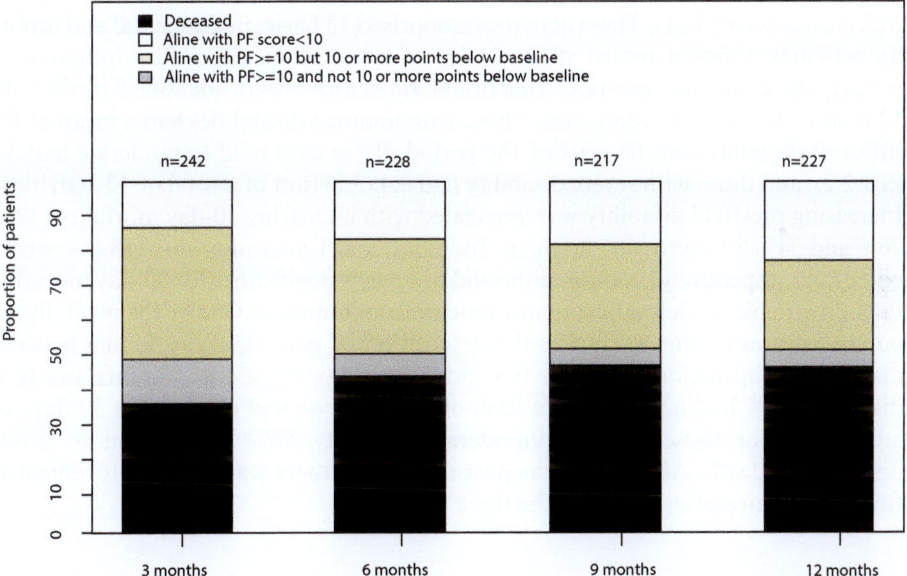

Fig. 13.2 Combined outcome of mortality and change of physical function from baseline at different time points during follow-up. (From Heyland et al. [79])

13.4.2 Changes in Pre-illness Functional Status as a Predictor of Outcomes

Measuring functional status at a single time point before critical illness is relatively easy to ascertain, although assessors need to consider the duration of the pre-illness period and ascertain status before this (often 2 weeks to 2 months before critical illness). However, a change in physical function before admission may also highlight poor outcomes. In a two-centre study conducted in the UK, pre-ICU admission change in function was simply defined as patient- or family-reported worsening in functional status in the preceding year, analysed as a binary variable [83]. Those with a decline in pre-admission functional status experienced higher 1-year mortality than those with stable pre-admission function (59.4% vs 33.0%). However, there were systematic differences in baseline characteristics between the two groups which may have accounted for this differential mortality. For example, those with a functional deterioration were older and had more organ dysfunction on admission, and more comorbidities, and higher frailty. As no multivariable analysis was undertaken, it is unclear if a worsening in functional status is independently associated with mortality.

A more sophisticated approach is to use repeated measures of functional status in longitudinal data which allows trajectories of functional status over time to be identified. Ferrante and colleagues used such a study design [84]. They used the number of activities of daily living that a person needed help with as a measure of functional trajectories before ICU. These activities comprised 13 basic, instrumental and mobility activities. Using a robust study design of repeated measures in a longitudinal cohort, three distinct pre-ICU functional trajectories were identified during the 12 months before ICU admission. Those with minimal disabilities had a mean of 0.6 (SD 1.0) disabilities at the start of the period, those with mild to moderate had 3.1 (SD 2.2), and those with severe disability had 8.4 (3.2) (out of a total of 13 activities). Increasing pre-ICU disability was associated with increasing 30-day mortality (12%, 26% and 34% for increasing levels of disability) and 1-year mortality (18.6%, 44.5% and 67.5% respectively), although this did not reach significance for 30-day mortality in multivariable models adjusting for potential confounders. One of the most illuminating features of this study was the description of patients transitioning between disability groups before and after ICU admission. For those with minimal pre-ICU disability, 51% had a more severe level of disability or had died within 30 days of admission. For those with mild/moderate disability, 66% transitioned to severe disability or death. After 6 months post-admission, there was little improvement in functional trajectories in any of the three groups.

13.4.3 Functional Status and ICU Triage

While much of the focus in the literature relates to outcomes after ICU admission, there is a smaller, albeit important, literature on ICU triage in the older adult. Functional status plays an important role in this process. The ICE-CUB group reported factors associated with non-referral to the ICU of patients aged 80 or older by emergency physicians [85]. In multivariable analysis, worse functional status, measured by the Katz Index of Activities of Daily Living, was independently associated with non-referral. For each additional activity of daily living which a patient was able to undertake independently, there was a 7% reduction in odds of non-referral (OR 0.93; 95% CI 0.88, 0.99; $p = 0.02$). The importance of the influence of pre-admission functional status on decision-making was emphasised in a randomised controlled trial of systematic ICU triage in people aged 75 and older, for which entry criteria included preserved functional status, determined by an Index of Independence in Activities of Daily Living of at least 4 [86].

Pre-illness functional status has a demonstrable impact on both ICU triage and patient outcomes. A greater understanding of the evidence base will allow clinicians to have informed conversations with patients and families to ensure that the consequences of ICU admission are aligned with a patient's priorities and treatment preferences. It also highlights the necessity for comprehensive rehabilitation services for older patients who survive ICU to maximise their chance of recovery.

> **Practical Implications**
>
> - When evaluating functional status, it is necessary to consider the range of instruments available, such as measurements relying on self-report which are relatively easy to administer, and those that require clinical supervision, such as the 6-Minute Walk Test. For research purposes, investigators should only use instruments that are validated in ICU populations and await publication of the agreed core outcome set for functional status.
> - There are substantial societal and public health gains to be made from the growing literature relating to healthy ageing. Public health interventions which promote preservation of activity levels in older people, careful management of long-term health conditions and lifestyle interventions earlier in adulthood can realise substantial societal benefit by compressing morbidity to a shorter period at the end of life.
> - At the time of assessment for ICU admission, clinicians should take an accurate history relating to functional status and activities of daily living. If a patient is incapacitated, this history should be clarified with a family member. Those with poor pre-existing functional status, or those who are on a declining functional trajectory, are likely to have worse outcomes. Following a careful exploration of treatment preferences, clinicians should use this information to weigh the benefits and burdens of critical care therapies to arrive at a person-centred decision.
> - In the context of rehabilitation within and after ICU, a careful assessment of functional status is required to track progress and establish realistic goals for patients.

Conclusion

Pre-illness functional status is an important consideration in ICU triage and has a demonstrable impact on patient outcomes. There are a range of validated tools which can be used to objectively assess functional status, both before ICU admission, and to track recovery. This will become increasingly important given the dramatic increase in the age-specific prevalence of chronic degenerative diseases in older populations.

A greater understanding of the evidence base presented in this chapter will allow clinicians to have informed conversations with patients and families to ensure that the consequences of ICU admission are aligned with a patient's treatment preferences. Furthermore, the importance placed by older people on functional independence highlights the necessity for comprehensive rehabilitation services for older patients who survive ICU to maximise their chance of recovery.

> **Take-Home Messages**
> - Risk factors for a decline in functional status in older adults include non-modifiable characteristics, such as age, sex and socioeconomic status, and potentially modifiable factors, such as low physical activity, smoking and obesity. Interventions which can promote preservation of functional status include careful control of multimorbid conditions, lifestyle interventions and promoting physical activity earlier in the life course.
> - There are a range of validated tools which can be used to objectively assess functional status, both before ICU admission, and to track recovery.
> - Pre-illness functional status is a key factor influencing decision-making relating to ICU admission. Poor functional status before ICU admission is associated with higher mortality and worse functional outcomes. Studies confirm that even simple measures of pre-illness functional status improve performance of sophisticated ICU risk prediction models for mortality used in benchmarking of care quality.

Conflict of Interest   The authors have no conflicts of interest to declare.

References

1. World Health Organization. World report on ageing and health. Geneva, Switzerland: World Health Organization; 2015.
2. World Health Organisation. Ageing: Healthy ageing and functional ability DOI. 2020
3. Kirch W. Functional ability. In: Kirch W, editor. Encyclopedia of public health. New York: Springer; 2008.
4. Ferrucci L, Guralnik JM, Cecchi F, Marchionni N, Salani B, Kasper J, Celli R, Giardini S, Heikkinen E, Jylha M, Baroni A. Constant hierarchic patterns of physical functioning across seven populations in five countries. Gerontologist. 1998;38:286–94.
5. Fleming DM, Cross KW, Barley MA. Recent changes in the prevalence of diseases presenting for health care. Br J Gen Pract. 2005;55:589–95.
6. Puts MT, Deeg DJ, Hoeymans N, Nusselder WJ, Schellevis FG. Changes in the prevalence of chronic disease and the association with disability in the older Dutch population between 1987 and 2001. Age Ageing. 2008;37:187–93.
7. Kingston A, Collerton J, Davies K, Bond J, Robinson L, Jagger C. Losing the ability in activities of daily living in the oldest old: a hierarchic disability scale from the Newcastle 85+ study. PLoS One. 2012;7:e31665.
8. Dunlop DD, Hughes SL, Manheim LM. Disability in activities of daily living: patterns of change and a hierarchy of disability. Am J Public Health. 1997;87:378–83.
9. Wloch EG, Kuh D, Cooper R. Is the hierarchy of loss in functional ability evident in midlife? Findings from a British birth cohort. PLoS One. 2016;11:e0155815.

10. Gore PG, Kingston A, Johnson GR, Kirkwood TBL, Jagger C. New horizons in the compression of functional decline. Age Ageing. 2018;47:764–8.
11. Phellas CN. Aging in European societies: healthy aging in Europe. New York: Springer; 2013.
12. Guralnik JM, Ferrucci L, Simonsick EM, Salive ME, Wallace RB. Lower-extremity function in persons over the age of 70 years as a predictor of subsequent disability. N Engl J Med. 1995;332:556–61.
13. Fried LP, Tangen CM, Walston J, Newman AB, Hirsch C, Gottdiener J, Seeman T, Tracy R, Kop WJ, Burke G, McBurnie MA, Cardiovascular Health Study Collaborative Research G. Frailty in older adults: evidence for a phenotype. J Gerontol A Biol Sci Med Sci. 2001;56:M146–56.
14. Cruz-Jentoft AJ, Bahat G, Bauer J, Boirie Y, Bruyère O, Cederholm T, Cooper C, Landi F, Rolland Y, Sayer AA, Schneider SM, Sieber CC, Topinkova E, Vandewoude M, Visser M, Zamboni M, Writing Group for the European Working Group on Sarcopenia in Older People 2 (EWGSOP2) atEGfE. Sarcopenia: revised European consensus on definition and diagnosis. Age Ageing. 2019;48:16–31.
15. Cruz-Jentoft AJ, Sayer AA. Sarcopenia. Lancet. 2019;393:2636–46.
16. Jonkman NH, Del Panta V, Hoekstra T, Colpo M, van Schoor NM, Bandinelli S, Cattelani L, Helbostad JL, Vereijken B, Pijnappels M, Maier AB. Predicting trajectories of functional decline in 60- to 70-year-old people. Gerontology. 2018;64:212–21.
17. Gill TM, Gahbauer EA, Han L, Allore HG. Trajectories of disability in the last year of life. N Engl J Med. 2010;362:1173–80.
18. Sun F, Park NS, Klemmack DL, Roff LL, Li Z. Predictors of physical functioning trajectories among Chinese oldest old adults: rural and urban differences. Int J Aging Hum Dev. 2009;69:181–99.
19. Freedman VA, Martin LG, Schoeni RF, Cornman JC. Declines in late-life disability: the role of early- and mid-life factors. Soc Sci Med. 2008;66:1588–602.
20. Black SA, Rush RD. Cognitive and functional decline in adults aged 75 and older. J Am Geriatr Soc. 2002;50:1978–86.
21. van der Vorst A, Zijlstra GA, Witte N, Duppen D, Stuck AE, Kempen GI, Schols JM, Consortium DS. Limitations in activities of daily living in community-dwelling people aged 75 and over: a systematic literature review of risk and protective factors. PLoS One. 2016;11:e0165127.
22. Morley JE, Vellas B, van Kan GA, Anker SD, Bauer JM, Bernabei R, Cesari M, Chumlea WC, Doehner W, Evans J, Fried LP, Guralnik JM, Katz PR, Malmstrom TK, McCarter RJ, Gutierrez Robledo LM, Rockwood K, von Haehling S, Vandewoude MF, Walston J. Frailty consensus: a call to action. J Am Med Dir Assoc. 2013;14:392–7.
23. Rockwood K. Conceptual models of frailty: accumulation of deficits. Can J Cardiol. 2016;32:1046–50.
24. Fried LP, Ferrucci L, Darer J, Williamson JD, Anderson G. Untangling the concepts of disability, frailty, and comorbidity: implications for improved targeting and care. J Gerontol A Biol Sci Med Sci. 2004;59:255–63.
25. Vermeulen J, Neyens JC, van Rossum E, Spreeuwenberg MD, de Witte LP. Predicting ADL disability in community-dwelling elderly people using physical frailty indicators: a systematic review. BMC Geriatr. 2011;11:33.
26. Smith GE, O'Brien PC, Ivnik RJ, Kokmen E, Tangalos EG. Prospective analysis of risk factors for nursing home placement of dementia patients. Neurology. 2001;57:1467–73.
27. Hebert R, Dubois MF, Wolfson C, Chambers L, Cohen C. Factors associated with long-term institutionalization of older people with dementia: data from the Canadian Study of Health and Aging. J Gerontol A Biol Sci Med Sci. 2001;56:M693–9.
28. Idland G, Pettersen R, Avlund K, Bergland A. Physical performance as long-term predictor of onset of activities of daily living (ADL) disability: a 9-year longitudinal study among community-dwelling older women. Arch Gerontol Geriatr. 2013;56:501–6.
29. Stuck AE, Walthert JM, Nikolaus T, Bula CJ, Hohmann C, Beck JC. Risk factors for functional status decline in community-living elderly people: a systematic literature review. Soc Sci Med. 1999;48:445–69.
30. Corona LP, Nunes DP, Alexandre Tda S, Santos JL, Duarte YA, Lebrao ML. Weight gain among elderly women as risk factor for disability: health, well-being and aging study (SABE study). J Aging Health. 2013;25:119–35.

31. Avlund K, Due P, Holstein BE, Sonn U, Laukkanen P. Changes in household composition as determinant of changes in functional ability among old men and women. Aging Clin Exp Res. 2002;14:65–74.
32. Cockerham WC, Hamby BW, Oates GR. The social determinants of chronic disease. Am J Prev Med. 2017;52:S5–S12.
33. Cesari M, Araujo de Carvalho I, Amuthavalli Thiyagarajan J, Cooper C, Martin FC, Reginster JY, Vellas B, Beard JR. Evidence for the domains supporting the construct of intrinsic capacity. J Gerontol A Biol Sci Med Sci. 2018;73:1653–60.
34. Depp CA, Jeste DV. Definitions and predictors of successful aging: a comprehensive review of larger quantitative studies. Am J Geriatr Psychiatry. 2006;14:6–20.
35. Tak E, Kuiper R, Chorus A, Hopman-Rock M. Prevention of onset and progression of basic ADL disability by physical activity in community dwelling older adults: a meta-analysis. Ageing Res Rev. 2013;12:329–38.
36. Hamer M, Lavoie KL, Bacon SL. Taking up physical activity in later life and healthy ageing: the English longitudinal study of ageing. Br J Sports Med. 2014;48:239–43.
37. Daskalopoulou C, Stubbs B, Kralj C, Koukounari A, Prince M, Prina AM. Physical activity and healthy ageing: a systematic review and meta-analysis of longitudinal cohort studies. Ageing Res Rev. 2017;38:6–17.
38. Michel JP, Dreux C, Vacheron A. Healthy ageing: evidence that improvement is possible at every age. Eur Geriatr Med. 2016;7:298–305.
39. Willis SL, Tennstedt SL, Marsiske M, Ball K, Elias J, Koepke KM, Morris JN, Rebok GW, Unverzagt FW, Stoddard AM, Wright E, Group AS. Long-term effects of cognitive training on everyday functional outcomes in older adults. JAMA. 2006;296:2805–14.
40. Sofi F, Valecchi D, Bacci D, Abbate R, Gensini GF, Casini A, Macchi C. Physical activity and risk of cognitive decline: a meta-analysis of prospective studies. J Intern Med. 2011;269:107–17.
41. Freiberger E, de Vreede P, Schoene D, Rydwik E, Mueller V, Frändin K, Hopman-Rock M. Performance-based physical function in older community-dwelling persons: a systematic review of instruments. Age Ageing. 2012;41:712–21.
42. Huisingh-Scheetz M, Kocherginsky M, Schumm PL, Engelman M, McClintock MK, Dale W, Magett E, Rush P, Waite L. Geriatric syndromes and functional status in NSHAP: rationale, measurement, and preliminary findings. J Gerontol B Psychol Sci Soc Sci. 2014;69(Suppl 2):S177–90.
43. Soto-Perez-de-Celis E, Li D, Yuan Y, Lau YM, Hurria A. Functional versus chronological age: geriatric assessments to guide decision making in older patients with cancer. Lancet Oncol. 2018;19:e305–16.
44. Wang T-J. Concept analysis of functional status. Int J Nurs Stud. 2004;41:457–62.
45. World Health Organization. Towards a common language for functioning, disability and health. 2002.
46. Duncan PW, Weiner DK, Chandler J, Studenski S. Functional reach: a new clinical measure of balance. J Gerontol. 1990;45:M192–7.
47. Nevitt MC, Cummings SR, Kidd S, Black D. Risk factors for recurrent nonsyncopal falls. A prospective study. JAMA. 1989;261(18):2663–8.
48. Csuka M, McCarty DJ. Simple method for measurement of lower extremity muscle strength. Am J Med. 1985;78:77–81.
49. Guralnik JM, Simonsick EM, Ferrucci L, Glynn RJ, Berkman LF, Blazer DG, Scherr PA, Wallace RB. A short physical performance battery assessing lower extremity function: association with self-reported disability and prediction of mortality and nursing home admission. J Gerontol. 1994;49:M85–94.
50. Melo TA, Duarte ACM, Bezerra TS, França F, Soares NS, Brito D. The five times sit-to-stand test: safety and reliability with older intensive care unit patients at discharge. Revista Brasileira De Terapia Intensiva. 2019;31:27–33.
51. Wade DT, Wood VA, Heller A, Maggs J, Langton Hewer R. Walking after stroke. Measurement and recovery over the first 3 months. Scand J Rehabil Med. 1987;19:25–30.
52. Guyatt GH, Thompson PJ, Berman LB, Sullivan MJ, Townsend M, Jones NL, Pugsley SO. How should we measure function in patients with chronic heart and lung disease? J Chronic Dis. 1985;38:517–24.
53. Podsiadlo D, Richardson S. The timed "up & go": a test of basic functional mobility for frail elderly persons. J Am Geriatr Soc. 1991;39:142–8.

54. Tinetti M. Performance-orientated assessment of mobility problems in elderly patients. J Am Geriat Soc. 1986;34:119–26.
55. Smith R. Validation and reliability of the elderly mobility scale. Physiotherapy. 1994;80:744–7.
56. Katz S, Downs TD, Cash HR, Grotz RC. Progress in development of the index of ADL. The Gerontologist. 1970;10:20–30.
57. Katz S, Ford AB, Moskowitz RW, Jackson BA, Jaffe MW. Studies of illness in the aged. The index of ADL: a standardized measure of biological and psychosocial function. JAMA. 1963;185:914–9.
58. Lawton MP, Brody EM. Assessment of older people: self-maintaining and instrumental activities of daily living. The Gerontologist. 1969;9:179–86.
59. Noelker LS, Browdie R. Sidney Katz, MD: a new paradigm for chronic illness and long-term care. The Gerontologist. 2014;54:13–20.
60. Mahoney FI, Barthel DW. Functional evaluation: the Barthel index. A simple index of independence useful in scoring improvement in the rehabilitation of the chronically ill. Md State Med J. 1965;14:61–5.
61. Keith RA, Granger CV, Hamilton BB, Sherwin FS. The functional independence measure: a new tool for rehabilitation. Adv Clin Rehabil. 1987;1:6–18.
62. Jolley SE, Bunnell AE, Hough CL. ICU-acquired weakness. Chest. 2016;150:1129–40.
63. Skinner EH, Berney S, Warrillow S, Denehy L. Development of a physical function outcome measure (PFIT) and a pilot exercise training protocol for use in intensive care. Crit Care Resusc. 2009;11:110–5.
64. Denehy L, de Morton NA, Skinner EH, Edbrooke L, Haines K, Warrillow S, Berney S. A physical function test for use in the intensive care unit: validity, responsiveness, and predictive utility of the physical function ICU test (scored). Phys Ther. 2013;93:1636–45.
65. Zanni JM, Korupolu R, Fan E, Pradhan P, Janjua K, Palmer JB, Brower RG, Needham DM. Rehabilitation therapy and outcomes in acute respiratory failure: an observational pilot project. J Crit Care. 2010;25:254–62.
66. McWilliams DJ, Atkins G, Hodson J, Boyers M, Lea T, Snelson C. Feasibility and reliability of the Manchester mobility score as a measure of physical function within the intensive care unit. J Assoc Chart Physiotherap Respirat Care. 2016;48:26–33.
67. Twose PW, Wise MP, Enright S. Critical care functional rehabilitation outcome measure: developing a validated measure. Physiother Theory Pract. 2015;31:474–82.
68. Corner EJ, Wood H, Englebretsen C, Thomas A, Grant RL, Nikoletou D, Soni N. The Chelsea critical care physical assessment tool (CPAx): validation of an innovative new tool to measure physical morbidity in the general adult critical care population; an observational proof-of-concept pilot study. Physiotherapy. 2013;99:33–41.
69. Perme C, Nawa RK, Winkelman C, Masud F. A tool to assess mobility status in critically ill patients: the Perme intensive care unit mobility score. Methodist Debakey Cardiovasc J. 2014;10:41–9.
70. Sommers J, Vredeveld T, Lindeboom R, Nollet F, Engelbert RHH, van der Schaaf M. de Morton mobility index is feasible, reliable, and valid in patients with critical illness. Phys Ther. 2016;96:1658–66.
71. Tipping CJ, Bailey MJ, Bellomo R, Berney S, Buhr H, Denehy L, Harrold M, Holland A, Higgins AM, Iwashyna TJ, Needham D, Presneill J, Saxena M, Skinner EH, Webb S, Young P, Zanni J, Hodgson CL. The ICU mobility scale has construct and predictive validity and is responsive. A Multicenter observational study. Ann Am Thorac Soc. 2016;13:887–93.
72. Williamson PR, Altman DG, Blazeby JM, Clarke M, Devane D, Gargon E, Tugwell P. Developing core outcome sets for clinical trials: issues to consider. Trials. 2012;13:132.
73. Connolly B, Denehy L, Hart N, Pattison N, Williamson P, Blackwood B. Physical rehabilitation core outcomes in critical illness (PRACTICE): protocol for development of a core outcome set. Trials. 2018;19:294.
74. Harrison DA, Ferrando-Vivas P, Shahin J, Rowan KM. Ensuring comparisons of health-care providers are fair: development and validation of risk prediction models for critically ill patients. Southampton (UK): NIHR Journals Library; 2015.
75. Krinsley JS, Wasser T, Kang G, Bagshaw SM. Pre-admission functional status impacts the performance of the APACHE IV model of mortality prediction in critically ill patients. Crit Care. 2017;21(1):10.
76. Needham DM, Wozniak AW, Hough CL, Morris PE, Dinglas VD, Jackson JC, Mendez-Tellez PA, Shanholtz C, Ely EW, Colantuoni E, Hopkins RO. Risk factors for physical impairment after acute lung injury in a national, multicenter study. Am J Respir Crit Care Med. 2014;189:1214–24.

77. Groll DL, To T, Bombardier C, Wright JG. The development of a comorbidity index with physical function as the outcome. J Clin Epidemiol. 2005;58:595–602.
78. Charlson M, Szatrowski TP, Peterson J, Gold J. Validation of a combined comorbidity index. J Clin Epidemiol. 1994;47:1245–51.
79. Heyland DK, Garland A, Bagshaw SM, Cook D, Rockwood K, Stelfox HT, Dodek P, Fowler RA, Turgeon AF, Burns K, Muscedere J, Kutsogiannis J, Albert M, Mehta S, Jiang X, Day AG. Recovery after critical illness in patients aged 80 years or older: a multi-center prospective observational cohort study. Intensive Care Med. 2015;41:1911–20.
80. Colantuoni E, Scharfstein DO, Wang C, Hashem MD, Leroux A, Needham DM, Girard TD. Statistical methods to compare functional outcomes in randomized controlled trials with high mortality. BMJ (Clinical Research Ed). 2018;360:j5748.
81. Fried TR, Tinetti ME, Iannone L, O'Leary JR, Towle V, Van Ness PH. Health outcome prioritization as a tool for decision making among older persons with multiple chronic conditions. Arch Intern Med. 2011;171:1854–6.
82. Ferrante LE, Pisani MA, Murphy TE, Gahbauer EA, Leo-Summers LS, Gill TM. Factors associated with functional recovery among older intensive care unit survivors. Am J Respir Crit Care Med. 2016;194:299–307.
83. Gross JL, Borkowski J, Brett SJ. Patient or family perceived deterioration in functional status and outcome after intensive care admission: a retrospective cohort analysis of routinely collected data. BMJ Open. 2020;10:e039416.
84. Ferrante LE, Pisani MA, Murphy TE, Gahbauer EA, Leo-Summers LS, Gill TM. Functional trajectories among older persons before and after critical illness. JAMA Intern Med. 2015;175:523.
85. Garrouste-Orgeas M, Boumendil A, Pateron D, Aergerter P, Somme D, Simon T, Guidet B, Group I-C. Selection of intensive care unit admission criteria for patients aged 80 years and over and compliance of emergency and intensive care unit physicians with the selected criteria: an observational, multicenter, prospective study. Crit Care Med. 2009;37:2919–28.
86. Guidet B, Leblanc G, Simon T, Woimant M, Quenot J-P, Ganansia O, Maignan M, Yordanov Y, Delerme S, Doumenc B, Fartoukh M, Charestan P, Trognon P, Galichon B, Javaud N, Patzak A, Garrouste-Orgeas M, Thomas C, Azerad S, Pateron D, Boumendil A, Network I-CS. Effect of systematic intensive care unit triage on long-term mortality among critically ill elderly patients in France: a randomized clinical trial. JAMA. 2017;318:1450–9.

13

Comprehensive Geriatric Assessment (CGA)

Hélène Vallet, Céline Bianco, and Caroline Thomas

Contents

> **Learning Objectives**
> - To know the definition of Comprehensive Geriatric Assessment (CGA)
> - To know the core elements of CGA
> - To know the impact of CGA on old patients' prognosis
> - To understand the limits of CGA
> - To understand the importance of CGA for management of old patients in emergency context and intensive care

14.1 Introduction

Definition of "old patient" is not consensual. Aging is a complex phenom including physiological modification due to genetic, epigenetic, and environmental factors. These modifications impact all organs and systems with large intra- and interindividual variations. Aging is also associated with an increased risk of comorbidities and functional disabilities that can impact prognosis of old patients.

For these reasons, the evaluation of this population is multimodal and complex. It needs to include:
- Medical aspect
- Functional aspect
- Social aspect
- Economic aspect

Furthermore, because of the great heterogeneity of the old population, this evaluation needs to be personalized, focused to the individual.

14.1.1 History of Comprehensive Geriatric Assessment (CGA)

The first notion of CGA takes place in the UK in the 1930s with three pioneer geriatricians who develop a multidimensional approach of old patients reviewing all their capacities and problems which can lead to functional health benefits [1, 2]. Geriatrics emerges as a specialty in the UK in 1948 and CGA becomes the "keystone" of this medical specialty [2]. Several years later, in 1988, experts from the National Institutes of Health Consensus Development Conference Statement conclude that CGA is effective when coupled with ongoing implementation of the resulting care plan [3].

In this chapter, we define CGA and explain its impact on older population prognosis. As we will see, this evaluation is time-consumed and difficult to be applied to emergency situation. We will propose an adaptation of this CGA before and during ICU stay of older patients.

14.2 What Is Comprehensive Geriatric Assessment (CGA)?

Definition of CGA has evolved with years. The concept is to (1) identify patients with higher risk of poor outcomes, (2) propose the most adequate treatment plan, and (3) allocate all available resources of the multidisciplinary team [4]. A recent umbrella review concludes that the most frequently used definition of CGA is "A multimodal, multidisciplinary process which identifies medical, social, functional needs, and the development of an integrated/coordinated care plan to meet those needs" [5].

The core dimensions of CGA are as follows [6, 7]:

- Medical dimension: comorbidities, polypharmacy, cognition, depression, geriatric syndrome (fall risk, delirium, urinary incontinence, dentition, visual, hearing impairments), frailty, nutrition
- Functional dimension: mobility, gait speed, activity of daily living, instrumental activity of daily living
- Social dimension: caregivers, social network, support needs, financial resources, environmental adequacy and safety

Several actors are systematically or if needed implicated in CGA such as [6]:
- Geriatricians
- Nurses
- Physiotherapists
- Social workers
- Pharmacists
- Dentists
- Occupational therapists
- Nutritionists
- Psychiatrists/psychologists
- Audiologists
- Podiatrists
- Opticians

CGA is applied in different kind of healthcare setting. In a meta-analysis, Stuck et al. describe for the first time several kinds of situations where CGA should be used in and out of hospital [8].

Inpatient CGA is divided into [8]:
- GEMU (Geriatric Evaluation and Management Unit): "a ward that admits frail older in-patients for a process of multidisciplinary assessment, review and therapy" [9]. It could be an acute geriatric center or a rehabilitation center.
- IGCS (Inpatient geriatrics Consultation Service): "a multidisciplinary team which assesses, discusses and recommends a plan of treatment for frail older in-patients" (mobile teams) [9].

Outpatient CGA is divided into [8]:
- HAS (home assessment service): "in-home CGA for community-dwelling elderly persons"
- HHAS (hospital home assessment service): "in-home CGA for patients recently discharged from hospital"
- OAS (outpatient assessment service): "CGA provided in an outpatient setting"

More recently, CGA is applied in specific condition such as oncogeriatrics [10] or ortho-geriatrics [11].

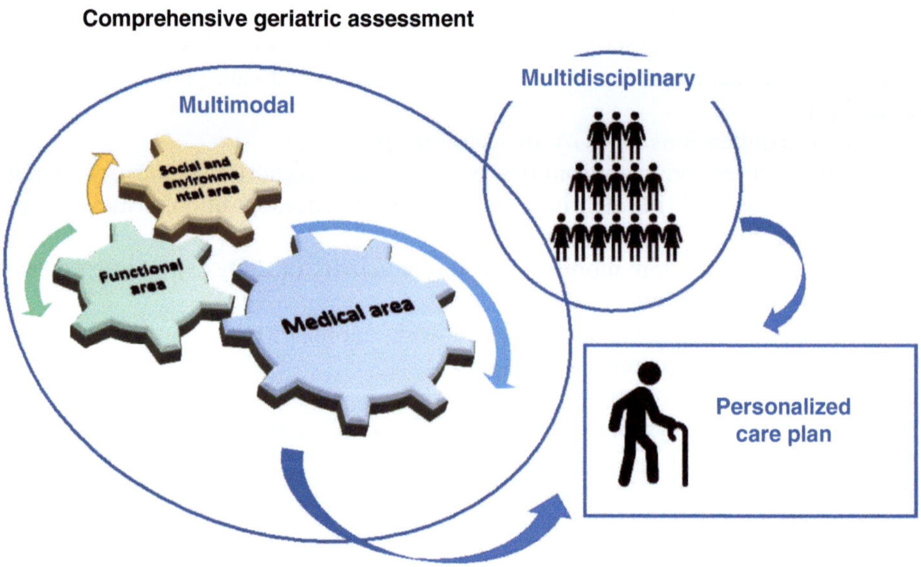

14.3 Scores and CGA

Many scores are used to evaluate each dimension of CGA. All these scores are validated in geriatric population. Some of them are described in previous specific chapter of the book. ☐ Table 14.1 presents the main scores used by CGA, but the list is non-exhaustive.

It is important to clarify that the CGA is not a list of scores, but a multidimensional evaluation that requires a real geriatric expertise acquired by practitioner over time. Scores are mainly useful for research and as screening tools to identify older patient requiring a real geriatric assessment.

14.4 Impact of CGA on Patient's Prognosis

Multiple studies have been interested about the effectiveness of CGA to improve prognosis of old patients. Results of these studies are contrasted for many reasons: first because of the complexity of CGA due to its multimodal aspects, second, because of the multiple possibilities of endpoint chosen for evaluation (short- and long-term mortality, loss of functional autonomy, new institutionalization, quality of life, etc.), and, third, because of great variety of healthcare setting and specific condition that could be evaluated. Because of these, we present in this part only the result of meta-analysis.

◘ Table 14.1 Example of scores

Dimensions	Scores
Comorbidities	Cumulative Illness Rating Scale (CIRS) [12] Charlson scale [13]
Cognition	Mini- Mental State Examination (MMSE) [14], Montreal Cognitive Assessment (MoCA) [15]
Depression	Geriatric Depression Scale (GDS) [16]
Delirium	Confusion Assessment Method (CAM) [17]
Mobility/sarcopenia/ risk of fall	Short Physical Performance Battery (SPPB) [18] Timed Up and Go Test [19] Handgrip [20]
Frailty	Frailty Index [21] Clinical Frailty Scale (CFS) [22]
Nutrition	Mini Nutritional Assessment (MNA) [23]
Functional status	Activity of Daily Living (ADL) [24] Instrumental Activity of Daily Living (IADL) [25]
Quality of life	SF-36, SF-12 Health Survey [26]
Caregiver's burden	Zarit Burden Interview (ZBI) [27]

14.4.1 Mortality

In 1993, a meta-analysis of 28 studies including 10,000 patients and controls concludes that CGA reduces mortality by 35% at 6 months for GEMU (OR 0.65; 95% CI 0.46–0.91) and by 14% at 36 months for HAS (OR 0.86; 95% CI 0.75–0.99) [8]. More recently, another meta-analysis of 17 trials including 4700 patients has evaluated the effects of inpatient rehabilitation specifically designed for geriatric patients. Mortality at discharge was reduced by 28% (OR 0.72; 95% CI 0.55–0.95), and long-term mortality (3–12 months) was reduced by 13% (OR 0.87; 95% CI 0.77–0.97) [28]. A meta-analysis evaluating the effectiveness of inpatient geriatric consultation team intervention concludes to a significant reduction of 6- and 8-month mortality (OR 0.66 and 95% CI 0.52–0.85 and OR 0.51 and 95% CI 0.31–0.85, respectively) [29]. On the other hand, a Cochrane meta-analysis published in 2011 concludes that CGA is associated with less mortality or deterioration (OR 0.76; 95% CI 0.64–0.90), but this effect is observed only for CGA ward and not for mobile team [30].

14.4.2 Functional Autonomy

The majority of meta-analysis about the impact of CGA on prognosis concludes to a significant effect on functional status. In hospital, Van Craen et al. found that admission to a GEMU has favorable effect with less decline in functional autonomy (RR 0.87, 95% CI 0.77–0.99) [7]. Admission in acute geriatric ward is also associated with a reduction of functional decline (RR 0.87; 95% CI 0.78–0.97) [31]. This positive effect is reinforced by Baztán et al. showing that compared with older people admitted to conventional care units, those admitted to acute geriatric units had a lower risk of functional decline at discharge (OR 0.82; 95% CI 0.68–0.99) [32]. For outpatient, preventive home visits have an impact to prevent functional decline only if the program includes a clinical examination (OR 0.64, 95% CI 0.48–0.87) [33].

14.4.3 Institutionalization

Several meta-analyses have evaluated the impact of CGA to prevent institutionalization. Hospitalization in geriatric acute care compared to conventional care unit reduces the risk to be discharged to a nursing home (RR = 0.82, 95% CI 0.68–0.99) [31] and give more chance to live at home after discharge (OR 1.30, 95% CI 1.11–1.52) [32]. Hospitalization in GEMU is also associated with lower rate of institutionalization 1 year after discharge (RR 0.78, 95% CI 0.66–0.92) [7]. Furthermore, CGA is associated with lower rate of institutionalization for CGA ward (OR 0.73, 95% CI 0.64–0.84) but not for CGA team (OR 1.16, 95% CI CI 0.83–1.63) [30].

14.5 Limits of CGA

The main limits of CGA are that it is time-consuming and it requires many actors. Because of dementia or delirium, many patients are non-informative or partially informative. To collect information about comorbidities and treatment, geriatricians need to often ask caregivers, attending physician, patient's usual pharmacist, or computerized medical records. Clinical examination and specific tests necessary to evaluate cognition, nutrition, frailty, mobility, and sarcopenia take often more time than in younger because of physical and mental limitations of geriatrics patients. Furthermore, the social and environmental evaluation sometimes look like a really "police investigation" and require a very long investigation by social workers.

14.6 CGA and ICU

In the context of ICU, there is no study evaluating the interest of CGA. However, due to the increase of old patients' admission in ICU, it seems to be necessary at different point of the patient trajectory.

14.6.1 At ICU Admission

ICU represents a great acute stress for old patient, because of the severity of the disease but also because of physical aggression represented by intubation, catheterization, or dialysis and because of environmental factors (light, noise). All old patients are not able to survive in good condition (without disability) to this stress. It's necessary to identify the most robust of them and for that to use CGA. Unfortunately, geriatricians are rarely associated to the decision of old patient admission in ICU. The first reason is probably there is no "culture" of collaboration between intensivist and geriatricians. The second (and not the least) is more pragmatic: decision of admission should be quick because of the severity of the patient, could occur 24/7 and geriatricians are not always available.

In this context, a detailed CGA is not possible, but it seems more and more important to adapt CGA to emergency context. Basic tools can be used to evaluate old patients' frailty like Clinical Frailty Scale (CFS). This pragmatic scale is associated with 1-month mortality in ICU (HR per point 1.1, 95% CI 1.05–1.15, $p < 0.001$) [34] and is repeatable whatever the assessor (ICU practitioner, nurse, dedicated study person) and the method of evaluation (information obtained from the patient, the family, or hospital records) with a weighted kappa for all measures of 0.86 and 95% CI 0.84–0.87 [35]. Nevertheless, this scale is probably insufficient even in emergency context and should be completed with an evaluation of comorbidities and polypharmacy.

14.6.2 During ICU Stay

A more complete CGA is probably feasible during ICU stay but requires a geriatrician. The role of the geriatrician could be to evaluate old patients in above dimensions but also their caregivers. Geriatrician could be helpful in ICU for delirium management, polypharmacy management, swallowing disorder management, or early rehabilitation, for example. It seems to be important that geriatricians integrate multidisciplinary team about withholding and withdrawing of life-sustaining therapy. In the past 15 years, specific geriatric emergency models have been developed as specific department [36] or multidisciplinary geriatric teams with encouraging results: decrease of ICU admission [37], functional decline [38], hospital admission rate [39, 40], and hospital readmission rate [40]. The top 10 of high-priority research questions for a European Research Agenda for Geriatric Emergency Medicine was recently published, highlighting the importance of this emergent specialty [41].

14.6.3 After ICU Discharge

After ICU discharge, management of geriatric patients is challenging. Indeed, many medical complications can occur in the few days post-ICU like infections, acute cardiac failure, or delirium. Furthermore, patients suffer often of swallowing disorder and critical illness neuromyopathy requiring early and specific rehabilitation.

Consideration around the clinical trajectory of old patients after ICU is necessary and CGA should take an important place. Specific geriatric post-ICU ward is lacking but could be very attractive to improve prognosis of these patients in the same model than ortho-geriatrics ward. Many publications highlight the effectiveness of ortho-geriatric unit to improve survival and functional autonomy post-hip fracture compared to standard of care in orthopedic unit. In a French cohort, survival of old patients 6 months after a hospitalization in ortho-geriatric unit for hip fracture was significantly higher than after a hospitalization in orthopedic unit (83.7% vs 74.6%; $p = 0.002$), and rehospitalizations were significantly reduced (26% vs 36%; $p < 0.001$) [42]. More recently, a prospective randomized study concluded that comprehensive geriatric care in a dedicated geriatric ward was associated with a greater mobility, functional autonomy, and quality of life 4 and 12 months after hip fracture compared to orthopedic care. Furthermore, comprehensive geriatric care had an 88% probability of being both less costly and more effective than orthopedic care [11]. Based on the ortho-geriatric model, dedicated geriatric post-ICU units should be developed as a clinical trajectory allowing an evaluation of the specific need of these patients and offering them a personalized, adapted program of care after ICU discharge.

Conclusion

Comprehensive geriatric assessment is the core of geriatric's care and is based on multidimensional and multi-professional care. Effectiveness of CGA has been proven particularly within dedicated geriatric wards. In emergency context, CGA could be adapted to be pragmatic and achievable by non-geriatricians. In ICU and especially after ICU discharge, CGA could improve prognosis of old patient and should be further developed in the future.

Take-Home Messages

- Comprehensive geriatric assessment is the core of geriatric's care.
- Comprehensive geriatric assessment is based on multidimensional and multi-professional care.
- Effectiveness of CGA has been proven in terms of improving survival, functional autonomy, and reduction of institutionalization.
- In emergency context, CGA could be adapted to be pragmatic and achievable by non-geriatricians.
- In ICU and especially after ICU discharge, CGA could improve prognosis of old patient and should be further developed in the future.

References

1. Matthews DA. Dr. Marjory Warren and the origin of British geriatrics. J Am Geriatr Soc. 1984;32(4):253–8.
2. Rubenstein LZ, Siu AL, Wieland D. Comprehensive geriatric assessment: toward understanding its efficacy. Aging (Milano). 1989;1(2):87–98.
3. National Institutes of Health Consensus Development Conference Statement: geriatric assessment methods for clinical decision-making. J Am Geriatr Soc. 1988;36(4):342–7.

4. Solomon DH. Geriatric assessment: methods for clinical decision making. JAMA. 1988;259(16):2450–2.
5. Parker SG, McCue P, Phelps K, McCleod A, Arora S, Nockels K, et al. What is comprehensive geriatric assessment (CGA)? An umbrella review. Age Ageing. 2018;47(1):149–55.
6. Pilotto A, Cella A, Pilotto A, Daragjati J, Veronese N, Musacchio C, et al. Three decades of comprehensive geriatric assessment: evidence coming from different healthcare settings and specific clinical conditions. J Am Med Dir Assoc. 2017;18(2):192.e1–192.e11.
7. Van Craen K, Braes T, Wellens N, Denhaerynck K, Flamaing J, Moons P, et al. The effectiveness of inpatient geriatric evaluation and management units: a systematic review and meta-analysis. J Am Geriatr Soc. 2010;58(1):83–92.
8. Stuck AE, Siu AL, Wieland GD, Adams J, Rubenstein LZ. Comprehensive geriatric assessment: a meta-analysis of controlled trials. Lancet. 1993;342(8878):1032–6.
9. Ellis G, Langhorne P. Comprehensive geriatric assessment for older hospital patients. Br Med Bull. 2004;71:45–59.
10. Extermann M, Aapro M, Bernabei R, Cohen HJ, Droz J-P, Lichtman S, et al. Use of comprehensive geriatric assessment in older cancer patients: recommendations from the task force on CGA of the International Society of Geriatric Oncology (SIOG). Crit Rev Oncol Hematol. 2005;55(3):241–52.
11. Prestmo A, Hagen G, Sletvold O, Helbostad JL, Thingstad P, Taraldsen K, et al. Comprehensive geriatric care for patients with hip fractures: a prospective, randomised, controlled trial. Lancet. 2015;385(9978):1623–33.
12. Linn BS, Linn MW, Gurel L. Cumulative illness rating scale. J Am Geriatr Soc. 1968;16(5):622–6.
13. Charlson ME, Pompei P, Ales KL, MacKenzie CR. A new method of classifying prognostic comorbidity in longitudinal studies: development and validation. J Chronic Dis. 1987;40(5):373–83.
14. Folstein MF, Folstein SE, McHugh PR. "Mini-mental state". A practical method for grading the cognitive state of patients for the clinician. J Psychiatr Res. 1975;12(3):189–98.
15. Nasreddine ZS, Phillips NA, Bédirian V, Charbonneau S, Whitehead V, Collin I, et al. The Montreal Cognitive Assessment, MoCA: a brief screening tool for mild cognitive impairment. J Am Geriatr Soc. 2005;53(4):695–9.
16. Yesavage JA, Brink TL, Rose TL, Lum O, Huang V, Adey M, et al. Development and validation of a geriatric depression screening scale: a preliminary report. J Psychiatr Res. 1982–1983;17(1):37–49.
17. Wei LA, Fearing MA, Sternberg EJ, Inouye SK. The Confusion Assessment Method: a systematic review of current usage. J Am Geriatr Soc. 2008;56(5):823–30.
18. Guralnik JM, Ferrucci L, Pieper CF, Leveille SG, Markides KS, Ostir GV, et al. Lower extremity function and subsequent disability: consistency across studies, predictive models, and value of gait speed alone compared with the short physical performance battery. J Gerontol A Biol Sci Med Sci. 2000;55(4):M221–31.
19. Podsiadlo D, Richardson S. The timed "Up & Go": a test of basic functional mobility for frail elderly persons. J Am Geriatr Soc. 1991;39(2):142–8.
20. Rijk JM, Roos PR, Deckx L, van den Akker M, Buntinx F. Prognostic value of handgrip strength in people aged 60 years and older: a systematic review and meta-analysis. Geriatr Gerontol Int. 2016;16(1):5–20.
21. Rockwood K, Stadnyk K, MacKnight C, McDowell I, Hébert R, Hogan DB. A brief clinical instrument to classify frailty in elderly people. Lancet. 1999;353(9148):205–6.
22. Rockwood K, Song X, MacKnight C, Bergman H, Hogan DB, McDowell I, et al. A global clinical measure of fitness and frailty in elderly people. CMAJ. 2005;173(5):489–95.
23. Vellas B, Guigoz Y, Garry PJ, Nourhashemi F, Bennahum D, Lauque S, et al. The Mini Nutritional Assessment (MNA) and its use in grading the nutritional state of elderly patients. Nutrition. 1999;15(2):116–22.
24. Katz S, Downs TD, Cash HR, Grotz RC. Progress in development of the index of ADL. The Gerontologist. 1970;10(1):20–30.
25. Lawton MP, Brody EM. Assessment of older people: self-maintaining and instrumental activities of daily living. The Gerontologist. 1969;9(3):179–86.
26. Gandek B, Ware JE, Aaronson NK, Apolone G, Bjorner JB, Brazier JE, et al. Cross-validation of item selection and scoring for the SF-12 Health Survey in nine countries: results from the IQOLA Project. International Quality of Life Assessment. J Clin Epidemiol. 1998;51(11):1171–8.
27. Zarit SH, Reever KE, Bach-Peterson J. Relatives of the impaired elderly: correlates of feelings of burden. The Gerontologist. 1980;20(6):649–55.

28. Bachmann S, Finger C, Huss A, Egger M, Stuck AE, Clough-Gorr KM. Inpatient rehabilitation specifically designed for geriatric patients: systematic review and meta-analysis of randomised controlled trials. BMJ. 2010;340:c1718.

29. Deschodt M, Flamaing J, Haentjens P, Boonen S, Milisen K. Impact of geriatric consultation teams on clinical outcome in acute hospitals: a systematic review and meta-analysis. BMC Med. 2013;11:48.

30. Ellis G, Whitehead MA, O'Neill D, Langhorne P, Robinson D. Comprehensive geriatric assessment for older adults admitted to hospital. Cochrane Database Syst Rev. 2011;(7):CD006211.

31. Fox MT, Persaud M, Maimets I, O'Brien K, Brooks D, Tregunno D, et al. Effectiveness of acute geriatric unit care using acute care for elders components: a systematic review and meta-analysis. J Am Geriatr Soc. 2012;60(12):2237–45.

32. Baztán JJ, Suárez-García FM, López-Arrieta J, Rodríguez-Mañas L, Rodríguez-Artalejo F. Effectiveness of acute geriatric units on functional decline, living at home, and case fatality among older patients admitted to hospital for acute medical disorders: meta-analysis. BMJ. 2009;338:b50.

33. Huss A, Stuck AE, Rubenstein LZ, Egger M, Clough-Gorr KM. Multidimensional preventive home visit programs for community-dwelling older adults: a systematic review and meta-analysis of randomized controlled trials. J Gerontol A Biol Sci Med Sci. 2008;63(3):298–307.

34. Guidet B, de Lange DW, Boumendil A, Leaver S, Watson X, Boulanger C, et al. The contribution of frailty, cognition, activity of daily life and comorbidities on outcome in acutely admitted patients over 80 years in European ICUs: the VIP2 study. Intensive Care Med. 2020;46(1):57–69.

35. Flaatten H, Guidet B, Andersen FH, Artigas A, Cecconi M, Boumendil A, et al. Reliability of the Clinical Frailty Scale in very elderly ICU patients: a prospective European study. Ann Intensive Care. 2021;11(1):22.

36. Hogan TM, Olade TO, Carpenter CR. A profile of acute care in an aging America: snowball sample identification and characterization of United States geriatric emergency departments in 2013. Acad Emerg Med Off J Soc Acad Emerg Med. 2014;21(3):337–46.

37. Grudzen C, Richardson LD, Baumlin KM, Winkel G, Davila C, Ng K, et al. Redesigned geriatric emergency care may have helped reduce admissions of older adults to intensive care units. Health Aff. 2015;34(5):788–95.

38. McCusker J, Verdon J, Tousignant P, de Courval LP, Dendukuri N, Belzile E. Rapid emergency department intervention for older people reduces risk of functional decline: results of a multicenter randomized trial. J Am Geriatr Soc. 2001;49(10):1272–81.

39. Harper KJ, Barton AD, Arendts G, Edwards DG, Petta AC, Celenza A. Controlled clinical trial exploring the impact of a brief intervention for prevention of falls in an emergency department. Emerg Med Australas. 2017;29(5):524–30.

40. Conroy SP, Ansari K, Williams M, Laithwaite E, Teasdale B, Dawson J, et al. A controlled evaluation of comprehensive geriatric assessment in the emergency department: the "Emergency Frailty Unit". Age Ageing. 2014;43(1):109–14.

41. Mooijaart SP, Nickel CH, Conroy SP, Lucke JA, van Tol LS, Olthof M, et al. A European Research Agenda for Geriatric Emergency Medicine: a modified Delphi study. Eur Geriatr Med. 2021;12(2):413–22.

42. Boddaert J, Cohen-Bittan J, Khiami F, Le Manach Y, Raux M, Beinis J-Y, et al. Postoperative admission to a dedicated geriatric unit decreases mortality in elderly patients with hip fracture. PLoS One. 2014;9(1):e83795.

Triage

Contents

Pre-ICU Triage: The Very Old Critically Ill Patient

Gavin M. Joynt

Contents

⊞ Learning Objectives

ICU resources are not unlimited, and in many circumstances frontline clinicians may be called upon to prioritize among patients who are referred for ICU care. When resources, manifested as ICU bed availability, are insufficient to offer ICU admission for all, some patients must be refused. There are concerns regarding this process of triage in the very elderly. On the one hand, some are concerned that the very elderly will be preferentially refused as a result of age discrimination, whereas others are concerned that the very elderly may receive inappropriately aggressive ICU care resulting in unnecessary suffering and pain, as well as consuming resources better redirected to the young.

This chapter will categorize the underlying reasons why very elderly patients may be refused ICU admission but focus on the process of triage in resource-restricted settings. A modified utilitarian approach will be used for justification of triage across all age groups, including the very elderly. Suggested methods of prioritization that avoid the need to directly and substantially consider chronological age will be described. A decision-making framework, coupled with a prioritization tool, is presented to inform the process of frontline triage.

15.1 Introduction

Intensive care is an expensive resource and, as a result, the availability of intensive care unit (ICU) beds is not unlimited [1]. The rapidly growing proportion of old patients in most countries is predicted to cause the unavailability of ICU resources worldwide [2]. In many countries, demand for beds outstrips supply, and processes to prioritize patients for access to the available resource have been developed. The term used to describe such prioritization is triage, and several national and international professional bodies and expert consensus groups have produced triage statements that justify currently agreed overarching principles of triage and sometimes propose methods of prioritization that offer practical advice for administrators and frontline healthcare workers [3–5]. The recent COVID-19 pandemic, by generating a substantial and often sustained need for more ICU resources, has brought the issue triage into immediate focus, even in those countries previously more generously supplied with ICU resources [6–8].

This chapter will focus on the triage of acute admissions in resource-limited settings. This implies the need for a rationing process as defined by the American Society of Critical Care Medicine task force on values, ethics and rationing in critical care "the allocation of potentially beneficial healthcare services to some individuals in the face of limited availability that necessarily involves the withholding of those services from other individuals" [4]. Resource-limited settings are those in which ICU bed availability is such that not all patients who may benefit from ICU admission can be admitted – thus prioritizing admissions is necessary. This may be a continuous situation in some countries where ICU is chronically under-resourced [3, 9–11], or may occur temporarily when systems are stressed, such as in many North American and European countries during the COVID pandemic [6–8, 12–14].

It is acknowledged that in many high-income countries with plentiful resources, and under normal circumstances, there may be few or no limitations regarding the ability to admit an individual patient. Much of the currently published ICU literature researching the admission and outcome characteristics of the very old is reported from such countries and in conditions where routine, daily rationing decisions are unusual. Regarding admission priority, the research questions set by these researchers have been focused on identifying which very old patients will benefit most from ICU admission and what meaningful short-, medium- and long-term outcomes for the very old may be expected in this patient group [15–17]. This information is important and informative, allows meaningful "goal of care" discussions with patients/ surrogates pre-ICU admission, advises the decision to admit or not, as well as potentially determines intensity and duration of intensive care provided. However, in this setting decision-making is focused on the needs and wishes of the individual patient and involves shared decision-making with the patient taking into account the benefits and burdens of ICU care. This contrasts with the meaning of triage, which specifically addresses the need for prioritization in the face of limited resources. It is triage in the face of limited resources, particularly in the context of an ageing population, that is the focus of this chapter.

15.2 Principles of Triage

When ICU resources, in this case available ICU beds, are insufficient to allow all requests for ICU admission, some patients must be refused admission. A minority of requests for ICU care may be refused because ICU admission would not result in additional benefit to the patient in comparison with alternatives such as continued general ward care, or alternative higher levels of care such as specialized care units, or high dependency units. These patients may be relatively well and not require ICU care to enhance survival, or other outcome benefits (the "too well" to benefit), or are so severely ill that ICU care would also not reasonably provide additional survival, or other outcome benefits (the "too sick" to benefit). Such "non-beneficial" or "futile" care can be reasonably refused [18, 19]. It should be highlighted, however, that these patients would be refused ICU admission, even in the presence of abundant resources, as there is no justification for the consumption of the additional costs associated with "non-beneficial" ICU care. However, what really concerns us is when we are faced with the need to refuse those patients who may reasonably be expected to derive some additional benefit from ICU admission and subsequent care. These patients are those correctly referred for ICU admission because they do have a realistic chance of benefit, even if this benefit may be relatively small. For these appropriately referred patients, a refusal to admit the patient results in likely harm [20–23]. Pre-ICU admission triage addresses the complex and difficult process of choosing among individual patients that would all likely benefit from admission; in other words, who will receive access to ICU care and who will not? This chapter will address the difficult process of triage, highlight some of the key and challenging issues specific to the very old and propose a guidance framework that may assist frontline ICU clinicians to fairly prioritize those very old patients referred to them for ICU admission.

A brief justification, using a principled approach and ethical reasoning, that underlies the purpose of triage follows. Doctors in general approach patient care with certain values uppermost in their minds. Such values include the desire to preserve human life, to protect or improve health and to use available resources effectively and efficiently while respecting personal dignity, maintaining the therapeutic relationship and protecting the least well-off [24]. However, when resources are limited, some generally accepted healthcare values such as autonomy, and fidelity to the individual patient, that are normally so much part of the doctor-patient relationship have to be have to be compromised [25]. The balancing of these values and establishing a hierarchy of necessity and/or importance, as to which values can be retained and which forgone or compromised, is essential. In the context of triage, some of the key arguments follow.

To begin with, ICU admission triage should only occur when ICU beds are insufficient to allow all referred patients who may benefit to be admitted (even if that benefit is small). Therefore all reasonable efforts to increase the resource (ICU bed availability) should have been exhausted, and some documentation of these efforts should be available [7, 10].

Given that all appropriately referred patients cannot be admitted, the triage (prioritization) must be achieved in a fair way and meet the requirements of the principle of justice [26]. It would, of course, be fair to all to admit on the basis of lottery, as each individual would have the same chance of admission. Simply choosing patients on the basis of "first come, first served" does represent a form of natural lottery. However, if this were done, some patients with very poor chance of benefiting from ICU care would still be admitted, while some patients with a very high chance of benefit would be refused, simply on the basis of the time point that they were referred for admission. Thus the efficient use of ICU would be compromised. To avoid this loss of utility of this expensive and limited resource, a pragmatically better use of ICU beds could be achieved by preferentially admitting those patients most likely to benefit from the available ICU resources. The utilitarian ethical approach justifies actions that will provide the greatest benefit to the greatest number of individuals in a society [27, 28]. Using a modified utilitarian approach, preferentially admitting those patients more likely to benefit, should result in a greater overall benefit to society from available resources. Clearly, the required consumption of ICU resources can be similarly considered, to provide a combined maximized cost-benefit assessment, thus optimizing the benefit derived from available ICU beds. Recent international consensus guidance documents addressing triage in the context of limited resources in the intensive care setting have favoured the approach of maximizing efficiency, utilizing the modified utilitarian justification for prioritizing admissions to intensive care [3, 4, 29, 30]. While this utilitarian justification underpins the approach to triage that follows, it should be acknowledged that it is not universally accepted and has been criticized by some [28, 31].

Finally, apart from the utilitarian consideration that all triage decisions should be made on medical health grounds only, no consideration for priority should be dependent on patient race, gender, age, religion, socio-economic importance, social standing or personal beliefs [10].

It remains important that proposed triage policies should respect the relationship between healthcare workers, patients and the wider public, and therefore it follows that they are justified and defensible when published and remain so over time. Policy implementation therefore requires transparency, accountability and mechanisms for review and appeal by affected stakeholders [32].

Because resources are, in the main, provided by society, and utilized by society's individual members, and the process of triage is complex, both in terms of moral justification and bedside implementation, triage should not be reliant on the solitary judgment of individuals, but should be guided by clear institutional policies. These policies require both relevant stakeholder review and validation from a broad spectrum of opinion [33].

15.3 Key Issues in the Very Old

15.3.1 Avoidance of Age Prejudice

Society increasingly expects that the aged are not unfairly prejudiced on the basis of their chronological age [34]. Additionally, as advanced age is associated with a reduction in physical and often mental ability, the old risk becoming increasingly vulnerable, and if identified as vulnerable, deserve the extra protections that are provided to the vulnerable in our societies [35]. A legitimate concern in countries with well-resourced medical facilities is that the aged may be unfairly excluded from ICU admission. There is evidence from several studies that triage decisions to refuse referred patients' ICU admission are associated with increasing chronological age [20–23]. This raises the question about unfair exclusion on the basis of age. A recent, well-constructed, cluster-randomized clinical trial sheds some light on the answer to this question. In this study, the promotion of the systematic ICU admission of critically ill very old patients was compared with usual practice, to establish whether increased ICU admission would benefit this very old group. Benefit was defined as the reduction of 6-month mortality. The result did show the expected increase in ICU admission in this group (almost by double), but 6-month mortality was not reduced, and neither functional status nor physical quality of life of those admitted was enhanced [36]. This and other recent similar findings raise many questions about current methods of assessing the appropriateness of admission to ICU for the old; however they do not provide evidence of the inappropriate withholding of ICU care to the old, at least in well-resourced medical systems [36, 37]. Nevertheless, as the numerical increase in the very old group of patients referred to ICU for care will continue to rise, even in the absence of critical ICU bed resource limitations, there remains a pressing need to establish robust admission criteria that are informed by accurate prognoses of relevant outcomes and costs. Such criteria are essential to prevent unnecessary burdens of ICU care being imposed on individuals and also to prevent excessive wastage of a very expensive resource.

If we return to circumstances where resources are limited and thus restrict admissions, which is the focus of this chapter, it is the objective that pre-ICU admission triage should be, as far as possible, fairly distributed among all ages.

15.3.2 The Effect of Age on Outcome Prognosis

While respecting the need to avoid age prejudice, a strong case can be made that age may have a legitimate influence on a triage decision for two objective reasons. The first relates to the reality that older patients, in general, have a shorter life expectancy than younger patients. Thus if benefit is quantified by the duration that that benefit may be enjoyed, for example, by life years gained, then older patients, all other things being equal, will necessarily derive less benefit than younger patients. This measure naturally has a greater magnitude when patients are toward the extreme of age, or the patients competing for the limited ICU beds are substantially younger than the very old. When considering quality of life, we need to be cautious. Although long-term quality of life after ICU discharge may appear relatively poor in the very old when compared with younger cohorts, it does appear to be similar to age-matched populations [38, 39]. Nevertheless, in regions where resources are an important consideration, it is revealing to consider outcomes in terms of quality-adjusted life years (QALYs). Data from Kaarlola et al. showed that the QALYs resulting from ICU admission in patients over 80 years would be a median of 4.1 years, in the 65–69-year-old group 10.2 years and in patients less than 65 years up to 22 years [38]. Exactly how much difference justifies a differential pre-ICU triage decision is a very difficult question to answer, and some have argued strongly that this type of calculation cannot be morally or legally justified [40, 41]. Because of this moral uncertainty, and no small controversy, it seems prudent to restrict the influence of life years or QALYs gained on triage decisions and, if used, to be a consideration of subsidiary importance. For example, either life years saved or QALYs gained could be considered only when directly competing patients otherwise have identical priority for admission, as described later.

The second reason age may reasonably influence a pre-admission triage decision, relates to the general effect of age on prognosis for survival and quality of life and thus negatively affects the benefit that may be derived from ICU admission. Regarding survival, there is overwhelming evidence that age, particularly extreme age, has a negative effect on short-, medium- and long-term prognosis. Crude mortality in the very old following ICU admission has been reported recently and ranged from 12–20% within the ICU, 24–26% within hospital, to 44–50% at 12 months and beyond [42–46]. Heyland et al. reported that only one quarter of very old patients who were admitted to ICU returned to pre-ICU admission of physical function at 1 year [15]. Another study reported similar findings and showed an association between poor functionality pre-ICU admission and poorer 1-year functional outcomes [45]. Not surprisingly, patient chronological age has been reported to be associated with triage decisions in resource-restricted settings [20, 22, 47, 48]; however there are many important problems with the use of a patient's chronological age as a criterion for triage. These include strong ethical arguments on the basis of age discrimination and criticisms of chronological age alone as a predictor of outcome in individual very old patients [34, 40, 41, 49].

15.3.3 Are There Better Alternative Prognosticators of Outcome than Age?

While age itself is clearly associated with relatively poor outcomes, both in terms of survival and quality of life, it is increasingly evident that not all patients of the same chronological age have the same outcome. In addition, the magnitude of this effect in an individual is sometimes difficult to measure and requires careful evaluation in individual cases. The effect of age on survival prognosis is complex. Factors such as co-morbidity resulting from chronic disease are known to increase with age and are associated with poorer prognoses. Other measures of pre-ICU admission health, such as frailty (a multi-faceted syndrome associated with the effects of age, but not fully determined by age), and measures of functional status are most likely to offer a more objective insights into likely prognosis for survival than the use of chronological age alone and are therefore more attractive to inform rationing decisions [50]. The use of such measures are also more attractive from an ethical and moral reasoning standpoint [41, 49].

There is a reasonable body of observational research that supports the potential use of frailty, most frequently and conveniently measured by the Clinical Frailty Scale (CFS) [51], as a prognostic marker at the time of referral to ICU. A systematic review and meta-analysis concluded that measures of increased frailty were associated with higher hospital and long-term mortality [52]. In the large multi-centre "VIP1" study, a positive linear relationship between the measured CFS of emergency ICU admissions and 30-day mortality from 30% with a CFS of 3 to 75% for a CFS of 9 was demonstrated [16]. More importantly, frailty also predicts survival in younger age groups. A large cohort study identified that increasing frailty was associated with increased long-term (median 7 years) mortality in middle-aged and older adults [53]. Brummel et al. also demonstrated that frailty in patients younger than 65 was associated with lower survival [54] and that approximately half of all frail patients were <65 years old. Similarly, a prospective cohort of patients from North America demonstrated that in those patients admitted to ICU aged 50–65, frailty remained associated with adjusted 12-month mortality risk [55]. Thus utilizing frailty, for example, in the form of the CFS, to prioritize prognosis is attractive, as it can be used across age groups and is a reasonably good predictor of short- to medium-term mortality. The CFS is, however, not a universally robust predictor by itself [56], and as a result it still appears necessary that when individual prognostication is required to make an on the spot triage decision, such prognostication should be informed by more than one category of predictor [57] and be made by experienced frontline ICU clinicians [7, 11]. Other known categories of prognostic indicators that can be rapidly assessed at the bedside include number of organ failures (or SOFA score), functional ability or co-morbidity by a simple score such as a modified ASA score, etc [58–60]. Intuitive survival prognostication by clinicians is also important and has been shown to be at least equivalent to individual prognostic scores [61, 62].

15.3.4 Quality of Life as an Outcome

Quality of life is a largely personal assessment, and unless the predicted future quality of life is likely to be extremely poor (e.g. end-stage dementia or minimally conscious state), it is not recommended as a justification of a triage decision to decline ICU care [10]. This cautious approach is taken for the following reason. An important distinction must be made between functional restriction and perceived quality of life. It has been shown that objective functional restrictions in the old do not necessarily impact on reported quality of life [38]. It is not easy to discuss the patient's perception of quality of life at the time of an emergency admission, and an error frequently made by healthcare providers is the assumption that functional health restrictions are automatically associated with reduced quality of life. Understanding that this is frequently not a valid association is critical to recognize, so that appropriate caution is exercised when invoking a reduction of quality of life to justify a triage decision to refuse or limit ICU care.

15.3.5 Respecting Individual Autonomy

As the very old have an increased incidence of severe co-morbidity and extreme frailty, as well as cognitive decline, the patient may themselves wish to avoid the burdens of ICU care and rehabilitation or limit their exposure to such burdens. Therefore, while an honest evaluation and clear communication with the patient and/or surrogate of likely prognosis, and the benefits and burdens of ICU care, forms an important part of a "goals of care" discussion in all patients, it is especially important in the very old. Some patients who have been offered ICU care may therefore elect to exercise their autonomy at the time of referral by declaring their preference to refuse ICU admission [63]. Sensitivity regarding the timing of a "goals of care discussion" is required, and such discussions should generally be avoided until after a final triage decision to admit/or not is made. This is because modified utilitarian triage prioritizes distributive justice (and societal good) over autonomy and patient preference. It can then be anticipated that a patient or surrogate who, after a discussion, elects to accept ICU care would likely be distressed if then advised they are not eligible as a result of a negative triage decision.

15.4 The Potential Use of the "Time-Limited Trial" at Pre-admission Triage

Being relatively compared, there is no consistent objective evidence that the very old are more likely than younger patients to have a prolonged ICU length of stay (LOS) after an individual ICU admission [52]. Nevertheless, for all patients admitted to ICU, LOS is an important consideration if maximum benefit from available ICU resources is to be achieved [10].

The concept of time-limited trials of therapy is gaining ground as an acceptable way to set limits to invasive treatments when individual patients fail to respond to initially aggressive therapy. They are also potentially useful to mitigate medical uncertainty about the likely response to intensive care treatment and the subsequent outcomes, in that doctors may feel more comfortable to prognosticate after seeing whether there is an initial response to therapy. Medical decision-makers may sometimes be overwhelmed by the potential consequence of the illness facing them, and this may make them unable to make rapid, thoughtful decisions. In the face of this uncertainty, the use of a time-limited trial is sometimes useful to provide more time to better assess patient's chances of a meaningful recovery, more thoroughly establish a trusting relationship with the family and allow more time for treating doctors to reach a considered consensus about prognosis. Briefly, a time-limited trial establishes an agreement between the healthcare team and the patient/surrogate, prior to admission, to apply the necessary intensive care therapies for a fixed period of time. The treatment team keeps the family informed of progress, and when the pre-agreed time limit is reached, life support therapies are either continued if the patient has responded positively to therapy, or withdrawn if therapy is failing [64]. Setting an appropriate time period for the trial is challenging, and dependent on careful clinical assessment of the patient's specific condition, balanced with resource availability. Some general guidance has been published, and it has been suggested that from 3 to 7 days would be appropriate for hypoxic-ischaemic encephalopathy, end-stage cardiac failure and other similar conditions, while longer (1–2 weeks) may be required for conditions such as stroke [64]. A recent review suggested a time limit of at least 24–72 h for acute conditions in potentially terminal patients [65]. This overview recommended that the end points of time-limited trials be categorized into narrowly and broadly defined goals [65]. Narrowly defined goals are focused on specific trends in laboratory values (e.g. lactate concentrations), organ failure scores (e.g. changes in SOFA scores [59]), dependence on circulatory support (e.g. vasopressor dose), weaning efforts, etc. and are suited to acute conditions such as severe pneumonia, abdominal infections and septic shock. On the other hand, more broadly defined goals such as wakefulness, mobility, responsiveness and potential future independence are more suited to patients with traumatic brain injury, stroke or infectious brain injury. While there is currently little high-quality evidence of the benefit of time-limited trials compared to routine practice, if conducted well, time-limited trials have the potential to reduce the length of ICU stay and improve patient/surrogate satisfaction.

The concept of the time-limited trial was born out of patient-centred end-of-life considerations but may potentially be applied to the pre-ICU triage decision-making process in a constructive way. As discussed earlier, a key consideration in making the triage decision to admit or refuse admission is an assessment of the anticipated resource utilization of a referred patient with an only moderate medium- or long-term prognosis. If, once admitted, the patient's access to ICU resources is unlimited, and their clinical condition one that is known to likely require a long ICU stay, with many potential complications, and thus a high cost of ICU resources, refusal on the basis of anticipated resource use and thus a relatively poor incremental cost-benefit gain could be justified. However, uncertainty remains. Some patients may respond rapidly to therapy, without suffering complications, and obtain an acceptable outcome with little resource use. At the moment of admission, it is unknown if the patient will fall into the subgroup of patients who will do unexpectedly well in a short time, or those who will consume many days or weeks of resources, for occasionally good, or more often much poorer outcomes. In this setting, an agreed time-limited trial would allow the triage decision-maker to recommend ICU admission, with greater certainty about the upper limit of the resource cost, and perhaps greater certainty of ultimate patient outcome after a limited trial of ICU care.

15.5 Practical Implications: An Overall Approach to Triage Including the Very Old

15.5.1 Proposed Framework and Bedside Advisory Tool

Taking into account the specific issues discussed above leads us to adapt triage policies and guidelines to accommodate, in a direct way, a number of the key factors that apply to the very old. For example, by incorporating measures of function, frailty and co-morbidity into prognosis estimation, the potentially direct relationship between chronological age and a triage decision can be de-emphasized, and fairness across all ages becomes more attainable. With this principle in mind, the following approach to triage seeks to accommodate fairness to the very old while remaining a universal framework applicable to all ages and proposes an example of how a front-line triage tool may be constructed.

A key foundation of the tool is that pre-ICU triage should be fair to all patients, regardless of age. Therefore all patients of all ages may be considered part of the same triage "pool" and are be prioritized accordingly. Prioritization for admission should be based on a comparative incremental medical cost-benefit assessment. Thus patients with the greatest benefit relative to cost should receive priority to maximize efficiency of the available ICU beds. Incremental benefit means the extra benefit likely gained in comparison with likely outcome if the patient were left at the highest available alternative level of care (e.g. general ward, high care unit). An overall decision-making framework is shown schematically in ◘ Fig. 15.1 [11, 66].

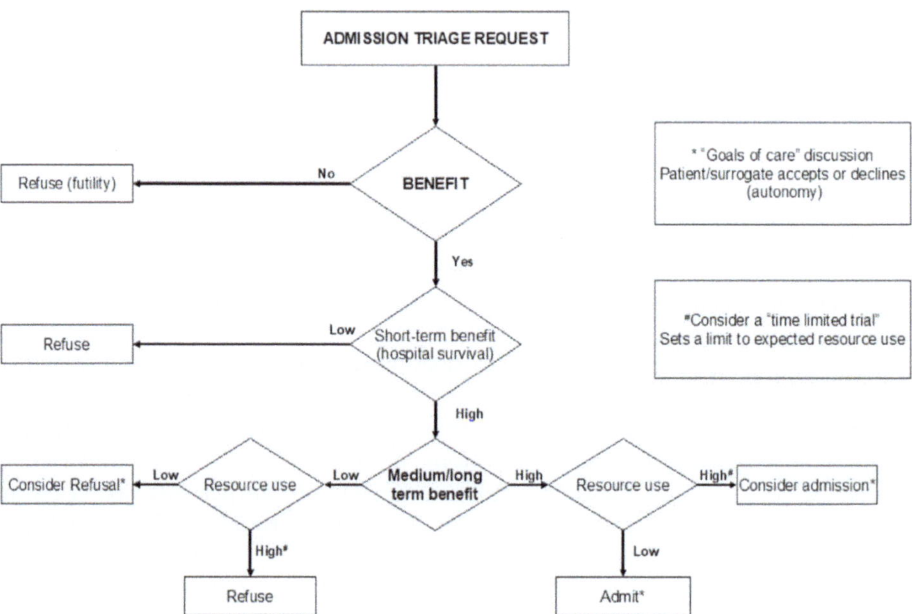

◘ **Fig. 15.1** Triage (prioritization) decisions are complex clinical decisions enforced by the lack of sufficient ICU beds to accommodate all appropriate referrals. A transparent decision-making process is necessary to improve decision-making consistency. Estimating likely benefit (comparing likely outcome after ICU admission against the likely outcomes if the patient remained in the ward/other high care area) prioritizes patients who will benefit most. This conceptual algorithm outlines the decision-making process for triage. Decision thresholds are relevant for the particular setting, and stricter thresholds may be utilized during substantial surges of referrals (e.g. pandemics) or reduction in resources (e.g. closure of ICU beds). Long-term benefit (≥6-month survival) may include an assessment of expected quality of life, if considered appropriate. Notes: Prior to ICU admission, patient preference for admission should be explored during a "goals of care" discussion. Resource use is most practically predicted by estimating ICU length of stay, and this may be prospectively determined by agreeing a reasonable upper limit of duration of aggressive therapy through the process of a "time-limited trial". (Figure adapted and modified from [11, 66])

As no single, validated, objective prognostication score or tool to accurately prognosticate ICU survival (or duration of survival post-ICU admission) exists [67], prognostication should be based on a combination of rapidly available clinical information that incorporates aspects of co-morbidity, baseline function and physiological reserve, as well as the severity of the acute illness. An example of a bedside priority advisory tool is shown. It has been adapted and modified from one initially proposed for COVID-19 triage and is shown in ◘ Fig. 15.2 [7, 11].

Once inclusion and exclusion criteria are satisfied, prognosis is determined by assessing a combination of frailty (CFS), co-morbidity (modified ASA score as shown in ◘ Table 15.1) and acute disease severity (number of organ failures, assessed by clinical judgment, or by SOFA score). While the priorities focus on prognosis for short- to medium-term survival, the resource cost of an admission to ICU must also be considered. The cost of ICU care is many orders of magnitude greater than the cost of ward care, and directly proportional to the number of days the patient spends in ICU. Thus incremental resource cost may reasonably be estimated by considering the anticipated ICU LOS, and incorporated into final decision-making (◘ Fig. 15.2), bearing in mind that mean ICU LOS, while varying on the basis of diagnosis, co-morbidity and severity of acute illness, is generally not affected by age itself [52].

The magnitude of incremental cost-benefit (triage threshold) required for a referred patient to achieve sufficient priority for admission should be determined by local circumstances and protocols. In the interests of fairness, and to demonstrate consistency of decision-making to referring medical teams, an attempt to maintain a constant triage threshold over time has advantages. However, during periods when resources are critically limited, triage thresholds may be higher, whereas when resources are more plentiful, the triage thresholds may be lowered. Triage exclusion decisions may be made when ICU beds are available, allowing consistency and sufficient bed availability to accommodate daily fluctuations in demand for admission. As local circumstances change over time, triage thresholds require revision from time to time, e.g. during temporary bed closures, or during the acute phases of the COVID-19 pandemic. When adjustments are made, they should be made by appropriate institutional committees and transparently communicated to frontline doctors and healthcare staff.

It should be noted that the percentage survival predictions that appear on the tool are absolute prognoses. The inclusion criteria set in the tool are such that it may be reasonably anticipated that patient mortality, if not admitted to ICU, would be >90%. Thus the estimated incremental mortality gained should be estimated to be 10% less than the absolute prognostic percentage given. This particular tool is thus approximately aligned with the estimates of incremental benefit required to receive priority for admission that were set in a recent South African consensus meeting on triage. South Africa has a moderate to severe shortfall of ICU resources in publicly funded ICUs, and an incremental survival benefit of >20–30% at 3–6 months was set, by consensus, as an example of an admission threshold for an average urban ICU [5].

Final bedside triage decisions should be made by, or directly supervised by, a senior intensive care specialist, who is generally the least conflicted by previous association with individual patients, has the best understanding of expected ICU outcomes and current ICU resource limitations and is best positioned to estimate the resource implications of potential admissions. Because of the high level of responsi-

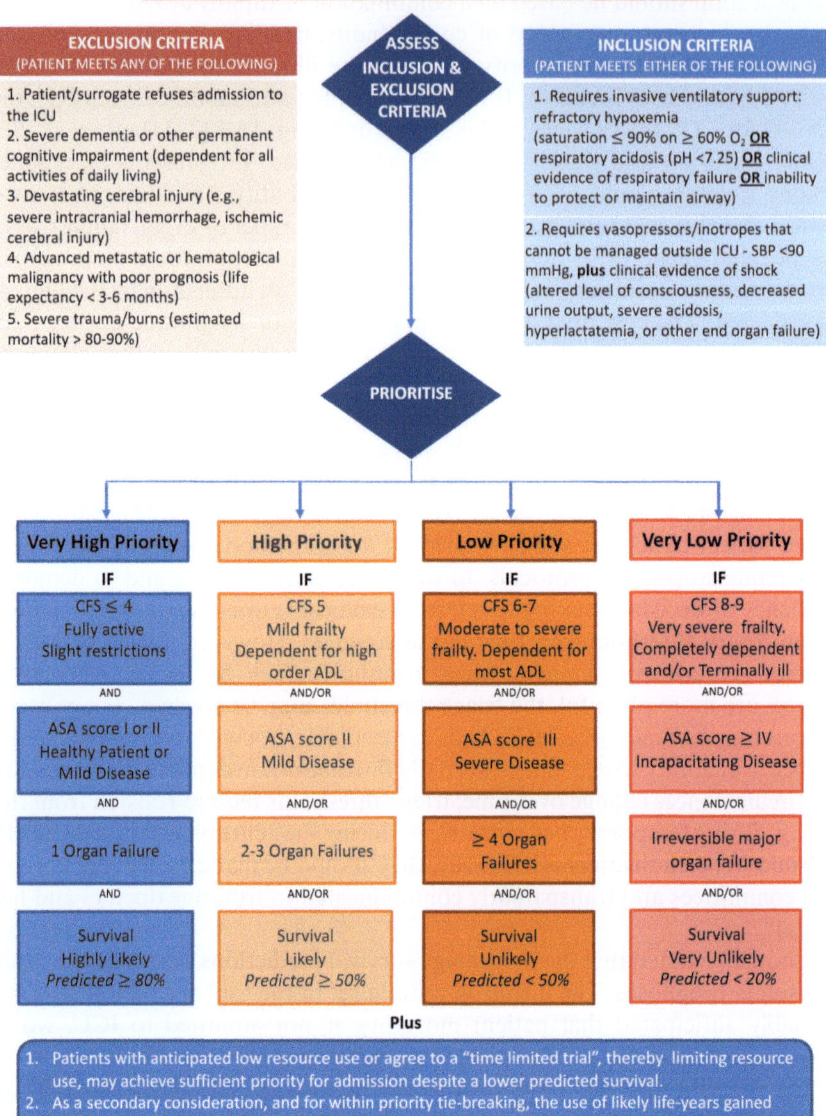

Fig. 15.2 An example of an ICU triage tool that may be considered (with the necessary modifications for local use) for use in ICU settings with limited available ICU beds. Such units are those that are forced to refuse admission to one or more appropriately referred patients on a daily basis [5]. In such a unit, it may be justified that admission should usually follow for patients assessed to be very high or high priority, regardless of anticipated length of stay (LOS) in ICU. Low-priority assignation should usually result in admission being declined, unless anticipated LOS is short and/or a "time-limited trial" has been agreed. In most circumstances those patients assessed as very low priority will be declined admission. Note that specific local policy should set/reset the triage threshold from time to time depending on the degree of resource availability (e.g. change in number of available ICU beds, or systematic change in number of patients queuing). (Adapted and modified from [7, 11])

◼ Table 15.1   Modified American Society of Anesthesiologists Score for use with the pre-ICU triage tool for use in ICUs with limited resources

American Society of Anesthesiologists (ASA) Score		
Class	Description	Example
I	Previously healthy and fit	Normal effort tolerance (comparison with peers)
II	Mild systemic controlled co-morbidity	No substantial functional limitations (examples are well-controlled diabetes/hypertension, mild pulmonary disease, effort tolerance $\geq$1–2 flights of stairs at normal pace)
III	Severe but not incapacitating co-morbidity	Measurable functional limitations (examples are poorly controlled diabetes/hypertension, COPD, reduction of cardiac ejection fraction, effort tolerance < flight of stairs at normal pace, end-stage renal disease, previous myocardial infarction, stroke, TIA, or coronary artery disease)
IV	Incapacitating co-morbidity	Severe functional limitations (examples include ongoing cardiac ischemia or severe valve dysfunction, severe reduction of ejection fraction, or effort tolerance restricted to short distances on level ground)
V	Moribund	Not expected to survive 24 h (massive trauma, severe intracranial bleed with substantial mass effect, extensive ischemic bowel, end-stage cardiac failure, multiple or irreversible organ system failures)

Adapted and simplified from: ▶ https://www.asahq.org/standards-and-guidelines/asa-physical-status-classification-system
Modified and adapted from [60]

bility attached to triage decisions, and their complexity, all doctors responsible for triage decisions should receive appropriately supervised training.

Disagreements between referring teams and the ICU triage supervisor should be dealt with by formal mechanisms involving senior hospital management structures. Finally, it must be remembered, to ensure fairness between competing individual patients, triage decisions should be made without patient/surrogate consent [68].

Practical Implications

While final decisions remain the task of senior ICU clinicians, the framework and tool should serve to encourage understanding, communication, consistency and transparency among key stakeholders.

15.5.2   Justification and Limitations

Although it has been previously recommended that the pre-ICU triage process for very old patients should differ from processes for the less old, and should ideally be informed by different tools than those used for younger patients [69, 70], an opposite approach has been described. It is hoped that the use of a single decision-making process and triage tool for all ages will minimize age-related prejudice and negate the need to specifically consider age alone as a factor in triage decisions. Although age is related to prognosis, and thus the likelihood of benefiting from ICU, if we instead focus on age-related deterioration in function, cognition and physiological reserve, and directly assess these factors, it should serve to eliminate chronological age as the dominant factor in triage decisions.

As no single scoring system is capable of integrating prognosis if admitted to ICU, prognosis at the alternative available level of care, predict ICU LOS, and quality of life considerations, it is necessary for the senior ICU triage decision-maker to make a clinical decision after taking these factors into account. The methods proposed provide a framework and tool firstly to outline the components of the decision and secondly to direct the decision-maker to the factors that may predict prognosis while including the provision for assessing predicted LOS. It is expected that these aids will improve the consistency of decision-making and perhaps the reliability of the ultimate decisions. The combination of multiple predictive components in the tool, reflecting prognostic predictors based on factors prior to the acute illness, the acute illness, and factors that predict outcome independent of age, should serve to mitigate the deficiencies of individual scores/components [57].

It must again be stressed that the contents of the triage tool example provided here are indicative only and should be modified for individual circumstances and changing knowledge and conditions. New and better prognostic scores can be added or replace existing components when they become available. Furthermore, while the framework principles remain constant, the triage tool is modifiable, both in terms of setting admission thresholds at stricter, or less strict, levels and in terms of substituting scores/components to suit local conditions. If triage thresholds are kept relatively consistent, it is expected that both ICU and referring clinicians can better understand the rationale and implementation of triage and become accustomed to consistent decision-making.

Several limitations must be acknowledged. The predicted survival percentages are designed to be in line with the interpretation of the results of the largely objective scores/components in the corresponding column. However, individual overriding factors, not captured by the tool components, may exist. Thus the key prognostic decision-making factor placing the patient in a priority group is the percentage expected survival. There must be open acknowledgement regarding the uncertainties inherent in prognostication, nevertheless decision-making consistency relies on a best attempt to achieve the most accurate prognosis possible, and it is anticipated that the provision of a framework and tool will ultimately assist the triage decision to be more consistent and reliable. The experience and training of the senior supervising triage decision-maker therefore should be an essential component of the implementation of the proposed method. Neither the proposed decision-making framework nor the triage tool has been prospectively tested for efficacy. The decision-making framework appears to be intuitively sound and formally underlies the triage protocols practised across public hospitals in Hong Kong. More recently the decision framework has been adopted by the Critical Care Society of Southern Africa to inform the development of frontline triage policy. However, in both cases individual units are encouraged to create local triage policies that adhere to the framework principle. The triage tool is relatively novel and, although the previously published tools on which it is based were formed through expert consensus [7, 11], has yet to be formally tested in practice. Thus any implementation of these or similar tools should be preceded by carefully considered development and modification, and transparent implementation in the institution and society where they will be applied.

The last limitation worthy of mention is the inability of the above triage process to provide guidance for prioritizing those patients that require "elective" ICU admission. This largely refers to those patients requiring post-operative care after elective interventional medical or surgical procedures. Such procedures can be considered life-saving, or at least life-changing interventions and of benefit to both the individual and society at large. Therefore, considerations should be made by individual units to reasonably accommodate elective surgery, recognizing that ICU length of stay post-operatively is generally short and resource use relatively small [71]. Nevertheless, it must be explicitly acknowledged that, from time to time, resource constraints imposed by the need to accommodate emergency cases may result in cancellation or delay of elective cases.

Conclusion

Many retrospective studies of triage have identified age as an important factor affecting admission, with older patients less likely to be admitted. The lower rate of admission may be related to several factors that limit the benefit that the very old may gain from admission, and the need to conserve resources that would benefit younger patients with better prognoses. However, extreme care must be exercised in maintaining fairness of distribution of resources and assessment of benefit, such that age itself only justifies exclusion because of the objective relationship that exists between age and prognosis. In this regard chronological age by itself is not a justification for supporting a triage decision, and benefit should be assessed equitably across all age groups. The approach to triage taken in this chapter attempts to place all ages on an equal footing, with medical prognosis and predicted resource being the only factor determining priorities. Thus the utilization of markers of prognosis such as frailty, co-morbidity, organ function and pre-admission function should be utilized so that priority for admission may be compared across age boundaries. Future research needs to seek even better markers of medical prognosis, and identifying a rapid, objective, cheap and accessible score(s) or physiological marker(s) remains the holy grail of prognostication. There is evidence from some well-conducted studies that poorer post-ICU admission function alone in the very old does not necessarily predict perceived quality of life, and extreme care should be taken in assessing a patient's likely quality of life post-ICU admission, especially if it has made a consideration during the triage decision. Regarding the assessment of the resource cost of ICU admission, when perceived likely benefits for admission to ICU are small, consideration could be made of offering limited trials of care, so that response to therapy may be observed and limited resources redistributed if therapeutic failure occurs.

Finally, those of us who are forced to triage regularly are acutely aware that triage decisions are never easy and often emotionally tough to implement. However much of a challenge they are for us, the patients and their doctors who are exposed to triage likely suffer more. It is our responsibility to be honest, fair, consistent and clear when making decisions and above all always communicate the outcome of decisions with empathy and sensitivity.

> **Take-Home Messages**
> — Studies of triage have identified age as an important factor affecting admission, with older patients less likely to be admitted.
> — Extreme care should be exercised in maintaining fairness of distribution of resources and assessment of benefit across all age groups, such that age itself only indirectly justifies exclusion because of the objective relationship that exists between age and prognosis in any particular individual.
> — Triage decisions are best made by senior ICU clinicians, and in a way that maximizes the overall incremental benefit received by the cohort of patients referred for ICU admission.
> — Markers of prognosis that are required to facilitate prioritization such as frailty, co-morbidity, organ function and pre-admission function should be used so that priority for admission may be compared across age boundaries.
> — The framework provided outlines the components of the triage decision, and the tool directs the decision-maker to the factors that may predict prognosis while including the provision for assessing predicted LOS.
> — It is expected that decision-making aids such as this one provided will improve the consistency of decision-making and possibly improve reliability of the ultimate decisions.
> — The combination of multiple predictive components in the tool, reflecting prognostic predictors based on factors prior to the acute illness, the acute illness, and factors that predict outcome independent of age, should serve to mitigate the deficiencies of individual scores/components.

References

1. Chin-Yee N, D'Egidio G, Thavorn K, Heyland D, Kyeremanteng K. Cost analysis of the very elderly admitted to intensive care units. Crit Care. 2017;21(1):109. https://doi.org/10.1186/s13054-017-1689-y.
2. Flaatten H, de Lange DW, Artigas A, Bin D, Moreno R, Christensen S, Joynt GM, Bagshaw SM, Sprung CL, Benoit D, Soares M, Guidet B. The status of intensive care medicine research and a future agenda for very old patients in the ICU. Intensive Care Med. 2017;43(9):1319–28. https://doi.org/10.1007/s00134-017-4718-z.
3. Blanch L, Abillama FF, Amin P, et al. Triage decisions for ICU admission: report from the Task Force of the World Federation of Societies of Intensive and Critical Care Medicine. J Crit Care. 2016;36:301–5. https://doi.org/10.1016/j.jcrc.2016.06.014.
4. Nates JL, Nunnally M, Kleinpell R, et al. ICU admission, discharge, and triage guidelines: a framework to enhance clinical operations, development of institutional policies, and further research. Crit Care Med. 2016;44(8):1553–602. https://doi.org/10.1097/ccm.0000000000001856.
5. Joynt GM, Gopalan DP, Argent AA, Chetty S, Wise R, Lai VKW, Hodgson E, Lee A, Joubert I, Mokgokong S, Tshukutsoane S, Richards GA, Menezes C, Mathivha RL, Espen B, Levy B, Asante K, Paruk F. The Critical Care Society of Southern Africa Consensus Guideline on ICU triage and rationing (ConICTri). S Afr Med J. 2019;109(8b):630–42. https://doi.org/10.7196/SAMJ.2019.v109i8b.13.
6. White DB, Lo B. A framework for rationing ventilators and critical care beds during the COVID-19 pandemic. JAMA. 2020;323(18):1773–4. https://doi.org/10.1001/jama.2020.5046.
7. Sprung CL, Joynt GM, Christian MD, Truog RD, Rello J, Nates JL. Adult ICU triage during the coronavirus disease 2019 pandemic: who will live and who will die? Recommendations to improve

survival. Crit Care Med. 2020;48(8):1196–202. https://doi.org/10.1097/CCM.0000000000004410. PMID: 32697491; PMCID: PMC7217126.

8. Maves RC, Downar J, Dichter JR, Hick JL, Devereaux A, Geiling JA, Kissoon N, Hupert N, Niven AS, King MA, Rubinson LL, Hanfling D, Hodge JG Jr, Marshall MF, Fischkoff K, Evans LE, Tonelli MR, Wax RS, Seda G, Parrish JS, Truog RD, Sprung CL, Christian MD, ACCP Task Force for Mass Critical Care. Triage of scarce critical care resources in COVID-19: an implementation guide for regional allocation: an expert panel report of the Task Force for Mass Critical Care and the American College of Chest Physicians. Chest. 2020;158(1):212–25. https://doi.org/10.1016/j.chest.2020.03.063.

9. Sprung CL, Baras M, Iapichino G, Kesecioglu J, Lippert A, Hargreaves C, Pezzi A, Pirracchio R, Edbrooke DL, Pesenti A, Bakker J, Gurman G, Cohen SL, Wiis J, Payen D, Artigas A. The Eldicus prospective, observational study of triage decision making in European intensive care units: part I--European Intensive Care Admission Triage Scores. Crit Care Med. 2012;40(1):125–31. https://doi.org/10.1097/CCM.0b013e31822e5692. PMID: 21926598.

10. Joynt GM, Gopalan DP, Argent AA, Chetty S, Wise R, Lai VKW, Hodgson E, Lee A, Joubert I, Mokgokong S, Tshukutsoane S, Richards GA, Menezes C, Mathivha RL, Espen B, Levy B, Asante K, Paruk F. The Critical Care Society of Southern Africa Consensus Statement on ICU triage and rationing (ConICTri). S Afr Med J. 2019;109(8b):613–29. https://doi.org/10.7196/SAMJ.2019.v109i8b.13947.

11. Joynt GM, Leung AKH, Ho CM, So D, Shum HP, Chow FL, Yeung AWT, Lee KL, Tang GKY, Yan WW. Admission triage tool for adult intensive care unit admission in Hong Kong during the COVID-19 outbreak. Hong Kong Med J. 2021; https://doi.org/10.12809/hkmj209033. Epub ahead of print.

12. Leclerc T, Donat N, Donat A, Pasquier P, Libert N, Schaeffer E, D'Aranda E, Cotte J, Fontaine B, Perrigault PF, Michel F, Muller L, Meaudre E, Veber B. Prioritisation of ICU treatments for critically ill patients in a COVID-19 pandemic with scarce resources. Anaesth Crit Care Pain Med. 2020;39(3):333–9. https://doi.org/10.1016/j.accpm.2020.05.008. Epub 2020 May 17. PMID: 32426441; PMCID: PMC7230138.

13. Valiani S, Terrett L, Gebhardt C, Prokopchuk-Gauk O, Isinger M. Development of a framework for critical care resource allocation for the COVID-19 pandemic in Saskatchewan. CMAJ. 2020;192(37):E1067–73. https://doi.org/10.1503/cmaj.200756.

14. Herreros B, Gella P, Real de Asua D. Triage during the COVID-19 epidemic in Spain: better and worse ethical arguments. J Med Ethics. 2020;46(7):455–8. https://doi.org/10.1136/medethics-2020-106352.

15. Heyland DK, Garland A, Bagshaw SM, Cook D, Rockwood K, Stelfox HT, Dodek P, Fowler RA, Turgeon AF, Burns K, Muscedere J, Kutsogiannis J, Albert M, Mehta S, Jiang X, Day AG. Recovery after critical illness in patients aged 80 years or older: a multi-center prospective observational cohort study. Intensive Care Med. 2015;41(11):1911–20. https://doi.org/10.1007/s00134-015-4028-2.

16. Flaatten H, De Lange DW, Morandi A, Andersen FH, Artigas A, Bertolini G, Boumendil A, Cecconi M, Christensen S, Faraldi L, Fjølner J, Jung C, Marsh B, Moreno R, Oeyen S, Öhman CA, Pinto BB, Soliman IW, Szczeklik W, Valentin A, Watson X, Zaferidis T, Guidet B, VIP1 Study Group. The impact of frailty on ICU and 30-day mortality and the level of care in very elderly patients (≥ 80 years). Intensive Care Med. 2017;43(12):1820–8. https://doi.org/10.1007/s00134-017-4940-8.

17. Guidet B, de Lange DW, Boumendil A, Leaver S, Watson X, Boulanger C, Szczeklik W, Artigas A, Morandi A, Andersen F, Zafeiridis T, Jung C, Moreno R, Walther S, Oeyen S, Schefold JC, Cecconi M, Marsh B, Joannidis M, Nalapko Y, Elhadi M, Fjølner J, Flaatten H, VIP2 Study Group. The contribution of frailty, cognition, activity of daily life and comorbidities on outcome in acutely admitted patients over 80 years in European ICUs: the VIP2 study. Intensive Care Med. 2020;46(1):57–69. https://doi.org/10.1007/s00134-019-05853-1.

18. Schneiderman LJ, Jecker NS, Jonsen AR. Medical futility: its meaning and ethical implications. Ann Intern Med. 1990;112(12):949–54.

19. Bosslet GT, Pope TM, Rubenfeld GD, Lo B, Truog RD, Rushton CH, Curtis JR, Ford DW, Osborne M, Misak C, Au DH, Azoulay E, Brody B, Fahy BG, Hall JB, Kesecioglu J, Kon AA, Lindell KO, White DB, American Thoracic Society ad hoc Committee on Futile and Potentially Inappropriate Treatment; American Thoracic Society; American Association for Critical Care Nurses; American College of Chest Physicians; European Society for Intensive Care Medicine; Society of Critical

Care. An official ATS/AACN/ACCP/ESICM/SCCM policy statement: responding to requests for potentially inappropriate treatments in intensive care units. Am J Respir Crit Care Med. 2015;191(11):1318–30. https://doi.org/10.1164/rccm.201505-0924ST.

20. Sprung CL, Geber D, Eidelman LA, Baras M, Pizov R, Nimrod A, Oppenheim A, Epstein L, Cotev S. Evaluation of triage decisions for intensive care admission. Crit Care Med. 1999;27(6):1073–9.
21. Azoulay E, Pochard F, Chevret S, Vinsonneau C, Garrouste M, Cohen Y, Thuong M, Paugam C, Apperre C, De Cagny B, Brun F, Bornstain C, Parrot A, Thamion F, Lacherade JC, Bouffard Y, Le Gall JR, Herve C, Grassin M, Zittoun R, Schlemmer B, Dhainaut JF, PROTOCETIC Group. Compliance with triage to intensive care recommendations. Crit Care Med. 2001;29(11):2132–6.
22. Joynt GM, Gomersall CD, Tan P, Lee A, Cheng CA, Wong EL. Prospective evaluation of patients refused admission to an intensive care unit: triage, futility and outcome. Intensive Care Med. 2001;27(9):1459–65. https://doi.org/10.1007/s001340101041.
23. Iapichino G, Corbella D, Minelli C, Mills GH, Artigas A, Edbooke DL, Pezzi A, Kesecioglu J, Patroniti N, Baras M, Sprung CL. Reasons for refusal of admission to intensive care and impact on mortality. Intensive Care Med. 2010;36(10):1772–9. https://doi.org/10.1007/s00134-010-1933-2.
24. Dougherty CJ. Ethical values at stake in health care reform. JAMA. 1992;268(17):2409–12.
25. Moskop JC, Iserson KV. Triage in medicine, part II: underlying values and principles. Ann Emerg Med. 2007;49(3):282–7. https://doi.org/10.1016/j.annemergmed.2006.07.012.
26. Beauchamp TL, Childress JF. Moral principles. Principles of biomedical ethics. New York: Oxford University Press; 2013.
27. Sanders JT. Why the numbers should sometimes count. Philos Publ Aff. 1988;17:3–14.
28. Baker R, Strosberg M. Triage and equality: an historical reassessment of utilitarian analyses of triage. Kennedy Inst Ethics J. 1992;2:103–23.
29. Christian MD, Joynt GM, Hick JL, Colvin J, Danis M, Sprung CL, European Society of Intensive Care Medicine's Task Force for intensive care unit triage during an influenza epidemic or mass disaster. Chapter 7. Critical care triage. Recommendations and standard operating procedures for intensive care unit and hospital preparations for an influenza epidemic or mass disaster. Intensive Care Med. 2010;36 Suppl 1(Suppl 1):S55–64. https://doi.org/10.1007/s00134-010-1765-0.
30. Christian MD, Sprung CL, King MA, Dichter JR, Kissoon N, Devereaux AV, Gomersall CD, Task Force for Mass Critical Care; Task Force for Mass Critical Care. Triage: care of the critically ill and injured during pandemics and disasters: CHEST consensus statement. Chest. 2014;146(4 Suppl):e61S–74S. https://doi.org/10.1378/chest.14-0736.
31. American Thoracic Society Bioethics Task Force. Fair allocation of intensive care unit resources. Am J Respir Crit Care Med. 1997;156(4):1282–301. https://doi.org/10.1164/ajrccm.156.4.ats7-97.
32. Daniels N. Accountability for reasonableness. BMJ. 2000;321(7272):1300–1.
33. Tomlinson T, Czlonka D. Futility and hospital policy. Hast Cent Rep. 1995;25(3):28–35.
34. Bowling A. Honour your father and mother: ageism in medicine. Br J Gen Pract. 2007;57(538):347–8.
35. Bozzaro C, Boldt J, Schweda M. Are older people a vulnerable group? Philosophical and bioethical perspectives on ageing and vulnerability. Bioethics. 2018;32(4):233–9. https://doi.org/10.1111/bioe.12440.
36. Guidet B, Leblanc G, Simon T, Woimant M, Quenot JP, Ganansia O, Maignan M, Yordanov Y, Delerme S, Doumenc B, Fartoukh M, Charestan P, Trognon P, Galichon B, Javaud N, Patzak A, Garrouste-Orgeas M, Thomas C, Azerad S, Pateron D, Boumendil A, ICE-CUB 2 Study Network. Effect of systematic intensive care unit triage on long-term mortality among critically ill elderly patients in France: a randomized clinical trial. JAMA. 2017;318(15):1450–9. https://doi.org/10.1001/jama.2017.13889.
37. Boumendil A, Angus DC, Guitonneau AL, Menn AM, Ginsburg C, Takun K, Davido A, Masmoudi R, Doumenc B, Pateron D, Garrouste-Orgeas M, Somme D, Simon T, Aegerter P, Guidet B, ICE-CUB Study Group. Variability of intensive care admission decisions for the very elderly. PLoS One. 2012;7(4):e34387. https://doi.org/10.1371/journal.pone.0034387. Epub 2012 Apr 11. PMID: 22509296; PMCID: PMC3324496.
38. Kaarlola A, Tallgren M, Pettila V. Long-term survival, quality of life, and quality-adjusted life-years among critically ill elderly patients. Crit Care Med. 2006;34(8):2120–6.
39. Andersen FH, Flaatten H, Klepstad P, Romild U, Kvåle R. Long-term survival and quality of life after intensive care for patients 80 years of age or older. Ann Intensive Care. 2015;5(1):53. https://doi.org/10.1186/s13613-015-0053-0.

40. Erasmus N. Age discrimination in critical care triage in South Africa: the law and the allocation of scarce health resources in the COVID-19 pandemic. S Afr Med J. 2020;110(12):1172–5.
41. den Exter A. View. The Dutch critical care triage guideline on Covid-19: not necessarily discriminatory. Eur J Health Law. 2020;27:495–8. https://doi.org/10.1163/15718093-bja10028.
42. Heyland D, Cook D, Bagshaw SM, Garland A, Stelfox HT, Mehta S, Dodek P, Kutsogiannis J, Burns K, Muscedere J, Turgeon AF, Fowler R, Jiang X, Day AG, Canadian Critical Care Trials Group; Canadian Researchers at the End of Life Network. The very elderly admitted to ICU: a quality finish? Crit Care Med. 2015;43(7):1352–60. https://doi.org/10.1097/CCM.0000000000001024.
43. Boumendil A, Maury E, Reinhard I, Luquel L, Offenstadt G, Guidet B. Prognosis of patients aged 80 years and over admitted in medical intensive care unit. Intensive Care Med. 2004;30(4):647–54.
44. Bagshaw SM, Webb SA, Delaney A, George C, Pilcher D, Hart GK, Bellomo R. Very old patients admitted to intensive care in Australia and New Zealand: a multi-centre cohort analysis. Crit Care. 2009;13(2):R45. https://doi.org/10.1186/cc7768.
45. Ferrante LE, Pisani MA, Murphy TE, Gahbauer EA, Leo-Summers LS, Gill TM. Functional trajectories among older persons before and after critical illness. JAMA Intern Med. 2015;175(4):523–9. https://doi.org/10.1001/jamainternmed.2014.7889.
46. Hoffman KR, Loong B, Haren FV. Very old patients urgently referred to the intensive care unit: long-term outcomes for admitted and declined patients. Crit Care Resusc. 2016;18(3):157–64.
47. Garrouste-Orgeas M, Boumendil A, Pateron D, Aergerter P, Somme D, Simon T, Guidet B, ICE-CUB Group. Selection of intensive care unit admission criteria for patients aged 80 years and over and compliance of emergency and intensive care unit physicians with the selected criteria: an observational, multicenter, prospective study. Crit Care Med. 2009;37(11):2919–28.
48. Garrouste-Orgeas M, Tabah A, Vesin A, Philippart F, Kpodji A, Bruel C, Grégoire C, Max A, Timsit JF, Misset B. The ETHICA study (part II): simulation study of determinants and variability of ICU physician decisions in patients aged 80 or over. Intensive Care Med. 2013;39(9):1574–83. https://doi.org/10.1007/s00134-013-2977-x.
49. Wilkinson DJC. Frailty triage: is rationing intensive medical treatment on the grounds of frailty ethical? Am J Bioeth. 2020;8:1–22. https://doi.org/10.1080/15265161.2020.1851809.
50. Cuthbertson BH, Wunsch H. Long-term outcomes after critical illness. The best predictor of the future is the past. Am J Respir Crit Care Med. 2016;194(2):132–4. https://doi.org/10.1164/rccm.201602-0257ED. PMID: 26953728.
51. Rockwood K, Song X, MacKnight C, Bergman H, Hogan DB, McDowell I, Mitnitski A. A global clinical measure of fitness and frailty in elderly people. CMAJ. 2005;173(5):489–95. https://doi.org/10.1503/cmaj.050051.
52. Muscedere J, Waters B, Varambally A, Bagshaw SM, Boyd JG, Maslove D, Sibley S, Rockwood K. The impact of frailty on intensive care unit outcomes: a systematic review and meta-analysis. Intensive Care Med. 2017;43(8):1105–22. https://doi.org/10.1007/s00134-017-4867-0.
53. Hanlon P, Nicholl BI, Jani BD, Lee D, McQueenie R, Mair FS. Frailty and pre-frailty in middle-aged and older adults and its association with multimorbidity and mortality: a prospective analysis of 493 737 UK Biobank participants. Lancet Public Health. 2018;3(7):e323–32. https://doi.org/10.1016/S2468-2667(18)30091-4.
54. Brummel NE, Bell SP, Girard TD, Pandharipande PP, Jackson JC, Morandi A, Thompson JL, Chandrasekhar R, Bernard GR, Dittus RS, Gill TM, Ely EW. Frailty and subsequent disability and mortality among patients with critical illness. Am J Respir Crit Care Med. 2017;196(1):64–72. https://doi.org/10.1164/rccm.201605-0939OC.
55. Bagshaw M, Majumdar SR, Rolfson DB, Ibrahim Q, McDermid RC, Stelfox HT. A prospective multicenter cohort study of frailty in younger critically ill patients. Crit Care. 2016;20(1):175. https://doi.org/10.1186/s13054-016-1338-x. Erratum in: Crit Care. 2016;20(1):223.
56. Darvall JN, Bellomo R, Bailey M, Paul E, Young PJ, Rockwood K, Pilcher D. Frailty and outcomes from pneumonia in critical illness: a population-based cohort study. Br J Anaesth. 2020;125(5):730–8. https://doi.org/10.1016/j.bja.2020.07.049. Epub 2020 Sep 3. PMID: 32891413; PMCID: PMC7467940.
57. Flaatten H, Beil M, Guidet B. Prognostication in older ICU patients: mission impossible? Br J Anaesth. 2020;125(5):655–7. https://doi.org/10.1016/j.bja.2020.08.005.
58. Knaus WA, Draper EA, Wagner DP, Zimmerman JE. Prognosis in acute organ-system failure. Ann Surg. 1985;202:685–93. https://doi.org/10.1097/00000658-198512000-00004.

59. Ferreira FL, Bota DP, Bross A, Mélot C, Vincent JL. Serial evaluation of the SOFA score to predict outcome in critically ill patients. JAMA. 2001;286:1754–8. https://doi.org/10.1001/jama.286.14.1754.

60. ASA Physical Status Classification System. American Society of Anaesthesiologists House of Delegates/Executive Committee. 2019. Available at: https://www.asahq.org/standards-and-guidelines/asa-physical-status-classification-system. Accessed March 22, 2021.

61. Sinuff T, Adhikari NK, Cook DJ, Schünemann HJ, Griffith LE, Rocker G, Walter SD. Mortality predictions in the intensive care unit: comparing physicians with scoring systems. Crit Care Med. 2006;34(3):878–85. https://doi.org/10.1097/01.CCM.0000201881.58644.41.

62. Detsky ME, Harhay MO, Bayard DF, Delman AM, Buehler AE, Kent SA, Ciuffetelli IV, Cooney E, Gabler NB, Ratcliffe SJ, Mikkelsen ME, Halpern SD. Discriminative accuracy of physician and nurse predictions for survival and functional outcomes 6 months after an ICU admission. JAMA. 2017;317(21):2187–95. https://doi.org/10.1001/jama.2017.4078.

63. Bernacki RE, Block SD. Communication about serious illness care goals: a review and synthesis of best practices. JAMA Intern Med. 2014;174(12):1994–2003. https://doi.org/10.1001/jamainternmed.2014.5271.

64. Quill TE, Holloway R. Time-limited trials near the end of life. JAMA. 2011;306(13):1483–4.

65. Vink EE, Azoulay E, Caplan A, Kompanje EJO, Bakker J. Time-limited trial of intensive care treatment: an overview of current literature. Intensive Care Med. 2018;44:1369–77.

66. Joynt GM, Gomersall C. Integrating elective workloads into an emergency setting in the intensive care unit. In: Flaatten H, Moreno RP, Putensen C, Rhodes A, editors. Organisation and management of intensive care. Berlin: Medizinisch Wissenschaftliche Verlagsgesellschaft; 2010. p. 53–64.

67. Guidet B, Hejblum G, Joynt G. Triage: what can we do to improve our practice? Intensive Care Med. 2013;39(11):2044–6. https://doi.org/10.1007/s00134-013-3063-0. Epub 2013 Aug 28. PMID: 23982726.

68. Sprung CL, Danis M, Iapichino G, Artigas A, Kesecioglu J, Moreno R, Lippert A, Curtis JR, Meale P, Cohen SL, Levy MM, Truog RD. Triage of intensive care patients: identifying agreement and controversy. Intensive Care Med. 2013;39(11):1916–24. https://doi.org/10.1007/s00134-013-3033-6.

69. Nguyen YL, Angus DA, Boumendil A, Guidet B. The challenge of admitting the very elderly to intensive care. Ann Intensive Care. 2011;1:29. https://doi.org/10.1186/2110-5820-1-29.

70. Flaatten H, Oeyen S, deLange DW. Predicting outcomes in very old ICU patients: time to focus on the past? Intensive Care Med. 2018;44(8):1344–5. https://doi.org/10.1007/s00134-018-5262-1.

71. Lupei MI, Chipman JG, Beilman GJ, Oancea SC, Konia MR. The association between ASA status and other risk stratification models on postoperative intensive care unit outcomes. Anesth Analg. 2014;118(5):989–94. https://doi.org/10.1213/ane.0000000000000187.

Decision-Making Under Resource Constraints

Michael Beil, P. Vernon van Heerden, and Sigal Sviri

Contents

Learning Objectives

Seasonal or continuous resource constraints are evident in many healthcare systems and necessitate restrictions on admissions to intensive care units (ICUs). When the demand for ICU beds exceeds capacity, patients who are expected to benefit most are prioritised for admission and continuation of intensive care. In addition to survival, the benefit of intensive care in old patients strongly depends on the quality of life that can be achieved after discharge. In this chapter, we will discuss the challenges of predicting outcome for this patient population as well as the medical and ethical issues which may arise during triage.

16.1 Introduction

Limitations of intensive care resources imposed by economic or other constraints, such as lack of sufficiently trained staff, make an efficient utilisation of intensive care units (ICUs) mandatory. This especially concerns the admission of old patients with complex conditions on the background of long-term multi-morbidity and progressive functional decline. Although the relative survival benefit of treatment in ICU was found to be the largest for the cohort of old patients [1], it remains to be evaluated and confirmed in the individual case whether admission to ICU is likely to provide any benefit other than survival that is also concordant with the individual's personal view about quality of life [2]. Prognostication has to be reassessed when deciding about continuation or escalation of treatment in ICU. Whenever the demand for intensive care substantially exceeds capacity, triage procedures have to be implemented to select those patients who might gain the most from admission to ICU. Some degree of triage regularly occurs in regions with very limited healthcare resources [3] or during periods of seasonal strain [4]. In times of rapidly increasing pressure on intensive care resources, e.g. during exponential growth of a pandemic, pre-admission triage might not be sufficient to optimise short-term utilisation of ICU capacity according to utilitarian principles. Hence, patients already admitted to the ICU might be included in triage decisions which may eventually lead to withdrawal of life-sustaining treatment in patients with otherwise favourable prognosis [5]. The fundamental uncertainty of prognostication in general [6] and in particular when comparing outcome predictions between individual patients [7] then results in ethical dilemmas and legal controversies [8]. Involving other stakeholders from outside the medical community in developing guidelines for triage could help to mitigate the impact of these problems and ease the burden of difficult decision-making on clinicians.

16.2 Availability and Utilisation of ICU Resources Under Constraints

Access to intensive care depends on the availability of beds, equipment and specialised staff. The amount of these resources differs significantly between countries which created substantial inequalities with regard to access to intensive care throughout Europe [9]. The number of formally designated ICU beds is a frequent

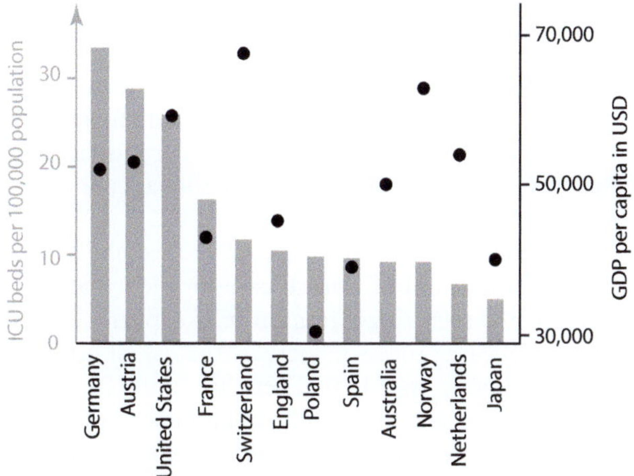

Fig. 16.1 Number of ICU beds per 100,000 population as documented between 2017 and 2020 (grey columns) and gross domestic product (GDP) per capita in US dollar in 2017 (black dots) for selected countries based on OECD data (► www.oecd.org). Please note that the definition of ICU beds may vary between countries [10]

benchmark and ranges up to 34 beds per 100,000 population in Western European countries [10]. Of note, there is no strong correlation between this benchmark and the gross domestic product (■ Fig. 16.1) despite intensive care being one of the most expensive components of healthcare. The definition of intensive care and the set of intensive care equipment considered essential at the bedside varies between countries [11]. Thus, the number of registered ICU beds needs to be put into the context of national standards and availability of staff. For example, within the overall ICU bed number of 34 per 100,000 population reported for Germany, less than half of that capacity was available for invasive ventilation or extracorporeal membrane oxygenation (ECMO) in April 2021 [12]. ICU staffing is a crucial parameter that determines the actual availability of ICU beds in the context of outcome quality [13]. In France, the risk of death was found to be increased by a factor of 3.5 when the patient-to-nurse ratio was greater than the standard of 2.5 and doubled when the patient-to-physician ratio exceeded 14 [14].

Recent years have seen an increase of both the total number and percentage of old patients in the critical care environment [15]. Moreover, the onset of severe and terminal diseases has shifted further towards an even more advanced age. Consequently, the population of ICU patients has changed, with more old and very old patients, with complex multi-morbidity and multi-organ failure treated in ICUs [16]. In several countries though, this upward trend in demand has faced a stagnation of ICU capacity, mainly due to austerity measures over the past decade [17]. Staffing levels have become a variable for economic adjustments. In some healthcare systems though, misguided incentives within the reimbursement system for invasive interventions have resulted in overtreatment of patients in ICU [18], associated with a persisting scarcity of alternative care pathways, notably palliative care. This threat of under- as well as overutilisation of ICU resources especially affects the cohort of old patients who are in need for holistic treatment approaches [2, 19].

When healthcare systems come under pressure, the cohort of old patients becomes an easy target to be deselected from accessing scarce ICU resources because of the incorrect perception that these patients generally have poorer outcome [20]. Of note, quality-adjusted life years (QALY) after ICU admission are approximately 4 QALY on average for patients aged 80 years or older [21]. Interestingly, limitations of life-sustaining treatment for older ICU patients are most prevalent in high-income countries indicating a stronger impact of cultural factors in comparison to economic restrictions [22]. Also of note, there are new concepts aiming at alleviating these problems by creating acute and critical care facilities designated for geriatric patients which focus on the special needs of older individuals in a more comprehensive way. This includes staged approaches to critical care in accordance with advanced directives and care plans [23, 24].

The above issues have affected the capability of ICUs to absorb unscheduled changes in demand of critical care for older patients. That problem has been illustrated by the recurring strain on ICU capacity caused by seasonal influenza. These surges alter care processes, increase the risk of adverse events for patients and impact the wellbeing of staff [25]. There are limits to expanding ICU uptake in the short term as well as downstream hospital facilities later on. The planning for crisis situations is hampered by the probabilistic nature of model projections which may lead to expensive resources being unutilised for most of the time. Regardless of these constraints, situations occur when an unexpected surge of critically ill patients surpasses ICU capacity without much advance notice [26]. Cancelation of elective activities and imposing stricter rules for ICU admission constitutes the first levels of response [27]. These measures are intended to keep ICU resources available for those patients whose survival depends on invasive organ support, at least to the moment when the expansion and reorganisation of critical care services have sufficiently progressed to accommodate more patients. In Australia, such an expansion of ICU services was reported to be able to provide a 191% increase of bed capacity [28]. If these measures do not create sufficient ICU capacity, triage needs to be implemented on ICU admissions [29].

In the year 2020, the outbreak of a highly contagious respiratory infection (COVID-19) that required extended periods of invasive ventilation in many critically ill individuals rapidly saturated and overwhelmed ICU resources in several countries [17]. A larger than average ICU baseline capacity can delay that time point only by a small offset when there is fast exponential growth of case numbers, with the doubling time larger than the length of stay in ICU [30]. In a realistic scenario, groups of non-distinct patients arrive in hospitals in respiratory failure with the total number of critically ill individuals exceeding the available ICU capacity even after expansion. Triage rules for selecting patients fail, and the process of pre-admission triage becomes insufficient to ensure access to intensive care for all those cases deemed appropriate for invasive ventilation with equal justification. Patients already admitted to ICU may then be included in the triage processes with the option to withdraw life-sustaining treatment in individuals with relatively poor prognosis. Consequently, prognostic assessment in ICU will have to shift from an independent evaluation of individuals to quantitative predictions used for comparisons between two or more patients or with system-wide thresholds for discontinuation of life-sustaining treatment [27]. However, even such measures may become insufficient in a rapidly escalating crisis with large and non-distinct groups of people affected within a short period in time. This might eventually lead to triage based on non-medical criteria [31] or a random selection of ICU patients [32], such as by order of admission to hospital ('first come, first served').

16.3 Prognostication for Individual Patients

Decision-making for patients in ICU hinges on predicting the individual response to interventions and prognosticating outcome. Interventions are considered futile if they are not expected to accomplish a physiological goal, such as restoring circulation in the short term [19]. Functional disabilities and cognitive impairment are well-known consequences of intensive care with functional outcomes in older ICU patients being generally poorer than in younger cohorts [33]. Older patients with multi-morbidity are at an increased risk for complications in ICU, and post-ICU recovery is inversely correlated with the duration of organ support [34]. Thus, survival is not the only outcome important to old patients. Other meaningful outcome measures encompass quality of life and the level of functional independence that can be achieved in the future [35]. However, the interpretation and weight of these measures depend on the patient's personal experience as well as the social and economic support available after discharge from hospital. It is therefore crucial to take the self-perceived quality of life into account for decision-making about the appropriateness of interventions in ICU. For example, having a 'good' life means living independently with a high level of social functioning for some patients, whilst being alive and supported by caregivers might be acceptable to other individuals. Mental wellbeing showed a stronger association with self-reported unacceptable outcome than the physical health [36]. Thus, personalised outcome predictions are highly desirable for older ICU patients and might require repeated adjustments according to the duration and intensity of treatment in ICU.

The uncertainty of prognostication for individual patients constitutes a fundamental challenge in healthcare [37] and in intensive care in particular because of the latter's considerable burden on patients. There is a significant variation among intensivists in the assessment of individual patients which may eventually lead to oppositional decisions [38]. When asked for outcome predictions in ICU, the error rate of specialists' prognostication even when pooled is substantial, e.g. >10% for survival [39]. Thus, survival rates after withholding or withdrawing life-sustaining treatment in ICU are surprisingly high [40]. The traditional way for medical professionals to make predictions for patients has been heuristics involving rules built on their past experience. Intuition is especially helpful for decision-making under time constraints and with insufficient information [41]. However, humans may have a different experience, and even experts are vulnerable to cognitive biases [42, 43] which cause a substantial variability of decision-making even in cases classified as straightforward [44]. With the amount of information growing in more complex cases and environments, prognostication based on heuristics becomes more prone to errors, i.e. an inappropriate judgement was made when a more appropriate alternative should have been chosen when determined in retrospect [45].

Disease severity scores or other regression models of patient characteristics do not add much value to individual prognostication and are not recommended for triage decisions [46]. This is especially relevant for older patients in which many of these models have not been sufficiently validated so far [47]. Moreover, there are methodological problems, including issues with cross-sectional data sampling and the probabilistic nature of many models based on cohort data with overlapping distributions [7]. Thus, statistical models are considered inappropriate to determine irreversible decisions for individual patients [48]. For example, there is no practical difference between a predicted survival of 10% or 90% for an individual, i.e. sample size of 1. In the absence of alternatives, however, disease severity scores are still used for decision-making [49]. In most scenarios, however, the requirement to impose a threshold on patient characteristics for deciding about interventions inevitably results in false-positive or false-negative decisions [50], even when the set of observable characteristics of an individual patient match those of the training cohort for the model perfectly [51]. This way, patients with a favourable but falsely calculated negative prognosis might be assigned a low priority for treatment in ICU during triage. On the other hand, patients with a negative prognosis might get a high priority for ICU due to a false-positive prognosis. Some demographic features are important for prognostication but are not included in most models. For example, ethnicity is not part of scoring systems but has a significant impact on their discriminatory performance [52]. The fundamental problems of statistical discrimination have also been illustrated by simulations of triage decisions with historical cohorts showing a substantial number of patients surviving 5 years or longer if not excluded from ICU admission [6]. These issues need to be taken into account when considering the use of such models for triage. Of note, new techniques from the field of artificial intelligence and machine learning have not yet abolished these problems, but rather added new issues, notably lack of transparency and adversarial examples [53].

Although predictive uncertainty in individuals is inevitable, its magnitude can be reduced by extending the time frame for assessments. In old patients, long-term trajectories of functional disabilities prior to ICU admission were shown to contain more prognostic information for long-term outcome than the severity of the acute illness [54]. After admission to ICU, the analysis of time-dependent changes of organ physiology adds significant value in predicting survival [55]. Prognostication based on aggregation of these data with information about the patients' past medical history outperformed predictions by disease severity scores [56]. However, model discrimination with regard to outcome after ICU still is insufficient to be used for personalised predictions. The current ceiling of precision as measured by the area under the receiver operating characteristic curve (AUROC) appears to be 0.9 [57]. That translates into a substantial number of false-positive and false-negative predictions and, therefore, appears unsuitable for triage decisions about withholding or withdrawing life-sustaining treatment.

Time-limited treatment trials in ICU were used to provide more robust estimates for individual prognosis by obtaining longitudinal data in response to treatment [58]. This concept resembles the N-of-1 trial design that was developed to tackle heterogeneous treatment effects due to interindividual variability in clinical studies [59]. In both settings, patients are exposed to various interventions and the cumulative response over time is used for predictions. This setup also provides time series data for fitting mathematical models of organ physiology, which can then be employed for predicting recovery or deterioration of organ failure in deterministic ways [60]. However, time is a precious asset in crisis situations. Contrary to the potential benefit of improved prognostication during triage, the time available for individual assessments will actually become shorter in this situation and time-limited trials impossible.

16.4 Triage in ICU

There are various approaches to triage based on conflicting principles and criteria as well as different ways of endorsement and implementation (�‣ Table 16.1). Several professional societies and expert groups [5, 61] recommend including patients already treated in ICU into triage decisions during a surge situation when all options to expand ICU capacity and optimise patient flow are exhausted. Of note, this concerns all ICU patients regardless of their illness. Some ethicists and intensivists also advocate abolishing the distinction between withholding and withdrawing life-sustaining treatment in general [62]. Based on these views, ICU patients have to be included into all triage decisions from the beginning of a crisis to ensure equal access to critical care for all individuals with comparable clinical needs irrespective of the time of presentation to hospital. These recommendations are being justified by the utilitarian goal to save the most people or the lives most valued in a population according to

�‣ **Table 16.1** Framework to guide triage in ICU

	Options
Principles	Utilitarian vs egalitarian concepts
	All patients vs only patients before admission to ICU
	All patients vs preference for certain social groups (e.g. key workers)
	All patients vs only patients with single conditions (e.g. pandemic infection)
	Non-discriminatory regarding age, gender, ethnicity, chronic disabilities
Criteria	Short-term vs long-term prognosis
	Clinical improvement vs steady state vs deterioration in condition
	Prediction of short vs extended stay in ICU
	Physiological vs chronological age
	Comorbidities and frailty
	Expected quality of life and functional abilities after ICU
Endorsement	Democratic institutions vs professional societies
	Judicial review vs none
	Time-limited vs permanent
Implementation	Multiprofessional team vs single person
	External professionals vs ICU staff
	Medical vs medical and non-medical decision-makers
	Local decision-making vs regional or national coordination
	Supervision and legal accountability

various medical and non-medical criteria. These criteria range from thresholds for age or remaining life expectancy to professional qualifications considered essential for society. They can vary over time with changing demand and supply levels for ICU beds or according to social, political and economic considerations and, thus, make decisions for individual patients dependent on the dynamics of social rules that are beyond medical reasoning.

Predicted outcome is the criterion for triage in ICU that gained the broadest consensus among medical professionals. Triage based on this measure leads to withdrawal of life-sustaining treatment in individuals whose prognoses are favourable in general but less so in comparison to that of a newly arriving patient or adjustable thresholds for predicted outcome. Since such comparisons are based on human (expert) opinion or statistical models, they propagate the fundamental uncertainty of individual prognostication to decisions about withdrawing life-sustaining treatment [50]. Importantly, the inevitable constraints on the time of decision-making during a surge situation further increase the uncertainty of predictions. Moreover, there still is a debate about the time horizon most suitable for prognostication, e.g. short- vs long-term prognosis [63], adding another layer of uncertainty to triage decisions. Even independent of crisis situations, predictive uncertainty causes considerable variations of decisions to withdraw life-sustaining treatment at various levels ranging from medical teams within the same ICU to geographic regions with different healthcare systems and cultures [64].

Regardless of the extent of predictive uncertainty, triage of ICU patients is considered unlawful in various countries [8, 65], because it violates the rights of individuals by terminating life support without consent and is against medical reasoning when applied to the level of individual patients. Moreover, constitutional provisions about human dignity in some countries prohibit comparing the value of individuals for this type of administrative decision-making. Of note, the opposite of utilitarian triage as described above is an egalitarian approach that would result in a random selection of patients that is blinded with regard to individual characteristics, such as physiological reserve and prognosis. The concept of 'first come, first served' is a rude implementation of egalitarian principles. Many intensivists and other stakeholders do not consider that method to be an ethical ideal either [66]. Moreover, this rule also provides incentives for unwanted behaviour within the population. It appears fair to expect that the dilemmas of triage, especially between providing best care for individual patients and utilitarian interests during a crisis, cannot be fully resolved. Even outside triage situations, the rate of objections by medical professionals against withdrawing life-sustaining treatment without the patient's consent varies considerably between countries (0–41%) and medical specialties (up to 42% in geriatric medicine) [67]. The ethical and legal discourse about the principles for triage will continue. That includes the discussion about conflicting roles of stakeholders in the decision-making process and the consequences for the mental wellbeing of ICU staff responsible for the triage [17].

Importantly, there are substantial disagreements between different triage models when applied to the same population of critically ill patients [68, 69] causing confusion about ethical and legal implications. Other issues in the discussion about triage involve the need for special rules to deal with previously disadvantaged communities as well as long-term biases in healthcare [70]. In this context, triage guidelines need to adhere to laws protecting people with chronic conditions and disabilities or at an advanced age from being discriminated against with respect to allocation of health-care resources [71]. Patients in need for intensive care who do not suffer from the condition causing a crisis situation, such as individuals with long-term cardiovascular or respiratory conditions, should be guaranteed equal access to ICU [72].

Pragmatic protocols for triage have taken regional and cultural preferences into account [73]. They are aimed at maintaining public trust and social coherence which strongly depend on the belief systems and views of lay people. Two surveys in the UK and in Germany among the general population have revealed similar attitudes towards the role of chronological age as a triage criterion [74, 75]. Contrary to legislation against discrimination in both countries, more than two thirds of the respondents would prefer a younger to an older patient for admission to ICU. In Japan, which has one of the demographically oldest populations, more than three quarters of respondents expressed a preference for younger patients [76]. Regarding other triage criteria, only one fourth of lay people in Germany would give patients who work in healthcare preference over other patients, whereas approximately two thirds of people in the UK would do so. These findings illustrate the variability of opinions and, thus, emphasise the need to consider the input by stakeholders from outside professional communities to mitigate controversies when developing and implementing triage guidelines (□ Table 16.1). Moreover, sharing individual triage decisions with patients' families and caregivers, although difficult to implement in crisis situations, could help to alleviate the impact of these problems [77].

16.5 The Role of Age and Geriatric Conditions for Triage Decisions

Regardless of the ethical and legal concerns mentioned above, the need for triaging ICU patients may occur during an escalating crisis. The most robust prognosticators should then be used to guarantee equitable decisions in selecting patients for continuation or withdrawal of life-sustaining treatment [78]. Chronological age is not considered an appropriate prognosticator due the diversity of the ageing process [79], albeit thresholds for chronological age have been used to triage or as a tiebreaker in recent crisis situations [17, 69]. At an advanced age, medically relevant similarities in disease trajectories are better determined by quantifying the extent of chronic disorders and functional disabilities [80, 81]. These interrelated characteristics are considered geriatric conditions and associated with reduced resilience and increased vulnerability to physical and cognitive stress. Thus, these features are expected to strongly correlate with poor outcome in critically ill old patients. In fact, they were shown to outperform features of the acute illness in predicting long-term outcome [56]. Nevertheless, the discriminatory power of these features is less than ideal, and there will be a substantial number of false-positive or false-negative predictions for outcome during triage.

The prognostic value of frailty [82] in ICU patients aged 80 years or older has been confirmed by large multicentre studies [83, 84]. In the year 2020, frailty as assessed by the Clinical Frailty Scale [80] was recommended to be considered for triaging patients above the age of 65 years on admission to ICU in the UK and other countries [85]. Even before that time, frailty was found to significantly contribute to the decision-making about withdrawing life-sustaining treatment in old ICU patients [22]. Importantly, the Clinical Frailty Scale has been found to be a highly reproducible tool to quantify frailty in ICU [86]. There was, however, a debate whether this tool accurately measures the vulnerability of patients with chronic but stable conditions [87], and the recommendations for triage have been modified accordingly.

The concurrence of multiple, usually two or more, chronic conditions in an individual is called multi-morbidity [88]. The combination of some diseases and its sequelae, notably polypharmacy, can trigger super-additive interactions [89] resulting in an enhanced effect of these comorbidities on functional disabilities, quality of life as well as life expectancy [90]. Thus, multi-morbidity is regarded as a condition in itself. A detailed analysis of multi-morbidity in 440,000 older ICU patients that included disease-specific survival rates to account for their variable impact on outcome provided a good prediction of survival that outperformed biomarkers of acute physiology [91]. Specific clusters of multi-morbidity are known to be associated with different outcome in ICU [92]. Thus, multi-morbidity was suggested to be included into triage protocols, although not as a stand-alone feature [66]. However, there still is no uniform standard to evaluate and quantify multi-morbidity [93] compromising its value for fair and transparent triage decisions.

Conclusions

Balancing supply and demand of intensive care resources belongs to the skill set of intensivists. Whilst the focus usually remains on providing the best medical care to individual patients, surge situations overwhelming resources in a short period of time may force medical professionals to divert from that objective. Although many countries have adopted egalitarian principles to guide medical decision-making in general, utilitarian rules aimed at an overall benefit for the population appear to be the preferred approach to medical decisions during disasters and pandemics. This shift causes fundamental ethical and legal dilemmas, notably when life-sustaining treatment in ICU is withdrawn from a patient only to provide care for another patient who happens to better match a set of prognostic criteria. Despite the multitude of predictive models with good accuracy at the cohort level, there is no method that abolishes the burden of uncertainty when making decisions for individuals. Thus, guidelines for triage decisions in ICU leading to withdrawal of life-sustaining treatment in individual patients require the contribution by stakeholders from outside the medical community.

Practical Implications

Preparation for surges of patients overwhelming the available ICU capacity encompasses:

- Comprehensive plans to extend ICU bed numbers as well as step-down and palliative care facilities on short notice
- Triage protocols based on legal and ethical requirements and a thorough understanding of prognostic uncertainty
- Liaising with other stakeholders and the general public to prepare for difficult scenarios when decisions about withholding or withdrawing life-sustaining treatment can no longer be justified by medical reasons alone

> **Clinical Protocols**
>
> - Follow the law and professional guidelines; seek advice when they conflict with each other.
> - Share decision-making with other stakeholders.
> - Document and audit the decision-making process.

> **Take-Home Messages**
>
> During periods of significant resource contraints, decision-making about initiation, continuation and withdrawal of intensive care suffers from substantial uncertainty and requires a holistic approach considering medical, legal as well as social aspects.

References

1. Sprung CL, Artigas A, Kesecioglu J, Pezzi A, Wiis J, Pirracchio R, Baras M, Edbrooke DL, Pesenti A, Bakker J, et al. The Eldicus prospective, observational study of triage decision making in European intensive care units. Part II: intensive care benefit for the elderly. Crit Care Med. 2012;40:132–8.
2. Turnbull AE, Bosslet GT, Kross EK. Aligning use of intensive care with patient values in the USA: past, present, and future. Lancet Respir Med. 2019;7:626–38.
3. Siow WT, Liew MF, Shrestha BR, Muchtar F, See KC. Managing COVID-19 in resource-limited settings: critical care considerations. Crit Care. 2020;24:167.
4. Rowan KM, Harrison DA, Walsh TS, McAuley DF, Perkins GD, Taylor BL, Menon DK. The Swine Flu Triage (SwiFT) study: development and ongoing refinement of a triage tool to provide regular information to guide immediate policy and practice for the use of critical care services during the H1N1 swine influenza pandemic. Health Technol Assess. 2010;14:335–492.
5. Emanuel EJ, Persad G, Upshur R, Thome B, Parker M, Glickman A, Zhang C, Boyle C, Smith M, Phillips JP. Fair allocation of scarce medical resources in the time of Covid-19. N Engl J Med. 2020;382:2049–55.
6. Darvall JN, Bellomo R, Bailey M, Anstey J, Pilcher D. Long-term survival of critically ill patients stratified according to pandemic triage categories: a retrospective cohort study. Chest. 2021;160:538–48.
7. Beil M, Sviri S, Flaatten H, De Lange DW, Jung C, Szczeklik W, Leaver S, Rhodes A, Guidet B, van Heerden PV. On predictions in critical care: the individual prognostication fallacy in elderly patients. J Crit Care. 2021;61:34–8.
8. Liddell K, Martin S, Palmer S. Allocating medical resources in the time of Covid-19. N Engl J Med. 2020;382:e79.
9. Bauer J, Brüggmann D, Klingelhöfer D, Maier W, Schwettmann L, Weiss DJ, Groneberg DA. Access to intensive care in 14 European countries: a spatial analysis of intensive care need and capacity in the light of COVID-19. Intensive Care Med. 2020;46:2026–34.
10. OECD. Beyond containment: health systems responses to COVID-19 in the OECD. 2020. https://www.oecd.org/coronavirus/en/.
11. Phua J, Hashmi M, Haniffa R. ICU beds: less is more? Not sure. Intensive Care Med. 2020;46:1600–2.
12. DIVI-Intensivregister. Intensivmedizinischer Behandlungskapazitäten – Tagesreport vom April 3, 2021. www.intensivregister.de.
13. Rimmelé T, Pascal L, Polazzi S, Duclos A. Organizational aspects of care associated with mortality in critically ill COVID-19 patients. Intensive Care Med. 2021;47:119–21.

14. Neuraz A, Guérin C, Payet C, Polazzi S, Aubrun F, Dailler F, Lehot JJ, Piriou V, Neidecker J, Rimmelé T, Schott AM, Duclos A. Patient mortality is associated with staff resources and workload in the ICU: a multicenter observational study. Crit Care Med. 2015;43:1587–94.

15. Glattacker M, Kanat M, Schaefer J, Motschall E, Kivelitz L, Voigt-Radloff S, Dirmaier J. Availability and quality of assessment instruments on patient-centredness in the multimorbid elderly (AQuA-PCE): a study protocol of a systematic review. BMJ Open. 2020;10:e033273.

16. Damluji AA, Forman DE, van Diepen S, Alexander KP, Page RL 2nd, Hummel SL, Menon V, Katz JN, Albert NM, Afilalo J, Cohen MG. Older adults in the cardiac intensive care unit. Circulation. 2020;141:e6–e32.

17. Faggioni MP, González-Melado FJ, Di Pietro ML. National health system cuts and triage decisions during the COVID-19 pandemic in Italy and Spain: ethical implications. J Med Ethics. 2021;47(5):300–7.

18. Michalsen A, Neitzke G, Dutzmann J, Rogge A, Seidlein AH, Jöbges S, Burchardi H, Hartog C, Nauck F, Salomon F, et al. Overtreatment in intensive care medicine-recognition, designation, and avoidance. Med Klin Intensivmed Notfmed. 2021;116:281–94.

19. Kon AA, Shepard EK, Sederstrom NO, Swoboda SM, Marshall MF, Birriel B, Rincon F. Defining futile and potentially inappropriate interventions. Crit Care Med. 2016;44:1769–74.

20. Fowler RA, Yarnell CJ, Nayfeh A, Kiiza P. Challenging the pessimism in providing critical care for elderly patients. JAMA Netw Open. 2019;2:e193201.

21. Kaarlola A, Tallgren M, Pettilä V. Long-term survival, quality of life, and quality-adjusted life-years among critically ill elderly patients. Crit Care Med. 2006;34:2120–6.

22. Guidet B, Flaatten H, Boumendil A, Morandi A, Andersen FH, Artigas A, Bertolini G, Cecconi M, Christensen S, Faraldi L, Fjølner J, Jung C, Marsh B, Moreno R, Oeyen S, Öhman CA, Pinto BB, Soliman IW, Szczeklik W, Valentin A, Watson X, Zafeiridis T, De Lange DW, VIP1 Study Group. Withholding or withdrawing of life-sustaining therapy in older adults (≥80 years) admitted to the intensive care unit. Intensive Care Med. 2018;44:1027–38.

23. Southerland LT, Lo AX, Biese K, Arendts G, Banerjee J, Hwang U, Dresden S, Argento V, Kennedy M, Shenvi CL, Carpenter CR. Concepts in practice: geriatric emergency departments. Ann Emerg Med. 2020;75:162–70.

24. Palmer RM. The acute care for elders unit model of care. Geriatrics (Basel). 2018;3:59.

25. Rewa OG, Stelfox HT, Ingolfsson A, Zygun DA, Featherstone R, Opgenorth D, Bagshaw SM. Indicators of intensive care unit capacity strain: a systematic review. Crit Care. 2018;22:86.

26. Sviri S, et al. Logistic challenges and constraints in intensive care during a pandemic. In: Flaatten H, et al., editors. The very old critically ill patients. Cham: Springer; 2022. (this volume).

27. Flaatten H, Van Heerden V, Jung C, Beil M, Leaver S, Rhodes A, Guidet B, deLange DW. The good, the bad and the ugly: pandemic priority decisions and triage. J Med Ethics. 2020;47(12):e75.

28. Litton E, Bucci T, Chavan S, Ho YY, Holley A, Howard G, Huckson S, Kwong P, Millar J, Nguyen N, Secombe P, Ziegenfuss M, Pilcher D. Surge capacity of intensive care units in case of acute increase in demand caused by COVID-19 in Australia. Med J Aust. 2020;212:463–7.

29. Joynt GM. Pre-ICU triage: the very old critically ill patient. In: Flaatten H, et al., editors. The very old critically ill patients. Cham: Springer; 2022. (this volume).

30. Ritter M, Ott DVM, Paul F, Haynes JD, Ritter K. COVID-19: a simple statistical model for predicting intensive care unit load in exponential phases of the disease. Sci Rep. 2021;11:5018.

31. Federatie Medisch Specialisten. Draaiboek Triage op basis van niet-medische overwegingen voor IC-opname ten tijde van fase 3 in de COVID-19 pandemie. 2020. https://nvic.nl/sites/nvic.nl/files/Draaiboek%20Triage%20op%20basis%20van%20niet-medische%20overwegingen%20voor%20IC-opname%20ten%20tijde%20van%20fase%203_COVID-19%20versie2.pdf.

32. Verweij M, van de Vathorst S, Schermer M, Willems D, de Vries M. Ethical advice for an intensive care triage protocol in the COVID-19 pandemic: lessons learned from the Netherlands. Public Health Ethics. 2020;13:157–65.

33. Brummel NE, Balas MC, Morandi A, Ferrante LE, Gill TM, Ely EW. Understanding and reducing disability in older adults following critical illness. Crit Care Med. 2015;43:1265–75.

34. Herridge MS, Chu LM, Matte A, Tomlinson G, Chan L, Thomas C, Friedrich JO, Mehta S, Lamontagne F, Levasseur M, et al. The RECOVER program: disability risk groups and 1-year outcome after 7 or more days of mechanical ventilation. Am J Respir Crit Care Med. 2016;194:831–44.

35. Gajic O, Ahmad SR, Wilson ME, Kaufman DA. Outcomes of critical illness: what is meaningful? Curr Opin Crit Care. 2018;24:394–400.

36. Kerckhoffs MC, Kosasi FFL, Soliman IW, van Delden JJM, Cremer OL, de Lange DW, Slooter AJC, Kesecioglu J, van Dijk D. Determinants of self-reported unacceptable outcome of intensive care treatment 1 year after discharge. Intensive Care Med. 2019;45:806–14.

37. Pate A, Emsley R, Ashcroft DM, Brown B, van Staa T. The uncertainty with using risk prediction models for individual decision making: an exemplar cohort study examining the prediction of cardiovascular disease in English primary care. BMC Med. 2019;17:134.

38. Reader TW, Reddy G, Brett SJ. Impossible decision? An investigation of risk trade-offs in the intensive care unit. Ergonomics. 2018;61:122–33.

39. Meadow W, Pohlman A, Frain L, Ren Y, Kress JP, Teuteberg W, et al. Power and limitations of daily prognostications of death in the medical intensive care unit. Crit Care Med. 2011;39:474–9.

40. Lobo SM, De Simoni FHB, Jakob SM, Estella A, Vadi S, Bluethgen A, Martin-Loeches I, Sakr Y, Vincent JL, ICON Investigators. Decision-making on withholding or withdrawing life support in the ICU: a worldwide perspective. Chest. 2017;152:321–9.

41. Adams E, Goyder C, Heneghan C, Brand L, Ajjawi R. Clinical reasoning of junior doctors in emergency medicine: a grounded theory study. Emerg Med J. 2017;34:70–5.

42. Kent DM, Steyerberg E, van Klaveren D. Personalized evidence based medicine: predictive approaches to heterogeneous treatment effects. BMJ. 2018;363:k4245.

43. Kahneman D, Slovic P, Tversky A. Judgment under uncertainty: heuristics and biases. Cambridge University Press; 1982.

44. Makridakis S, Kirkham R, Wakefield A, Papadaki M, Kirjkam J, Long L. Forecasting, uncertainty and risk – perspectives on clinical decision-making in preventive and curative medicine. Int J Forecast. 2019;35:659–66.

45. Kohn LT, Corrigan JM, Donaldson MS. To err is human. Washington, DC: Institute of Medicine. National Academies Press; 2000.

46. Aziz S, Arabi YM, Alhazzani W, Evans L, Citerio G, Fischkoff K, Salluh J, Meyfroidt G, Alshamsi F, Oczkowski S, Azoulay E, Price A, Burry L, Dzierba A, Benintende A, Morgan J, Grasselli G, Rhodes A, Møller MH, Chu L, Schwedhelm S, Lowe JJ, Bin D, Christian MD. Managing ICU surge during the COVID-19 crisis: rapid guidelines. Intensive Care Med. 2020;46:1303–25.

47. Flaatten H, de Lange DW, Artigas A, Bin D, Moreno R, Christensen S, Joynt GM, Bagshaw SM, Sprung CL, Benoit D, Soares M, Guidet B. The status of intensive care medicine research and a future agenda for very old patients in the ICU. Intensive Care Med. 2017;43:1319–28.

48. Nates JL, Nunnally M, Kleinpell R, Blosser S, Goldner J, Birriel B, Fowler CS, Byrum D, Miles WS, Bailey H, Sprung CL. ICU admission, discharge, and triage guidelines: a framework to enhance clinical operations, development of institutional policies, and further research. Crit Care Med. 2016;44:1553–602.

49. Grissom CK, Brown SM, Kuttler KG, Boltax JP, Jones J, Jephson AR, Orme JF Jr. A modified sequential organ failure assessment score for critical care triage. Disaster Med Public Health Prep. 2010;4:277–84.

50. White DB, Lo B. Reply to: social factors and critical care triage: right intentions, wrong tools. Am J Respir Crit Care Med. 2021; https://doi.org/10.1164/rccm.202103-0798LE.

51. Guptaa S, Batt J, Bourbeau J, Chapman KR, Gershon A, Hambly N, Hernandez P, Kolb M, Stephenson AL, Tullis DE, et al. Position statement from the Canadian Thoracic Society (CTS) on clinical triage thresholds in respiratory disease patients in the event of a major surge during the COVID-19 pandemic. Can J Respir Crit Care Sleep Med. 2020;4:214–25.

52. Sarkar R, Martin C, Mattie H, Gichoya JW, Stone DJ, Celi LA. Performance of intensive care unit severity scoring systems across different ethnicities in the USA: a retrospective observational study. Lancet Digit Health. 2021;3:e241–9.

53. Beil M, Proft I, van Heerden D, Sviri S, van Heerden PV. Ethical considerations about artificial intelligence for prognostication in intensive care. Intensive Care Med Exp. 2019;7:70.

54. Ferrante LE, Pisani MA, Murphy TE, Gahbauer EA, Leo-Summers LS, Gill TM. Functional trajectories among older persons before and after critical illness. JAMA Intern Med. 2015;175:523–9.

55. Lehmann LH, Nemati S, Moody GB, Heldt T, Mark RG. Uncovering clinical significance of vital sign dynamics in critical care. Comput Cardiol. 2014;41:1141–4.

56. Nielsen AB, Thorsen-Meyer HC, Belling K, Nielsen AP, Thomas EC, Chmura PJ, et al. Survival prediction in intensive-care units based on aggregation of long-term disease history and acute

physiology: a retrospective study of the Danish National Patient Registry and electronic patient records. Lancet Digit Health. 2019;1:e78–89.

57. Meiring C, Dixit A, Harris S, MacCallum NS, Brealey DA, Watkinson PJ, Jones A, Ashworth S, Beale R, Brett SJ, Singer M, Ercole A. Optimal intensive care outcome prediction over time using machine learning. PLoS One. 2018;13:e0206862.

58. Vink EE, Azoulay E, Caplan A, Kompanje EJO, Bakker J. Time-limited trial of intensive care treatment: an overview of current literature. Intensive Care Med. 2018;44:1369–77.

59. Schork NJ. Personalized medicine: time for one-person trials. Nature. 2015;520:609–11.

60. Gillis A, Beil M, Halevi-Tobias K, van Heerden PV, Sviri S, Agur Z. Alleviation of exhaustion-induced immunosuppression and sepsis by immune checkpoint blockers sequentially administered with antibiotics-analysis of a new mathematical model. Intensive Care Med Exp. 2019;7:32.

61. Marckmann G, Neitzke G, Schildmann J, Michalsen A, Dutzmann J, Hartog C, Jöbges S, Knochel K, Michels G, Pin M, et al. Decisions on the allocation of intensive care resources in the context of the COVID-19 pandemic. Med Klin Intensivmed Notfmed. 2020;115(Suppl 3):115–22.

62. Wilkinson D, Savulescu J. A costly separation between withdrawing and withholding treatment in intensive care. Bioethics. 2014;28:127–37.

63. Wilson ME, Hopkins RO, Brown SM. Long-term functional outcome data should not in general be used to guide end-of-life decision-making in the ICU. Crit Care Med. 2019;47:264–7.

64. Mark NM, Rayner SG, Lee NJ, Curtis JR. Global variability in withholding and withdrawal of life-sustaining treatment in the intensive care unit: a systematic review. Intensive Care Med. 2015;41:1572–85.

65. Steinberg A, Levy-Lahad E, Karni T, Zohar N, Siegal G, Sprung CL. Israeli position paper: triage decisions for severely ill patients during the COVID-19 pandemic. Rambam Maimonides Med J. 2020;11:e0019.

66. Sprung CL, Joynt GM, Christian MD, Truog RD, Rello J, Nates JL. Adult ICU triage during the coronavirus disease 2019 pandemic: who will live and who will die? Recommendations to improve survival. Crit Care Med. 2020;48:1196–202.

67. Sprung CL, Jennerich AL, Joynt GM, Michalsen A, Curtis JR, Efferen LS, Leonard S, Metnitz B, Mikstacki A, Patil N, McDermid RC, Metnitz P, Mularski RA, Bulpa P, Avidan A. The influence of geography, religion, religiosity and institutional factors on worldwide end-of-life care for the critically ill: the WELPICUS study. J Palliat Care. 2021:8258597211002308. https://doi.org/10.1177/08258597211002308.

68. Wunsch H, Hill AD, Bosch N, Adhikari NKJ, Rubenfeld G, Walkey A, Ferreyro BL, Tillmann BW, Amaral ACKB, Scales DC, Fan E, Cuthbertson BH, Fowler RA. Comparison of 2 triage scoring guidelines for allocation of mechanical ventilators. JAMA Netw Open. 2020;3:e2029250.

69. Piscitello GM, Kapania EM, Miller WD, Rojas JC, Siegler M, Parker WF. Variation in ventilator allocation guidelines by US state during the coronavirus disease 2019 pandemic. JAMA Netw Open. 2020;3:e2012606.

70. Peterson A, Largent EA, Karlawish J. Ethics of reallocating ventilators in the covid-19 pandemic. BMJ. 2020;369:m1828.

71. Liddell K, Skopek JM, Palmer S, Martin S, Anderson J, Sagar A. Who gets the ventilator? Important legal rights in a pandemic. J Med Ethics. 2020;46:421–6.

72. Konrad-Adenauer-Stiftung. Who gets the last ventilator? 2020. https://www.kas.de/en/single-title/-/content/who-gets-the-last-ventilator.

73. Myers LC, Escobar G, Liu VX. Goldilocks, the three bears and intensive care unit utilization: delivering enough intensive care but not too much. Pulm Ther. 2020;6:23–33.

74. Wilkinson D, Zohny H, Kappes A, Sinnott-Armstrong W, Savulescu J. Which factors should be included in triage? An online survey of the attitudes of the UK general public to pandemic triage dilemmas. BMJ Open. 2020;10:e045593.

75. Forschungsgruppe g/d/p. 2020. https://www.gdp-group.com/fileadmin/ms/pressemeldung_triage.pdf.

76. Norisue Y, Deshpande GA, Kamada M, Nabeshima T, Tokuda Y, Goto T, Ishizuka N, Hara Y, Nakata R, Makino J, Matsumura M, Fujitani S, Hiraoka E. Allocation of mechanical ventilators during a pandemic: a mixed-methods study of perceptions among Japanese health-care workers and the general public. Chest. 2021;159(6):2494–502.

77. Anantham D, Chai-Lim C, Zhou JX, Phua GC. Operationalization of critical care triage during a pandemic surge using protocolized communication and integrated supportive care. J Intensive Care. 2020;8:59.
78. Christian MD, Joynt GM, Hick JL, Colvin J, Danis M, Sprung CL. Chapter 7. Critical care triage. Recommendations and standard operating procedures for intensive care unit and hospital preparations for an influenza epidemic or mass disaster. Intensive Care Med. 2010;36 Suppl 1:S55–64.
79. Belsky DW, Caspi A, Houts R, Cohen HJ, Corcoran DL, Danese A, Harrington H, Israel S, Levine ME, Schaefer JD, Sugden K, Williams B, Yashin AI, Poulton R, Moffitt TE. Quantification of biological aging in young adults. Proc Natl Acad Sci U S A. 2015;112:E4104–10.
80. Theou O, Brothers TD, Mitnitski A, Rockwood K. Operationalization of frailty using eight commonly used scales and comparison of their ability to predict all-cause mortality. J Am Geriatr Soc. 2013;61:1537–51.
81. Cuthbertson BH, Wunsch H. Long-term outcomes after critical illness. The best predictor of the future is the past. Am J Respir Crit Care Med. 2016;194:132–4.
82. Walford R, et al. Frailty. In: Flaatten H, et al., editors. The very old critically ill patients. Cham: Springer; 2022. (this volume).
83. Flaatten H, De Lange DW, Morandi A, Andersen FH, Artigas A, Bertolini G, Boumendil A, Cecconi M, Christensen S, Faraldi L, Fjølner J, Jung C, Marsh B, Moreno R, Oeyen S, Öhman CA, Pinto BB, Soliman IW, Szczeklik W, Valentin A, Watson X, Zaferidis T, Guidet B, VIP1 Study Group. The impact of frailty on ICU and 30-day mortality and the level of care in very elderly patients (80 years). Intensive Care Med. 2017;43:1820–8.
84. Guidet B, de Lange DW, Boumendil A, Leaver S, Watson X, Boulanger C, Szczeklik W, Artigas A, Morandi A, Andersen F, Zafeiridis T, Jung C, Moreno R, Walther S, Oeyen S, Schefold JC, Cecconi M, Marsh B, Joannidis M, Nalapko Y, Elhadi M, Fjølner J, Flaatten H, VIP2 Study Group. The contribution of frailty, cognition, activity of daily life and comorbidities on outcome in acutely admitted patients over 80 years in European ICUs: the VIP2 study. Intensive Care Med. 2020;46:57–69.
85. Wilkinson DJC. Frailty triage: is rationing intensive medical treatment on the grounds of frailty ethical? Am J Bioeth. 2020;8:1–22.
86. Flaatten H, Guidet B, Andersen FH, Artigas A, Cecconi M, Boumendil A, Elhadi M, Fjølner J, Joannidis M, Jung C, Leaver S, Marsh B, Moreno R, Oeyen S, Nalapko Y, Schefold JC, Szczeklik W, Walther S, Watson X, Zafeiridis T, de Lange DW, VIP2 Study Group. Reliability of the Clinical Frailty Scale in very elderly ICU patients: a prospective European study. Ann Intensive Care. 2021;11:22.
87. Newdick C, Sheehan M, Dunn M. Tragic choices in intensive care during the COVID-19 pandemic: on fairness, consistency and community. J Med Ethics. 2020;46:646–51.
88. The Academy of Medical Sciences. Multimorbidity: a priority for global health research. 2018. https://acmedsci.ac.uk/file-download/99630838.
89. Mujica-Mota RE, Roberts M, Abel G, Elliott M, Lyratzopoulos G, Roland M, Campbell J. Common patterns of morbidity and multi-morbidity and their impact on health-related quality of life: evidence from a national survey. Qual Life Res. 2015;24:909–18.
90. Yarnall AJ, Sayer AA, Clegg A, Rockwood K, Parker S, Hindle JV. New horizons in multimorbidity in older adults. Age Ageing. 2017;46:882–8.
91. Min H, Avramovic S, Wojtusiak J, Khosla R, Fletcher RD, Alemi F, Kheirbek RE. A comprehensive multimorbidity index for predicting mortality in intensive care unit patients. J Palliat Med. 2017;20:35–41.
92. Zador Z, Landry A, Cusimano MD, Geifman N. Multimorbidity states associated with higher mortality rates in organ dysfunction and sepsis: a data-driven analysis in critical care. Crit Care. 2019;23:247.
93. Stirland LE, González-Saavedra L, Mullin DS, Ritchie CW, Muniz-Terrera G, Russ TC. Measuring multimorbidity beyond counting diseases: systematic review of community and population studies and guide to index choice. BMJ. 2020;368:m160.

The Very Old Critically Ill Patients Risk Scores for the Very Old, Achievable?

Rui Moreno

Contents

⌂ Learning Objectives

Learning objectives of this chapter is to review existent risk score applicable to the very old patient. Problems, challenges and ongoing developments are discussed, with particular emphasis on the importance of previous health status over the presence and degree of physiological derangements in this particular population when developing or applying one of these methods.

17.1 Introduction

Since 1981, with the publication of the first general severity scores such as the APACHE (Acute Physiology and Chronic Health Evaluation) [1], followed in 1983 by the SAPS (Simplified Acute Physiology Score) I [2] and in 1985 by the APACHE II [3], many attempts have been made by the researchers to stratify intensive care patients by severity of illness and later on to predict vital status at hospital discharge.

However, this field of science faces some unique challenges. First, outcome of critical illnesses that will inexorably lead to death in a short period of time has improved greatly. Nowadays, both in young and specially in old patients, survival rates are several times greater than they were a few decades ago.

Driven by the developments in the knowledge of the physiopathology, therapeutic options and support care, the impact of deranged physiology responsible for the clinical syndromes we learned to recognize, changes in the baseline characteristics of populations, driven mainly by changes in lifestyle and early recognition and long-time control of chronic diseases more than by true (genetic) changes in our patients, changes in the way we organize and deliver healthcare and in the way we prevent, diagnose and treat major diseases all have a strong impact on the accuracy of our instruments [4].

One of the consequences of these changes is a continuous pressure on the representativeness of our patient databases and in the way we model the outcome of our patients based on a set of predictive variables. Life is made of change, and with regard to intensive care medicine (ICM), most of the changes have been positive. However, in this process, those involved on the development of severity scores and outcome models faced a major challenge: are the major determinants of outcome in critically ill patients still the same than in 1981? And if so, have we been able to cope with these changes and incorporating them in our models?

One of these major changes has been the changing demography of the population and the increase in life span in most countries, as well as the major changes in ICU referral, assessment and treatment of patients with critical illness or with an acute, severe, decompensation of a chronic disease. In 1991, when the APACHE III was published [5], acute physiological derangement explained around 73% of the prognostic value of the model while age (7%) and chronic diseases (3) only 10% of the prognostic value of the model.

When we published the general SAPS 3 model in 2005 [6], acute physiological derangement was reduced to 27.4% of the explanatory power of the model, with chronic health status increased to 49.9%. If this is true, and this incredible change – exhaustively explored by our group – seems not to be explained by statistical or other methodological factors [7], it represents possibly one of the best evidences we have nowadays about the increasing success of ICM in dealing with deranged physiology and being able to achieve survival in many diseases and syndromes that until now have been hopeless.

As we wrote more than 10 years ago, "*When we compare the case mix of a modern ICU nowadays with the one we had 20 years ago, it is evident that an increase in the mean age of the admitted patients, an increase in the number and severity of chronic diseases presented by our patients, a change in diagnosis and a huge change in the complexity of the interventions is being made. These processes lead to an emphasis on the early detection and correction of physiological derangements (because of the fact that globally the degree of physiological reserve of our patients is lower nowadays compared with what it used to be) and the need of multidisciplinary approaches for care, with more focus on the effectiveness and safety of our practices*" [4].

However, this evolution raised as many questions as it provided answers:

- Are our databases still representative of the actual population, as demographics change quickly?
- Are we still using in the building and development of our models the most important variables, specially in what concerns age and chronic health status?

17.2 The Prognostic Determinants of General Severity Scores and General Prognostic Models

Most general severity scores build until now are composed essentially of two groups of variables:

(a) Those accessing the presence and degree of physiological dysfunction (e.g. hypoxaemia, hypotension, hypothermia, leucocytosis, anaemia, urinary output)
(b) Those assessing the health status of the patient before critical illness (age, some co-morbid diseases and age-related factors like frailty)

Apart from these two groups, some (not all) of the general severity scores use other kind of variables, such as time since hospital admission, location in the hospital before ICU admission, diagnoses, etc. Given their specificity to each model I will not review it here.

17.3 Presence and Degree of Physiological Dysfunction

Most – if not all – of the major general severity scores used today use a combination of the most deranged values of physiological variables (or a surrogate of this, like the need for organ support) to access the presence and degree of organ dysfunction/failure. Overall, despite that the variables and their limits differ among them, they assign points to each variable according to their impact on mortality (correcting all other variables in the model). This approach was later on simplified by the development of organ failure scores such as the Sequential Organ Failure Assessment (SOFA) score [8], later proved to correlate quite well with the progress of the patient [9, 10]. Designed to describe and not to predict the presence and severity of organ dysfunction/failure over time, the interaction of these scores with age and chronic health status has been studied in some specific settings (e.g. the interaction among age, disease, severity of disease and chronic health status on survival from an acute illness [11]). It is interesting to see that, in very recent manuscripts about the infection by SARS-CoV-2 virus, which mortality is strongly (but not exclusively) influenced by age, the SOFA score demonstrated only a moderate discriminative accuracy to predict survival in ICU patients with sepsis. Despite the claims by the authors that this fact may be due to the poor accuracy of SOFA score in patients requiring mechanical ventilation for COVID-19 pneumonia because such patients generally have severe single-organ dysfunction and less variation in SOFA scores [12], we are probably quite far away from a definitive explanation of this fact.

Also, despite the fact that the normal values of several (if not all) physiological variables changes with age, no general severity score or organ dysfunction/failure score build up to know used different cut-offs for variables according to age. This fact can compromise the prognostic impact on mortality of several important variables used to quantify physiologic dysfunction.

17.4   Health Status of the Patient Before Critical Illness

Up to now, health status of the patient before critical illness has been accessed mainly based on (chronological) age and the presence or absence of a very limited list of co-morbid diseases. Many other demographic facts, possibly important in this context, have been left out, such as gender [13].

From these, chronological age has been the most consistent among all the variables used to quantify the prognostic impact of the patient's health status before critical illness. As shown in ▣ Figs. 17.1 and 17.2, in all of the graphs, we can see an increase in the number of points assigned to the model (and consequently on mortality) with increasing chronological age, when this variable is controlled for all the

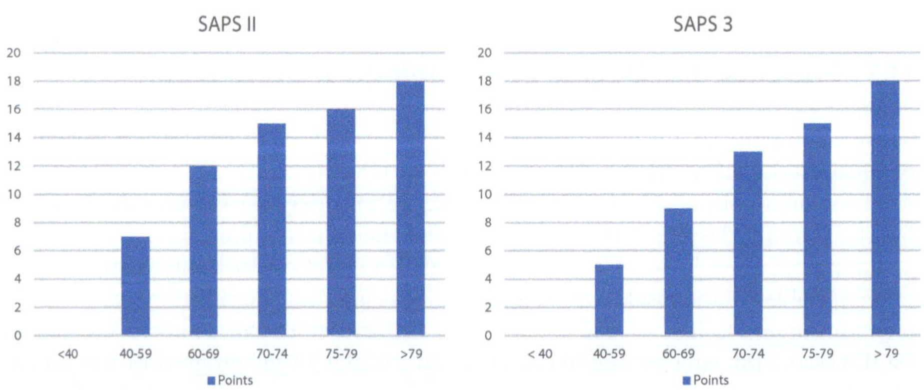

▣ **Fig. 17.1**   SAPS II (left) and SAPS 3 (right) points assigned to the model according to patient age at ICU admission [6, 35]

APACHE II vs APACHE III

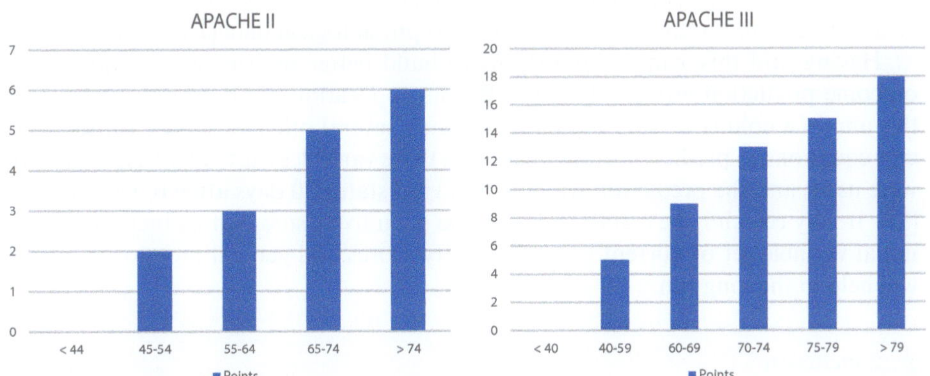

Fig. 17.2 APACHE II (left) and APACHE III (right) points assigned to the model according to patient age at ICU admission [3, 5]

other variables on the model. This stresses the impact and the importance of this variable on the explanatory power of the models. However, since its inclusion, criticisms have been raised to the use of chronologic versus physiological age. Difficult to define and measure, with an impact on mortality that changes significantly with time, gender and many more variables, the measurement of age has hampered further developments on the field of severity evaluation and outcome prediction in intensive care.

For this reason, *frailty*, a concept that was first applicable to the critically ill patient around 2011 [14], soon was developed and provided with an easy way to measure it, even from data given by the next of kin or other people who know the patient, with the development of an easy to use scale for its quantification [15]. Defined as *"a state of vulnerability to poor resolution of homeostasis after a stressor event"* [16] and strongly associated with adverse outcomes in different settings (and not only in critical care), this becomes an essential part of evaluation of the old patient [17], despite some criticism when extracted automatically and not collected by interviewing patient's relatives [18]. What is now called by some the "frailty syndrome" [19] can also allow the researcher or the clinician to follow the path of frailty during the last years of life, a significant information when ICU triage and the option for palliative care are open options [20].

Able to be collected in a quite reliable way in critically ill patients [21], it seems clear now that frailty is associated with a worst health even across the spectrum of frailty domains, in particular functional dependence, malnutrition and prior hospital admissions [22]. These results have been demonstrated clearly by our research group (VIP) on patients over 80 years of age [23, 24] and others [16, 25].

It does not replace entirely chronological age (that remains significant in multivariate analysis but adds explanatory power to the analysis), and neither it has reached already the primetime to decide on triage issues, despite being relevant to resource allocation through its impact on probability of survival, longevity and quality of life [26].

The recent pandemic of COVID-19 demonstrated that, in a very vulnerable group of patients, the elderly, frailty was an integrative marker of physiological vulnerability [27] and prognosis [28], but not perfect without tracking the trajectories of disease, especially when applied to individual patients [29], a mission still impossible to be achieved without taking into account also physiological data [12, 30–32].

Having said this, can *frailty* help us to build better severity scores and general outcome prediction models? Possibly. But its application has been only tested with this aim in a cohort of very old patients, using several other variables, without specific equations to predict mortality based on these variables (instead different cut-offs were used) and the prediction window was vital status 30 days after ICU admission [33]. It may certainly be a start, but it is too soon to be sure that its inclusion in the initial variable set of current general severity scores and general prognostic models will help in the long run.

> **Conclusion**
>
> It is certainly that, in the future, our emphasis on accessing the prognosis (both in the short term and in the long term) will incorporate a more exhaustive characterization of the patient background (in terms of genetic variations in the inflammatory and anti-inflammatory response to an acute or acute-on-chronic insult), available in most ICUs in a very short time, meaning a better characterization of the effects of decades of interaction between that genetic background with a certain lifestyle and prior diseases that conditionate a certain immune response and a certain physiological reserve – mainly neurological and cardiovascular reserve – and its possible/probable interactions with the acute insult that results to the development of organ dysfunction/failure and – at the end – mortality.
>
> As our knowledge of deranged physiology and how to cope with it on a personalised way, these issues, seem by many today as belonging to science-fiction, will be in our frontier of knowledge in order to provide care to those who we can decrease morbidity and mortality saving important resources and causing important morbidity to the patients and their loved ones.
>
> Finally, to finish where I have started, "Do we need dedicated risk scores for the very old ICU patients?". I think maybe never, certainly not at this time; the definition of a "very old" patient is different among different cultures and is prone to an increase with time as life spam changes, and the main arguments to build such instruments: different predisposition (chronological age and frailty), different physiological response to insults as immune, neurological, cardiovascular (and possibly other) physiological reserve will decease and that will became exhausted at a certain age (or by genetics, by disease, or by a combination of all) and will be addressed with different methods of therapy, personalised to age but also to other factors, will came into life. Also, people would then start asking for a "perfect" severity score or outcome prediction model to "young patients" or to "patients of a certain age, gender, or skin colour" – something that we cannot deliver with 100% certainty until we will be able to know all the prognostic information about a certain patient – something that Gödel's incompleteness theorems demonstrated: that it is impossible to be made and impossible for the consistency to be demonstrated [34]. It remains for our generation to be certain tand to cope hat all general severity scores and general outcome prediction models will not be perfect and carry with them a certain level of uncertainty that we must accept and cope with, no matter the sub-group of interest.

> **Take-Home Messages**
> From this review it seems clear that in the future, our emphasis on accessing the prognosis of very old patients must incorporate a more exhaustive characterization of the patient. This means a better characterization of the effects of decades of interaction between that genetic background with a certain lifestyle and prior diseases that conditionate a certain immune and physiological response and their possible/probable interactions with the acute insult that leads to the development of organ dysfunction/failure and – at the end – mortality.
>
> This is crucial to help us to provide care to those patients in which we can decrease morbidity and mortality, optimizing the use of resources and decreasing morbidity and healthcare-related stress to the patients and their loved ones.
>
> This author claims that this is achievable without the need for dedicated risk scores for the very old ICU patients. In the meanwhile, we must be aware of the limitations of existent instruments and learn to accept and cope with their application in sub-groups of interest – in this case the very old patients.

References

1. Knaus W, Zimmerman J, Wagner D, Draper E, Lawrence D. APACHE - Acute Physiology and Chronic Health Evaluation: a physiologically based classification system. Crit Care Med. 1981;9:591–7.
2. Le Gall J-R, Loirat P, Alperovitch A. Simplified acute physiological score for intensive care patients. Lancet. 1983;ii:741.
3. Knaus WA, Draper EA, Wagner DP, Zimmerman JE. APACHE II: a severity of disease classification system. Crit Care Med. 1985;13:818–29.
4. Moreno RP. Outcome prediction in intensive care: why we need to reinvent the wheel. Curr Opin Crit Care. 2008;14:483–4.
5. Knaus WA, Wagner DP, Draper EA, et al. The APACHE III prognostic system. Risk prediction of hospital mortality for critically ill hospitalized adults. Chest. 1991;100:1619–36.
6. Moreno RP, Metnitz PG, Almeida E, et al. SAPS 3. From evaluation of the patient to evaluation of the intensive care unit. Part 2: development of a prognostic model for hospital mortality at ICU admission. Intensive Care Med. 2005;31:1345–55.
7. Moreno R, Jordan B, Metnitz P. The changing prognostic determinants in the critically ill patient. In: Vincent JL, editor. 2007 yearbook of intensive care and emergency medicine. Springer-Verlag; 2007. p. 899–907.
8. Vincent J, Moreno R, Takala J, et al. The SOFA (Sepsis-related Organ Failure Assessment) score to describe organ dysfunction/failure. On behalf of the Working Group on Sepsis-Related Problems of the European Society of Intensive Care Medicine. Intensive Care Med. 1996;22:707–10.
9. Vincent J-L, de Mendonça A, Cantraine F, et al. Use of the SOFA score to assess the incidence of organ dysfunction/failure in intensive care units: results of a multicentric, prospective study. Crit Care Med. 1998;26:1793–800.
10. Moreno R, Vincent J-L, Matos R, et al. The use of maximum SOFA score to quantify organ dysfunction/failure in intensive care. Results of a prospective, multicentre study. Intensive Care Med. 1999;25:686–96.
11. Knaus WA. Prognosis with mechanical ventilation. The influence of disease, severity of disease, age, and chronic health status on survival from an acute illness. Am Rev Respir Dis. 1989;140:S8–13.
12. Raschke RA, Agarwal S, Rangan P, Heise CW, Curry SC. Discriminant accuracy of the SOFA score for determining the probable mortality of patients with COVID-19 pneumonia requiring mechanical ventilation. JAMA. 2021;325:1469.
13. Wernly B, Bruno RR, Kelm M, et al. Sex-specific outcome disparities in very old patients admitted to intensive care medicine: a propensity matched analysis. Sci Rep. 2020;10:18671.

14. McDermid RC, Stelfox HT, Bagshaw SM. Frailty in the critically ill: a novel concept. Crit Care. 2011;15:301.
15. Clegg A, Young J, Iliffe S, Rikkert MO, Rockwood K. Frailty in elderly people. Lancet. 2013;381:752–62.
16. So RKL, Bannard-Smith J, Subbe CP, et al. The association of clinical frailty with outcomes of patients reviewed by rapid response teams: an international prospective observational cohort study. Crit Care. 2018;22:227.
17. Rockwood K, Howlett SE. Fifteen years of progress in understanding frailty and health in aging. BMC Med. 2018;16:220.
18. Bruno RR, Wernly B, Flaatten H, Schölzel F, Kelm M, Jung C. The hospital frailty risk score is of limited value in intensive care unit patients. Crit Care. 2019;23:239.
19. Whitlock EL, Whittington RA. The frailty syndrome: anesthesiologists must understand more and fear less. Anesth Analg. 2020;130:1445–8.
20. Stow D, Matthews FE, Hanratty B. Frailty trajectories to identify end of life: a longitudinal population-based study. BMC Med. 2018;16:171.
21. Flaatten H, Guidet B, Andersen FH, et al. Reliability of the Clinical Frailty Scale in very elderly ICU patients: a prospective European study. Ann Intensive Care. 2021;11:22.
22. Darvall JN, Greentree K, Braat MS, Story DA, Lim WK. Contributors to frailty in critical illness: multi-dimensional analysis of the Clinical Frailty Scale. J Crit Care. 2019;52:193–9.
23. de Lange DW, Guidet B, Moreno R, Christensen S, Flaatten H, on behalf of the VIP1 Study Group. Huge variation in obtaining ethical permission for a non-intervention observational study in Europe. Intensive Care Med Exp. 2017;5:44.
24. Guidet B, de Lange DW, Boumendil A, et al. The contribution of frailty, cognition, activity of daily life and comorbidities on outcome in acutely admitted patients over 80 years in European ICUs: the VIP2 study. Intensive Care Med. 2019;46:57.
25. Muessig JM, Nia AM, Masyuk M, et al. Clinical Frailty Scale (CFS) reliably stratifies octogenarians in German ICUs: a multicentre prospective cohort study. BMC Geriatr. 2018;18:162.
26. Wilkinson DJC. Frailty triage: is rationing intensive medical treatment on the grounds of frailty ethical? Am J Bioeth. 2020:1–22.
27. Xue Q-L. Frailty as an integrative marker of physiological vulnerability in the era of COVID-19. BMC Med. 2020;18:333.
28. Jung C, Flaatten H, Fjølner J, et al. The impact of frailty on survival in elderly intensive care patients with COVID-19: the COVIP study. Crit Care. 2021;25:149.
29. Beil M, Sviri S, Flaatten H, et al. On predictions in critical care: the individual prognostication fallacy in elderly patients. J Crit Care. 2021;61:34–8.
30. Khan Z, Hulme J, Sherwood N. An assessment of the validity of SOFA score based triage in H1N1 critically ill patients during an influenza pandemic. Anaesthesia. 2009;64:1283–8.
31. Wunsch H, Hill AD, Bosch N, et al. Comparison of 2 triage scoring guidelines for allocation of mechanical ventilators. JAMA Netw Open. 2020;3:e2029250–e.
32. Flaatten H, Beil M, Guidet B. Prognostication in older ICU patients: mission impossible? Br J Anaesth. 2020;125:655–7.
33. de Lange DW, Brinkman S, Flaatten H, et al. Cumulative prognostic score predicting mortality in patients older than 80 years admitted to the ICU. J Am Geriatr Soc. 2019;67:1263–7.
34. Gödel K. Über formal unentscheidbare Sätze der Principia Mathematica und verwandter Systeme, I. Monatshefte für Mathematik und Physik. 1931;38:173–98.
35. Le Gall JR, Lemeshow S, Saulnier F. A new simplified acute physiology score (SAPS II) based on a European / North American multicenter study. J Am Med Assoc. 1993;270:2957–63.

Usual ICU Procedures

Contents

Ventilation

Marta Lorente-Ros, Antonio Artigas, and José A. Lorente

Contents

💬 Learning Objectives

In this chapter the reader will learn the physiological effects and the commonly accepted indications for noninvasive respiratory support (high flow nasal cannulae [HFNC], noninvasive mechanical ventilation [NIMV]) and invasive mechanical ventilation (IMV), with special consideration to the elderly patient, whenever there is specific information in the literature regarding this age group.

Practical Implications

HFNC are increasingly used for the treatment of acute hypoxemic respiratory failure (AHRF), acute exacerbation of chronic obstructive pulmonary disease (AECOPD), and other conditions associated with risk of hypoxemia.

Unlike standard oxygen therapy (SOT), HFNC provide a higher airflow rate, higher fraction of inspired oxygen (FiO_2), and effectively heated and humidified air.

Physiological effects include provision of some level of positive end expiratory pressure, improved oxygenation, reduced anatomical dead space, better patient comfort, and less dryness.

When compared to SOT, HFNC decreases the need for intubation and escalation of respiratory support in AHRF.

Patients with AHRF being treated with HFNC should be closely monitored to identify signs of failure and the need for intubation. There are studies supporting the use of the ROX index ($[SpO_2/FiO_2]/RR$) to predict the likelihood of intubation in patients requiring HFNC.

NIMV is used for the treatment of AECOPD. In elderly patients it has been shown that NIMV, as compared to standard medical treatment, is associated with a significant decrease in the proportion of patients meeting criteria for tracheal intubation.

NIMV is also used for the treatment of acute cardiogenic pulmonary edema (ACPE) where, as compared to SOT, it is associated with a reduction in hospital mortality, intubation rate and ICU length of stay, and a quicker symptomatic improvement and better tolerance.

In AHRF, NIMV reduces the intubation rate and hospital mortality, as compared to SOT.

In ARDS, success rates of NIMV in mild, moderate, and severe ARDS are 78%, 58%, and 53%, respectively, according to the LUNG SAFE study. The use of NIMV was in that study independently associated with increased ICU (but not hospital) mortality. Using propensity score, ICU mortality was greater in the NIMV versus the IMV group only in patients with PaO_2/FiO_2 ratio <150. Thus, consideration should be given to the high mortality rate of patients with ARDS failing treatment with NIMV, and to the association between the initial use of NIMV and mortality in ARDS, at least for patients with more impaired oxygenation (e.g., PaO_2/FiO_2 < 150). The conclusions of the LUNG SAFE study may partly pertain to the elderly, as median age was between 66 and 63 years.

18.1 Introduction

Different forms of respiratory support can be used to treat oxygenation and ventilation failure of the lungs. We will discuss here the role of HFNC, NIMV, and IMV for the treatment of acute respiratory failure (ARF) in the elderly. We will also address ventilation issues in patients with AHRF and COVID-19 pertaining to elderly patients. Most of the published literature does not deal directly with elderly patients, but often a large proportion of patients included in the different studies are >65 years of age, and conclusions can to some extent be applied to the treatment of the elderly patient population.

18.2 High Flow Nasal Cannulae

HFNC are increasingly used for the treatment of AHRF and AECOPD and prevention of post-extubation respiratory failure, preintubation oxygenation, sleep apnea, acute heart failure, and hypoxemia in the context of do-not-intubate (DNI) orders [1].

Unlike standard oxygen therapy (SOT), HFNC provide a higher airflow rate, higher fraction of inspired oxygen (FiO2), and effectively heated and humidified air.

Physiological effects include provision of some level of positive end expiratory pressure (PEEP), improved oxygenation, reduced anatomical dead space, better patient comfort, and less dryness [2–4]. Due to the higher airflow rate delivered, the FiO2 provided is more predictable than with SOT [5–7]. As a result of providing high FiO2 and low level of PEEP, oxygenation increases with HFNC [4, 7–15]. HFNC also increases tidal volume (Vt) and decreases respiratory rate (RR) [11], thus decreasing the work of breathing.

18.3 HFNC in AHRF

A number of studies have shown that HFNC improves oxygenation and enhances patient comfort, but whether its use attains other benefits as compared to SOT or NIMV is less clear. The outcome benefits of treatment with HFNC have been analyzed in different meta-analysis.

Nedel et al. evaluated nine studies that assessed HFNC in critically ill subjects with AHRF or at risk for this complication [16]. They found that HFNC was associated with nonsignificant reduction in the incidence of IMV compared with NIMV (odds ratio [OR] 0.83, 95% confidence interval [CI] 0.57–1.20) or SOT (OR 0.49, 95% CI 0.22–1.08), nor was it associated with reduction in ICU mortality compared with NIMV (OR 0.72, 95% CI 0.23–2.21) or with SOT (OR 0.69, 95% CI 0.33–1.42). There was a trend toward better oxygenation compared with SOT but a worse gas exchange compared with NIMV.

Another meta-analysis of randomized controlled trials that compared HFNC and SOT or nasal continuous positive airway pressure (nCPAP) in children with acute lower respiratory infection reported treatment failure as an outcome [17]. HFNC significantly reduced treatment failure (risk ratio [RR] 0.49, 95% CI 0.40–0.60) in children with mild hypoxemia (arterial pulse oximetry [SpO_2] >90% on room air), but in infants of 1–6 months of age with severe hypoxemia (SpO_2 < 90% on room air or SpO_2 > 90% on supplemental oxygen), HFNC was associated with an increased risk of treatment failure compared with nCPAP (risk ratio [RR] 1.77, 95% CI 1.17–2.67). No significant differences were found in intubation rates or mortality between HFNC and SOT or nCPAP. HFNC had a significantly lower risk of nasal trauma compared with nCPAP (RR 0.35, 95% CI 0.16–0.77).

In a more recent meta-analysis, Lewis et al. [18] included 51 studies in which treatment was initiated either after extubation or before mechanical ventilation in adults admitted to the ICU. The authors concluded that HFNC, versus SOT, may lead to less treatment failure (low-certainty evidence) but probably with little or no difference in mortality (moderate-certainty evidence). HFNC versus NIMV found no evidence of a difference in treatment failure, either being used post-extubation or before IMV (low-certainty evidence), nor was it associated with difference in in-hospital mortality (low-certainty evidence).

Thus, HFNC has been shown to enhance patient comfort and improve oxygenation, and may lead to less treatment failure when compared to SOT, but probably makes little or no difference when compared to NIMV, conclusions supported in general by low or very low certainty. There is not enough evidence to support the use of HFNC to achieve other benefits such as decrease in mortality or decrease in intubation rates.

The recommendation based on the available evidence is that HFNC is preferred to SOT for the treatment of AHRF [18]. When compared to SOT, HFNC decreases the need for intubation and escalation of respiratory support. It also has a greater improvement in oxygenation, but it provides no benefit in mortality, length of stay, dyspnea, or patient comfort [19–24]. There is not enough data to compare HFNC with NIMV for treatment of AHRF [18]. Patient comfort is greater with HFNC, but there is not enough evidence to support a benefit in other outcomes such as intubation rate, mortality, or length of stay [25, 26].

18.4   Other Indications for HFNC

HFNC is used for preoxygenation before and during intubation. However, studies have not shown consistent benefit in clinically relevant outcomes [27–30], and therefore practice guidelines give no recommendation as to the use of HFNC for the intubation procedure [1].

HFNC is also used in post-extubation respiratory failure. In patients at low risk for extubation failure, SOT often suffices to maintain oxygenation. One clinical trial showed reduction in re-intubation rate as compared to SOT [31], but no difference was reported in another study [32]. Thus, HFNC is not routinely recommended for the prevention of post-extubation respiratory failure in patients with low risk for re-intubation.

In patients at high risk for re-intubation, clinical trials show that HFNC is superior to SOT for the prevention of post-extubation respiratory failure [4, 33–36]. However, no differences are shown when HFNC is compared to NIMV [36–38]. Current guidelines thus indicate a conditional recommendation for the use of HFNC (versus SOT) in patients at high risk for re-intubation. NIMV should be used instead according to routine practice of the particular institution [1].

In the postoperative setting, HFNC can be used for the treatment or prevention of respiratory failure. Some patients, but not all, should receive HFNC in the postoperative period, such as obese and high-risk patients following cardiothoracic surgery [1, 11, 18, 32, 39–48].

Other common uses of HFNC include oxygenation during bronchoscopy, in patients with tracheostomy being weaned off the ventilator, and in combination with NIMV for oxygenation support.

18.5 Failure of HFNC in AHRF

Patients with AHRF being treated with HFNC should be closely monitored to identify signs of failure and the need for intubation. There are studies supporting the use of the ROX index to predict the likelihood of intubation in patients requiring HFNC [15]. The acronym ROX stands for respiratory rate and oxygenation. It is calculated as the ratio of (SpO_2/FiO_2) to respiratory rate (RR): ($[SpO_2/FiO_2]/RR$). The ROX index remains to be validated and is not currently routinely used to guide the clinical decision of intubation.

Roca et al. studied 157 patients with severe pneumonia treated with HFNC, of whom 44 (28.0%) required MV [49]. The ROX index measured at 12 hours after initiation of HFNC had the best accuracy (area under the receiver operating characteristic curve [AUC] 0.74) for the prediction of the need for MV, with the best cut-off value of 4.88. In a more recent multicenter prospective observational cohort study of patients with pneumonia treated with HFNC [50], among the 191 patients treated with HFNC in the validation cohort, 68 (35.6%) required intubation. The prediction accuracy of the ROX index increased over time. ROX index $\geq$4.88 measured at 2 (hazard ratio [HR] 0.434; 95% CI 0.264–0.715), 6 (HR 0.304; 95% CI 0.182–0.509), or 12 hours (HR 0.291; 95% CI 0.161–0.524) after HFNC initiation was consistently associated with a lower risk for intubation. ROX indices <2.85, < 3.47, and <3.85 at 2, 6, and 12 hours of HFNC initiation, respectively, were predictors of HFNC failure. Patients who failed presented a lower increase in the values of the ROX index over the 12 hours. Among the components of the index, SpO_2/FiO_2 was more predictive than RR. In a retrospective analysis of patients with COVID-19 pneumonia, the ROX index was tested in 120 patients receiving HFNC [51], of whom 35 patients (29%) failed HFNC and required intubation. ROX index at 12 h was the best predictor of intubation, with an AUC of 0.792 and a cut-off value of 5.99, with specificity 96% and sensitivity 62%. The ROX index has also been tested in other conditions. For instance, in 171 chest trauma patients receiving SOT, 49 (28.6%) of whom required endotracheal intubation, a threshold value of 12.85 (sensitivity 82, specificity 89) over the first 24 h predicted endotracheal intubation [52]. According to these data, the ROX index may be useful in assessing treatment failure in patients with different conditions, but different threshold values may be optimal in different conditions.

18.6 Development of NIMV

First used as the iron lung in the polio epidemics [53], NIMV later evolved when delivering intermittent positive pressure ventilation, and continuous positive airway pressure via a rubber face mask to treat different respiratory conditions became feasible [54, 55]. In 1981 Sullivan et al. described the successful use of continuous positive airway pressure (CPAP) via nasal mask in the management of obstructive sleep apnea [56] that was later used to treat respiratory failure from neuromuscular disease and nocturnal hypoventilation [57]. Subsequently, a Consensus Conference agreed on the role of NIMV in the management of patients with ARF [58–61]. NIMV is currently recommended for the treatment of various forms of ARF as detailed below. Specific indications for the elderly, when available, will be commented.

18.7 NIMV for the Treatment of AECOPD

AECOPD is one of the leading causes of hospitalizations. Pathophysiological changes during AECOPD include increased airflow resistance resulting in incomplete expiration, dynamic hyperinflation, and subsequent reduced diaphragm strength and respiratory muscle fatigue [62–64]. Reduced respiratory reserve in the elderly aggravates these physiological changes. NIMV is not the first line of treatment in AECOPD, but it is rather used in severe cases to prevent progression of the respiratory failure [65]. NIMV unloads the respiratory muscles and improves oxygenation and ventilation [25].

A trial of NIMV is recommended for AECOPD since it has shown a significant decrease in mortality, length of stay, intubation rate, and improvement in gas exchange [18, 59, 60, 66–76]. The recommended modality in this setting is bilevel positive airway pressure (BPAP). The benefit of BPAP in AECOPD extends from mild to severe COPD exacerbation and therefore should be used in all range of severities [69].

A national audit by Roberts et al. [77] of 10,000 COPD admissions showed that in patients with acidosis, mortality was higher if they received NIMV versus those who did not. However, this could be due to the late use of NIMV in patients already deteriorated or to the use of NIMV in cases of non-respiratory acidosis.

Whereas NIMV is recommended in the management of AECOPD, little evidence existed at the time of those recommendations [78, 79] to advocate its use in the elderly, and the guidelines had little evidence for the use of NIMV in the elderly with AECOPD [80].

Later studies proved the safety and efficacy of NIMV for the treatment of AECOPD in elderly patients. In a clinical trial on the treatment of AECOPD with NIMV, 82 patients aged >75 years [81] were randomized to receive NIMV or standard medical treatment (SMT). Treatment was associated with a significant decrease in the proportion of patients meeting criteria for tracheal intubation (7.3 versus 63.4%, in the treated and control groups, respectively), and a reduction in mortality rate (OR 0.40; 95% CI 0.19–0.83). Interestingly, 22 of 41 patients in the SMT group and DNI orders received NIMV as a rescue therapy. The mortality rate in this subgroup was comparable to the group receiving NIMV (OR 0.60, 95% CI 0.18–1.92), and significantly lower when compared with patients receiving intubation (OR 4.03,

95% CI 2.35–6.94). Balami et al. conducted a prospective study of 36 patients >65 years of age with AECOPD [82]. Mean age was 77.4 years. Only 2 patients (6%) could not be started on NIMV because of lack of tolerance, and treatment was successful in 27 of 34 patients treated (79%), whereas it did not succeed in 21%. Another indirect evidence that NIMV is effective in elderly patients is the finding that when patients ≥75 years of age are compared to younger patients, there are no differences in intubation or mortality rates [83], suggesting that NIMV is also safe and effective in the elderly population.

It is important to underline the clinical impact of a specialized NIMV team to optimize treatment success. A lower risk of death and intubation and a shorter ICU and hospital stay have been shown in patients treated with a dedicated NIMV team compared to management by ICU doctors and nurses working independently [84].

18.8 NIMV for the Treatment of Acute Cardiogenic Pulmonary Edema

Acute cardiogenic pulmonary edema (ACPE) is a leading cause of hospitalization for the elderly [85] and is associated with a high mortality rate. Reported in-hospital and 1-year mortality rates are 12% and 40%, respectively [86, 87]. In ACPE, the increase in extravascular lung fluid results in reduced lung volume and respiratory system compliance, increased airway resistance, and increased work of breathing. Noninvasive ventilation in ACPE prevents alveolar collapse, reduces alveolar edema, improves lung compliance [87], and decreases preload and afterload, thus reducing the work of breathing, increasing cardiac output, and improving oxygenation [65, 87, 88].

Systematic reviews and meta-analysis demonstrated a reduction in the rate of intubation and mortality in patients that received NIM [89]. Although a non-inferiority study questioned the role of NIMV in the management of ACPE, showing no difference in short-term mortality or need for intubation between the NIMV and standard therapy groups, several subsequent studies concluded that the use of NIMV in treating ACPE decreased the rate of intubation and in-hospital mortality [90–94]. However, results regarding mortality have not been entirely consistent between clinical trials [89, 90, 95–101].

There are few studies focused specifically on the elderly population, but given that the mean age of patients admitted for acute heart failure is greater than 70 years, many of the previous studies are thought to be applicable to this population. A study designed to investigate the clinical efficacy of NIMV in ACPE in patients greater than 75 years of age demonstrated early clinical improvement with a reduction in the rate of intubation and 48-hour mortality without sustained benefit during their hospital stay [101].

18.9 NIMV for the Treatment of AHRF

There is conflicting evidence about whether NIMV is beneficial to patients with AHRF not due to ACPE [102–110]. A prospective observational study on the use of NIMV in patients with AHRF reported a failure rate of 61% in patients with septic shock and 23% in patients without sepsis [111]. A meta-analysis of 11 studies (excluding patients with AECOPD or ACPE) showed that NIMV reduced the intubation rate (RR 0.59, 95% CI 0.44–0.79) and hospital mortality (RR 0.46; 95% CI 0.24–0.87) compared with SOT [109]. The wide confidence intervals reported suggest variable benefit among patients. A network meta-analysis studied 25 clinical trials comparing noninvasive treatments (NIMV or HFNC) with SOT in patients with AHRF [25]. Mortality was lower in patients treated with helmet or face mask NIMV compared with SOT. All three noninvasive modalities (helmet NIMV, face mask NIMV, HFNC) reduced intubation rates. High heterogeneity and risk of bias suggest caution when interpreting the results of this meta-analysis. In addition, a mortality benefit was not observed in patients with more severe impairment of oxygenation (PaO2/FiO2 < 200 mm Hg). In another meta-analysis of 29 randomized trials of mixed population of patients with AHRF comparing NIMV versus HFNC [112], it was found that HFNC resulted in lower mortality (RR 0.44, 95% CI 0.24–0.79), intubation rate (RR 0.71, 95% CI 0.53–0.95), and possibly hospital-acquired pneumonia (RR 0.46, 95% CI 0.15–1.45) and improved patient comfort.

The LUNG SAFE study provided important insights into the effects of treatment with NIMV in patients with ARDS [113]. Of 2813 patients with ARDS, 436 (15.5%) were managed with NIMV on days 1 and 2 following fulfillment of diagnostic criteria. The use of NIMV in moderate and severe forms of ARDS was surprising as the recommendations for NIMV in ARDS suggest that its use be restricted to mild ARDS [114]. However, success rates of NIMV in mild, moderate, and severe ARDS were not low (78%, 58%, and 53%, respectively). Hospital mortality in patients with NIMV success and failure was 16.1% and 45.4%, respectively. Importantly, the use of NIMV was independently associated with increased ICU (HR 1.446, 95% CI, 1.159–1.805), but not hospital, mortality. However, using propensity score, ICU mortality was greater in the NIMV versus the IMV group only in patients with PaO_2/FiO_2 ratio <150 (36.2% with NIMV compared with 24.7% with IMV). Thus, consideration should be given to the high mortality rate of patients with ARDS failing treatment with NIMV, and to the association between the initial use of NIMV and mortality in ARDS, at least for patients with more impaired oxygenation (e.g., $PaO2/FiO_2$ < 150). The conclusions of the LUNG SAFE study do not pertain necessarily to the elderly patient population. However the median (IQR) age of patients with NIMV success or failure was, respectively, 66.5 [52–77] and 63.0 [53–73] years, indicating that elderly patients were notably represented in this study.

In immunocompromised patients, NIMV is suggested as first option for treatment of patients with mild or moderate AHRF [115–117]. Several studies [118–122], but not all [123], have suggested improved mortality by using NIMV in these patients.

18.10   Noninvasive Mechanical Ventilation for Weaning from Mechanical Ventilation

Different clinical trials and a meta-analysis have shown that patients weaned with NIMV after extubation demonstrate reduced mortality, less ventilator-associated pneumonia, and shorter ICU and hospital stay, without increasing the risk of weaning failure or re-intubation [124–131].

In a Cochrane systematic review, 16 trials comparing extubation and immediate application of NIMV with continued invasive weaning in adults on mechanical ventilation were studied, involving 994 participants, most of them with COPD [132]. The use of NIMV was associated with reduced mortality (RR 0.53, 95% CI 0.36–0.80), weaning failure (RR 0.63, 95% CI 0.42–0.96), ventilator-associated pneumonia (RR 0.25, 95% CI 0.15–0.43), length of stay in the ICU (mean difference [MD] −5.59 days, 95% CI −7.90 to −3.28) and in hospital (MD -6.04 days, 95% CI −9.22 to −2.87), and total duration of mechanical ventilation (MD −5.64 days, 95% CI −9.50 to −1.77). This indication for NIMV mainly applies to hypercapnic respiratory failure, and patients included in the studies are generally old. For instance, in the study by Ferrer et al. [126], mean age was 70 years.

18.11   NIMV for Post-extubation Support

NIMV can be used after extubation in patients at low risk for post-extubation respiratory failure. In this scenario, NIMV provides no benefit compared to SOT. In patients at high risk for post-extubation respiratory failure, some studies do not show reduction in re-intubation rate or mortality [133–136], whereas others suggest a decrease in the re-intubation rate [131, 132, 136–140].

18.12   NIMV in the Postoperative Setting

Changes in respiratory function in the postoperative period, including depressed respiratory drive, decreased Vt because of postoperative pain, recumbent atelectasis, etc., place the patient at increased risk of ARF. The elderly is at increased risk for these changes, as muscle function may already be deteriorated.

NIMV is not recommended in all postoperative patients for the prevention of ARF. The general indication of NIMV in the postoperative period is for the treatment of patients who develop AHRF and fail to respond to HFNC [141–143].

18.13   Invasive Mechanical Ventilation

ARDS represents a high proportion of patients receiving mechanical ventilation in the ICU. Among 29,144 ICU patients, 10.4% fulfilled the criteria for the diagnosis of ARDS, and ARDS represented 23.4% of patients requiring mechanical ventilation [144]. In line with those results [144], in a large prospective study, among 7944 patients requiring mechanical ventilation for >24 hours, 986 (12.3%) had hypoxemic respiratory failure (PaO_2/FiO_2 < 300), and 731 (9.1%) met criteria for ARDS [145].

Mortality of AHRF and ARDS is high. In the LUNG SAFE study, hospital mortality was 34.9%, 40.3%, and 46.1% for patients with mild, moderate, and severe ARDS, respectively [144]. Parhar et al. reported that hospital mortality for mild, moderate, and severe ARDS was, respectively, 26.5%, 31.8%, and 60.0%, whereas 3-year mortality was 43.5%, 46.9%, and 71.1% [145].

How ARDS is diagnosed and managed seems to be suboptimal. First, the syndrome is recognized only in part of the patients fulfilling the diagnostic criteria, ranging from 51.3% in mild to 79% in severe ARDS [144]. Second, modifiable mortality risk factors related with mechanical ventilation settings are not always measured or set according to current recommendations. In 18,302 patients receiving mechanical ventilation for various indications [146], Vt decreased over time from a mean (SD) of 9.3 (2.3) to 8.2 (2.0) mL/kg predicted body weight between 2004 and 2010. However, in the more recent LUNG SAFE study [144], less than two-thirds of 2377 patients with ARDS received a tidal volume ≤8 mL/kg of predicted body weight. Plateau airway pressure was measured only in 40.1% of patients with ARDS, and prone positioning was used in 16.3% of patients with severe ARDS [144]. In addition, it has been shown that mechanical power is associated with increased 28-day hospital and 3-year mortality [145]. This finding is of importance, since modifiable determinants of mechanical power associated with lower survival include plateau pressure and driving pressure.

Description on how mechanical ventilation is used may apply to the elderly population only to some extent. For instance, in a large prospective study of 731 patients with ARDS [145], median (IQR) age was 60 (49–69) years; in 3022 ARDS patients [144], mean (95% CI) age was 61.5 (60.9–62.1). In another study of 18,302 patients [146], mean (SD) age was 59 (17), 59 (17), and 61 (17) years in three different study periods (1998, 2004, and 2010, respectively). However, it seems reasonable to assume that conclusions as to under recognition of ARDS and suboptimal treatment in terms of attaining low plateau and delta pressures, and low tidal volume, and using prone positioning as indicated, will also apply to the elderly patient population.

18.14 Invasive Versus Noninvasive Ventilation for Patients with COVID-19 and ARF

Clinical experience indicates that many patients can be supported with noninvasive oxygen therapy (either HFNC or NIMV) only to require tracheal intubation and IMV some time later in worse clinical conditions. Whether late intubation worsens prognosis is not known. Mortality of patients with COVID-19 and AHRF seems to be decreasing over time [147, 148], and it has been proposed that the decrease in mortality could be related to less frequency in the use of tracheal intubation as first therapy in patients with COVID-19 and AHRF. Other factors can certainly contribute to the decreased mortality, including routine use of corticosteroids, the use of HFNC, lung-protective ventilation strategies, better sedation, better attention to the treatment of delirium, and avoidance of unproven therapies [149].

In an ancillary analysis of the COVID-ICU study, Dres et al. [150] studied 1199 elderly patients admitted to the ICU, 62% of whom were intubated on day 1 and an additional 16% were intubated during their ICU stay. Those two groups did not differ in their PaO2/FiO2 ratio or other characteristics, suggesting that the decision to intubate was based just on clinical judgment. However, using Inverse Probability Weighting Treatment and propensity score analysis, mortality was higher in patients intubated on day 1 (42% versus 28%).

In a large multicenter cohort of 13,301 patients with the diagnosis of COVID-19 admitted to 126 ICUs in Brazil, younger age, absence of frailty, and the use of noninvasive respiratory support (NIRS) as first support strategy were independently associated with improved outcomes [151]. Among all patients, 18% received some form of NIRS (either NIMV, HFOT, or both), and 13% received IMV. However, there was a time pattern from the first to the last period of time analyzed: some form of NIRS (NIMV or HFOT) increased from 8.3% to 25%, whereas only IMV decreased markedly from 25% to 6.5% of all patients. Among those patients receiving some form of NIRS, there were significant changes: only NIMV from 92% to 79%, only HFOT from 4.4% to 6%, and both NIVM and HFOT from 3.3% to 15.0%. Thus, patients were less often intubated to receive IMV, and among those not intubated, the use of only NIMV decreased, whereas the use of HFOT or a combination of NIMV and HFOT increased over time. In addition, patients who suffered failure of NIRS did not show a greater mortality in comparison to those intubated directly [151]. In conclusion, HFNC has been used during the COVID-19 outbreak [51, 152–154]. The use of first some form of NIRS, probably HFNC, rather than quickly deciding IMV in patients with COVID-19 and AHRF, does not seem to be unwarranted, even in elderly patients [150, 151].

If HFNC is chosen, close monitoring is required for the early identification of signs of failure that would indicate the requirement of IMV [152]. Roca et al. [49] identified patients at high risk of HFNC failure if ROX <4.88 at 12 hours. This threshold was confirmed also in COVID-19 patients [155, 156] who showed, however, higher intubation rates than in other studies [153, 154, 157]. Panadero et al. conducted a retrospective, observational single-center study of 196 patients with COVID-19 and bilateral pneumonia, 40 of whom were treated with HFNC [156]. The intubation rate at day 30 was 52.5%, and overall mortality was 22.5%. Patients that required intubation, as compared to patients who did not, presented a significantly lower PaO2/FiO2 (93.7 ± 6.7 vs. 113.4 ± 6.6) and a significantly lower ROX index (4.0 ± 1.0 vs. 5.0 ± 1.6). A ROX index <4.94 measured 2 to 6 h after the start of therapy was associated with increased risk of intubation (HR 4.03, 95% CI 1.18–13.7). In another study, Vega et al. [51] tested whether the ROX index is an accurate predictor of HFNC failure for COVID-19 patients treated outside the ICU. In a multicenter retrospective observational study, 120 patients with confirmed COVID-19 treated with HFNC were included, of whom 35 (29%) failed HFNC and required intubation. The 12-hour ROX index was the best predictor of intubation according to an area under the ROC curve of 0.792 (95% CI 0.691–0.893), with a threshold of 5.99 (specificity 96%, sensitivity 62%). Thus, the ROX index seems useful to predict failure of treatment with HFNC, although the best discriminative value differs from the previously reported for patients with other types of AHRF. Previous small single-center studies in patients with COVID-19, probably with greater disease severity, reported lower values for the ROX index (4.95 and 5.40) during the first 6 hours of treatment [155, 156].

18.15 Liberation from Mechanical Ventilation in the Elderly

Physiological and anatomical respiratory peculiarities in the elderly make the weaning process different as compared to younger adults. Different studies have investigated factors involved in weaning in patients ≥ 75 years of age. Decreased elastic recoil of the lung and the chest wall, ventilation-perfusion mismatch, and diminished muscle strength are among the age-related respiratory physiological changes in the elderly. Of interest, studies reviewing weaning in the elderly did not identify age in itself as an independent risk factor for difficult weaning, but severity of acute illness instead influences weaning [158–163].

It has been shown that the probability of meeting weaning criteria and successful weaning decreases with age [159], but independent predictors of weaning were comorbidity, severity of illness, rapid shallow breathing (the ratio between the respiratory frequency to the tidal volume), and lung static compliance, not age. Negative fluid balance and lower central venous pressure have also been shown to be related to weaning success [162].

In another study [163], after adjusting for the APACHE II score, patients ≥75 years of age passed a spontaneous breathing trial earlier than younger patients, further indicating that age in itself is not a risk factor for delayed extubation. Same results on the lack of independent relationship between age and weaning were obtained by Hifumi et al. [158] in a retrospective study in patients with community-acquired pneumonia. Another study [160] found that the presence of emphysematous changes in chest CT and low serum albumin concentration, but not age, were associated with difficult weaning.

A number of measures have been proposed to expedite weaning, including less use of benzodiazepines to decrease the risk of delirium [164, 165], and early rehabilitation and prevention of immobility [166]. Daily spontaneous breathing trial to test for readiness for extubation (one the inciting event has resolved) is crucial to shorten the time spent on mechanical ventilation [167]. Daily awakening trials have been associated with fewer days on mechanical ventilation, better cognitive function, and decreased long-term mortality [164, 165]. Cader et al. [161] studied 41 elderly intubated patients who had been mechanically ventilated for at least 48 h and showed that providing inspiratory muscle training resulted in increased maximal inspiratory pressure and reduction in the weaning time by 1.7 days. In addition, physical therapy and occupational therapy during spontaneous awakening trials to patients who had been intubated for more than 48 hours had beneficial effects and found decreased incidence of delirium and shortened time spent in mechanical ventilation [166, 168].

Conclusions

Recommendations for the use of various form of respiratory support (NIMV, HFNC, IMV) exist for different forms of ARF. However, studies in elderly patients are scarce and insufficient to emit recommendations for this specific age group. Patients included in studies on NIMV for the treatment of AECOPD and ACPE represent to some extent the aged group and could reasonably be extrapolated to the elderly. This is less the case for studies on the use of IMV for the treatment of AHRF and ARDS. Thus, studies on respiratory support for the elderly are required, particularly for the treatment of AHRF.

Take-Home Message

- Different forms of respiratory support (SOT, CPAP, HFNC, NIMV, IMV) are available to treat ARF of different etiologies.
- It is important to know the specific indications (and the supporting evidence) of these therapies in the various conditions associated with (or risk of) ARF.
- Early identification of signs of failure of any of these therapies is crucial for optimal patient management, to make timely decisions to escalate therapy. Failure to do so is associated with increased mortality.

> – The elderly population is often underrepresented in clinical trials; thus the physiological peculiarities of the elderly patient should be considered when applying the results of clinical trials to the elderly.

References

1. Rochwerg B, Einav S, Chaudhuri D, et al. The role for high flow nasal cannula as a respiratory support strategy in adults: a clinical practice guideline. Intensive Care Med. 2020;46(12):2226–37.
2. Roca O, Riera J, Torres F, Masclans JR. High-flow oxygen therapy in acute respiratory failure. Respir Care. 2010;55(4):408–13.
3. Tiruvoipati R, Lewis D, Haji K, Botha J. High-flow nasal oxygen vs high-flow face mask: a randomized crossover trial in extubated patients. J Crit Care. 2010;25(3):463–8.
4. Rittayamai N, Tscheikuna J, Rujiwit P. High-flow nasal cannula versus conventional oxygen therapy after endotracheal extubation: a randomized crossover physiologic study. Respir Care. 2014;59(4):485–90.
5. Sim MA, Dean P, Kinsella J, et al. Performance of oxygen delivery devices when the breathing pattern of respiratory failure is simulated. Anaesthesia. 2008;63(9):938–40.
6. Ritchie JE, Williams AB, Gerard C, Hockey H. Evaluation of a humidified nasal high-flow oxygen system, using oxygraphy, capnography and measurement of upper airway pressures. Anaesth Intensive Care. 2011;39(6):1103–10.
7. Wagstaff TA, Soni N. Performance of six types of oxygen delivery devices at varying respiratory rates. Anaesthesia. 2007;62(5):492–503.
8. Parke RL, McGuinness SP. Pressures delivered by nasal high flow oxygen during all phases of the respiratory cycle. Respir Care. 2013;58(10):1621–4.
9. Parke RL, Eccleston ML, McGuinness SP. The effects of flow on airway pressure during nasal high-flow oxygen therapy. Respir Care. 2011;56(8):1151–5.
10. Groves N, Tobin A. High flow nasal oxygen generates positive airway pressure in adult volunteers. Aust Crit Care. 2007;20(4):126–31.
11. Parke R, McGuinness S, Dixon R, Jull A. Open-label, phase II study of routine high-flow nasal oxygen therapy in cardiac surgical patients. Br J Anaesth. 2013;111(6):925–31.
12. Corley A, Caruana LR, Barnett AG, et al. Oxygen delivery through high-flow nasal cannulae increase end-expiratory lung volume and reduce respiratory rate in postcardiac surgical patients. Br J Anaesth. 2011;107(6):998–1004.
13. Frat JP, Brugiere B, Ragot S, et al. Sequential application of oxygen therapy via high-flow nasal cannula and noninvasive ventilation in acute respiratory failure: an observational pilot study. Respir Care. 2015;60(2):170–8.
14. Schwabbauer N, Berg B, Blumenstock G, et al. Nasal high-flow oxygen therapy in patients with hypoxic respiratory failure: effect on functional and subjective respiratory parameters compared to conventional oxygen therapy and non-invasive ventilation (NIV). BMC Anesthesiol. 2014;14:66. https://doi.org/10.1186/1471-2253-14-66. eCollection 2014.
15. Nishimura M. High-flow nasal cannula oxygen therapy in adults: physiological benefits, indication, clinical benefits, and adverse effects. Respir Care. 2016;61(4):529–41.
16. Nedel WL, Deutschendorf C, Moraes Rodrigues Filho E. High-flow nasal cannula in critically ill subjects with or at risk for respiratory failure: a systematic review and meta-analysis. Respir Care. 2017;62(1):123–32.
17. Luo J, Duke T, Chisti MJ, Kepreotes E, Kalinowski V, Li J. Efficacy of high-flow nasal cannula vs standard oxygen therapy or nasal continuous positive airway pressure in children with respiratory distress: a meta-analysis. J Pediatr. 2019;215:199–208.
18. Lewis SR, Baker PE, Parker R, Smith AF. High-flow nasal cannulae for respiratory support in adult intensive care patients. Cochrane Database Syst Rev. 2021;3(3):CD010172. https://doi.org/10.1002/14651858.CD010172.pub3. PMID: 33661521; PMCID: PMC8094160.
19. Azoulay E, Lemiale V, Mokart D, et al. Effect of high-flow nasal oxygen vs standard oxygen on 28-day mortality in immunocompromised patients with acute respiratory failure: the HIGH randomized clinical trial. JAMA. 2018;320(20):2099–107.

20. Bell N, Hutchinson CL, Green TC, Rogan E, Bein KJ, Dinh MM. Randomised control trial of humidified high flow nasal cannulae versus standard oxygen in the emergency department. Emerg Med Austr EMA. 2015;7(6):537–41.
21. Frat JP, Thille AW, Mercat A, et al. High-flow oxygen through nasal cannula in acute hypoxemic respiratory failure. N Engl J Med. 2015;372(23):2185–96.
22. Jones PG, Kamona S, Doran O, Sawtell F, Wilsher M. Randomized controlled trial of humidified high-flow nasal oxygen for acute respiratory distress in the emergency department: the HOT-ER study. Respir Care. 2016;61(3):291–9.
23. Lemiale V, Mokart D, Mayaux J, et al. The effects of a 2-h trial of high-flow oxygen by nasal cannula versus Venturi mask in immunocompromised patients with hypoxemic acute respiratory failure: a multicenter randomized trial. Crit Care. 2015;19:380.
24. Makdee O, Monsomboon A, Surabenjawong U, et al. High-flow nasal cannula versus conventional oxygen therapy in emergency department patients with cardiogenic pulmonary edema: a randomized controlled trial. Ann Emerg Med. 2017;70(4):465–72.
25. Ferreyro BL, Angriman F, Munshi L, et al. Association of Noninvasive Oxygenation Noninvasive ventilation in adults with acute respiratory failure: strategies with all-cause mortality in adults with acute hypoxemic respiratory failure: a systematic review and meta-analysis. JAMA. 2020;324(1):57–67.
26. Grieco DL, Menga LS, Raggi V, Bongiovanni F, Anzellotti GM, Tanzarella ES, Bocci MG, Mercurio G, Dell'Anna AM, Eleuteri D, Bello G, Maviglia R, Conti G, Maggiore SM, Antonelli M. Physiological comparison of high-flow nasal cannula and helmet noninvasive ventilation in acute hypoxemic respiratory failure. Am J Respir Crit Care Med. 2020;201(3):303–12.
27. Jaber S, Monnin M, Girard M, et al. Apnoeic oxygenation via high-flow nasal cannula oxygen combined with non-invasive ventilation preoxygenation for intubation in hypoxaemic patients in the intensive care unit: the single-Centre, blinded, randomized controlled OPTINIV trial. Intensive Care Med. 2016;42(12):1877–87.
28. Miguel-Montanes R, Hajage D, Messika J, et al. Use of high-flow nasal cannula oxygen therapy to prevent desaturation during tracheal intubation of intensive care patients with mild-to-moderate hypoxemia. Crit Care Med Crit Care Med. 2015;43(3):574–83.
29. Vourc'h M, Asfar P, Volteau C, et al. High-flow nasal cannula oxygen during endotracheal intubation in hypoxemic patients: a randomized controlled clinical trial. Intensive Care Med. 2015;41:1538.29.
30. Semler MW, Janz DR, Lentz RJ, et al. Randomized trial of Apneic oxygenation during endotracheal intubation of the critically ill. Am J Respir Crit Care Med. 2016;193(3):273–80.
31. Hernandez G, Vaquero C, Gonzalez P, et al. Effect of postextubation high-flow nasal cannula vs conventional oxygen therapy on reintubation in low-risk patients: a randomized clinical trial. JAMA. 2016;315(13):1354–61.
32. Futier E, Paugam-Burtz C, Godet T, et al. Effect of early postextubation high-flow nasal cannula vs conventional oxygen therapy on hypoxaemia in patients after major abdominal surgery: a French multicentre randomised controlled trial (OPERA). Intensive Care Med. 2016;42(12):1888–98.
33. Maggiore SM, Idone FA, Vaschetto R, et al. Nasal high-flow versus Venturi mask oxygen therapy after extubation. Effects on oxygenation, comfort, and clinical outcome. Am J Respir Crit Care Med. 2014;190(3):282–8.
34. Fernandez R, Subira C, Frutos-Vivar F, et al. High-flow nasal cannula to prevent postextubation respiratory failure in high-risk non-hypercapnic patients: a randomized multicenter trial. Ann Intensive Care. 2017;7(1):47. https://doi.org/10.1186/s13613-017-0270-9. Epub 2017 May 2. PMID: 28466461; PMCID: PMC5413462.
35. Song HZ, Gu JX, Xiu HQ, Cui W, Zhang GS. The value of high-flow nasal cannula oxygen therapy after extubation in patients with acute respiratory failure. Clinics (Sao Paulo). 2017;72(9):562–7.
36. Hernandez G, Vaquero C, Colinas L, et al. Effect of postextubation high-flow nasal cannula vs noninvasive ventilation on reintubation and postextubation respiratory failure in high-risk patients: a randomized clinical trial. JAMA. 2016;316(15):1565–74.
37. Theerawit PN, Sutherasan Y. The efficacy of the Whisperflow CPAP system versus high flow nasal cannula in patients at high risk for postextubation failure. J Crit Care. 2021;63:117–23.

38. Jing G, Li J, Hao D, et al. Comparison of high flow nasal cannula with noninvasive ventilation in chronic obstructive pulmonary disease patients with hypercapnia in preventing postextubation respiratory failure: a pilot randomized controlled trial. Res Nurs Health. 2019;42(3):217–25.
39. Stephan F, Barrucand B, Petit P, et al. High-flow nasal oxygen vs noninvasive positive airway pressure in hypoxemic patients after cardiothoracic surgery: a randomized clinical trial. JAMA. 2015;313(23):2331–9.
40. Lu Z, Chang W, Meng S, et al. The effect of high-flow nasal oxygen therapy on postoperative pulmonary complications and hospital length of stay in postoperative patients: a systematic review and meta-analysis. J Intensive Care Med. 2020;35:1129–40.
41. Ansari BM, Hogan MP, Collier TJ, et al. A randomized controlled trial of high-flow nasal oxygen (Optiflow) as part of an enhanced recovery program after lung resection surgery. Ann Thorac Surg. 2016;101(2):459–64.
42. Brainard J, Scott BK, Sullivan BL, et al. Heated humidified high-flow nasal cannula oxygen after thoracic surgery—a randomized prospective clinical pilot trial. J Crit Care. 2017;40:225–8.
43. Corley A, Bull T, Spooner AJ, Barnett AG, Fraser JF. Direct extubation onto high-flow nasal cannulae post-cardiac surgery versus standard treatment in patients with a BMI >/=30: a randomised controlled trial. Intensive Care Med. 2015;41(5):887–94.
44. Pennisi MA, Bello G, Congedo MT, et al. Early nasal high-flow versus Venturi mask oxygen therapy after lung resection: a randomized trial. Crit Care (Lond Engl). 2019;23(1):68. https://doi.org/10.1186/s13054-019-2361-5.
45. Sahin M, El H, Akkoc I. Comparison of mask oxygen therapy and high-flow oxygen therapy after cardiopulmonary bypass in obese patients. Can Respir J. 2018;2018:1039635. https://doi.org/10.1155/2018/1039635. PMID: 29623135; PMCID: PMC5829344
46. Tatsuishi W, Sato T, Kataoka G, Sato A, Asano R, Nakano K. High-flow nasal cannula therapy with early extubation for subjects undergoing off-pump coronary artery bypass graft surgery. Respir Care. 2020;65(2):183–90.
47. Yu Y, Qian X, Liu C, Zhu C. Effect of high-flow nasal cannula versus conventional oxygen therapy for patients with thoracoscopic lobectomy after extubation. Can Respir J. 2017;2017:7894631. https://doi.org/10.1155/2017/7894631. Epub 2017 Feb 19
48. Zochios V, Collier T, Blaudszun G, et al. The effect of high-flow nasal oxygen on hospital length of stay in cardiac surgical patients at high risk for respiratory complications: a randomised controlled trial. Anaesthesia. 2018;73(12):1478–88.
49. Roca O, Messika J, Caralt B, et al. Predicting success of high-flow nasal cannula in pneumonia patients with hypoxemic respiratory failure: the utility of the ROX index. J Crit Care. 2016;35:200–5.
50. Roca O, Caralt B, Messika J, et al. An index combining respiratory rate and oxygenation to predict outcome of nasal high-flow therapy. Am J Respir Crit Care Med. 2019;199(11):1368–76.
51. Vega ML, Dongilli R, Olaizola G, Colaianni N, Sayat MC, Pisani L, Romagnoli M, Spoladore G, Prediletto I, Montiel G, Nava S. COVID-19 pneumonia and ROX index: time to set a new threshold for patients admitted outside the ICU. Pulmonology. 2021;S2531-0437(21)00092-1 https://doi.org/10.1016/j.pulmoe.2021.04.003.
52. Cornillon A, Balbo J, Coffinet J, Floch T, Bard M, Giordano-Orsini G, Malinovsky JM, Kanagaratnam L, Michelet D, Legros V. The ROX index as a predictor of standard oxygen therapy outcomes in thoracic trauma. Scand J Trauma Resusc Emerg Med. 2021;29(1):81. https://doi.org/10.1186/s13049-021-00876-4.
53. Drinker PA, McKhann CF 3rd. Landmark perspective: the iron lung. First practical means of respiratory support. JAMA. 1986;255(11):1476–80.
54. Motley HL, Cournand A, et al. Intermittent positive pressure breathing; a means of administering artificial respiration in man. JAMA. 1948;137(4):370–82.
55. Motley HL, Lang LP, Gordon B. Use of intermittent positive pressure breathing combined with nebulization in pulmonary disease. Am J Med. 1948;5(6):853–6.
56. Sullivan CE, Issa FG, Berthon-Jones M, Eves L. Reversal of obstructive sleep apnoea by continuous positive airway pressure applied through the nares. Lancet. 1981;1(8225):862–5.
57. Kerby GR, Mayer LS, Pingleton SK. Nocturnal positive pressure ventilation via nasal mask. Am Rev Respir Dis. 1987;135(3):738–40.

58. Bersten AD, Holt AW, Vedig AE, Skowronski GA, Baggoley CJ. Treatment of severe cardiogenic pulmonary edema with continuous positive airway pressure delivered by face mask. N Engl J Med. 1991;325(26):1825–30.
59. Bott J, Carroll MP, Conway JH, et al. Randomised controlled trial of nasal ventilation in acute ventilatory failure due to chronic obstructive airways disease. Lancet. 1993;341(8860):1555–7.
60. Brochard L, Mancebo J, Wysocki M, et al. Noninvasive ventilation for acute exacerbations of chronic obstructive pulmonary disease. N Engl J Med. 1995;333(13):817–22.
61. British Thoracic Society Standards of Care Committee. Non-invasive ventilation in acute respiratory failure. Thorax. 2002;57(3):192–211.
62. Antonelli M, Conti G. Noninvasive positive pressure ventilation as treatment for acute respiratory failure in critically ill patients. Crit Care. 2000;4(1):15–22.
63. Stevenson NJ, Walker PP, Costello RW, Calverley PM. Lung mechanics and dyspnea during exacerbations of chronic obstructive pulmonary disease. Am J Respir Crit Care Med. 2005;172(12):1510–6.
64. O'Donnell DE, Parker CM. COPD exacerbations. 3: pathophysiology. Thorax. 2006;61(4):354–61.
65. Organized jointly by the American Thoracic Society, the European Respiratory Society, the European Society of Intensive Care Medicine, and the Société de Réanimation de Langue Française, and approved by ATS Board of Directors, December 2000. International Consensus Conferences in Intensive Care Medicine: noninvasive positive pressure ventilation in acute Respiratory failure. Am J Respir Crit Care Med. 2001;163(1):283–91.
66. Williams JW Jr, Cox CE, Hargett CW, et al. Noninvasive Positive-Pressure Ventilation (NPPV) for Acute Respiratory Failure [Internet]. Rockville (MD): Agency for Healthcare Research and Quality (US); 2012 Jul. Report No.: 12-EHC089-EF. PMID: 22876372.
67. Diaz O, Iglesia R, Ferrer M, et al. Effects of noninvasive ventilation on pulmonary gas exchange and hemodynamics during acute hypercapnic exacerbations of chronic obstructive pulmonary disease. Am J Respir Crit Care Med. 1997;156(6):1840–5.
68. Lindenauer PK, Stefan MS, Shieh MS, Pekow PS, Rothberg MB, Hill NS. Outcomes associated with invasive and noninvasive ventilation among patients hospitalized with exacerbations of chronic obstructive pulmonary disease. JAMA Intern Med. 2014;174(12):1982–93.
69. Osadnik CR, Tee VS, Carson-Chahhoud KV, Picot J, Wedzicha JA, Smith BJ. Non-invasive ventilation for the management of acute hypercapnic respiratory failure due to exacerbation of chronic obstructive pulmonary disease. Cochrane Database Syst Rev. 2017;7(7):CD004104. https://doi.org/10.1002/14651858.CD004104.pub4. PMID: 28702957; PMCID: PMC6483555.
70. Conti G, Antonelli M, Navalesi P, et al. Noninvasive vs. conventional mechanical ventilation in patients with chronic obstructive pulmonary disease after failure of medical treatment in the ward: a randomized trial. Intensive Care Med. 2002;28(12):1701–7.
71. Kramer N, Meyer TJ, Meharg J, Cece RD, Hill NS. Randomized, prospective trial of noninvasive positive pressure ventilation in acute respiratory failure. Am J Respir Crit Care Med. 1995;151(6):1799–806.
72. Angus RM, Ahmed AA, Fenwick LJ, Peacock AJ. Comparison of the acute effects on gas exchange of nasal ventilation and doxapram in exacerbations of chronic obstructive pulmonary disease. Thorax. 1996;51(10):1048–50.
73. Celikel T, Sungur M, Ceyhan B, Karakurt S. Comparison of noninvasive positive pressure ventilation with standard medical therapy in hypercapnic acute respiratory failure. Chest. 1998;114(6):1636–42.
74. Plant PK, Owen JL, Elliott MW. Early use of non-invasive ventilation for acute exacerbations of chronic obstructive pulmonary disease on general respiratory wards: a multicentre randomised controlled trial. Lancet. 2000;355(9219):1931–5.
75. Mehta S, Hill NS. Noninvasive ventilation. Am J Respir Crit Care Med. 2001;163(2):540–77.
76. Wedzicha JA Ers Co-Chair, Miravitlles M, Hurst JR, Calverley PM, Albert RK, Anzueto A, Criner GJ, Papi A, Rabe KF, Rigau D, Sliwinski P, Tonia T, Vestbo J, Wilson KC, Krishnan JA Ats Co-Chair. Management of COPD exacerbations: a European Respiratory Society/American Thoracic Society guideline. Eur Respir J. 2017;49(3):1600791. https://doi.org/10.1183/13993003.00791-2016. PMID: 28298398.
77. Roberts CM, Stone RA, Buckingham RJ, Pursey NA, Lowe D, National Chronic Obstructive Pulmonary Disease Resources and Outcomes Project Implementation Group. Acidosis, non-invasive ventilation and mortality in hospitalised COPD exacerbations. Thorax. 2011;66(1):43–8.

78. National Collaborating Centre for Chronic Conditions. Chronic obstructive pulmonary disease. National clinical guideline on management of chronic obstructive pulmonary disease in adults in primary and secondary care. Thorax. 2004;59(Suppl 1):1–232.
79. National Clinical Guideline Centre. Chronic obstructive pulmonary disease: management of chronic obstructive pulmonary disease in adults in primary and secondary care. London: National Clinical Guideline Centre. 2010. Available at: http://guidance.nice.org.uk/CG101/Guidance/pdf/English.
80. Connolly MJ. Acute non-invasive ventilation in older patients: medical evolution and improvement in survival of the un-fittest. Age Ageing. 2011;40(4):414–6.
81. Nava S, Grassi M, Fanfulla F, et al. Non-invasive ventilation in elderly patients with acute hypercapnic respiratory failure: a randomised controlled trial. Age Ageing. 2011;40(4):444–50.
82. Balami JS, Packham SM, Gosney MA. Non-invasive ventilation for respiratory failure due to acute exacerbations of chronic obstructive pulmonary disease in older patients. Age Ageing. 2006;35(1):75–9.
83. Nicolini A, Santo M, Ferrera L, Ferrari-Bravo M, Barlascini C, Perazzo A. The use of non-invasive ventilation in very old patients with hypercapnic acute respiratory failure because of COPD exacerbation. Int J Clin Pract. 2014;68(12):1523–9.
84. Vaudan S, Ratano D, Beuret P, Hauptmann J, Contal O, Garin N. Impact of a dedicated noninvasive ventilation team on intubation and mortality rates in severe COPD exacerbations. Respir Care. 2015;60(10):1404–8.
85. Siirilä-Waris K, Lassus J, Melin J, Peuhkurinen K, Nieminen MS, Harjola VP, FINN-AKVA Study Group. Characteristics, outcomes, and predictors of 1-year mortality in patients hospitalized for acute heart failure. Eur Heart J. 2006;27(24):3011–7.
86. Girou E, Brun-Buisson C, Taillé S, Lemaire F, Brochard L. Secular trends in nosocomial infections and mortality associated with noninvasive ventilation in patients with exacerbation of COPD and pulmonary edema. JAMA. 2003;290(22):2985–91.
87. Nieminen MS, Böhm M, Cowie MR, ESC Committee for Practice Guideline (CPG). Executive summary of the guidelines on the diagnosis and treatment of acute heart failure: the Task Force on Acute Heart Failure of the European Society of Cardiology. Eur Heart J. 2005;26(4):384–416.
88. Gray A, Goodacre S, Newby DE, Masson M, Sampson F, Nicholl J. 3CPO Trialists. Noninvasive ventilation in acute cardiogenic pulmonary edema. N Engl J Med. 2008;359(2):142–51.
89. Masip J, Roque M, Sánchez B, Fernández R, Subirana M, Expósito JA. Noninvasive ventilation in acute cardiogenic pulmonary edema: systematic review and meta-analysis. JAMA. 2005;294(24):3124–30.
90. Potts JM. Noninvasive positive pressure ventilation: effect on mortality in acute cardiogenic pulmonary edema: a pragmatic meta-analysis. Pol Arch Med Wewn. 2009;119:349–53.
91. Goodacre SW, Gray A, Newby D. Errors in meta-analysis regarding the 3CPO trial. Ann Intern Med. 2010;153(4):277–8.
92. Bello G, De Santis P, Antonelli M. Non-invasive ventilation in cardiogenic pulmonary edema. Ann Transl Med. 2018;6(18):355. https://doi.org/10.21037/atm.2018.04.39. PMID: 30370282; PMCID: PMC6186545.
93. Weng CL, Zhao YT, Liu QH, et al. Meta-analysis: noninvasive ventilation in acute cardiogenic pulmonary edema. Ann Intern Med. 2010;152(9):590–600.
94. Mariani J, Macchia A, Belziti C, et al. Noninvasive ventilation in acute cardiogenic pulmonary edema: a meta-analysis of randomized controlled trials. J Card Fail. 2011;17(10):850–9.
95. Nava S, Carbone G, DiBattista N, Bellone A, Baiardi P, Cosentini R, Marenco M, Giostra F, Borasi G, Groff P. Noninvasive ventilation in cardiogenic pulmonary edema: a multicenter randomized trial. Am J Respir Crit Care Med. 2003;168(12):1432–7.
96. Nouira S, Boukef R, Bouida W, et al. Non-invasive pressure support ventilation and CPAP in cardiogenic pulmonary edema: a multicenter randomized study in the emergency department. Intensive Care Med. 2011;37(2):249–56.
97. Masip J, Betbesé AJ, Páez J, et al. Non-invasive pressure support ventilation versus conventional oxygen therapy in acute cardiogenic pulmonary oedema: a randomised trial. Lancet. 2000;356(9248):2126–32.
98. Cabrini L, Landoni G, Oriani A, et al. Noninvasive ventilation and survival in acute care settings: a comprehensive systematic review and metaanalysis of randomized controlled trials. Crit Care Med. 2015;43(4):880–8.

99. Mehta S, Al-Hashim AH, Keenan SP. Noninvasive ventilation in patients with acute cardiogenic pulmonary edema. Respir Care. 2009;54(2):186–95.

100. Winck JC, Azevedo LF, Costa-Pereira A, Antonelli M, Wyatt JC. Efficacy and safety of non-invasive ventilation in the treatment of acute cardiogenic pulmonary edema--a systematic review and meta-analysis. Crit Care. 2006;10(2):R69. https://doi.org/10.1186/cc4905. PMID: 16646987; PMCID: PMC1550884.

101. L'Her E, Duquesne F, Girou E, et al. Noninvasive continuous positive airway pressure in elderly cardiogenic pulmonary edema patients. Intensive Care Med. 2004;30(5):882–8.

102. Ferrer M, Esquinas A, Leon M, Gonzalez G, Alarcon A, Torres A. Noninvasive ventilation in severe hypoxemic respiratory failure: a randomized clinical trial. Am J Respir Crit Care Med. 2003;168(12):1438–44.

103. Martin TJ, Hovis JD, Costantino JP, et al. A randomized, prospective evaluation of noninvasive ventilation for acute respiratory failure. Am J Respir Crit Care Med. 2000;161:807–13.

104. Antonelli M, Conti G, Rocco M, et al. A comparison of noninvasive positive-pressure ventilation and conventional mechanical ventilation in patients with acute respiratory failure. N Engl J Med. 1998;339(7):429–35.

105. Delclaux C, L'Her E, Alberti C, et al. Treatment of acute hypoxemic nonhypercapnic respiratory insufficiency with continuous positive airway pressure delivered by a face mask: a randomized controlled trial. JAMA. 2000;284(18):2352–60.

106. Keenan SP, Sinuff T, Cook DJ, Hill NS. Does noninvasive positive pressure ventilation improve outcome in acute hypoxemic respiratory failure? A systematic review. Crit Care Med. 2004;32(12):2516–23.

107. Hernandez G, Fernandez R, Lopez-Reina P, et al. Noninvasive ventilation reduces intubation in chest trauma-related hypoxemia: a randomized clinical trial. Chest. 2010;137(1):74–80.

108. Faria DA, da Silva EM, Atallah ÁN, Vital FM. Noninvasive positive pressure ventilation for acute respiratory failure following upper abdominal surgery. Cochrane Database Syst Rev. 2015;2015(10):CD009134. https://doi.org/10.1002/14651858.CD009134.pub2. PMID: 26436599; PMCID: PMC8080101.

109. Xu XP, Zhang XC, Hu SL, et al. Noninvasive ventilation in acute hypoxemic Nonhypercapnic respiratory failure: a systematic review and meta-analysis. Crit Care Med. 2017;45(7):e727–33. https://doi.org/10.1097/CCM.0000000000002361. PMID: 28441237; PMCID: PMC5470860.

110. Schettino G, Altobelli N, Kacmarek RM. Noninvasive positive-pressure ventilation in acute respiratory failure outside clinical trials: experience at the Massachusetts General Hospital. Crit Care Med. 2008;36(2):441–7.

111. Duan J, Chen L, Liang G, et al. Noninvasive ventilation failure in patients with hypoxemic respiratory failure: the role of sepsis and septic shock. Ther Adv Respir Dis. 2019;13:1753466619888124. https://doi.org/10.1177/1753466619888124. PMID: 31722614; PMCID: PMC6856973.

112. Baldomero AK, Melzer AC, Greer N, et al. Effectiveness and harms of high-flow nasal oxygen for acute respiratory failure: an evidence report for a clinical guideline from the American College of Physicians. Ann Intern Med. 2021;174(7):952–66.

113. Bellani G, Laffey JG, Pham T, LUNG SAFE Investigators, ESICM Trials Group, et al. Noninvasive ventilation of patients with acute respiratory distress syndrome. Insights from the LUNG SAFE study. Am J Respir Crit Care Med. 2017;195(1):67–77.

114. Ferguson ND, Fan E, Camporota L, et al. The Berlin definition of ARDS: an expanded rationale, justification, and supplementary material. Intensive Care Med. 2012;38(10):1573–82.

115. Antonelli M, Conti G, Bufi M, et al. Noninvasive ventilation for treatment of acute respiratory failure in patients undergoing solid organ transplantation: a randomized trial. JAMA. 2000;283(2):235–41.

116. Adda M, Coquet I, Darmon M, Thiery G, Schlemmer B, Azoulay E. Predictors of noninvasive ventilation failure in patients with hematologic malignancy and acute respiratory failure. Crit Care Med. 2008;36(10):2766–72.

117. Squadrone V, Massaia M, Bruno B, et al. Early CPAP prevents evolution of acute lung injury in patients with hematologic malignancy. Intensive Care Med. 2010;36(10):1666–74.

118. Gristina GR, Antonelli M, Conti G, GiViTI (Italian Group for the Evaluation of Interventions in Intensive Care Medicine), et al. Noninvasive versus invasive ventilation for acute respiratory failure in patients with hematologic malignancies: a 5-year multicenter observational survey. Crit Care Med. 2011;39(10):2232–9.

119. Lemiale V, Resche-Rigon M, Mokart D, et al. Acute respiratory failure in patients with hematological malignancies: outcomes according to initial ventilation strategy. A groupe de recherche respiratoire en réanimation onco-hématologique (Grrr-OH) study. Ann Intensive Care. 2015;5(1):28. https://doi.org/10.1186/s13613-015-0070-z. Epub 2015 Sep 30. PMID: 26429355; PMCID: PMC4883632.

120. Azoulay E, Mokart D, Pène F, et al. Outcomes of critically ill patients with hematologic malignancies: prospective multicenter data from France and Belgium–a groupe de recherche respiratoire en réanimation onco-hématologique study. J Clin Oncol. 2013;31(22):2810–8.

121. Conti G, Marino P, Cogliati A, et al. Noninvasive ventilation for the treatment of acute respiratory failure in patients with hematologic malignancies: a pilot study. Intensive Care Med. 1998;24(12):1283–8.

122. Depuydt PO, Benoit DD, Roosens CD, Offner FC, Noens LA, Decruyenaere JM. The impact of the initial ventilatory strategy on survival in hematological patients with acute hypoxemic respiratory failure. J Crit Care. 2010;25(1):30–6.

123. Lemiale V, Mokart D, Resche-Rigon M, Groupe de Recherche en Réanimation Respiratoire du patient d'Onco-Hématologie (GRRR-OH), et al. Effect of noninvasive ventilation vs oxygen therapy on mortality among immunocompromised patients with acute respiratory failure: a randomized clinical trial. JAMA. 2015;314(16):1711–9.

124. Nava S, Ambrosino N, Clini E, et al. Noninvasive mechanical ventilation in the weaning of patients with respiratory failure due to chronic obstructive pulmonary disease. A randomized, controlled trial. Ann Intern Med. 1998;128(9):721–8.

125. Girault C, Daudenthun I, Chevron V, Tamion F, Leroy J, Bonmarchand G. Noninvasive ventilation as a systematic extubation and weaning technique in acute-on-chronic respiratory failure: a prospective, randomized controlled study. Am J Respir Crit Care Med. 1999;160(1):86–92.

126. Ferrer M, Esquinas A, Arancibia F, et al. Noninvasive ventilation during persistent weaning failure: a randomized controlled trial. Am J Respir Crit Care Med. 2003;168(1):70–6.

127. Vaschetto R, Turucz E, Dellapiazza F, et al. Noninvasive ventilation after early extubation in patients recovering from hypoxemic acute respiratory failure: a single-Centre feasibility study. Intensive Care Med. 2012;38(10):1599–606.

128. Trevisan CE, Vieira SR, Research Group in Mechanical Ventilation Weaning. Noninvasive mechanical ventilation may be useful in treating patients who fail weaning from invasive mechanical ventilation: a randomized clinical trial. Crit Care. 2008;12(2):R51. https://doi.org/10.1186/cc6870. Epub 2008 Apr 17. PMID: 18416851; PMCID: PMC2447605.

129. Collaborating Research Group for Noninvasive Mechanical Ventilation of Chinese Respiratory, S., Pulmonary infection control window in treatment of severe respiratory failure of chronic obstructive pulmonary diseases: a prospective, randomized controlled, multi-centred study. Chin Med J. 2005;118(19):1589–94.

130. Prasad SB, Chaudhry D, Khanna R. Role of noninvasive ventilation in weaning from mechanical ventilation in patients of chronic obstructive pulmonary disease: an Indian experience. Indian J Crit Care Med. 2009;13(4):207–12.

131. Girault C, Bubenheim M, Abroug F, VENISE Trial Group, et al. Noninvasive ventilation and weaning in patients with chronic hypercapnic respiratory failure: a randomized multicenter trial. Am J Respir Crit Care Med. 2011;184(6):672–9.

132. Burns KE, Meade MO, Premji A, Adhikari NK. Noninvasive ventilation as a weaning strategy for mechanical ventilation in adults with respiratory failure: a Cochrane systematic review. CMAJ. 2014;186(3):E112–22.

133. Keenan SP, Powers C, McCormack DG, Block G. Noninvasive positive-pressure ventilation for postextubation respiratory distress: a randomized controlled trial. JAMA. 2002;287(24):3238–44.

134. Esteban A, Frutos-Vivar F, Ferguson ND, et al. Noninvasive positive-pressure ventilation for respiratory failure after extubation. N Engl J Med. 2004;350(24):2452–60.

135. Lin C, Yu H, Fan H, Li Z. The efficacy of noninvasive ventilation in managing postextubation respiratory failure: a meta-analysis. Heart Lung. 2014;43(2):99–104.

136. Nava S, Gregoretti C, Fanfulla F, Squadrone E, Grassi M, Carlucci A, Beltrame F, Navalesi P. Noninvasive ventilation to prevent respiratory failure after extubation in high-risk patients. Crit Care Med. 2005;33(11):2465–70.

137. Ferrer M, Valencia M, Nicolas JM, Bernadich O, Badia JR, Torres A. Early noninvasive ventilation averts extubation failure in patients at risk: a randomized trial. Am J Respir Crit Care Med. 2006;173(2):164–70.

138. El-Solh AA, Aquilina A, Pineda L, Dhanvantri V, Grant B, Bouquin P. Noninvasive ventilation for prevention of post-extubation respiratory failure in obese patients. Eur Respir J. 2006;28(3):588–95.

139. Ferrer M, Sellarés J, Valencia M, Carrillo A, Gonzalez G, Badia JR, Nicolas JM, Torres A. Non-invasive ventilation after extubation in hypercapnic patients with chronic respiratory disorders: randomised controlled trial. Lancet. 2009;374(9695):1082–8.

140. Khilnani GC, Galle AD, Hadda V, Sharma SK. Non-invasive ventilation after extubation in patients with chronic obstructive airways disease: a randomised controlled trial. Anaesth Intensive Care. 2011;39(2):217–23.

141. Jaber S, Lescot T, Futier E, NIVAS Study Group, et al. Effect of noninvasive ventilation on tracheal reintubation among patients with hypoxemic respiratory failure following abdominal surgery: a randomized clinical trial. JAMA. 2016;315(13):1345–53.

142. Jaber S, Chanques G, Jung B. Postoperative noninvasive ventilation. Anesthesiology. 2010;112(2):453–61.

143. Chiumello D, Chevallard G, Gregoretti C. Non-invasive ventilation in postoperative patients: a systematic review. Intensive Care Med. 2011;37(6):918–29.

144. Bellani G, Laffey JG, Pham T, LUNG SAFE Investigators, ESICM Trials Group, et al. Epidemiology, patterns of care, and mortality for patients with acute respiratory distress syndrome in intensive care units in 50 countries. JAMA. 2016;315(8):788–800.

145. Parhar KKS, Zjadewicz K, Soo A, et al. Epidemiology, mechanical power, and 3-year outcomes in acute respiratory distress syndrome patients using standardized screening. An observational cohort study. Ann Am Thorac Soc. 2019;16(10):1263–72. https://doi.org/10.1513/AnnalsATS.201812-910OC. PMID: 31247145; PMCID: PMC6812172.

146. Esteban A, Frutos-Vivar F, Muriel A, et al. Evolution of mortality over time in patients receiving mechanical ventilation. Am J Respir Crit Care Med. 2013;188(2):220–30.

147. Dennis JM, McGovern AP, Vollmer SJ, Mateen BA. Improving survival of critical care patients with coronavirus disease 2019 in England: a National Cohort Study, March to June 2020. Crit Care Med. 2021;49(2):209–14.

148. COVID-ICU Group on behalf of the REVA Network and the COVID-ICU Investigators. Clinical characteristics and day-90 outcomes of 4244 critically ill adults with COVID-19: a prospective cohort study. Intensive Care Med. 2021;47:60–73.

149. Prescott HC, Levy MM. Survival from severe coronavirus disease 2019: is it changing? Crit Care Med. 2021;49(2):351–3.

150. Dres M, Hajage D, Lebbah S, COVID-ICU Investigators, et al. Characteristics, management, and prognosis of elderly patients with COVID-19 admitted in the ICU during the first wave: insights from the COVID-ICU study: prognosis of COVID-19 elderly critically ill patients in the ICU. Ann Intensive Care. 2021;11(1):77.

151. Kurtz P, Bastos LSL, Dantas LF, et al. Evolving changes in mortality of 13,301 critically ill adult patients with COVID-19 over 8 months. Intensive Care Med. 2021;47(5):538–48.

152. Fernández R, González de Molina FJ, Batlle M, Fernández MM, Hernandez S, Villagra A, Grupo Semicríticos Covid. Non-invasive ventilatory support in patients with COVID-19 pneumonia: a Spanish multicenter registry. Med Intensiva (Engl Ed). 2021;45(5):315–7.

153. Franco C, Facciolongo N, Tonelli R, et al. Feasibility and clinical impact of out-of-ICU noninvasive respiratory support in patients with COVID-19-related pneumonia. Eur Respir J. 2020;56(5):2002130.

154. Patel M, Gangemi A, Marron R, et al. Retrospective analysis of high flow nasal therapy in COVID-19-related moderate-to-severe hypoxaemic respiratory failure. BMJ Open Respir Res. 2020;7(1):e000650. https://doi.org/10.1136/bmjresp-2020-000650. PMID: 32847947; PMCID: PMC7451488.

155. Zucman N, Mullaert J, Roux D, Roca O, Ricard JD, Contributors. Prediction of outcome of nasal high flow use during COVID-19- related acute hypoxemic respiratory failure. Intens Care Med. 2020;46(10):1924–6.

156. Panadero C, Abad-Fernández A, Rio-Ramirez MT, et al. High-flow nasal cannula for Acute Respiratory Distress Syndrome (ARDS) due to COVID-19. Multidiscip Respir Med. 2020;15(1):693. https://doi.org/10.4081/mrm.2020.693. PMID: 32983456; PMCID: PMC7512942.
157. Vianello A, Arcaro G, Molena B, et al. High-flow nasal cannula oxygen therapy to treat patients with hypoxemic acute respiratory failure consequent to SARS- CoV-2 infection. Thorax. 2020;75(11):998–1000.
158. Hifumi T, Jinbo I, Okada I, et al. The impact of age on outcomes of elderly ED patients ventilated due to community acquired pneumonia. Am J Emerg Med. 2015;33(2):277–81.
159. Frengley JD, Sansone GR, Shakya K, Kaner RJ. J Am Geriatr Soc. 2014;62(1):1–9.
160. Fujii M, Iwakami S, Takagi H, et al. Factors influencing weaning from mechanical ventilation in elderly patients with severe pneumonia. Geriatr Gerontol Int. 2012;12(2):277–83.
161. Cader SA, Vale RG, Castro JC, et al. Inspiratory muscle training improves maximal inspiratory pressure and may assist weaning in older intubated patients: a randomised trial. J Physiother. 2010;56(3):171–7.
162. Epstein CD, Peerless JR. Weaning readiness and fluid balance in older critically ill surgical patients. Am J Crit Care. 2006;15(1):54–64.
163. Ely EW, Evans GW, Haponik EF. Mechanical ventilation in a cohort of elderly patients admitted to an intensive care unit. Ann Int Med. 1999;131(2):96–104.
164. Kher S, Roberts RJ, Garpestad E, et al. Development, implementation, and evaluation of an institutional daily awakening and spontaneous breathing trial protocol: a quality improvement project. J Intensive Care Med. 2013;28(3):189–97.
165. Jackson DL, Proudfoot CW, Cann KF, Walsh T. A systematic review of the impact of sedation practice in the ICU on resource use, costs and patient safety. Crit Care. 2010;14(2):R59. https://doi.org/10.1186/cc8956. Epub 2010 Apr 9. PMID: 20380720; PMCID: PMC2887180.
166. Schweickert WD, Pohlman MC, Pohlman AS, et al. Early physical and occupational therapy in mechanically ventilated, critically ill patients: a randomised controlled trial. Lancet. 2009;373(9678):1874–82.
167. MacIntyre NR, Cook DJ, Ely EW, et al. Evidence-based guidelines for weaning and discontinuing ventilatory support: a collective task force facilitated by the American College of Chest Physicians; the American Association for Respiratory Care; and the American College of Critical Care Medicine. Chest. 2001;120(6 suppl):375S–95S.
168. Barr J, Fraser GL, Puntillo K, et al. Clinical practice guidelines for the management of pain, agitation, and delirium in adult patients in the intensive care unit. Crit Care Med. 2013;41(1):263–306.

Vasoactive Drugs

Dylan de Lange

Contents

Learning Objective

The aging heart and vessels are less able to adapt to changing needs. To keep cardiac output at an acceptable level, the heart needs to increase in frequency. In contrast to younger patients, the aging heart reacts less to beta-adrenergic stimulation, and the first step in resuscitation is adequate fluid resuscitation. However, older patients are more prone to fluid overload. The evidence to opt for one vasopressor above the others is limited, and particularly in older patients, evidence is lacking. The optimal blood pressure targets in older patients are lacking, but some trials showed that permissive hypotension (MAP 60–65 mmHg) is acceptable and does not cause more organ dysfunction.

19.1 Introduction

When patients become older, there are various (patho)physiologic changes and adaptations in the heart and the vessels that might necessitate higher blood pressure targets. Within the heart there are a decrease in the number of myocytes and an increase in myocardial connective tissue and fat [1]. Additionally, fibrosis causes conduction abnormalities. These combined changes result in a decrease in left ventricular ejection fraction and an overall decline in ventricular compliance. Arterial distensibility decreases with advancing age and this results in increased cardiac afterload. The heart adapts to this by maintaining the resting cardiac output, but maximal heart rate, ejection fraction, and cardiac output decrease with aging. Ventricular relaxation becomes impaired with aging, and diastolic dysfunction is therefore much more common in the elderly, particularly in those patients with hypertension [2, 3]. The result of these changes is that the heart is less responsive to β-adrenergic stimulation. Some have coined the term "hyposympathetic state" in which the heart becomes less responsive to sympathetic stimulation and does not increase heart rate. The aging heart, therefore, increases cardiac output by increasing ventricular filling (preload) and stroke volume rather by an increase in heart rate. Because of this dependence of preload, even minor hypovolemia can result in significant decrease in cardiac output. This dependence on preload to maintain cardiac output is even more important because of the diastolic dysfunction that is associated with aging. Atrial fibrillation is therefore poorly tolerated by elderly patients.

Of course, the abovementioned cardiac changes are exacerbated by a high incidence of cardiac comorbidities, like coronary artery disease. Particularly coronary artery disease may go unrecognized in the elderly, as myocardial ischemia may present with nonspecific symptoms [4, 5].

Practical Implication

Rhythm disturbances are not well tolerated by older patients and they might have a profound effect upon cardiac output. These rhythm disturbances should be corrected immediately with a particular focus on preload and filling pressures.

19.2 **Fluid Resuscitation**

Elderly patients with hypotension will react less to β-adrenergic stimulation and are more preload dependent than their younger counterparts. Therefore, the first thing to adjust in elderly patients presenting with hypotension is to correct hypovolemia. Unfortunately, the titration of fluids in the elderly patient is particularly challenging. Rapid fluid administration might lead to pulmonary venous congestion and pulmonary edema. Fluid boluses of 250–500 ml are recommended with close monitoring of the patients' blood pressure, heart rate, respiratory rate, urine output, and arterial oxygen saturation. In the setting of an ICU, all these parameters can be closely monitored by pulmonary artery catheters, cardiac ultrasonography, pulse wave contour measurements, etc. However, in elderly patients the application of all these devices is devoid of supportive data. Indeed, irrespective of the age of the patients, multiple studies have confirmed that both the central venous pressure and pulmonary capillary wedge pressure are unable to predict the hemodynamic response to a fluid challenge [6, 7].

19.3 **Vasoactive Medication**

When an adequate fluid resuscitation of approximately 30 ml/kg has not resulted in the targeted mean arterial blood pressure (MAP) of >65 mmHg, the next step will be to restore organ perfusion by initiation of a vasopressor. Elderly patients with sepsis have a markedly abnormal ventricular response to volume infusion, with a significantly smaller increase in left ventricular stroke work index than in controls in response to fluid challenges [8]. Sepsis is characterized by biventricular dysfunction: there are systolic depressed ejection fraction and diastolic decreased chamber compliance. Myocardial depression together with peripheral vasodilation and a reduced systemic vascular resistance are the characteristic hemodynamic features found in patients with sepsis. There is sometimes a certain reluctance to optimize hemodynamics with vasopressors because vasopressors produce vasoconstrictive effects that might hamper peripheral circulation. However, failure to restore organ perfusion may lead to progressive multi-organ failure and subsequent death [9]. However, despite years of research, the optimal choice of inotropic agents in patients with sepsis has not been determined. Currently norepinephrine remains the first-choice vasopressor agent in patients with septic shock [10–16]. The initiation of low dose vasopressin (0.01–0.04 units/min) should be considered as a second-line vasopressor in patients receiving norepinephrine. In septic patients low dose vasopressin markedly increases arterial pressure [14, 17].

Dopamine has been used to increase cardiac output and increase vascular tone. However, a randomized controlled trial in patients with shock showed that dopamine was roughly equivalent to norepinephrine in the reversal of shock. There was no significant difference in 28-day mortality between the dopamine-treated arm and the norepinephrine-treated arm. However, the number of side effects, particularly arrhythmias, was higher in the dopamine-treated patient group [18]. Given the fact that elderly patients are not able to cope with such rhythm disturbances, dopamine should be avoided.

Levosimendan is a calcium-sensitizing drug that increases the intracellular calcium concentration, and this adds to the contractility of cardiomyocytes. It is a drug with inotropic and vasodilator properties and has been used to treat decompensated heart failure. However, in septic shock the addition of levosimendan to standard of care (often treatment with norepinephrine) did not result in better outcomes. On the contrary, 28-day mortality was nonsignificantly higher than in the standard of care group (34.5% versus 30.9%). Other, more intermediate outcomes, like chances in SOFA score, were also not different between these two treatment arms [19].

The overall conclusion is that, despite several years of research, there is no clear benefit of one vasopressor over the other, although dopamine and levosimendan are not often prescribed for septic shock [20].

In none of these studies, the elderly patients were specifically investigated. The median age of the research population was often equivalent to the median age of patients with sepsis or septic shock: roughly 65–70 years old. The truly elderly patient population (e.g., >80 years old) is extremely underrepresented in all these randomized clinical trials.

> **Practical Implication**
>
> The optimal vasopressor for older patients has not been determined, a vasopressor that with limited beta-adrenergic effect (risk of rhythm disturbances) seems logical.

19.4 Blood Pressure Targets in Elderly ICU Patients

Elderly patients in general have a less compliant vascular system and often, but not always, have higher median blood pressures. It is, therefore, very straightforward to think that elderly patients should have higher blood pressure targets when treated with vasopressors.

This research has been performed albeit not in the very elderly patient population [21]. In a randomized controlled trial, patients with septic shock were assigned to a mean arterial blood pressure of 65–70 mmHg or a mean arterial blood pressure of 80–85 mmHg [22]. The patients were, as always, aged 65 years (i.e., mean age, standard deviation of 13 years) meaning that very few patients were actually >80 years old. However, the outcome was not much different between these groups: mortality was 36.6% versus 34.0%, and the distribution of side effects of vasopressors was similar in both groups. A systematic review of all blood pressure trials in critically ill adult patients with shock did not support higher blood pressure targets in older patients [23]. However, the difference in blood pressure targets was small (a target MAP >65 mmHg versus a MAP >70 mmHg), and, again, the definition of "older patients" was >65 years.

Another question that is still open for debate is whether patients with hypertension before their current period of illness need higher target blood pressures. The most recent guidelines suggested a treatment goal of 130/80 mmHg in patients older than 65 years. However, many factors need to be considered to reach this goal, and clinical judgment and team-based approach is recommended [24]. Individual tailoring of targets seems necessary. Adhering to guidelines, which currently advocate a

MAP >65 mmHg for all, might lead to longer treatment with vasopressors and higher dosages for patients that have low premorbid blood pressures [25, 26].

One of the most recent studies looking into "higher" versus "lower" blood pressure targets took it one step further and looked at MAP >60 mmHg versus MAP >65 mmHg in patients with vasodilatory shock. This "65 study" showed that further reduction of the target blood pressure in patients older than 65 years reduced the 90-day mortality in comparison to a target blood pressure of MAP >65 mmHg [27]. This was one of the first studies that clearly showed an age distribution at randomization and showed a post hoc analysis in various age groups. Quite counterintuitive the effect of lower blood pressure in older age patients was associated with lower odds for 90-day mortality: the higher the age, the lower the odds of 90-day mortality. This effect was, however, not statistically significant. Of note, the mortality difference between the two groups took a rather long time to diverge – it was only after hospital discharge that potentially significant differences emerged. Post hoc analysis showed that permissive hypotension seemed to be the most beneficial among patients with chronic hypertension, a group that is expected to be at the greatest risk of harm from low blood pressure. There are no signals that organ damage caused by vasopressors is the result of the late, post-discharge mortality benefit. Intermediary endpoints, like renal function, respiratory function, ICU length of stay, and fluid balance, were quite similar in both study arms. As such, it remains unclear why a lower vasopressor dose should reduce mortality in elderly patients. Several hypotheses have arisen.

First, lower pressures are not equal to less perfusion. The systemic perfusion pressure is the difference between MAP and central venous pressure (CVP). If you target for a higher MAP, then you have to transfuse more fluids which will simultaneously increase the CVP. Higher or lower target MAPs might actually yield similar systemic perfusion pressures.

One of the potential dangers of the "65 trial" is that patients will have a MAP <60 mmHg for a substantial period of time which might be detrimental for these patients.

Second, patients with a lower target blood pressure received less vasopressors than the normal target blood pressure group. Previous research has shown that the use of vasopressors is associated with ICU-acquired weakness [28]. Such muscle wasting might result in prolonged recovery periods and vulnerability to secondary complications, resulting in a higher 90-day mortality in the higher vasopressor group.

Third, potentially detrimental effect of catecholamines appears to be mediated through the stimulation of the β-adrenergic receptor: elevated heart rate, increased rates of arrhythmias, myocardial ischemia, and direct toxic effects on cardiac myocytes leading to apoptosis and fibrosis [18, 29–32]. In addition, there is a growing body of evidence supporting the potentially detrimental immunomodulatory effects of norepinephrine [33, 34] and induction of a hypercoagulable state [30, 35]. The metabolic system is also affected, with catecholamines affecting various metabolic pathways and inducing hyperglycemia [36].

Although these studies provide biologic plausibility for an independent detrimental effect of excessive β-adrenergic stimulation on skeletal muscle, further studies are clearly needed in this area to confirm the association between specific vasoactive medication use and the development of neuromuscular weakness in elderly critically ill patients.

> **Conclusion**
>
> The elderly patient population has a lot of pathophysiological changes to the heart and vessels requiring another target blood pressure when severely ill. It is, however, not clear what the optimal blood pressure is for the elderly critically ill patient. Most studies do not specifically analyze this age group. One of the latest studies showed, rather counterintuitively, that a lower target blood pressure was better than a normal blood pressure. However, more research is needed to elucidate which target blood pressure is needed in specific diseases.

> **Take-Home Messages**
>
> The evidence for fluid resuscitation, the application of vasopressors, and the optimal blood pressure targets in older patients are lacking. Permissive hypotension in older patients does not seem to result in organ failure and appears justified. However, individualized treatment targets are advised.

References

1. Pugh KG, Wei JY. Clinical implications of physiological changes in the aging heart. Drugs Aging. 2001;18(4):263–76. https://doi.org/10.2165/00002512-200118040-00004. PMID: 11341474
2. Sanders D, Dudley M, Groban L. Diastolic dysfunction, cardiovascular aging, and the anesthesiologist. Anesthesiol Clin. 2009;27(3):497–517.
3. Chang WT, Chen JS, Hung YK, Tsai WC, Juang JN, Liu PY. Characterization of aging-associated cardiac diastolic dysfunction. PLoS One. 2014;9(5):e97455.
4. Qureshi WT, Zhang ZM, Chang PP, et al. Silent myocardial infarction and long-term risk of heart failure: the ARIC study. J Am Coll Cardiol. 2018;71(1):1–8. https://doi.org/10.1016/j.jacc.2017.10.071.
5. Zhang ZM, Rautaharju PM, Prineas RJ, Tereshchenko L, Soliman EZ. Electrocardiographic QRS-T angle and the risk of incident silent myocardial infarction in the atherosclerosis risk in communities study. J Electrocardiol. 2017;50(5):661–6. https://doi.org/10.1016/j.jelectrocard.2017.05.001.
6. Velissaris D, Karamouzos V, Kotroni I, Pierrakos C, Karanikolas M. The use of pulmonary artery catheter in sepsis patients: a literature review. J Clin Med Res. 2016;8(11):769–76. https://doi.org/10.14740/jocmr2719w.
7. Ospina-Tascón GA, Cordioli RL, Vincent JL. What type of monitoring has been shown to improve outcomes in acutely ill patients? Intensive Care Med. 2008;34(5):800–20. https://doi.org/10.1007/s00134-007-0967-6. Epub 2008 Jan 5
8. Ognibene FP, Parker MM, Natanson C, Shelhamer JH, Parrillo JE. Depressed left ventricular performance. Response to volume infusion in patients with sepsis and septic shock. Chest. 1988;93(5):903–10. https://doi.org/10.1378/chest.93.5.903.
9. Singer M, Deutschman CS, Seymour CW, Shankar-Hari M, Annane D, Bauer M, Bellomo R, Bernard GR, Chiche JD, Coopersmith CM, Hotchkiss RS, Levy MM, Marshall JC, Martin GS, Opal SM, Rubenfeld GD, van der Poll T, Vincent JL, Angus DC. The third international consensus definitions for sepsis and septic shock (Sepsis-3). JAMA. 2016;315(8):801–10. https://doi.org/10.1001/jama.2016.0287. PMID: 26903338; PMCID: PMC4968574
10. Hamzaoui O, Scheeren TWL, Teboul JL. Norepinephrine in septic shock: when and how much? Curr Opin Crit Care. 2017;23(4):342–7. https://doi.org/10.1097/MCC.0000000000000418.
11. Permpikul C, Tongyoo S, Viarasilpa T, Trainarongsakul T, Chakorn T, Udompanturak S. Early use of norepinephrine in septic shock resuscitation (CENSER). A randomized trial. Am J Respir Crit Care Med. 2019;199(9):1097–105. https://doi.org/10.1164/rccm.201806-1034OC.

12. Menich BE, Miano TA, Patel GP, Hammond DA. Norepinephrine and vasopressin compared with norepinephrine and epinephrine in adults with septic shock. Ann Pharmacother. 2019;53(9):877–85. https://doi.org/10.1177/1060028019843664. Epub 2019 Apr 8

13. Myburgh JA, Higgins A, Jovanovska A, Lipman J, Ramakrishnan N. Santamaria J; CAT study investigators. A comparison of epinephrine and norepinephrine in critically ill patients. Intensive Care Med. 2008;34(12):2226–34. https://doi.org/10.1007/s00134-008-1219-0. Epub 2008 Jul 25

14. Russell JA, Walley KR, Singer J, Gordon AC, Hébert PC, Cooper DJ, Holmes CL, Mehta S, Granton JT, Storms MM, Cook DJ, Presneill JJ, Ayers D, Investigators VASST. Vasopressin versus norepinephrine infusion in patients with septic shock. N Engl J Med. 2008;358(9):877–87. https://doi.org/10.1056/NEJMoa067373.

15. Annane D, Vignon P, Renault A, Bollaert PE, Charpentier C, Martin C, Troché G, Ricard JD, Nitenberg G, Papazian L, Azoulay E, Bellissant E; CATS Study Group. Norepinephrine plus dobutamine versus epinephrine alone for management of septic shock: a randomised trial. Lancet. 2007;370(9588):676–84. https://doi.org/10.1016/S0140-6736(07)61344-0. Erratum in: Lancet. 2007 Sep 22;370(9592):1034.

16. Hajjar LA, Zambolim C, Belletti A, de Almeida JP, Gordon AC, Oliveira G, Park CHL, Fukushima JT, Rizk SI, Szeles TF, Dos Santos Neto NC, Filho RK, Galas FRBG, Landoni G. Vasopressin versus norepinephrine for the Management of Septic Shock in cancer patients: the VANCS II randomized clinical trial. Crit Care Med. 2019;47(12):1743–50. https://doi.org/10.1097/CCM.0000000000004023.

17. Gordon AC, Mason AJ, Thirunavukkarasu N, Perkins GD, Cecconi M, Cepkova M, Pogson DG, Aya HD, Anjum A, Frazier GJ, Santhakumaran S, Ashby D, Brett SJ, Investigators VANISH. Effect of early vasopressin vs norepinephrine on kidney failure in patients with septic shock: the VANISH randomized clinical trial. JAMA. 2016;316(5):509–18. https://doi.org/10.1001/jama.2016.10485.

18. De Backer D, Biston P, Devriendt J, Madl C, Chochrad D, Aldecoa C, Brasseur A, Defrance P, Gottignies P, Vincent JL, SOAP II Investigators. Comparison of dopamine and norepinephrine in the treatment of shock. N Engl J Med. 2010;362(9):779–89. https://doi.org/10.1056/NEJMoa0907118.

19. Gordon AC, Perkins GD, Singer M, McAuley DF, Orme RM, Santhakumaran S, Mason AJ, Cross M, Al-Beidh F, Best-Lane J, Brealey D, Nutt CL, McNamee JJ, Reschreiter H, Breen A, Liu KD, Ashby D. Levosimendan for the prevention of acute organ dysfunction in sepsis. N Engl J Med. 2016;375(17):1638–48. https://doi.org/10.1056/NEJMoa1609409. Epub 2016 Oct 5.

20. Ospina-Tascón GA, Calderón-Tapia LE. Inodilators in septic shock: should these be used? Ann Transl Med. 2020;8(12):796. https://doi.org/10.21037/atm.2020.04.43. PMID: 32647721; PMCID: PMC7333155.

21. D'Aragon F, Belley-Cote EP, Meade MO, Lauzier F, Adhikari NK, Briel M, Lalu M, Kanji S, Asfar P, Turgeon AF, Fox-Robichaud A, Marshall JC, Lamontagne F. Canadian critical care trials group. Blood pressure targets for vasopressor therapy: a systematic review. Shock. 2015;43(6):530–9. https://doi.org/10.1097/SHK.0000000000000348.

22. Asfar P, Meziani F, Hamel JF, Grelon F, Megarbane B, Anguel N, Mira JP, Dequin PF, Gergaud S, Weiss N, Legay F, Le Tulzo Y, Conrad M, Robert R, Gonzalez F, Guitton C, Tamion F, Tonnelier JM, Guezennec P, Van Der Linden T, Vieillard-Baron A, Mariotte E, Pradel G, Lesieur O, Ricard JD, Hervé F, du Cheyron D, Guerin C, Mercat A, Teboul JL, Radermacher P, SEPSISPAM Investigators. High versus low blood-pressure target in patients with septic shock. N Engl J Med. 2014;370(17):1583–93. https://doi.org/10.1056/NEJMoa1312173. Epub 2014 Mar 18

23. Hylands M, Moller MH, Asfar P, Toma A, Frenette AJ, Beaudoin N, Belley-Côté É, D'Aragon F, Laake JH, Siemieniuk RA, Charbonney E, Lauzier F, Kwong J, Rochwerg B, Vandvik PO, Guyatt G, Lamontagne F. A systematic review of vasopressor blood pressure targets in critically ill adults with hypotension. Can J Anaesth. 2017;64(7):703–15. https://doi.org/10.1007/s12630-017-0877-1. English. Epub 2017 May 11.

24. Alsarah A, Alsara O, Bachauwa G. Hypertension management in the elderly: what is the optimal target blood pressure? Heart Views. 2019;20(1):11–16. https://doi.org/10.4103/HEARTVIEWS.HEARTVIEWS_28_18. PMID: 31143381; PMCID: PMC6524422.

25. Russell JA. Personalized blood pressure targets in shock: what if your normal blood pressure is "low"? Am J Respir Crit Care Med. 2020;202(1):10–2. https://doi.org/10.1164/rccm.202004-1124ED. PMID: 32352319; PMCID: PMC7328338.

26. Gershengorn HB, Stelfox HT, Niven DJ, Wunsch H. Association of Premorbid Blood Pressure with vasopressor infusion duration in patients with shock. Am J Respir Crit Care Med. 2020;202(1):91–9. https://doi.org/10.1164/rccm.201908-1681OC.
27. Lamontagne F, Richards-Belle A, Thomas K, Harrison DA, Sadique MZ, Grieve RD, Camsooksai J, Darnell R, Gordon AC, Henry D, Hudson N, Mason AJ, Saull M, Whitman C, Young JD, Rowan KM, Mouncey PR; 65 Trial Investigators. Effect of reduced exposure to vasopressors on 90-day mortality in older critically ill patients with vasodilatory hypotension: a randomized clinical trial. JAMA. 2020;323(10):938–49. https://doi.org/10.1001/jama.2020.0930. Epub ahead of print. PMID: 32049269; PMCID: PMC7064880.
28. Wolfe KS, Patel BK, MacKenzie EL, et al. Impact of vasoactive medications on ICU-acquired weakness in mechanically ventilated patients. Chest. 2018;154(4):781–7. https://doi.org/10.1016/j.chest.2018.07.016.
29. Schmittinger CA, Torgersen C, Luckner G, Schröder DCH, Lorenz I, Dünser MW. Adverse cardiac events during catecholamine vasopressor therapy: a prospective observational study. Intensive Care Med. 2012;38(6):950–8.
30. Dünser MW, Hasibeder WR. Sympathetic overstimulation during critical illness: adverse effects of adrenergic stress. J Intensive Care Med. 2009;24(5):293–316.
31. Iwai-Kanai E, Hasegawa K, Araki M, Kakita T, Morimoto T, Sasayama S. α- and β-adrenergic pathways differentially regulate cell type-specific apoptosis in rat cardiac myocytes. Circulation. 1999;100(3):305–11.
32. Todd GL, Baroldi G, Pieper GM, Clayton FC, Eliot RS. Experimental catecholamine-induced myocardial necrosis. II. Temporal development of isoproterenol-induced contraction band lesions correlated with ECG, hemodynamic and biochemical changes. J Mol Cell Cardiol. 1985;17(7):647–56.
33. Stolk RF, van der Poll T, Angus DC, van der Hoeven JG, Pickkers P, Kox M. Potentially inadvertent immunomodulation: norepinephrine use in sepsis. Am J Respir Crit Care Med. 2016;194(5):550–8.
34. Stolk RF, van der Pasch E, Naumann F, Schouwstra J, Bressers S, van Herwaarden AE, Gerretsen J, Schambergen R, Ruth MM, van der Hoeven JG, van Leeuwen H, Pickkers P, Kox M. Norepinephrine dysregulates the immune response and compromises host Defense during sepsis. Am J Respir Crit Care Med. 2020;202(6):830–42. https://doi.org/10.1164/rccm.202002-0339OC.
35. de Montmollin E, Aboab J, Mansart A, Annane D. Bench-to-bedside review: β-adrenergic modulation in sepsis. Crit Care. 2009;13(5):230.
36. Trager K, DeBacker D, Radermacher P. Metabolic alterations in sepsis and vasoactive drug-related metabolic effects. Curr Opin Crit Care. 2003;9(4):271–8.

Acute Kidney Injury and Renal Replacement Therapy in the Very Old Critically Ill Patient

Antoine Lamblin, Florent Sigwalt, and Thomas Rimmele

Contents

© The Author(s), under exclusive license to Springer Nature Switzerland AG 2022
H. Flaatten et al. (eds.), *The Very Old Critically Ill Patients*, Lessons from the ICU,
https://doi.org/10.1007/978-3-030-94133-8_20

> **Learning Objectives**
> - AKI is very frequent in very old critically ill patients, hitting up to 75% of them.
> - Polymedication and drug interactions favor the occurrence of these episodes of AKI.
> - Renal replacement therapy in this subpopulation represents both a clinical and an ethical challenge.
> - In terms of ethics, the following rules are crucial: collegiality for the decision to initiate or not initiate RRT, respect of the patient advance healthcare directives, patient autonomy, beneficence, and distributive justice.
> - Extreme caution should be taken during the RRT session in order to optimize patient hemodynamics.
> - CRRT should be administered when the patient is hemodynamically unstable, whereas intermittent hemodialysis seems very appropriate during the rehabilitation phase of critical care.

20.1 Introduction

Between 50 and 75% of critically ill patients develop acute kidney injury (AKI) during their intensive care unit (ICU) stay [1]. Approximately 10% of ICU patients undergo renal replacement therapy [1]. Among all these patients, some of them are very old, and it seems important to make a focus on this subgroup of the ICU population when it comes to AKI and RRT in the ICU. Are AKI characteristics the same in this subgroup of critically ill patients? What are the ethical questions to be discussed when renal replacement therapy (RRT) is needed in one of these very old patients? When RRT is finally decided, are there any specific points to highlight regarding the RRT prescription?

20.2 Acute Kidney Injury in the Very Old Critically Ill Patient

20.2.1 AKI Epidemiology in the ICU

Aging population leads to more comorbidities and complications such as AKI in the ICU. Aging leads to physiologic renal modifications with the decrease of the glomerular filtration flow rate, tubular dysfunctions, and the increase of renal resistances. AKI is extremely frequent in the ICU, ranging from 50 to 75% of the whole ICU population, and this is particularly true in the very old critically ill patient [1, 2].

Several risk factors have been specifically reported in the elderly population, such as polymedication, chronic cardiovascular diseases such as hypertension, diabetes mellitus, and chronic kidney disease. Moreover, exposure to nephrotoxic molecules such as some antibiotics and immunosuppressive therapies also increases the risk of developing AKI. Importantly, AKI and age are strongly associated (incidence and severity of AKI). In the geriatric population, AKI is also associated with a higher risk of mortality, a higher risk of dependence, and a higher risk of developing end-stage renal disease and chronic dialysis [3]. However, very old patients with AKI (as compared to old patients with AKI) do not necessarily exhibit a worse prognosis. This confirms that age, as a stand-alone criterion, is irrelevant for assessment of risk mortality and progression to end-stage renal disease [4].

20.2.2 AKI Etiologies in the Very Old Patient

AKI etiologies in the very old population are overall the same as in the general adult population although some age-related specificities can be underlined. Prerenal AKI, sometimes referred as transient AKI, is frequently reported in this population [5]. Transient AKI is related to macro- and microcirculatory hemodynamic failure which leads to renal perfusion defect. This AKI state is qualified as transient because rapid correction of these hemodynamic disturbances usually allows for rapid improvement of the renal function. One of the reasons why transient AKI is particularly frequent in very old patients stands with the fact that 50% of patients with hypertension receive angiotensin converting enzyme inhibitors or angiotensin II receptor blockers [6]. These drugs are known to directly impact renal hemodynamics through the inhibition of vasoconstriction of the efferent arteriole when this vasoconstriction may be needed. Moreover, those patients are also much more affected by situations of hypovolemia due to the frequent impaired sensation of thirst and/or other situations which may lead to hypovolemia such as post-chemotherapy diarrhea and vomiting, bowel obstruction, diuretics use, and dysregulation of water and sodium reabsorption.

Chronic kidney disease (CKD) is strongly associated with age and is one of the main risk factors to develop AKI (named AKI on CKD). AKI in the ICU is mostly multifactorial with hemodynamic disturbances, sepsis, and/or nephrotoxic medications (antibiotics, immunosuppressive therapies) being common in this population. Acute tubular necrosis (ATN) is known to be the following state of transient AKI when hemodynamic impairment subsists (continuum between transient AKI and ATN) [3]. Importantly, two causes of intrinsic AKI need to be underlined in the geriatric population:

- Glomerulonephritis (e.g., rapidly progressive glomerulonephritis with anti-neutrophil cytoplasmic antibodies (ANCA) and glomerulonephritis associated with renal amyloidosis (AL or AA))
- Acute vascular nephritis (e.g., cholesterol-embolization syndrome, thrombotic microangiopathy)

Postrenal AKI, also named obstructive AKI, is more frequent in elderly patients due to the higher prevalence of pelvic cancers. Obstructive prostatic causes in elderly males (prostate cancer, benign prostatic hyperplasia) are also often involved in postrenal AKI [7].

20.3 Renal Replacement Therapy in the ICU: Should This Therapy be Initiated in the Elderly?

20.3.1 A Clinical But Also an Ethical Dilemma

To initiate RRT in a very old critically ill patient is always a difficult decision to make. When the question arises in a patient previously admitted to the ICU, physicians often discuss whether or not they should withhold or withdraw this life-sustaining therapy. In terms of epidemiology, a French multicenter retrospective matched cohort study reported that critically ill patients over 80 years of age did receive RRT with a lower rate as compared to a cohort of patients aged 65–79 years (adjusted odds ratio (95%), 0.52 (0.41–0.66); $p < 0.001$) [8].

To provide RRT in the ICU in the elderly is indeed not only a clinical dilemma regarding which modality to be used and how the therapy will be administered (see III) but also an ethical dilemma. In other words, the question is not only "How to start RRT in this patient?" but also and above all "Should RRT be initiated in this very old patient?".

Age alone does not seem to be a sufficient determinant although, in some studies, it appears to be closely related to the risk of long-term mortality [9]. However, one would argue that it would not be ethically acceptable to use this only criterion for the decision-making process. This would be easily experienced as discrimination on the grounds of a person's age, sometimes referred as "ageism."

When it comes to medical condition, it is obvious and well accepted that an important inter-individual variability between patients of the same age can be observed. Like for ICU admission decision, the presence of comorbidities, the assessment of the nutritional status, the patient autonomy before ICU admission, and the patient frailty (assessed by the Rockwood clinical frailty scale) seem to be, taken all together, robust criteria to decide whether or not to undertake RRT in one very old patient [10, 11]. Of course, the severity of the ongoing acute disease must also be taken into account.

Prognostic scores can also help the clinician to make the decision, even if these scores have not been specifically validated for critically ill patients. For example, the Couchoud score is a prognostic tool predicting mortality at 3 months in patients over 75 years of age with end-stage renal disease (ESRD). It is composed of 15 items including age, gender, presence of specific comorbidities, nutritional status assessed by serum albuminemia, and mobility. This score, ranging from 0 to 25 points, allows the physician to stratify the short-term mortality risk into three groups: low risk (score < 12 points, mortality less than 20%), intermediate risk (score between 12 and 16 points, mortality between 20 and 40%), and high risk (score > 16 points, mortality >40%) [12].

The ethical reflection takes a prominent place in this context. It is part of an individualized, holistic approach, considering the clinical, biological, psychological, and social dimensions while considering the patient as a fully-fledged actor of the decision.

20.3.2 Temporality and Principle of Collegiality for the Decision-Making Process

When RRT must be urgently initiated, for instance, in case of severe pulmonary edema in an anuric patient unresponsive to diuretics, the temporality of the emergency does not always allow for a structured and collegial ethical reflection process. The same applies during night shifts, when the physician is usually alone to make decisions. The absence of clear instructions regarding the level of care to be undertaken for a given patient can lead to difficult feelings such as intense distress or significant anxiety for the lonely physician who clearly faces the uncertainty of his/her decisions. The risk here for the practitioner is to subsequently develop a feeling of guilt, which may even lead to a psychic or psychosomatic disorder such as the burnout syndrome, particularly when this situation occurs several times [13]. It is now well established that the level of care to be provided to a very old patient should ideally be discussed beforehand. A clear therapeutic strategy should be defined from the moment the patient is admitted to the ICU, and, importantly, this includes the strategy/procedure to be followed in case RRT becomes necessary.

The collegiality of these decisions is also a crucial aspect. This means that the intensivists but also the paramedical staff of the ICU, the general practitioner, the geriatrician, eventually the nephrologist, and any other external consultant physician have to be involved with the decisions to withhold or withdraw specific treatments and therapies. As the French National Academy of Medicine underlines, "The destiny of a life requires a moment's reflection that cannot be performed by one person alone." The collective effort of the group to handle the situation helps professionals to alleviate or even prevent moral distress [14].

In case of doubt regarding the relevance of initiating RRT, especially in the context of an emergency situation in a patient for whom nothing has been discussed beforehand, a "RRT trial" can be proposed, following the example of the "ICU Trial" for ICU admission decision [15]. The doubt must benefit the patient as it is always possible to reassess the need to continue or stop the RRT session.

20.3.3 The Patient's Role in the Decision: The Principle of Autonomy

The authors of a French study questioned 100 patients over 80 years of age, who needed several major or invasive organ support therapies, on their wish to benefit from them. They were shown videos of those therapies, and only 21% of respondents claimed they would like to benefit from RRT (47% for mechanical ventilation) [16]. This raised the question of the autonomy of very old patients, which rarely seems to be taken into account in decisions in Europe [17].

The possibility of RRT should therefore be considered at an early stage and, if possible, discussed with patients beforehand if they are still conscious. If they are unable to express their wishes, the advance healthcare directives, if they have been drawn up, also apply and must be respected. In France, they have even become prescriptive and are imposed on physicians, outside the context of a life-threatening emergency, for the time it takes to fully assess the situation. In the absence of advance healthcare directives, or if the RRT issue is not mentioned, the family or relatives must be consulted in order to ascertain the patient's wishes, having informed them of the risks of subsequent chronic dialysis. In order to make a conscious decision, the patient must be informed of the medium- and long-term risks associated with AKI, in particular, the risk of end-stage renal disease (ESRD), which is known to increase in very elderly patients due to reduced physiological reserves and the presence of comorbidities [18]. Elderly patients with AKI in the ICU are twice as likely to develop ESRD requiring RRT. This raises questions about the future quality of life (QoL) of patients who will have to benefit from ESRD treatments: either RRT (hemodialysis or peritoneal dialysis) or conservative care. Dialysis can radically change the autonomy and functional capacity of these patients in the form of transport inconveniences, and a rapid decline in the functional capacity of hemodialysis patients has been demonstrated in institutionalized patients [19, 20].

Renal transplantation can only be considered in elderly patients with few or no comorbidities. The maximum age recommended by health authorities to be registered on the kidney transplant waiting list in France is 85 years old. Beyond 80 years of age, however, this practice remains exceptional. Conservative care, whose objective is to reduce the impact of the symptoms encountered in ESRD (pain, pruritus, nausea, fatigue, anxiety, depression), seems to show good results in terms of survival compared to dialysis but requires regular monitoring, which has a significant impact on patients' QoL [21].

20.3.4 Principles of Beneficence, Non-maleficence, and Distributive Justice

In Western societies, the aging of the population and the reduction in the resources allocated to healthcare in certain countries lead us to question the rationalization of the resources available to ICU physicians. The principle of egalitarianism that prevailed until the 1980s and 1990s would require that human and material means of life-sustaining treatments be used for any patient who needs it. However, given the increase in the number of elderly patients admitted to the ICU, is it possible to propose maximum care, including RRT, for all those who need it from a strictly medical point of view? RRT is a highly technical procedure that implies considerable human and material costs in the acute phase, but also in the long term, if dialysis is required after discharge from hospital.

The principle of distributive justice therefore applies in addition to that of egalitarianism, physicians having a duty to preserve expensive medical resources and avoid unreasonable therapeutic obstinacy. The challenge is to avoid costly, potentially invasive care or sources of physical or moral pain in patients for whom such care would have no other effect than to temporarily supply one or more organ failures, with no hope of survival. It is an individualized approach, essentially centered on the benefit of the patient and the respect for their dignity (deontologist approach) and balanced by the criterion of distributive justice, avoiding inconsiderate expenses to society.

The assessment of the risk/benefit balance is essential before initiating RRT in an ICU. RRT requires a chain of interventions at the risk of human errors and material failures. An iatrogenic risk exists at all stages of the procedure: when inserting the dialysis catheter (risks of arterial puncture, catheter malposition, infection, catheter thrombosis) but also during treatment (risk linked to anticoagulation, risk of gas embolism). Recommendations for securing RRT were drawn up by learning medical societies [22, 23]. Each department must have a clear protocol to reduce the risk of human error. Practitioners must therefore be aware of the risks to the patient if such treatment is initiated and weigh these against the expected benefits. Here once again, it is an individualized approach in which the principle of non-maleficence plays an essential role.

20.4 How to Provide RRT in the Very Old Critically Ill Patient?

20.4.1 Dialysis Catheter

Optimal dialysis catheter management is crucial for efficient RRT delivery. Like in other adults, the preferential anatomic site for the oldest critically ill subpopulation remains the right intern jugular vein, followed by the femoral vein (right or left) and then the left intern jugular vein. Subclavian access is still not recommended, like in other adults. However, due to the greater prevalence of malnourished patients with BMI < 18 kg/m2 in the elderly population, some authors recommend the femoral site as the preferential site for dialysis catheters. Indeed, in this subpopulation, the jugular approach may be more complex due to the prominent bone relief [24]. Importantly, the right internal jugular site remains the one preferred in case of overweight/obesity.

Hemorrhagic complications related to the insertion of dialysis catheters are more frequent in elderly patients due to the frequent use of anticoagulant or antiplatelet medications in this context. Indeed, comorbidities requiring curative anticoagulation increase with advanced age [25]. Moreover, anticoagulant drug overdoses are also more frequent in this patient population (polymedication with drug interferences), particularly in case of AKI. However, this hemorrhagic risk is nowadays markedly reduced by the systematic use of vascular ultrasound for dialysis catheter insertion.

Importantly, the high prevalence of delirium in the ICU (80% of very old patients with mechanical ventilation) in the elderly should be taken into account for the choice of the vascular site for the dialysis catheter [26]. The non-desired removal of the dialysis catheter during a state of delirium can indeed lead to serious adverse events including gas embolism, hemorrhage, or death. The risk is even more important in case of *superior vena cava* territory catheters due to the higher risk of gas embolism, especially in the semi-seated position (negative pressure, higher during inspiration). Moreover, in case of delirium in this population, the septic risk is also increased due to the involuntary or voluntary manipulations of the catheter by the patient. Advanced age is an independent risk factor for catheter infection among other factors such as immunosuppression, malnutrition, mechanical ventilation, and multiple organ failure [27].

20.4.2　Which RRT Modality for the Elderly Population in the ICU?

De novo hemodynamic instability (perdialytic hypotension) defined by a 20% drop in blood pressure or hypotension requiring specific management (vasopressors, vascular filling, net ultrafiltration stop) is estimated at 15–30% [28]. Although the scientific literature does not report any superiority of continuous renal replacement therapy over intermittent modalities in terms of hemodynamic stability, some authors nevertheless suggest that the variation in plasma osmolarity is much more progressive with continuous modalities, leading to a better hemodynamic tolerance [29, 30]. In addition, net ultrafiltration over a period of 24 h is very likely to be better tolerated than the same net ultrafiltration occurring during a period of 4–6 h.

Importantly, when RRT is initiated, blood is replaced within the patient blood circulation by a crystalloid solution. This replacement, occurring at the very beginning of the session, should be performed with a low blood flow rate which will be progressively increased, in order to preserve patient hemodynamics. Of note, we do remind the reader here that, contrary to popular belief, the blood flow rate has no impact on hemodynamic tolerance, except during the first 3 to 5 minutes of the session, as just stated above.

The theoretical better hemodynamic tolerance of continuous modalities should therefore be one of the "criteria of choice" in this elderly population with blood pressure regulation mechanisms altered either by drug intake (beta-blockers, angiotensin converting enzyme inhibitors), by dysautonomia, or by processes related to the ongoing disease (e.g., septic shock). Furthermore, due to the frequent malnutrition and hypoalbuminemia observed in these elderly patients, associated to the aggressive fluid administration during the acute phase of resuscitation, fluid overload is a common problem (low oncotic pressure causing edematous state). Continuous modalities are known to provide an easier control of fluid overload.

To date, no study has ever demonstrated any superiority of a continuous convective modality (CVVH) over a continuous diffusive modality (CVVHD) and vice versa [31]. Having said that, CVVHD seems much more adaptable in the event of a metabolic complication related to the use of regional citrate anticoagulation, thanks to the removal of the citrate-calcium complexes through diffusion in the dialysate and thanks to the use of lower blood flow rates with CVVHD and therefore lower citrate administration [32]. For the record, like in other critically ill patients, regional citrate anticoagulation is recommended as the first-line anticoagulation modality, whether or not a bleeding risk situation is identified [2].

Last but not least, the high prevalence of polymedication in the elderly population requires close pharmacokinetic monitoring in case of AKI. Drug clearance is influenced by molecular weight, plasma protein binding, specific renal clearance, and volume of distribution. During RRT, the use of a continuous modality is interesting because of the limited and slow variations of the volume of distribution as compared to IHD, even when the pharmacokinetic profile of the drug is well known in chronic dialysis. In fact, CVVH and CVVHD allow for a progressive and constant purification and thus a better prediction of the pharmacokinetic variations of the drugs, potentially resulting in fewer drug dosage adjustments [33].

20.4.3 Optimization of the Critical Care Rehabilitation Phase: Impact of the RRT Modality Choice

During the critical care rehabilitation phase, when hemodynamics is restored, intermittent hemodialysis (IHD) and sustained low-efficiency dialysis (SLED) can be of great interest. Indeed, dialyzing elderly patients during only few hours makes time optimization doable with, for example, some periods of time dedicated to patient mobilization or physiotherapy. Interestingly, IHD also allows for the use of the same machine for several patients on the same day. Furthermore, IHD can be performed with no circuit anticoagulation, which thus limits the risk of bleeding in this population at greater risk.

In addition to the undesired removal of a large amount of low molecular weight molecules (amino acids, vitamins, trace elements), RRT increases protein catabolism and leads to the production of free radicals. These molecular losses and metabolic issues worsen the nutritional status of these old patients. Thus, the longer the duration of the RRT session is, the greater the loss of these low molecular weight molecules will be. The use of IHD in the rehabilitation phase is therefore supposed to decrease these metabolic consequences although supplementation with trace elements, vitamins, and amino acids may still be necessary.

Conversely, continuous modalities are associated with better long-term renal recovery, potentially reducing the need for subsequent chronic hemodialysis [30, 34]. This finding is of crucial importance in this patient population with frequent significant advanced chronic kidney disease, already at high risk for chronic hemodialysis.

> **Conclusion**
>
> Like in the general ICU population, AKI is extremely frequent in very old critically ill patients. Among other standard risk factors of AKI, polymedication and drug interactions need to be underlined. Initiating RRT in a very old patient is always a complex decision to make. Ethically speaking, this decision should follow several important rules and concepts: collegiality for the decision, respect of the patient advance healthcare directives, patient autonomy, beneficence, and distributive justice. When the decision to start RRT is finally taken, a particular attention has to be paid regarding hemodynamic management of the session. CRRT should be administered when hemodynamics is impaired, but IHD is also very interesting in the rehabilitation phase of critical care.

> **Take-Home Messages**
> - Age alone cannot be the only determinant to decide whether or not RRT should be initiated in a very old critically ill patient.
> - The presence of comorbidities, the assessment of the nutritional status, the patient autonomy before ICU admission, the patient frailty, and the severity of the ongoing acute disease must also be taken into account.
> - For the decision-making process regarding RRT initiation, healthcare providers' collegiality, respect of the patient advance healthcare directives, patient autonomy, beneficence, and distributive justice are mandatory.

20

References

1. Hoste EA, Bagshaw SM, Bellomo R, et al. Epidemiology of acute kidney injury in critically ill patients: the multinational AKI-EPI study. Intensive Care Med. 2015;41:1411–23.
2. KDIGO AKI Work Group. KDIGO clinical practice guideline for acute kidney injury. Kidney Int Suppl. 2012;17:1–138.
3. Rosner MH, La Manna G, Ronco C. Acute kidney injury in the geriatric population. Contrib Nephrol. 2018;193:149–60.
4. Pascual J, Liano F. Causes and prognosis of acute renal failure in the very old. J Am Geriatr Soc. 1998;46:721–5.
5. Li Q, Zhao M, Du J, et al. Outcomes of renal function in elderly patients with acute kidney injury. Clin Interv Aging. 2017;12:153–60.
6. Formica M, Politano P, Marazzi F, et al. Acute kidney injury and chronic kidney disease in the elderly and polypharmacy. Blood Purif. 2018;46:332–6.
7. Commereuc M, Rondeau E, Ridel C. Acute kidney injury in elderly patient: diagnostic and therapeutic aspects. Presse Med. 2014;43:341–7.
8. Boumendil A, Aegerter P, Guidet B. CUB-Rea Network. Treatment intensity and outcome of patients aged 80 and older in intensive care units: a multicenter matched-cohort study. J Am Geriatr Soc. 2005;53:88–93.
9. Bouchard J, Acharya A, Cerda J, et al. A prospective international multicenter study of AKI in the intensive care unit. Clin J Am Soc Nephrol. 2015;10:1324–31.
10. Church S, Rogers E, Rockwood K, et al. A scoping review of the Clinical Frailty Scale. BMC Geriatr. 2020;20:393.
11. Guidet B, de Lange DW, Boumendil A, et al. VIP2 study group. The contribution of frailty, cognition, activity of daily life and comorbidities on outcome in acutely admitted patients over 80 years in European ICUs: the VIP2 study. Intensive Care Med. 2020;46:57–69.
12. Couchoud CG, Beuscart JB, Aldigier JC, et al. Development of a risk stratification algorithm to improve patient-centered care and decision making for incident elderly patients with end-stage renal disease. Kidney Int. 2015;88:1178–86.
13. Basile B, Mancini F, Macaluso E, et al. Deontological and altruistic guilt: evidence for distinct neurobiological substrates. Hum Brain Mapp. 2011;32:229–39.
14. Pagani V, Alla F, Cambon L, et al. Elaboration of prevention norms: need for ethical reflection? Sante Publique. 2018;1:121–31.
15. Scherer JS, Holley JL. The role of time–limited trials in dialysis decision making in critically ill patients. Clin J Am Soc Nephrol. 2016;11:344–53.
16. Philippart F, Vesin A, Bruel C, et al. The ETHICA study (part I): elderly's thoughts about intensive care unit admission for life-sustaining treatments. Intensive Care Med. 2013;39:1565–73.
17. Guidet B, De Lange DW, Christensen S, et al. Attitudes of physicians towards the care of critically ill elderly patients - a European survey. Acta Anaesthesiol Scand. 2018;62:207–19.
18. Singh S, Patel S, Doley PK, et al. Outcomes of hospital-acquired acute kidney injury in elderly patients: a single-centre study. Int Urol Nephrol. 2019;51:875–83.
19. Hole B, Tonkin-Crine S, Caskey FJ, et al. Treatment of end-stage kidney failure without renal replacement therapy. Semin Dial. 2016;29:491–506.
20. Kurella Tamura M, Covinsky KE, Chertow GM, et al. Functional status of elderly adults before and after initiation of dialysis. N Engl J Med. 2009;361:1539–47.
21. Levy JB, Chambers EJ, Brown EA. Supportive care for the renal patient. Nephrol Dial Transplant. 2004;19:1357–60.
22. Brochard L, Abroug F, Brenner M, et al. ATS/ERS/ESICM/SCCM/SRLF Ad Hoc Committee on Acute Renal Failure. An official ATS/ERS/ESICM/SCCM/SRLF statement: prevention and management of acute renal failure in the ICU patient: an international consensus conference in intensive care medicine. Am J Respir Crit Care Med. 2010;181:1128–55.
23. Vinsonneau C, Allain-Launay E, Blayau C, et al. Renal replacement therapy in adult and pediatric intensive care: recommendations by an expert panel from the French Intensive Care Society (SRLF) with the French Society of Anesthesia Intensive Care (SFAR) French Group for Pediatric Intensive Care Emergencies (GFRUP) the French Dialysis Society (SFD). Ann Intensive Care. 2015;5:58.
24. Huriaux L, Costille P, Quintard H, et al. Haemodialysis catheters in the intensive care unit. Anaesth Crit Care Pain Med. 2017;36:313–9.

25. Garwood CL, Corbett TL. Use of anticoagulation in elderly patients with atrial fibrillation who are at risk for falls. Ann Pharmacother. 2008;42:523–32.
26. Ely EW, Shintani A, Truman B, et al. Delirium as a predictor of mortality in mechanically ventilated patients in the intensive care unit. JAMA. 2004;291:1753–62.
27. Cheng S, Xu S, Guo J, et al. Risk factors of central venous catheter-related bloodstream infection for continuous renal replacement therapy in kidney intensive care unit patients. Blood Purif. 2019;48:175–82.
28. Palevsky PM, Zhang JH, O'Connor TZ, et al. Intensity of renal support in critically ill patients with acute kidney injury. N Engl J Med. 2008;359:7–20.
29. Tandukar S, Palevsky PM. Continuous renal replacement therapy: who, when, why, and how. Chest. 2019;155:626–38.
30. Wald R, Shariff SZ, Adhikari NK, et al. The association between renal replacement therapy modality and long-term outcomes among critically ill adults with acute kidney injury: a retrospective cohort study. Crit Care Med. 2014;42:868–77.
31. Friedrich JO, Wald R, Bagshaw SM, et al. Hemofiltration compared to hemodialysis for acute kidney injury: systematic review and meta-analysis. Crit Care. 2012;16:R146.
32. Sigwalt F, Bouteleux A, Dambricourt F, et al. Clinical complications of continuous renal replacement therapy. Contrib Nephrol. 2018;194:109–17.
33. Thompson A, Li F, Kendall GA. Considerations for medication management and anticoagulation during continuous renal replacement therapy. Adv Crit Care. 2017;28:51–63.
34. Bonnassieux M, Duclos A, Schneider AG, et al. Renal replacement therapy modality in the ICU and renal recovery at hospital discharge. Crit Care Med. 2018;46:e102–10.

Sedation and Analgesia

Michelle Chew

Contents

© The Author(s), under exclusive license to Springer Nature Switzerland AG 2022
H. Flaatten et al. (eds.), *The Very Old Critically Ill Patients*, Lessons from the ICU,
https://doi.org/10.1007/978-3-030-94133-8_21

21

🎓 Learning Objectives

The main objective of this chapter is to obtain an understanding of the interaction between pain, sedation, and delirium. Specifically, the reader should be able to identify the unique challenges for their management taking into account that the very old are a particularly vulnerable group with often conflicting treatment priorities. This chapter will discuss implications for short- and long-term ICU outcomes including mortality, time on mechanical ventilation, and increased ICU and hospital lengths of stay, as well long-term cognitive impairment. Finally, the reader should be able to formulate a plan for sedation, pain, and delirium management for the very old ICU patient using ABCDEF principles.

Practical Implications

- Non-pharmacological interventions are an important part of the management plan and should be implemented prior to, and always in conjunction with, pharmacological treatment
- The contribution of dementia to ICU delirium is frequently neglected and has substantial implications for improving practice patterns for older patients in the ICU.
- The ABCDEF strategy should be used with increased vigilance for underlying comorbidities, drug interactions against a background of polypharmacy, and altered pharmacokinetic and pharmacodynamic profiles.

Suggested Clinical Management Strategy

- Assess pre-ICU frailty and cognitive function, including the presence of dementia.
- Assess pain using the BPS or CPOT.
- Assess delirium using CAM-ICU or ICDSC.
- Assess the need for sedation and its level.
- Document targets for pain relief and sedation daily.
- Have a plan for delirium prevention and management.
- Avoid at-risk medications such as anticholinergics, antihistamines, tricyclic antidepressants, and benzodiazepines.
- Non-pharmacological:
  - Talk calmly and nurse in a quiet, well-lit environment.
  - Regular orientation.
  - Use hearing aids and glasses.
  - Avoid at risk maneuvers such as restraints, moving beds, and excessive noise levels.
  - Consider additional staffing to help manage delirious patients.
  - Involve family members.
- Pharmacological
  - Consider analgesia first and sedation-free strategy
  - Start low and titrate up sedatives and hypnotics.
  - Note contraindications, and monitor response and side effects

21.1 Introduction

The triad of sedation, analgesia, and delirium is inextricably linked, and extensive evidence demonstrates the deleterious effects of their inadequate management in critically ill patients. Adherence to best practice treatment strategies has important impacts on patient-centered outcomes [1].

Although evidence-based guidelines [1–3] and management bundles have been developed, none have specifically addressed the very old critically ill patient. Many of these recommendations also apply to the very old patient, paying meticulous attention to this group of particularly vulnerable patients with reduced biological reserve. This vulnerability extends through all aspects of care, from more challenging assessments of pain and delirium to increased risk of experiencing adverse effects related to even the best of management strategies. In this chapter we will consider how pain, sedation, and delirium should be managed in the very old critically ill patient.

21.2 Pain

21.2.1 Scope of the Problem

Most critically ill patients will experience pain during their stay. Pain occurs commonly, even at rest and during routine ICU care [4–7]. Procedural pain is common in adult ICU patients and varies with age [1, 5, 7–10]. Yet, less than 20% of patients receive opioid analgesics before painful procedures in ICU [7, 10]. The inability to self-report is a major challenge for all critically ill patients but particularly in the very old due to higher incidences of neurocognitive dysfunction, hearing and speech impairment among many other limitations. This reinforces the burden of duty for carers to assess pain and provide pain relief.

21.2.2 Assessment

Self-reporting of pain is considered the golden standard, with the 0–10 NRS considered the most valid and reliable tool [1]. However, self-reporting is particularly challenging in the elderly and very old, who may suffer from a variety of cognitive problems and are at increased risk of delirium. Both interfere with the ability to self-report. Although pain intensity does not differ between the elderly (>65 years old) and younger ICU patients, the proportion of patients receiving analgesics for procedural pain is greater for younger patients [8, 10]. The use of vital signs as a marker of procedural pain is unreliable [1, 11] and may be masked by decreased cardiovascular reserve and concurrent medications such as antihypertensives and beta-blockers that are common in the elderly and very old populations.

The challenge of reliably assessing pain in patients who cannot self-report is mitigated by the availability of valid and reliable bedside pain assessment tools that concentrate primarily on patients' behaviors as indicators of pain and may be particularly useful in the elderly who may have difficulties verbalizing their pain experience. Current guidelines recommend the Behavioral Pain Scale (BPS) and the Critical Care

Pain Observation Tool (CPOT) as the most valid and reliable behavioral pain scales for monitoring pain in medical, postoperative, or trauma (except for brain injury) adult ICU patients who are unable to self-report and in whom motor function is intact and behaviors are observable [1, 5]. A BPS score ≥5 or CPOT score ≥3 indicates significant pain. Implementing behavioral pain scales improves both ICU pain management and clinical outcomes, including better use of analgesic and sedative agents and shorter durations of mechanical ventilation and ICU stay [12–14].

21.2.3 Treatment

Opioids remain the mainstay of non-neuropathic pain. However, in very old adults special pharmacokinetic/pharmacodynamic considerations may apply due to altered protein binding, volumes of distribution, and elimination. Polypharmacy and drug-to-drug interactions may be significant. Potentially inappropriate medication use in older adults may be evaluated using the Beers Criteria [15].

A multimodal and protocol-based approach to pain management in ICU patients has been recommended [1], with an analgesia-first approach to analgosedation (i.e., prioritizing analgesia to reach sedation goals). Few studies have been published on the effectiveness of non-pharmacological interventions in these patients [16]. Latest guidelines recommend the use of non-opioid analgesics such as nefopam, ketamine, and paracetamol to reduce the amount and side effects of opioids [1]. Although it may benefit subgroups of patients, the routine use of nonsteroidal anti-inflammatory drugs in the critically ill is not recommended due to safety concerns (e.g., bleeding and kidney injury), and this would be particularly applicable to very old critically ill patients. A recent study suggested that multimodal pain therapy is underutilized in elderly patients in the ICU [17]. The importance of assessment and implementation pain management protocols is demonstrated by improvements in ICU outcome [18, 19].

21.3 Sedation

21.3.1 Scope of the Problem

A large body of evidence shows that a strategy of minimal sedation has demonstrable short-term and long-term benefits in mechanically ventilated patients, such as reduced duration of mechanical ventilation, ICU length of stay, mortality, and improved psychological outcomes. Current guidelines recommend both Spontaneous Awakening Trials (SAT) and Spontaneous Breathing Trials (SBT) [1]. This may be achieved using a daily sedation interruption (DSI) or nurse-driven protocol [20– 22], noting that the use of DSI may be associated with deeper sedation for the rest of the day and thus counterproductive. An important issue for all critically ill patients, but particularly in the very old population who have an increased burden of care, is the availability of nurse-driven protocols and how sedation management impacts nursing workload. While light sedation, defined as RASS −2 to +1, is commonly accepted to be the current standard of care, there are still no consensus definitions of light and deep sedation [1]. Data evaluating clinical outcomes are equivocal, and no study has evaluated the effect of light vs. deep sedation on cognitive function [1]. In a further extension to the question of the depth of sedation, a recent study investigated light sedation and DSI vs. no sedation. The median age of participants was 70–72 years, and 90-day mortality was not different between the groups. There were no important differences in the number of ventilator-free days or in the length of ICU or hospital stay [23].

21.3.2 Assessment

The Richmond Agitation-Sedation Scale (RASS) and the Riker Sedation-Agitation Scale (SAS) are the most valid and reliable sedation assessment tools. Guidelines do not recommend that objective measures of brain function such as the Bispectral Index (BIS) may have a role in sedation titration in deeply sedated patients and those on neuromuscular blockade. However, the underlying literature is heterogeneous, and a wide range of study designs applied. Therefore, it is currently not common practice nor recommended to use these tools to monitor depth of sedation in non-comatose, non-paralyzed critically ill adult patients. Where monitoring nonconvulsive seizure activity is required, EEG monitoring is indicated.

21.3.3 Treatment: Choice of Sedative

Current guidelines suggest that sedation strategies using non-benzodiazepine sedatives (either propofol or dexmedetomidine) may be preferred over sedation with benzodiazepines (either midazolam or lorazepam) to improve clinical outcomes in mechanically ventilated adult ICU patients [1, 24, 25]. This was also recommended in a recent review of the care of very old critically ill patients [26]. In a large, randomized trial in a population with a median age of 65 years, dexmedetomidine was not inferior to midazolam or propofol for maintaining light-moderate sedation and reduced the duration of mechanical ventilation. However, bradycardia and hypotension occurred more frequently in dexmedetomidine-treated patients despite the exclusion of patients with risk factors such as bradycardia and AV block at the outset of the study [27]. There is still no unequivocal evidence for the use of dexmedetomidine, and studies indicate that cardiovascular side effects may be a significant limiting factor especially in the very old population [24, 25, 27]. Light sedation and/or DSI is associated with increased stress response and oxygen consumption [28, 29] but not associated with myocardial ischemia [28, 30]. How this may be extrapolated to the very old population is still unknown.

21.4 Delirium

21.4.1 Scope of the Problem

Delirium is defined as an acute, fluctuating syndrome of altered attention, awareness, and cognition and may present as hypoactive and hyperactive (agitated) or mixed forms. While hyperactive delirium may be more obvious, it affects only a minority of

21

patients in the ICU. Hypoactive delirium is common [31, 32] and associated with decreased survival, but those who do survive may have better long-term function than those with agitated or mixed delirium [33].

Estimates for the incidence of delirium among adult patients in the ICU range from 11% to 91% [1, 5, 34], with the large variation likely explained by differences in the underlying population and method of detection. Very old ICU patients are a vulnerable group that are exposed to multiple predisposing risks and precipitating factors for delirium (Table 21.1) including polypharmacy, sleep deprivation, inactivity, and dementia [31, 35–37]. They have higher overall rates of delirium than younger patients, with a predominance of the hypoactive type [32, 35]. The association between older age and delirium is independent of severity of illness, mechanical ventilation, and use of sedatives. This is of interest because hypoactive delirium is often missed by the treating team unless systematic screening is done. In patients >65 years of age, 47% have delirium persisting beyond ICU stay [38].

Pain is thought to have a role in precipitating delirium; however, an increased delirium risk may also be attributed to analgesics [39, 40]. Signs and symptoms of pain and delirium may overlap and complicate detection. Finally, the coexistence of dementia and delirium is not uncommon in the very old critically ill patient, and dementia independently predicts the risk of delirium in the ICU and extends even to the post-ICU period [38]. The relative contributions of predisposing and precipitating factors are however unknown. These findings, along with the predominance of the hypoactive subtype, highlight the importance of routine assessment of every patient in the ICU.

21.4.1.1 Pathophysiology

The pathophysiology of delirium during critical illness is likely multifactorial. Proinflammation, cerebral bioenergetic failure, microcirculatory, and neurovascular dysfunctions have been proposed [35]. The observation that delirium is associated with the use of $GABA_A$ agonists and anticholinergic drugs suggests a role for these substrates [5, 35, 39–41]. Excess dopaminergic activity and direct neurotoxic effects of inflammatory cytokines are also offered as possible pathophysiological mechanisms. The importance of the circadian rhythm is suggested by the finding that sleep deprivation is associated with development and severity of delirium. Although none of these hypotheses have been proven or have led to strategic pharmacological management, a number of non-pharmacological interventions may be implemented.

21.4.2 Assessment

Delirium remains a clinical diagnosis. The hypoactive type is particularly difficult to detect and is often confused with depression or coma. Routine monitoring of delirium in adult ICU patients is therefore required in order to decrease the risk of under-detection.

The two validated and recommended scales [1] are the Confusion Assessment Method for the ICU (CAM-ICU) [42] and the Intensive Care Delirium Screening Checklist (ICDSC) [43]. The CAM-ICU relies on a combination of four features: (1) acute/fluctuating course, (2) inattention (3) altered level of consciousness, and (4) disorganized thinking to detect delirium with high sensitivity and specificity. CAM-

◼ Table 21.1 Predisposing and precipitating factors for delirium

Predisposing factors	
	Advanced age
	Multimorbidity
	Neurological disease
	Dementia
	Depression
	Alcoholism
	Malnutrition
	Poor functional status
Precipitating factors	
Acute illness	
	Increased severity of illness
	Hypoxia
	Shock
	Dehydration
	Infection
	Surgery
	Metabolic disturbances
	Coma
	Multiple organ failure
ICU treatment	
	Mechanical ventilation
	Benzodiazepines
	Deep sedation
	Anticholinergics
	Dopamine agonists
	Steroids
	Polypharmacy
	Constipation and urinary retention
	Inadequately treated pain
	Sleep deprivation
	Lack of mobilization
	Noise and other environmental disturbances

ICU is positive if the patient has both features 1 and 2, plus either feature 3 or 4. When combined with the RASS, it can also reliably detect hypoactive delirium (=CAM-ICU positive, RASS negative range) which is often missed and may be especially useful in the very old population. The ICDSC is an eight-item screening tool and has the advantage of being extractable from medical records or via reports from the treating team [43]. It is slightly less sensitive and specific compared to the CAM-ICU but will also detect subsyndromal delirium. In contrast to the CAM-ICU that provides a "snapshot," the ICDSC scores the patient over an entire 8-hour shift or over the previous 24 hours. A score >4 suggests delirium. Both scales are feasible in clinical practice [6].

21.4.3 Outcomes

Delirium is associated with increased short- and long-term mortalities, prolonged ICU and hospital lengths of stay, and a longer time on mechanical ventilation [1, 34, 44]. Delirium is also associated with cognitive dysfunction after ICU discharge [1, 34, 45–47].

Delirium is a frequent event that is underdetected in critically ill patients without regular assessment and is associated with poor short- and long-term outcomes. Very old ICU patients are particularly vulnerable due to exposure to multiple preexisting and precipitating risk factors. Surveillance and meticulous management are therefore imperative in this population.

The use of benzodiazepines for sedation appears to be deleterious, increasing the incidence and length of delirium [1, 24, 25, 34, 41]. Sedation with dexmedetomidine compared to benzodiazepines may reduce the prevalence of delirium [24, 25, 27]; however, evidence for its use is still limited.

21.4.4 Prevention and Treatment

21.4.4.1 Non-pharmacological

Non-pharmacological interventions are an important cornerstone of delirium management. Noise reduction, reorientation, cognitive stimulation, vision and hearing aids, and early mobilization can reduce the incidence of delirium in hospitalized patients [1, 41]. Although not specific for the ICU population, the Hospital Elder Life Program (HELP) is an interdisciplinary model of care tailored to prevent delirium in hospitalized patients that may be applied to very old patients post-ICU discharge. Interventions include therapeutic activities, limiting the use of psychoactive drugs, reorientation, sleep promotion, attention to hydration and nutritional needs, and early mobilization [48, 49]. Among patients in the ICU, early mobilization and interruptions in sedation significantly reduce delirium [50].

When incorporated into a care bundle, non-pharmacological approaches also decrease the duration of delirium [51–53]. The **A**ssess, prevent, and manage pain, **B**oth Spontaneous Awakening Trials and Spontaneous Breathing Trials, **C**hoice of analgesia and sedation, **D**elirium: assess, prevent, and manage, **E**arly mobility and exercise, and **F**amily engagement and empowerment (ABCDEF) bundle is an evidence-based guide for a wholistic approach to management of delirium and is the standard of care for delirium management for adult critically ill patients [6, 54].

21.4.4.2 Pharmacological

For the prevention of delirium, a strategy based on avoidance of benzodiazepines and daily sedation breaks are the mainstay of management. This does not apply to alcohol withdrawal where benzodiazepines are still the mainstay of treatment. Prophylactic cholinesterase inhibitors such as rivastigmine are not recommended due to futility and potential harm [55, 56]. Some studies suggest that antipsychotics such as low-dose haloperidol in elderly ICU patients [57], quetiapine [58], and risperidone [59] may reduce the incidence of delirium, decrease its severity and duration, increase the number of delirium-free days, or decrease ICU length of stay. Haloperidol prophylaxis also reduced the incidence and/or duration of delirium among adult high-risk patients in ICU [33, 60]. In the HOPE-ICU study, early treatment with haloperidol was safe, but it did not reduce the frequency and duration of delirium in a largely unselected critically ill population [61]. Although some of these studies have been conducted in the elderly and very old populations, there are few definitive data and guidelines that suggest against the use of prophylactic antipsychotics in the ICU due to lack of evidence. Very old patients are also more likely to suffer underlying cardiovascular diseases, predisposing them to conduction abnormalities such as long QT syndrome and torsade de pointes; therefore, the avoidance of these drugs seems prudent. General principles for the use of antipsychotics for the treatment and prevention of delirium include (1) a careful risk-benefit appraisal for the use of these drugs, (2) a baseline ECG to evaluate the QTc interval, (3) starting with a low dose with gradual upward titration, (4) using the lowest effective doses with a plan for de-escalation, (5) careful documentation, and (6) monitoring for responses and side effects.

No clear evidence exists regarding pharmacological strategies for the treatment of delirium. Cholinesterase inhibitors appear to be ineffective and are not recommended by PAD guidelines [1]. Although rivastigmine is used to treat elderly patients with dementia, the use of rivastigmine has not been associated with benefit among ICU patients with delirium, and there may even be a signal for harm [55]. Insufficient data exist to support the use of haloperidol. Limited data suggest that atypical antipsychotics such as quetiapine and olanzapine may reduce the duration of delirium when added onto haloperidol or may be a safer alternative to haloperidol [58, 59, 62]. Of note, the use of traditional antipsychotics such as haloperidol is contraindicated in patients with dementia with Lewy bodies, Parkinson's disease, neuroleptic malignant syndrome, and alcohol withdrawal.

Current data also suggest that dexmedetomidine may be more effective than haloperidol or placebo in reducing the duration of delirium, time to extubation, and hospital length of stay in patients with agitated delirium [63, 64], but these studies did not specifically study elderly and very old patients. Guidelines suggest using dexmedetomidine for the treatment of established delirium, where agitation is precluding weaning/extubation; however, there are no specific recommendations for very old patients. Bradycardia is an adverse effect that may limit the use of dexmedetomidine in this population at risk of cardiovascular disease and may already be on medications that predispose to conduction abnormalities.

21.5 Implementation of Pain, Analgesia, and Delirium Guidelines and the ABCDEF Bundle

Studies show that a multimodal approach to the management of pain, analgesia, and delirium (PAD) is effective and improves outcomes in critically ill patients. There are no studies specific for the very old critically ill population, but this does not preclude implementation of evidence-based guidelines and bundles. A recent nationwide audit [17] in critically ill patients >65 years of age showed that the prescription of sedatives and analgesics decreased with increasing age, suggesting increasing adherence to best practice guidelines. The use of benzodiazepines was still common in this group occurring in >70% of patients but decreasing with time concurrently with an increase in the use of analgesics, reflecting analgesia-based strategies. The use of fentanyl and remifentanil increased, also in line with recommendations of using drugs with short half-lives and non-active metabolites. However, the same study also reported the increased use of antipsychotics that was attributed to possibly higher incidences in delirium in an elderly population [17]. Large variations in implementation of the ABCDEF bundle exist worldwide, with data indicating an incomplete shift toward patient- and family-centered care according to recent PAD guidelines [54].

The ABCDEF bundle [6] (◻ Table 21.2) is an evidence-based guide that consists of six broad areas of management/treatments: **A**ssess, prevent, and manage pain, **B**oth Spontaneous Awakening Trials (SAT) and Spontaneous Breathing Trials (SBT), **C**hoice of analgesia and sedation, **D**elirium: assess, prevent, and manage, **E**arly mobility and exercise, and **F**amily engagement and empowerment.

◻ **Table 21.2**   Key elements of the ABCDEF bundle

Assess, prevent, and manage pain	Regular pain assessment by NRS. CPOT or BPS in patients not able to self-report
	Treat pain including administering opioids for non-neuropathic pain
	Opioids for non-neuropathic pain
	Non-opioids as adjunct to reduce opioid side effect and to reduce dose
Both Spontaneous Awakening Trials (SAT) and Spontaneous Breathing Trials (SBT)	SAT: Stop opioids if pain is controlled. Stop sedatives. Restart at half dose May also use a nurse-driven protocol Reassess after 24 hours
	SBT: Synchronize with SAT. Start if SAT passed. Use protocol
Choice of analgesia and sedation	Assess regularly using RASS or SAS
	Agree on and set target level
	Analgesia as above

◘ Table 21.2 (continued)

Delirium: assess, prevent, and manage	Assess serially, e.g., once per shift, using ICDSC or CAM-ICU
	Promote sleep hygiene and minimize disruptions
	Early and progressive mobilization
	No evidence for specific pharmacological prevention or treatment
Early mobility	Early physical therapy and mobilization
	Promote and use mobility team
	Feasible and safe even in patients on CRRT and ECMO
Family engagement	Family members and surrogates are part of multiprofessional decision-making and treatment planning
	Focus on communication
	Ethics and palliative care consults

Conclusion

The development of valid and reliable bedside assessment tools to measure pain, sedation, agitation, and delirium in ICU patients has allowed clinicians to manage patients better and to evaluate outcomes associated with both non-pharmacological and pharmacological interventions. The use of these tools is important for every critically ill patient but imperative for the very old patient in the ICU because of increased risk of poor outcomes related to multiple factors such as age, frailty, comorbidities, dementia, cognitive impairment, polypharmacy, and altered pharmacokinetic and pharmacodynamic profiles.

Ensuring that critically ill patients are free from pain, agitation, anxiety, and delirium may at times conflict with other clinical management goals. The very old ICU patient is particularly vulnerable to organ dysfunction and deterioration, and the risk-benefit ratio of some pharmacological treatments may be different compared to younger, healthier, and less fragile patients.

Worldwide variabilities in cultural and practice norms, and in the availability of manpower and resources, make widespread implementation of evidence-based practices challenging. The availability of standardized care plans and bundles such as ABCDEF provides a guide for clinicians involved in the care of the very old ICU patient.

21

> **Take-Home Messages**
> - Pain, delirium, and sedation are highly interlinked, and their codependency influences outcomes. The elderly are particularly vulnerable to poor detection and treatment of delirium.
> - Non-pharmacological interventions are an important part of the management strategy.
> - Pharmacological interventions should be carefully considered taking into account drug interactions and altered pharmacokinetic and pharmacodynamic profiles in the very old.
> - The ABCDEF bundle should be applied.

References

1. Devlin JW, Skrobik Y, Gelinas C, Needham DM, Slooter AJC, Pandharipande PP, et al. Clinical practice guidelines for the prevention and management of pain, sedation, delirium, immobility and sleep disruption in adult patients in the ICU. Crit Care Med. 2018;46:e825–73.
2. DAS-Taskforce 2015, Baron R, Binder A, Biniek R, Braune S, Buerkle H, Dall P et al. Evidence and consensus based guideline for the management of delirium, analgesia, and sedation in intensive care medicine. Revision 2015 (DASGuideline 2015) - short version. Ger Med Sci. 2015;13:Doc19.
3. Sauder P, Andreoletti M, Cambonie G, Capellier G, Feissel M, Gall O, et al. Sedation and analgesia in intensive care (with the exception of new-born babies). French Society of Anesthesia and Resuscitation. Ann Fr Anesth Reanim. 2008;27:541–51.
4. Stein-Parbury J, McKinley S. Patients' experiences of being in an intensive care unit: a select literature review. Am J Crit Care. 2000;9:20–7.
5. Reade MC, Finfer S. Sedation and delirium in the intensive care unit. N Engl J Med. 2014;370:444–54.
6. Marra A, Ely EW, Pandharipande P, Patel MB. The ABCDEF bundle in critical care. Crit Care Clin. 2017;33:225–43.
7. Stotts NA, Puntillo K, Stanik-Hutt J, et al. Does age make a difference in procedural pain perceptions and responses in hospitalized adults? Acute Pain. 2007;9:125–34.
8. Stotts NA, Puntillo K, Bonham Morris A, et al. Wound care pain in hospitalized adult patients. Heart Lung. 2004;33:321–32.
9. Arroyo-Novoa CM, Figueroa-Ramos MI, Puntillo KA, et al. Pain related to tracheal suctioning in awake acutely and critically ill adults: a descriptive study. Intensive Crit Care Nurs. 2008;24:20–7.
10. Puntillo KA, White C, Morris AB, et al. Patients' perceptions and responses to procedural pain: results from Thunder Project II. Am J Crit Care. 2001;10:238–51.
11. Siffleet J, Young J, Nikoletti S, et al. Patients' self-report of procedural pain in the intensive care unit. J Clin Nurs. 2007;16:2142–8.
12. Chanques G, Jaber S, Barbotte E, Violet S, Sebanne M, Perrigault PF, et al. Impact of systematic evaluation of pain and agitation in an intensive care unit. Crit Care Med. 2006;34:1691–9.
13. Payen JF, Bosson JL, Chanques G, Mantz J, Labarere J, Investigators DOLOREA, et al. Pain assessment is associated with decreased duration of mechanical ventilation in the intensive care unit: a post Hoc analysis of the DOLOREA study. Anesthesiology. 2009;111:1308–16.
14. Arbour C, Gélinas C, Michaud C. Impact of the implementation of the Critical-Care Pain Observation Tool (CPOT) on pain management and clinical outcomes in mechanically ventilated trauma intensive care unit patients: a pilot study. J Trauma Nurs. 2011;18:52–60.
15. American Geriatrics Society Beers Criteria® Update Expert Panel. American Geriatrics Society 2019 updated AGS beers criteria® for potentially inappropriate medication use in older adults. J Am Geriatr Soc. 2019;2019(67):674–94.
16. Erstad BL, Puntillo K, Gilbert HC, Grap MJ, Li D, Medina J, et al. Pain management principles in the critically ill. Chest. 2009;135:1075–86.

17. Jung S-Y, Lee HJ. Utilization of medications amongst elderly patients in intensive care units: a cross-sectional using a nationwide claims database. BMJ Open. 2019;9:e026605.
18. Skrobik Y, Ahern S, Leblanc M, Marquis F, Awissi DK, Kavanagh BP. Protocolized intensive care unit management of analgesia, sedation, and delirium improves analgesia and subsyndromal delirium rates. Anesth Analg. 2010;111:451–63.
19. Georgiou E, Hadjibalassi M, Lambrinou E, et al. The impact of pain assessment on critically ill patients' outcomes: a systematic review. Biomed Res Int. 2015;2015:503830.
20. Kress JP, Pohlman AS, O'Connor MF, Hall JB. Daily interruption of sedative infusions in critically ill patients undergoing mechanical ventilation. N Engl J Med. 2000;342:1471–7.
21. Girard TD, Kress JP, Fuchs BD, et al. Efficacy and safety of a paired sedation and ventilator weaning protocol for mechanically ventilated patients in intensive care (Awakening and Breathing Controlled trial): a randomised controlled trial. Lancet. 2008;371:126–34.
22. Mehta S, Burry L, Cook D, Ferguson D, Steinberg M, Devlin J, et al. Daily sedation interruption in mechanically ventilated critically ill patients cared for with a sedation protocol: a randomized controlled trial. JAMA. 2012;308:1985–92.
23. Olsen HT, Nedergaard HK, Strøm T, Oxlund J, Wian K-A, Ytrebo KM, et al. Nonsedation or light sedation in critically ill, mechanically ventilated patients. N Engl J Med. 2020;382:1103–11.
24. Riker RR, Shehabi Y, Bokesch PM, Wisemandel W, Koura F, Whitten P, et al. Dexmedetomidine vs midazolam for sedation of critically ill patients: a randomized trial. JAMA. 2009;301:489–99.
25. Pandharipande PP, Pun BT, Herr DL, Maze M, Girard TD, Miller RR, et al. Effect of sedation with dexmedetomidine vs lorazepam on acute brain dysfunction in mechanically ventilated patients: the MENDS randomized controlled trial. JAMA. 2007;298:2644–53.
26. Guidet B, Vallet H, Boddaert J, De Lange D, Morandi A, LeBlanc G, et al. Caring for the critically ill patients over 80: a narrative review. Ann Int Care. 2018;8:114.
27. Jakob SM, Ruokonen E, Grounds RM, Sarapohja T, Garatt S, Pocock SJ, et al. Dexmedetomidine vs midazolam or propofol for sedation during prolonged mechanical ventilation: two randomized controlled trials. JAMA. 2012;307:1151–60.
28. Kress JP, Vinayak AG, Levitt J, Schweikert WD, Gelbach BK, Zimmerman F, et al. Daily sedative interruption in mechanically ventilated patients at risk for coronary artery disease. Crit Care Med. 2007;35:365–71.
29. Terao Y, Miura K, Saito M, Sekino M, Fukusaki M, Sumikawa K. Quantitative analysis of the relationship between sedation and resting energy expenditure in postoperative patients. Crit Care Med. 2003;31:830–3.
30. Hall RI, MacLaren C, Smith MS, McIntyre AJ, Allen CT, Murphy JT, et al. Light versus heavy sedation after cardiac surgery: myocardial ischemia and the stress response. Anesth Analg. 1997;85:971–8.
31. Kalish VB, Gillham JE, Unwin BK. Delirium in older persons: evaluation and management. Am Fam Physician. 2014;90:150-158. J Am Geriatr Soc. 2003;51:591–8.
32. Peterson JF, Pun BT, Dittus RS, Thomasson JWW, Jackson JC, Shintani AK, Ely EW. Delirium and its motoric subtypes: a study of 614 critically ill patients. J Am Geriatr Soc. 2006;54:479–84.
33. Van den Boogaard M, Schoonhoven L, Evers AW, van der Hoeven JG, van Achterberg T, Pickkers P. Delirium in critically ill patients: impact on long-term health-related quality of life and cognitive functioning. Crit Care Med. 2012;40:112–8.
34. Salluh JIF, Wang H, Schneider EB, Nagaraja N, Yenokyan G, Damluji A, et al. Outcome of delirium in critically ill patients: systematic review and metaanalysis. BMJ. 2015;350:h2538.
35. Bellelli G, Brathwaite JS, Mazzola P. Delirium: a marker of vulnerability in older people. Front Aging Neurosci. 2021;13:626127.
36. Ahmed S, Leurent B, Sampson EL. Risk factors for incident delirium among older people in acute hospital medical units: a systematic review and meta-analysis. Age Ageing. 2014;43:326–33.
37. Zaal IJ, Devlin JW, Peelen LM, Slooter AJC. A systematic review of risk factors for delirium in the ICU. Crit Care Med. 2014;43:40–7.
38. McNicholl L, Pisani MA, Zhang Y, Wesley E, Siegel MMD, Inouye SK. Delirium in the intensive care unit: occurrence and clinical course in older patients. J Am Geriatr Soc. 2003;51:591–8.
39. Sampson EL, West E, Fischer T. Pain and delirium: mechanisms, assessment, management. Eur Geriatr Med. 2020;11:45–52.
40. Clegg A, Young JB. Which medications to avoid in people at risk of delirium: a systematic review. Age Ageing. 2011;40:23–9.

41. Hayhurst CJ, Pandradipande PP, Hughes CG. Intensive care unit delirium. A review of diagnosis, prevention, and treatment. Anesthesiology. 2016;125:1229–41.

42. Ely EW, Inouye SK, Bernard GR, Gordon S, Francis J, May L, et al. Delirium in mechanically ventilated patients: validity and reliability of the confusion assessment method for the intensive care unit (CAM-ICU). JAMA. 2001;286:2703–10.

43. Bergeron N, Dubois MJ, Dumont M, Dial S, Skrobik Y. Intensive care delirium screening checklist: evaluation of a new screening tool. Intensive Care Med. 2001;27:859–64.

44. Pisani MA, Kong SY, Kasl SV, Murphy TE, Araujo KL, Van Ness PH. Days of delirium are associated with 1-year mortality in an older intensive care unit population. Am J Respir Crit Care Med. 2009;180:1092–7.

45. Ely EW, Shintani A, Truman B, Speroff T, Gordon SM, Harell FE Jr, et al. Delirium as a predictor of mortality in mechanically ventilated patients in the intensive care unit. JAMA. 2004;291:1753–62.

46. Pandharipande PP, Girard TD, Jackson JC, Morandi A, Thompson JL, Pun BT, et al. BRAIN-ICU Study Investigators: long-term cognitive impairment after critical illness. N Engl J Med. 2013;369:1306–16.

47. Wolters AE, van Dijk D, Pasma W, Cremer OL, Looije MF, De Lange DW, et al. Long-term outcome of delirium during intensive care unit stay in survivors of critical illness: a prospective cohort study. Crit Care. 2014;18:R125.

48. Inouye S, Bogardus S, Charpentier P, Leo-Summers L, Acampora D, Holford T, et al. A multicomponent intervention to prevent delirium in hospitalized older patients. N Engl J Med. 1999;340:669–76.

49. Inouye SK, Bogardus ST, Baker DI, Leo-Summers L, Cooney LM. The Hospital Elder Life Program: a model of care to prevent cognitive and functional decline in older hospitalized patients. Hospital Elder Life Program. J Am Geriatr Soc. 2000;48:1697–706.

50. Schweickert WD, Pohlman MC, Pohlman AS, Nigos C, Pawlik AJ, Esbrook CL, et al. Early physical and occupational therapy in mechanically ventilated, critically ill patients: a randomised controlled trial. Lancet. 2009;373:1874–82.

51. Dale CR, Kannas DA, Fan VS, Daniel SL, Deem S, Yanez ND, et al. Improved analgesia, sedation, and delirium protocol associated with decreased duration of delirium and mechanical ventilation. Ann Am Thorac Soc. 2014;11:367–74.

52. Balas MC, Vasilevskis EE, Olsen KM, Schmid KK, Shostrom V, Cohen MZ, et al. Effectiveness and safety of the awakening and breathing coordination, delirium monitoring/management, and early exercise/mobility bundle. Crit Care Med. 2014;42:1024–36.

53. Hsieh SJ, Otusanya O, Gershengorn HB, Hope AA, Dayton C, Levi D, et al. Staged implementation of awakening and breathing, coordination, delirium monitoring and management, and early mobilization bundle improves patient outcomes and reduces hospital costs. Crit Care Med. 2019;47:885–93.

54. Morandi A, Piva S, Ely EW, Myatra SN, Salluh JIF, Amare D, et al. Worldwide survey of the "assessing pain, both spontaneous awakening and breathing trials, choice of drugs, delirium monitoring/management, early exercise/mobility, and family empowerment" (ABCDEF) bundle. Crit Care Med. 2017;45:e1111–22.

55. van Eijk MM, Roes KC, Honing ML, Kuiper MA, Karakus A, van der Jagt M, et al. Effect of rivastigmine as an adjunct to usual care with haloperidol on duration of delirium and mortality in critically ill patients: a multicentre, double-blind, placebo-controlled randomised trial. Lancet. 2010;376:1829–37.

56. Gamberini M, Bolliger D, Lurati Buse GA, Burkhart CS, Grapow M, Gagneux A, et al. Rivastigmine for the prevention of postoperative delirium in elderly patients undergoing elective cardiac surgery—a randomized controlled trial. Crit Care Med. 2009;37:1762–8.

57. Wang W, Li HL, Wang DX, Zhu X, Li SL, Yao GQ, Chen KS, Gu XE, Zhu SN. Haloperidol prophylaxis decreases delirium incidence in elderly patients after noncardiac surgery: a randomized controlled trial. Crit Care Med. 2012;40:731–9.

58. Devlin JW, Roberts RJ, Fong JJ, Skrobik Y, Riker RR, Hill NS, et al. Efficacy and safety of quetiapine in critically ill patients with delirium: a prospective, multicenter, randomized, double-blind, placebo-controlled pilot study. Crit Care Med. 2010;38:419–27.

59. Prakanrattana U, Prapaitrakool S. Efficacy of risperidone for prevention of postoperative delirium in cardiac surgery. Anaesth Intensive Care. 2007;35:714–9.

60. Kalisvaart KJ, de Jonghe JF, Bogaards MJ, Vreeswijk R, Egberts TC, Burger BJ, Eikelenboom P, van Gool WA. Haloperidol prophylaxis for elderly hip-surgery patients at risk for delirium: a randomized placebo-controlled study. J Am GeriatrSoc. 2005;53:1658–66.
61. Page VJ, Ely EW, Gates S, Zhao XB, Alce T, Shintani A, et al. Effect of intravenous haloperidol on the duration of delirium and coma in critically ill patients (Hope-ICU): a randomised, double-blind, placebo-controlled trial. Lancet Respir Med. 2013;1:515–23.
62. Skrobik YK, Bergeron N, Dumont M, Gottfried SB. Olanzapine vs haloperidol: treating delirium in a critical care setting. Intensive Care Med. 2004;30:444–9.
63. Reade MC, O'Sullivan K, Bates S, Goldsmith D, Ainslie WR, Bellomo R. Dexmedetomidine vs. haloperidol in delirious, agitated, intubated patients: a randomised open-label trial. Crit Care. 2009;13:R75.
64. Reade MC, Eastwood GM, Bellomo R, Bailey M, Bersten A, Cheung B, et al. Effect of dexmedetomidine added to standard care on ventilator- free time in patients with agitated delirium: a randomized clinical trial. JAMA. 2016;315:1460–8.

Nutrition: The Very Old Critically Ill Patients

Mette M. Berger, Claire Anne Hurni, and Olivier Pantet

Contents

⌂ Learning Objectives

The present chapter aims at raising the awareness about:
- The frequent prevalence of the geriatric syndrome, which includes frailty, sarcopenia and malnutrition.
- The importance of a very early screening upon ICU admission: the NRS score is an easily applicable screening tool, despite being less age specific than the MNA-SF.
- The importance of assessing the remaining muscle mass (lean body mass) using CT scan (thorax or L3) or bioimpedance analysis (BIA) with phase angle calculation.
- The frequently encountered practical difficulties in the very old.
- The existing tools for determination of energy, protein and micronutrient needs and the necessity of introducing early enteral nutrition or alternatively oral nutrition supplements.
- The high prevalence of refeeding syndrome, a potential deadly complication: importance of monitoring blood phosphate.

22.1 Introduction

The very old adults, generally defined by an age $\geq$ 80 years, are a group of ICU patients that has recently gained significant attention, given their rapidly growing number in Western countries. They pose multiple challenges: metabolic and nutritional management problems are ranking very high, due to the high prevalence of risk factors associated with the geriatric syndrome, which includes frailty, sarcopenia and pre-existing malnutrition – three conditions that frequently co-exist in older patients (see ▶ Chaps. 12, 13, and 14). Sarcopenia is highly prevalent in hospitalised elderly patients and is associated with an increased short-term mortality risk [1, 2]. Malnutrition is common in older age and is caused by low food intakes, monotonous diets and swallowing disorders [3, 4] and by intestinal function alterations which contribute to reduce absorption [5, 6]. Due to the globally reduced intakes, there is a corresponding decline in micronutrient intake, commonly resulting in vitamin and trace element deficiencies [7].

But the age cut-off for very old is susceptible to change, as shown by a Japanese longitudinal study, showing that the elderly population, although increasing, is also changing to the better with improved gait speed and grip strength over 10 years: the authors called this "rejuvenation" [8], and it reflects muscle function. Therefore, the perspectives are not all negative and point to the importance of detecting the patients who will benefit from an intervention. The aim of the present chapter is to discuss the screening tools and nutritional therapy options to be integrated into critical care of the very old patient.

22.2 Nutrition Therapy Improves Outcome

Are nutrition interventions futile, or alternatively, could they be effective? The good news is that targeted nutrition therapy in malnourished sarcopenic elderly patients does reduce weight loss and mortality [9, 10]. A Cochrane review and meta-analysis published in 2009 confirms that intervention in malnourished elderly is possible and successfully reduces both complications and mortality [11].

In non-critically ill patients, several randomised controlled trials (RCT) have proven the benefit of nutritional interventions. Already in 1984, a RCT including 122 elderly malnourished women admitted for femur neck fracture tested the delivery of 1000 kcal (28 g of protein) in addition to oral food [12]. This resulted in improvements not only in anthropometric and plasma protein measurements (prealbumin) but also in clinical outcome, with reduced length of hospital stay and mortality (8% in fed vs 22% in the controls): the results were the most significant in the very thin patients. More recently, the NOURISH trial was conducted in a large population of patients >65 years with malnutrition and showed that the daily provision of proteins for several weeks during and after an acute hospitalisation decreased mortality [10]. Another recent large Swiss RCT also supports the concept that the systematic nutritional screening of medical inpatients on hospital admission enables introducing an individualised nutritional support in patients assessed as malnourished, allowing a reduction of mortality [13].

22.3 Characteristics of the Very Old in a Multidisciplinary ICU

The specific challenges in the very old patients' ICU nutrition therapy being still little described, we analysed the ICU characteristics of the patients aged >80 years admitted over years 2016–2018 to the multidisciplinary ICU of Lausanne University Hospital to detect the difficulties. The >80 years patients accounted for 793/6130 admissions (12.9%). Probably as the result of selection criteria and pre-decided limitations, these very old patients stayed shorter in the ICU compared to the younger patients with a mean stay of 3.9 ± 5.8 days and 5.7 ± 9.9 days, respectively, but their ICU mortality was significantly higher with 27.9% versus 12.8%. Similarly, the hospital death rate was higher with 39.4% versus 17.8% in the younger.

Then, we focused on the analysis of the very old patients requiring >72 hours ICU treatment, in congruence with previous studies of the group [14], which is the minimal time required to allow a nutritional assessment and implement therapy. Over the 3-years, only 218 (27.5%) very old patients stayed longer than 3 days (■ Table 22.1). Importantly all were mechanically ventilated, 181 (83%) required intubation, 17% were on non-invasive mode (NIV). Forty-three died in the ICU (19.7%), twenty dying of neurological conditions (mainly post-cardiac arrest and severe brain injury). Of note, with a median BMI of 24.2 kg/m², their phenotype is falsely reassuring for the clinician, as shown by a median NRS of 5 points. BMI was abnormally low (BMI < 20) in 25 patients (11.5%) and abnormally high (BMI > 30) in 27 (12.4%). Sarcopenia is likely to have been present and gone undetected in most patients. Important to note that the low BMI cut-off is higher in old adults (WHO): a BMI < 20 kg/m² is associated with increased mortality.

22.4 Specific Clinical Difficulties

As a result of studies showing poor outcome in the very old requiring prolonged mechanical ventilation [15], every effort should be made to reduce sedation and to shorten time on mechanical ventilation and length of ICU stay. The use of non-invasive mechanical ventilation (NIV) or high-flow O2 is a widespread strategy,

22

Table 22.1 Characteristics of the Lausanne very old patient cohort requiring >72 hours of ICU treatment (*n* = 218) (median [IQR 25;75])

Age (years)	84 [82; 84]
Actual weight (kg)	70 [60; 80]
Ideal BW (kg)	66 [57; 70]
BMI (kg/m^2)	24.2 [22.3; 27.7]
SAPS II	56 [46; 68]
NRS score	5 [4; 6]
Length of intubation (*days*) *n* = 181	4.0 [1.9; 8.2]
LICU (days)	6.5 [4.5; 10.9]
Basal EE by the Harris and Benedict equation (kcal/day)	1310 [1155; 1440]
Prescribed energy (kcal/day)	1600 [1400; 1800]
Measured EE (*n* = 20) – Day 7 (kcal/day)	1732 [1542; 2299]

Abbreviations: *NRS* Nutritional Risk Screening score, *EE* energy expenditure

which is a problem on its own for feeding. In our cohort 17% were not intubated but required NIV or high-flow O2. Indeed, while feeding an intubated patient by the enteral route is easy, this is not always true in non-intubated patients, resulting in necessity of alternative strategies to cover the nutritional needs. A short ICU stay and NIV reduce the time for an individual evaluation of the needs and for implementation of an appropriate and individualised nutrition strategy.

The ICU nutrition recommendations for very old patients are the same as for other ICU patients: enteral nutrition (EN) using a nasogastric tube should be privileged, when oral nutrition is not feasible [16, 17]. But the latter, oral route, is not efficient. An Australian survey showed that oral intake in critically ill adult patients not requiring invasive mechanical ventilation was below the estimated needs [18]. Moreover, while swallowing disorders are frequent to start in the very old (part of the geriatric syndrome), acquired swallowing disorders are very common after extubation [19], compromising efficient oral feeding.

The feeding route of our cohort reflects these difficulties and was as follows: 13.8% nihil (combination of prescribed fasting and no feeding), oral 24.8%, enteral nutrition (EN) 39.5%, parenteral nutrition (PN) 18.8% and combined EN+PN 3.2%. The 13.8% patients without feeding (nihil) were intended to be on oral feeding – but never managed to eat. The nihil and the oral categories were associated with important cumulated energy deficits. Using Supplemental PN might have been a pragmatic Strategy to prevent the accumulation of large deficits. Of note, despite being recommended by protocol, oral nutrition supplements (ONSs) were used in only 13 patients (6%), and rarely during the first week. This failure stresses the importance of strict ONS routines in extubated patients that should probably be in the hands of the nurses.

22.5 Nutritional Status as Basis for Therapy

To be able to rapidly determine if nutrition therapy is required, and to optimise the feeding route and the goals, an early evaluation is essential. Different tools are available for nutrition assessment as described in previous chapters: the Subjective Global Assessment (SGA), Mini Nutritional Assessment-Short Form (MNA-SF) and the Nutritional Risk Screening (NRS). The SGA, although validated and widely used especially in the USA, is often difficult to apply in the critically ill. The MNA-SF is easier to carry out and has been shown to be easily convertible to an NRS equivalent [20]: the latter point is important as the availability of multiple scores increases the risk of none being used. The ESPEN-ICU guidelines therefore recommend the NRS [16], with a cut-off of 5 points to define high-risk patients. In our cohort 60.6% of our patients belonged to the high NRS category. This score is easy to calculate (■ Fig. 22.1), and although it is not specific of old age, it has the advantage of being known by most intensivists.

Obesity defined as BMI >30 kg/m^2 is also present in the very old [21]: 12.4% in our cohort. Besides, moderate overweight was frequent (BMI 25–30 kg/m^2). These patients are modestly overweight, due to an increase of the proportion of fat mass that occurs at the expense of lean body mass (LBM): as individuals age, the body composition changes with increase in fat mass and decrease in muscle mass [22]. Nevertheless in old adults, a modest overweight has been shown to be "protective".

The only tool easily available at the bedside for body composition determination is multiple frequency bioimpedance analysis (BIA). This painless and low-cost technique consists in measuring a current through the body, using electrodes applied on the hands and feet (■ Fig. 22.2). It measures resistance (R), reactance and impedance (Z) at several current frequencies, enabling the calculation of body composition (body water, fat and muscle mass), and phase angle: the latter reflects cell viability. Despite being influenced by fluid administration, the phase angle has been shown to

Nutritional status alteration - A		Points
None	Normal status	0
Light	- Weight loss > 5% in 3 months - Ingesta < 50 % of usual	1
Moderate	- Weight loss > 5% in 2 months - BMI 18,5-20,5 kg/m^2 - Ingesta: 25-50% of usual	2
Severe	- Weight loss > 5% in 2 months - BMI < 18,5 kg/m^2 - Ingesta < 25 % of usual	3

Severity of condition - B		Points
None	Healthy	0
Light	Femoral Fracture COPD, Diabetes	1
Moderate	Severe pneumonia Major surgery	2
Severe	**ICU patient** APACHE >10	3
Age C	< 70 years	0
	$\geq$ 70 years	1

NRS = A + B + C

■ Fig. 22.1 The Nutritional Risk Screening (NRS) score includes a nutritional appreciation (A), the severity of the disease (B) and age (C): the score is the total of the worst variables A+B+C. All old elderly patients score 1 point (C) + 2–3 points due to severity (B), the A component being variable

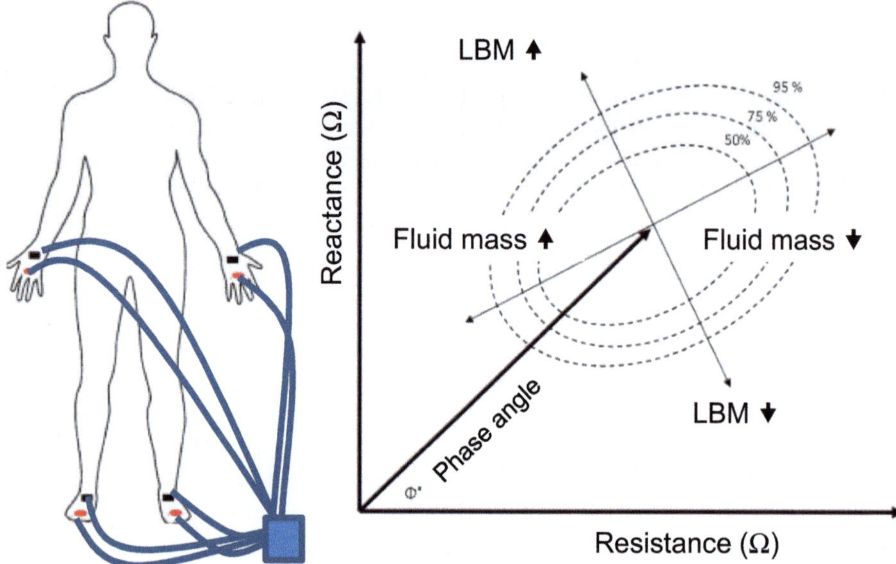

Fig. 22.2 Multiple-frequency bioimpedance can be carried out in the sitting or recumbent position, by applying four electrodes on the skin. (Adapted from Khalil et al. [42]): most devices use 5–1000 Hz and a small 1–10 µA current (not perceived by the patient) (LBM = Lean Body Mass)

accurately reflect viability [23]. BIA has been used in a few studies in elderly: the results confirm the facility of use and that narrow (low) phase angle is associated with frailty and mortality independent of age and comorbidity [24]. Phase angle is inversely related to muscle mass and strength in elderly subjects, and it is an easily available bioelectrical marker to identify elderly sarcopenic patients [25].

22.6 Energy, Protein and Micronutrient Needs

There is uncertainty as to the needs of the very old as evidence-based data are limited: the physiologic changes associated with normal aging process occur at different rates among individuals causing important variations. The 2018 ESPEN geriatric guidelines stress the fact that dehydration is frequent in old age, mainly due to the loss of thirst [17].

A series of age-related changes contribute to make requirements uncertain. The ageing gastrointestinal tract changes include a reduced mechanical disintegration of food, gastrointestinal motor dysfunction, food transit, chemical food digestion and functionality of the intestinal wall [5, 6]. The very frequent prescription of proton-pump inhibitors (PPIs) also reduces nutrient absorption [26]. These alterations progressively decrease the ability of the gastrointestinal tract to provide the ageing organism with adequate levels of nutrients, contributing to the development of malnutrition [6].

Energy

The geriatric guidelines propose to deliver 30 kcal/kg/day [17]. These recommendations are not ICU specific and do not consider the different illness phases. Predictive energy equations perform poorly in old adults [27], even worse than in younger patients. Among the equations, the Harris and Benedict (HB) equation performs best but underestimates energy expenditure (EE) in both sexes. This is particularly true in the frail elderly [28]. Obtaining the information about an exact "usual" body weight is often very difficult, and many ICUs do not weigh their patients. The effectiveness of predictive equations is even more limited in critically ill elderly patients as shown by a study including 97 critically ill elderly [29]. Segadilha et al. observed that the HB equation multiplied by a correction factor of 1.2 could be an option that avoided overfeeding. Another option is to use the ESPEN-ICU recommendation for the first week: 20 kcal/kg dry body weight (i.e. a preadmission weight before fluid resuscitation) to be achieved over the first 3–4 days. The comparison of these equations with indirect calorimetry values indicates that 20 kcal/kg/day during the first week is probably the best level of feeding in the absence of indirect calorimetry, which remains the gold standard for EE determination: but It is neither widely available yet, nor possible technically in patients who are non-intubated and oxygen dependent (◘ Table 22.2). ◘ Figure 22.3 shows the relation between the HB or the 20 kcal/kg predictions and indirect calorimetry measure EE in our cohort and confirms that HB underestimates the needs.

It is important to note that the needs increase after the first week and may increase to 30 kcal/kg already during the second week as shown by indirect calorimetry [30].

▬ Proteins

The geriatric guidelines recommend at least 1 g/kg/day protein [17]. A recent review summarised the recommendations: mild to moderate illness patients should receive 0.8–1.2 g/kg protein per day, while critically ill patients should receive higher doses of 1.2–1.5 g/kg protein per day [31]. The importance of proteins has been emphasised in recent years especially in the presence of low LBM: these patients have been shown to particularly benefit from high-protein feeding (>1.2 g/kg) [32].

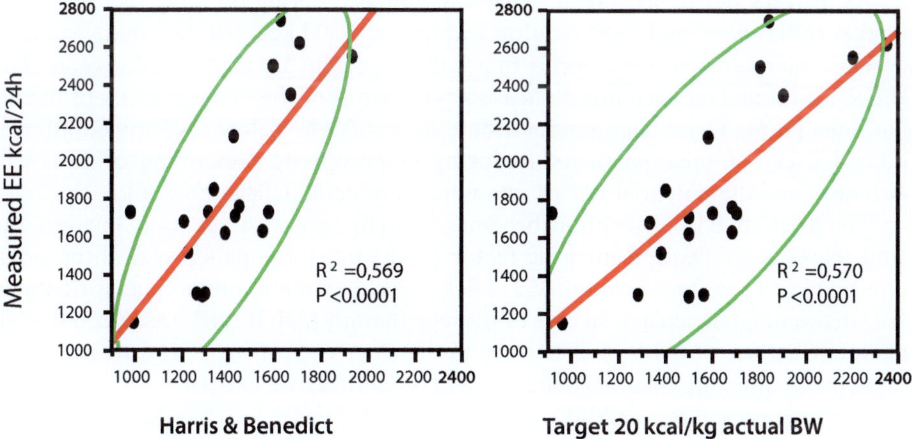

◘ **Fig. 22.3** Indirect calorimetry Energy expenditure (EE) values compared to the Harris and Benedict predictive equation or to the target 20 kcal/kg 95% ellipse confidence

Table 22.2 Strategies in the very old ICU patient

	Non-intubated	Intubated
Energy goal	Equation based: Harris and Benedict +10% Or 20 kcal/kg/day during the first week (25–30 kcal/kg/day thereafter)	Same targets in absence of Indirect calorimetry which should be privileged
Route	Oral: frequently little efficient. Swallowing disorders frequent (and worsened by intubation) Oral nutrition supplements: at least 400 kcal/day and 30 g proteins EN: efficient but feeding tubes poorly tolerated PN: central or peripheral if the previous is insufficient	EN: to be privileged – EN is efficient PN in case of insufficient EN, technical issues with enteral access or contraindication to EN
Proteins	1.2–1.3 g/day	
Micronutrients	Intravenous thiamine 100–200 mg, vitamin B12 plus intravenous multi-trace element and multivitamin doses daily from Day 1 for at least 3 days	

Looijaard et al. showed in large retrospective study including 739 ICU patients (mean age 58 years) that 60% of them had a low lean body mass based on data from the admission thorax CT scan. The delivery of >1.2 g/kg protein early during the ICU stay in the patients with very low lean body mass was associated with reduced 6-month mortality [32].

If patients are on oral feeding, the ONSs are strongly recommended because they enable covering the protein needs; they should be routinely prescribed on oral feeding.

Micronutrients

As the very old subjects tend to eat less, and as covering the daily recommended intakes (DRI) with oral food requires eating over 1500 kcal per day, many subjects develop micronutrient deficiencies that will be present upon ICU admission. The above-mentioned reduced intestinal absorption worsens the bioavailability of micronutrients [5, 6]. These changes contribute to justify the below encouraged intravenous delivery of micronutrients. Reducing inappropriate prescribing of PPIs will also minimise the potential risk of vitamin and mineral deficiencies [26].

The vitamin B12 absorption becomes less efficient with age as it involves the stomach (less acidity and intrinsic factor production), the pancreas and the small intestine [5]. Therefore, vitamin B12 deficiency is extremely common, as is thiamine (B1) deficiency, particularly in case of diuretic therapy [33]. It can be assumed that all micronutrients are at risk of deficiency in the elderly requiring ICU admission, the highest risk affecting thiamine, vitamin B12, vitamin D, Se and Zn.

The pragmatic way to address the potential deficiencies is to provide these micronutrients without blood determination from Day 1 (see §7) and to do blood tests only if an in-depth outwork is required.

22.7 Refeeding Syndrome

The risk of refeeding syndrome (RFS) is often underestimated, especially in the frail elderly population [34]. This partly relates to the unspecific clinical presentation and laboratory changes in the geriatric population. This complication affects a significant proportion of medical and surgical inpatients with malnutrition upon hospital admission. RFS is characterised by major electrolyte disturbances (low phosphate, magnesium and potassium), vitamin deficiency (thiamine), fluid overload and salt retention leading to organ dysfunction, cardiac arrhythmias and neurological disturbances [34]. A secondary analysis of a large RCT investigating the effects of nutritional support in malnourished medical inpatients screened patients for RFS and classified them as "RFS confirmed" and "RFS not confirmed" based on electrolyte shifts, clinical symptoms, clinical context and patient history [35]. Among 967 patients, RFS was confirmed in 141 (14.6%) patients. Compared to patients without, patients with confirmed RFS had significantly higher 180 days mortality rates (29.8% vs 21.9%, $P < 0.05$), an increased risk for ICU admission (4.3% vs 1.6%, $P < 0.05$) and a longer mean length of hospital stay (10.5 ± 6.9 vs 9.0 ± 6.6 days, $P = 0.01$).

In the critically ill, the usual clinical RFS criteria are particularly difficult to observe as they are largely non-specific: low values for phosphate, potassium and magnesium are often the only indication. In our cohort, neither BMI, nor weight, nor the NRS score was predictive of hypophosphataemia: 138/218 patients (63.3%) presented at least 1 episode of hypophosphataemia (Pi < 0.81 mmol/l), of which 79/218 (36.2%) presenting severe hypophosphataemia (Pi < 0.65 mmol/l). A daily determination of electrolytes and especially of phosphate is recommended to detect this complication [36], as hypophosphataemia is associated with increased mortality [37] and requires specific nutritional management with slow progression of feeding [16, 38].

22.8 Practical Issues

Oral nutrition supplement (ONS) administration should be systematic in the non-intubated elderly patients on oral feeding [17]. ONSs efficiently increase the protein intakes and improve wound healing after surgery or in the presence of pressure ulcers [39]. Our own data show that this recommendation is not sufficiently applied, resulting in energy deficits.

Tolerance for nasoenteric feeding tubes is often low in very old patients, who tend to rapidly tear off the feeding tubes. The frequent confusion and delirium contribute heavily. Reinserting them several times is for good reasons perceived as an "aggression" by patients and nursing team, questionable under an ethical standpoint, and moreover these actions increase the risk of misplacement [40]. Fighting to reinsert tubes increases the risk of underfeeding by delaying it. The use of sedation for feeding purpose is not considered acceptable in the geriatric ESPEN guidelines [17].

In this subgroup of patients, using parenteral nutrition may become an efficient alternative while waiting for return of efficient oral intake, thus preventing malnutrition: if a central line is available, it is easy, but peripheral PN may enable combined feeding complementing with 600–800 kcal, an insufficient oral intake. Particular attention should however be paid to fluid intake.

22.9 Monitoring Response to Feeding

The monitoring strategy can be reduced to very simple recommendations:

- Electrolytes: phosphate, potassium and magnesium determination on admission and daily thereafter should be routine [37].
- Blood glucose: the same ICU recommendations apply [16] while keeping in mind that a non-negligible portion of the elderly present with diabetes. The target blood glucose levels in the latter are 6–10 mmol/l.
- Energy delivery: daily verification of the really received feeds is of utmost importance, especially in the context of short stays – this is particularly true for patients on oral feeding, who are unlikely to cover their needs.
- Calculation of cumulated energy balance (difference between intake and prescription), especially during the first 7 days.
- Protein delivery: daily recording of delivery.
- Prealbumin determination weekly: this visceral protein was already shown in 1984 to indicate a response to protein and energy feeding [12]. A determination upon admission will enable analysis of the response to feeding: a simultaneous determination of C-reactive protein is required.

22.10 The Post-ICU Period

As done in the NOURISH trial, nutrition therapy should not stop at discharge [10]. As the patients are often rapidly discharged before full recovery, the post-ICU period is critical and should benefit from a close follow-up by the nurses and dieticians. Little is currently known about nutrition intake and energy requirements of this phase [30].

Prospective observational data are available from an Australian nested cohort study within a RCT in critically ill patients [30]. After discharge from ICU, energy and protein intake were quantified in 32 patients over 227 days: 12 patients had EE verified by indirect calorimetry. The median [IQR] estimated energy and protein requirements were 2000 [1650–2550] kcal and 112 [84–129] g, respectively. Oral nutrition either alone (55%) or in combination with EN (42%) was the predominant feeding mode. Patients received a median of 1240 kcal and 60 g of protein per day. In the 12 patients who had indirect calorimetry, the median measured daily EE was 1982 [1843–2345] kcal, and daily energy deficit was less than in the other patients with -95 [-1050–347] kcal, as if the measure had attracted attention to the needs. Energy and protein intake in the post-ICU period were below the estimated and measured energy requirements, worsening underfeeding, in a period where patients are supposed to recover.

Many barriers contribute to insufficient feeding after ICU discharge including patient barriers (poor appetite, persistent swallowing disorders, nausea, vomiting or diarrhoea) and clinical barriers (communication and resource issues such as lower nurse-to-patient ratio and knowledge deficits) [41].

Conclusion

The very old patients frequently present a high risk of malnutrition, frailty and sarcopenia, which worsens outcome [1]. We know that those who benefit most are those at highest risk, presenting with high NRS scores (≥5), or with demonstrated low lean body mass. An early assessment is required. If this is not possible due to lack of manpower, initiation of nutrition should be an automatic process, possibly best handled by the nurses. In the intubated patients, EN should be privileged with the alternative PN in case of EN contraindication. The most difficult cases are the non-intubated patients, where every effort should be made to over proteins needs using ONSs or supplemental PN.

The predominance of short ICU stays in the very old population shows the important of an early intervention. The nutrition process should be integrated during the entire hospital stay, starting for surgical cases in the preoperative period with preoperative nutritional assessment, or upon admission in the medical patients, and continuing after ICU discharge.

Note: Ethical issues are not addressed in this text, but the nutritional aspects involved in end-of-life decision and dementia management need to be integrated in the global ethical discussion.

Take-Home Messages

- Very old patients are characterised by a high prevalence of malnutrition, frailty and sarcopenia, which are associated with a higher mortality. The very old patients are even at higher risk of malnutrition than younger ICU patients: early evaluation is essential using e.g. NRS.
- Some ICU procedures are associated with prolonged periods of fasting and put the patients at additional risk of hospital malnutrition. Beware of fasting due to extubation attempts or NIV.
- Nutritional intervention in malnourished elderly has been shown to be efficient and to reduce complications and mortality.
- The very old are at a very high risk of refeeding syndrome: daily monitoring of phosphate, magnesium and potassium is required.
- Oral feeding is insufficient in most patients: ONS delivery should be part of oral feeding.
- Micronutrient deficiency is frequent; a pragmatic approach is to provide thiamine 100–200 mg/day, vitamin B12 and multi-trace element and vitamin products during the first 3–5 days of ICU stay.

References

1. Cruz-Jentoft AJ, Bahat G, Bauer J, et al. Sarcopenia: revised European consensus on definition and diagnosis. Age Ageing. 2019;48(1):16–31. https://doi.org/10.1093/ageing/afy169.
2. Cerri AP, Bellelli G, Mazzone A, et al. Sarcopenia and malnutrition in acutely ill hospitalized elderly: prevalence and outcomes. Clin Nutr. 2015;34(4):745–51. https://doi.org/10.1016/j.clnu.2014.08.015.
3. Robinson SM, Reginster JY, Rizzoli R, et al. Does nutrition play a role in the prevention and management of sarcopenia? Clin Nutr. 2018;37(4):1121–32. https://doi.org/10.1016/j.clnu.2017.08.016.

4. de Luis D, Lopez Guzman A. Nutrition Group of Society of C-L. Nutritional status of adult patients admitted to internal medicine departments in public hospitals in Castilla y Leon, Spain - a multi-center study. Eur J Intern Med. 2006;17(8):556–60. https://doi.org/10.1016/j.ejim.2006.02.030.

5. Stover PJ. Vitamin B12 and older adults. Curr Opin Clin Nutr Metab Care. 2010;13(1):24–7. https://doi.org/10.1097/MCO.0b013e328333d157.

6. Rémond D, Shahar DR, Gille D, et al. Understanding the gastrointestinal tract of the elderly to develop dietary solutions that prevent malnutrition. Oncotarget. 2015;6(16):13858–98. https://doi.org/10.18632/oncotarget.4030.

7. Marian M, Sacks G. Micronutrients and older adults. Nutr Clin Pract. 2009;24(2):179–95. https://doi.org/10.1177/0884533609332177.

8. Ouchi Y, Rakugi H, Arai H, et al. Redefining the elderly as aged 75 years and older: proposal from the Joint Committee of Japan Gerontological Society and the Japan Geriatrics Society. Geriatr Gerontol Int. 2017;17(7):1045–7. https://doi.org/10.1111/ggi.13118.

9. Guigoz Y. The Mini Nutritional Assessment (MNA) review of the literature--what does it tell us? J Nutr Health Aging. 2006;10(6):466–85. discussion 485-7. (In eng) (http://www.ncbi.nlm.nih.gov/pubmed/17183419)

10. Deutz N, Matheson E, Matarese L, et al. Readmission and mortality in malnourished, older, hospitalized adults treated with a specialized oral nutritional supplement: a randomized clinical trial. Clin Nutr. 2016;35(1):18–26. https://doi.org/10.1016/j.clnu.2015.12.010.

11. Milne AC, Potter J, Vivanti A, Avenell A. Protein and energy supplementation in elderly people at risk from malnutrition. Cochrane Database Syst Rev. 2009;(2):CD003288. https://doi.org/10.1002/14651858.CD003288.pub3.

12. Bastow M, Rawlings J, Allison S. Benefits of supplementary tube feeding after fractured neck of femur: a randomized controlled trial. BMJ. 1983;287:1589–92. https://pubmed.ncbi.nlm.nih.gov/6416514/

13. Schuetz P, Fehr R, Baechli V, et al. Individualised nutritional support in medical inpatients at nutritional risk: a randomised clinical trial. Lancet. 2019;393(10188):2312–21. https://doi.org/10.1016/S0140-6736(18)32776-4.

14. Soguel L, Revelly J, Schaller MD, Longchamp C, Berger MM. Energy deficit and length of hospital stay can be reduced by a two-step quality improvement of nutrition therapy: the intensive care unit dietitian can make the difference. Crit Care Med. 2012;40(2):412–9. (In eng). https://doi.org/10.1097/CCM.0b013e31822f0ad7.

15. Nabozny MJ, Barnato AE, Rathouz PJ, et al. Trajectories and prognosis of older patients who have prolonged mechanical ventilation after high-risk surgery. Crit Care Med. 2016;44(6):1091–7. https://doi.org/10.1097/CCM.0000000000001618.

16. Singer P, Reintam-Blaser A, Berger MM, et al. ESPEN guidelines: nutrition in the ICU. Clin Nutr. 2019;38:48–79. https://www.ncbi.nlm.nih.gov/pubmed/30348463.

17. Volkert D, Berner Y, Berry E, et al. ESPEN guidelines on enteral nutrition: geriatrics. Clin Nutr. 2006;25(2):330–360. (Consensus Development Conference Practice Guideline) (In eng). https://doi.org/10.1016/j.clnu.2006.01.012.

18. Chapple LA, Gan M, Louis R, Yaxley A, Murphy A, Yandell R. Nutrition-related outcomes and dietary intake in non-mechanically ventilated critically ill adult patients: a pilot observational descriptive study. Aust Crit Care. 2020;33(3):300–8. https://doi.org/10.1016/j.aucc.2020.02.008.

19. Macht M, King C, Wimbish T, et al. Post-extubation dysphagia is associated with longer hospitalization in survivors of critical illness with neurologic impairment. Crit Care. 2013;17(3):R119. https://doi.org/10.1186/cc12791.

20. Fournier J, Coutaz M, Hertzog H, Piccot P, Lamon J, Berger MM. Semi-automation of nutritional risk screening in the hospital results in systematic scoring. Clin Nutr Exp. 2016;8(1–8)

21. Ball L, Serpa Neto A, Pelosi P. Obesity and survival in critically ill patients with acute respiratory distress syndrome: a paradox within the paradox. Crit Care. 2017;21(1):114. https://doi.org/10.1186/s13054-017-1682-5.

22. Santanasto AJ, Goodpaster BH, Kritchevsky SB, et al. Body composition remodeling and mortality: the health aging and body composition study. J Gerontol A Biol Sci Med Sci. 2017;72(4):513–9. https://doi.org/10.1093/gerona/glw163.

23. Thibault R, Makhlouf A, Mulliez A, et al. Fat-free mass at admission predicts 28-day mortality in intensive care unit patients: the international prospective observational study phase angle project. Intensive Care Med. 2016;42(9):1445–53. https://www.ncbi.nlm.nih.gov/pubmed/27515162

24. Wilhelm-Leen ER, Hall YN, Horwitz RI, Chertow GM. Phase angle, frailty and mortality in older adults. J Gen Intern Med. 2014;29(1):147–54. https://doi.org/10.1007/s11606-013-2585-z.
25. Basile C, Della-Morte D, Cacciatore F, et al. Phase angle as bioelectrical marker to identify elderly patients at risk of sarcopenia. Exp Gerontol. 2014;58:43–6. https://doi.org/10.1016/j.exger.2014.07.009.
26. Heidelbaugh JJ. Proton pump inhibitors and risk of vitamin and mineral deficiency: evidence and clinical implications. Ther Adv Drug Saf. 2013;4(3):125–33. https://doi.org/10.1177/2042098613482484.
27. Melzer K, Karsegard VL, Genton L, Kossovsky M, Kayser B, Pichard C. Comparison of equations for estimating resting metabolic rate in healthy subjects over 70 years of age. Clin Nutr. 2007;26(4):498–505. http://www.ncbi.nlm.nih.gov/entrez/query.fcgi?cmd=Retrieve & db=PubMed & dopt=Citation & list_uids=17583391.
28. Gaillard C, Alix E, Salle A, Berrut G, Ritz P. Energy requirements in frail elderly people: a review of the literature. Clin Nutr. 2007;26(1):16–24. https://doi.org/10.1016/j.clnu.2006.08.003.
29. Segadilha N, Rocha EEM, Tanaka LMS, Gomes KLP, Espinoza REA, Peres WAF. Energy expenditure in critically ill elderly patients: indirect calorimetry vs predictive equations. JPEN J Parenter Enteral Nutr. 2017;41(5):776–84. https://doi.org/10.1177/0148607115625609.
30. Ridley EJ, Parke RL, Davies AR, et al. What happens to nutrition intake in the post-intensive care unit hospitalization period? An observational Cohort Study in critically ill adults. JPEN J Parenter Enteral Nutr. 2019;43(1):88–95. https://doi.org/10.1002/jpen.1196.
31. Deer RR, Volpi E. Protein requirements in critically ill older adults. Nutrients. 2018;10(3) https://doi.org/10.3390/nu10030378.
32. Looijaard W, Dekker IM, Beishuizen A, Girbes ARJ, Oudemans-van Straaten HM, Weijs PJM. Early high protein intake and mortality in critically ill ICU patients with low skeletal muscle area and -density. Clin Nutr. 2020;39(7):2192–201. https://doi.org/10.1016/j.clnu.2019.09.007.
33. Suter PM, Haller J, Hany A, Vetter W. Diuretic use: a risk for subclinical thiamine deficiency in elderly patients. J Nutr Health Aging. 2000;4(2):69–71. https://www.ncbi.nlm.nih.gov/pubmed/10842416
34. Aubry E, Friedli N, Schuetz P, Stanga Z. Refeeding syndrome in the frail elderly population: prevention, diagnosis and management. Clin Exp Gastroenterol. 2018;11:255–64. https://doi.org/10.2147/ceg.S136429.
35. Friedli N, Baumann J, Hummel R, et al. Refeeding syndrome is associated with increased mortality in malnourished medical inpatients: secondary analysis of a randomized trial. Medicine (Baltimore). 2020;99(1):e18506. https://doi.org/10.1097/MD.0000000000018506.
36. Koekkoek WAC, Van Zanten ARH. Is refeeding syndrome relevant for critically ill patients? Curr Opin Clin Nutr Metab Care. 2017;21(2):130–7. (In Eng)
37. Reintam Blaser A, Gunst J, Ichai C, et al. Hypophosphatemia in critically ill adults and children: a systematic review. Clin Nutr. 2021;40(4):1744–54. https://doi.org/10.1016/j.clnu.2020.09.045
38. Doig G, Simpson F, Heighes P, et al. Restricted versus continued standard caloric intake during the management of refeeding syndrome in critically ill adults: a randomised, parallel-group, multicentre, single-blind controlled trial. Lancet Respir Med. 2015;3(12):943–52. https://doi.org/10.1016/S2213-2600(15)00418-X.
39. Elia M, Normand C, Norman K, Laviano A. A systematic review of the cost and cost effectiveness of using standard oral nutritional supplements in the hospital setting. Clin Nutr. 2016;35(2):370–80. https://doi.org/10.1016/j.clnu.2015.05.010.
40. de Aguilar-Nascimento J, Kudsk K. Use of small-bore feeding tubes: successes and failures. Curr Opin Clin Nutr Metab Care. 2007;10(3):291–6. (Review) (In eng). https://doi.org/10.1097/MCO.0b013e3280d64a1d.
41. Ridley EJ, Chapple LS, Chapman MJ. Nutrition intake in the post-ICU hospitalization period. Curr Opin Clin Nutr Metab Care. 2020;23(2):111–5. https://doi.org/10.1097/MCO.0000000000000637.
42. Khalil SF, Mohktar MS, Ibrahim F. The theory and fundamentals of bioimpedance analysis in clinical status monitoring and diagnosis of diseases. Sensors (Basel). 2014;14(6):10895–928. https://doi.org/10.3390/s140610895.

Withhold and Withdraw Therapy

Contents

Limitation of Life-Sustaining Treatments

Bertrand Guidet and Hélène Vallet

Contents

🏠 Learning Objectives

- What are the limitations of life-sustaining treatment (LLST)?
- What are the determinants of LLST?
- How often such a decision occurs in old patients?
- What is the impact on mortality?
- Implication of patients and caregivers in the decision-making process
- How to deal with uncertainty: the concept of time-limited-trial
- What is the impact on caregivers?

23.1 Introduction

Old critically ill patients are increasing in Western countries. This translates in higher percentage of older patients admitted in ICUs although the prognosis is less favorable compared to younger patients, and the ability to recover after an ICU stay is reduced. Therefore, questions arose regarding the admission criteria [1] and level of care during the ICU stay. The life-sustaining treatment (LST) such as invasive mechanical ventilation and renal replacement therapy might not be started (withholding) or stopped (withdrawing). The determinants and consequences of such decision are of paramount importance to assess our current practice, since it has a profound impact on outcome, admission policy, level of care, family, and team satisfaction.

Decision to limit and/or to stop active treatment in any patient is probably one of the most difficult decisions for physicians. We are not trained to such exercise. Our goal is to save individual life and as many lives as possible. In one hand, it is important to avoid overutilization of ICU with potential detrimental effects for the patients, their relatives, and the ICU team and financial consequences for the society. However, on the other hand, we also want to avoid underutilization of ICU with critically ill old patient being denied ICU admission or treatments.

23.2 General Consideration in Old Critically Ill Old Population

Old patients are vulnerable. Vulnerability results from a combination of frailty, sarcopenia, cognitive decline, comorbidities, and polypharmacy. It reduces the ability to cope with an aggression like sepsis, trauma, and urgent surgery. In that perspective, in case of unfavorable response to treatment of organ failure, limiting LST is an option. The main objective of ICU treatment is to save lives but also to preserve long-term quality of life. In fact, almost 50% of old patients die or lose functional autonomy 6 months after ICU discharge.

Organ supports are often invasive and carry their own risk (hospital-acquired infection, delirium, etc.). Altogether, the question of limiting LST occurs frequently in the group of old critically ill patients. According to their age, the expected survival is much shorter than for younger patients with societal consequences. Therefore, decision to WH or WD treatment is of particular importance in critically ill old patients. However, in the constitution of many countries, discrimination is prohibited, and clearly, no choice should be based on age.

The life expectancy in many countries is steadily increasing. As a result, patients admitted to the hospital and ultimately to the ICU are older [2]. The proportion of "Very old Intensive care Patients" (VIPs) is estimated to increase up to 30% in 2050 [3] with a huge impact on total hospital expenditures [4]. Therefore, many ICUs across the globe must adapt their policies to increased demands. Some estimate that the need for ICU beds will increase 50% because of these developments [5].

In the last 15 years, there is a trend for more admission in ICU during the last month before death. Almost 30% of US Medicare patients were admitted in ICU during the last month before death with 3% being mechanically treated for at least 4 days [6].

Considering the high mortality [7], the increasing demand for intensive care in elderly, and the limited ICU resources, the society will face a challenge for matching increased spending in intensive care delivery in elderly and funding sustainability.

23.3　Limitation of Life-Sustaining Treatments

Limitation of treatments could occur at different steps of the patient pathway (■ Table 23.1). Triage at admission with refusal to admit in ICU an old patient is the first limitation but is beyond the scope of this chapter.

Several factors contribute to the decision to limit LST in Very old Intensive care Patients (VIP): expected survival and long-term outcomes such as functional decline, decrease of perceived quality of life, and expectation from patients and caregivers. External factors such as the economy and surge situation as with COVID-19 may also contribute even if individual ethical decision needs to be independent from collective pressure.

Unrestricted access to ICU treatment and/or lack of decision to forgo LST in old patient could lead to difficult access for younger patients as well as restrictions in other health services. Thus, it is imperative that appropriate allocation of ICU therapy (such as cardiopulmonary resuscitation, mechanical ventilation, renal replacement therapy,

■ **Table 23.1**　Limitation or optimization of ICU treatments

Prior to ICU admission	Advance directives	Living wills
Triage	Criteria	Alternative to ICU admission
Time-limited trial	How to deal with uncertainty?	Family conference
During the ICU stay	Withholding	Withdrawing
Discharge	Criteria	Location
Readmission	Yes/no	
Long-term follow-up	Prevention of new admission	Rehabilitation program

vasoactive drugs, and extra corporeal membrane oxygenation) should be considered in all cases. Trade-offs between different criteria and ethical principles will be unavoidable, and the principles of autonomy and distributive justice need to be balanced against each other.

Once a VIP has been admitted to the ICU for an acute medical reason, his/her expected short-term but also long-term mortality is high [7]. As a result, ICU physicians are increasingly faced with difficult decisions on continuation of life-sustaining treatment in VIPs. In these situations, decisions might be to withhold (WH) LST if patients deteriorate or even to withdraw (WD) already instigated LST if expected prognosis is poor.

Obviously, a collision of ethical, religious, conjectural, cultural, and personal issues is unavoidable partly explaining huge variation in LST limitation policies for VIPs across different countries [8–13].

Differences in admission policies and health care systems, together with insufficient information from the patients or their relatives (i.e., advanced directives), result in a huge variability in end-of-life (EOL) care in the ICU. In addition, there is a large variation in the proportion of deaths that occur after a decision to WH or WD life support, and this cannot solely be explained by patient characteristics or by patients' preferences.

Changes of end-of-life decision during the ICU stay have been elegantly shown in a study comparing 2 periods in 22 countries (Table 23.2) [14]. Compared with the patients included in the 1999–2000 cohort ($n = 2807$), the patients in 2015–2016 cohort were significantly older (median age, 70 years vs 67 years; $P < 0.001$). Significantly more treatment limitations occurred in the 2015–2016 cohort compared with the 1999–2000 cohort (89.7% vs 68.3%; $P < 0.001$), with more withholding of life-prolonging therapy (50.0% vs 40.7%; $P < 0.001$) and more withdrawing of life-prolonging therapy (38.8% vs 24.8%; $P < 0.001$). The composite ethical practice score doubled between the two periods suggesting a change in culture and organization of the participating ICUs. This score used 12 variables (routine family meetings, daily deliberation for the appropriate level of care, end-of-life discussions during meetings, written triggers for limitations, written end-of-life guidelines, written protocols, palliative care consultations, ethics consultations, staff taking communications, staff taking bioethics courses, each country's end-of-life guidelines, and each country's legislation). An important finding of this study was the higher survival rates after limitations in life-prolonging therapies in the second period. Limitations occur not only at the end of life but also earlier to respect patient wishes and to avoid invasive therapies likely to prolong the dying process or result in poor quality of life. Death occurred more often after the actual withdrawal of life-sustaining treatments than after withholding potential future or present life-prolonging therapies. In 2015–2016, more patients survived after withholding mechanical ventilation, vasopressor use, and renal replacement therapy, which may reflect improved ICU practices with more patients surviving acute illnesses [15].

◻ Table 23.2 Reporting of LLST in published studies

Year	First author	Country	Number of LLST	Total number whole population	% ICU stay with LLST
2017	Anderson	Norway	116	250	47
2015	Ferrão	Portugal	85	278	31
2017	Flaatten	Europe	1761	5021	35.1
2020	Guidet	Europe	1332	3920	34
2017	Le borgne	France	106	317	33.4
2014	Le Maguet	France	38	196	19
2018	Level	France	27	188	51
2017	Oeyen S	Belgium	34	131	25.9
2018	Pietilainen L	Finland	419	1827	22.9
2011	Roch A	France	69	299	23
2006	Rodriguez-Reganon I	Spain	9	100	9
2010	Tabah A	France	39	106	37.7
2012	Fuchs	USA	461	3003	15.4
2012	Fuchs	USA	496	1677	29.6
2015	Heyland	Canada	769	1671	46
2005	Pisani A	USA	132	395	33.4
2014	Al-dorzi HM	Saudi Arabia	103	748	13.8
2016	Kim	Korea	23	45	51.1
2017	Lee SH	Korea	23	106	21.7
2015	Sim YS	Korea	36	155	23
2014	Zampieri FG	Brazil	80	1129	7.1
2017	Auclin E	France	46	262	17.6
2014	Seder	USA	79	129	61
2017	Penasco Y	Spain	37	149	24.8
Total			6320	22102	29.7

Table 23.3 Changes in EOL decision over time (according to Sprung JAMA 2020)

Period	2015–2016	1999–2000
Patients (*n*)	13,625	2807
Age 70-96y (%)	51.5	43.5
WH decision (%)	50	40.7
WD decision (%)	38.8	24.8
Ethical practice score	5.6	2.9
Death with LLST	79.6	94.5
Time from ICU admission to first WH (days)	2.1	4
Time from WH decision until death (days)	29	14.1
Time from WD decision until death (days)	11.5	17.1

23.4 Reporting of Limitation of LST

It is important to emphasize that this information is lacking in most studies reporting mortality in old patients admitted in ICU. In a recent review focusing on mortality and including ICU patients ≥75 years, we retrieved 129 studies with only 23 studies with documented LLST (18%) [7]. This information was present in 6320/22,100 (29.7%) ICU stays (Table 23.3) [14, 16–37]. The absence of information on LLST is striking since this confounding/competing factor on mortality is documented in the past 20 years [38].

Since limitation of LST occurs more frequently among the most vulnerable or severely ill patients, this is a somewhat a self-fulfilling prophesy. Considering the huge heterogeneity of such decision, it is important to document this information [39]. This is particularly true for RCT when mortality is the primary endpoint. In a study analyzing 65 trials, LLST were documented in only 6 (9.2%) [40]. The exclusion of patients who die following LLST from benchmarking efforts leads to a major change in hospital ranks. Potentially preventable deaths, such as those following a major complication, should not be excluded [41].

23.5 Determinants of LLST

The factors usually reported as determinants of LLST are numerous, including origin (direct admission vs transfer from ward), type of patients (medical vs surgical or planned admission vs acute), comorbidities, and severity of the disease. Some structural aspects are also involved such as those described with the SAPS-3 database. A higher number of nurses per bed was associated with increased incidence of LLST, while availability of an emergency department in the same hospital, presence of a full-time ICU-specialist, and doctors' presence during nights and weekends were associated with a decreased incidence of LLST [42].

Age is usually reported as one of the factors used by clinicians for decision-making when deciding to limit LST.

We performed a survey with a panel of 22 international ICU physicians from 13 countries responding to a questionnaire related to withholding (WH) and withdrawing (WD) LST in elderly patients [43]. Most experts disagree or strongly disagree (77%) that age should be used as the sole criterion for WH or WD LST, and almost all disagree (91%) that there should be a specific age for such decision-making. However, the vast majority (91%) acknowledge that age should be an important consideration in conjunction with other factors.

Several studies have documented a higher rate of treatment limitations in aged patients compared to younger patients. In a study including 9000 ICU patients in the USA, LST limitation occurred in 2% of patients younger than 50 years and 25% in patients older than 80 years [44]. In the study by Hakim et al. [45], the rate of DNR orders increased with age (21% <54 years; 27% 55–65 years; 33% 65–74 years; 42% 75–84 years, and 55% for patients > 84 years). DNR orders were also decided earlier in elderly than in younger patients. In the SUPPORT study, the rate of decisions to withdraw treatment increased for every increase in patient's age of 10 years: 15% for mechanical ventilation, 19% for surgery, and 12% for RRT [45]. In a study from Australia and New Zealand, the length of stay (LOS) of elderly non-survivors was shorter than survivors suggesting that end-of-life (EOL) decisions were made sooner in patients older than 80 years [46]. In a matched-cohort study, 2299 patients over 80 years were matched (severity, organ failure, type of ICU stay, gender, Charlson Comorbidity Index) to 2299 patients aged from 65 to 79 years [47]. The oldest patients had a lower LOS and lower workload, were less often mechanically ventilated, and had less renal support and tracheostomy than matched "young old patients."

Age and specific geriatric scores are commonly reported as independent factors for deciding to forgo LST. In a prospective observational study, we examined the incidence and determinants of LST limitation decision (WH and/or WD) in VIP patients admitted to ICUs in European countries [48]. LST limitation was identified in 1356/5021 (27.2%) of patients of which 15% had a WH and 12.2% a WD (including those with a previous WH) decision. The patients with no LST limitation were younger, less frail, less severely ill, and more frequently electively admitted. Patients with WD of LST were more frequently male and had a longer ICU length of stay. The ICU mortality was 29.1% in the WH group and 82.2% in the WD group. The 30-day mortality was 53.1% in the WH group and 93.1% in the WD group. LST were less frequently limited in Eastern and Southern European countries compared to the ICUs located in the northern part(s) of Europe. The patient independent factors associated with LST limitation were "acute ICU admission," followed by the "Clinical Frailty Scale" (CFS), increased age, and SOFA score. Percentage of LST limitation was higher in countries with high GDP and lower when inhabitants considered God as very important.

In 2014, worldwide consensus definitions and statements about end-of-life practices for the majority of participating ICUs were developed. There was a very high consensus that preadmission state of health and mental functioning before the entrance to the hospital contributes to the patient's prognosis (93%) [49].

23.6 Implication of Patients and Caregivers in the Decision-Making Process

Advance directives include living wills and durable powers of attorney. Living wills are written by competent persons providing requests for specific medical treatments to be given or not in the event that these individuals no longer have decision-making capacity. They should take precedence over any other non-medical opinion expressed. However, these documents are very rarely available, poorly updated, and not precise enough regarding the desired level of care. In the ICE-CUB1 study with inclusion of 2646 patients older than 80 and visiting ED for a potential ICU admission [50], the family was present in 41% of the cases, but their opinion about ICU admission was asked in only 10% of the cases. In Germany, advance directive with living and therapeutic wills were available in less than 10% of the cases [51]. In the Ethicus study, performed in 17 European countries, the primary reason given by physicians for end-of-life decisions was the living will in only 1% of cases [52]. A review on the subject stressed "that the success of advance care planning should not be defined on the basis of completed paper work alone" [53], emphasizing the importance of communication and building trust over time [54]. In a prospective study involving patients aged 80 or more, it was shown that advance care planning was able to improve end-of-life care and patient and family satisfaction while reducing stress, anxiety, and depression among surviving relatives [55]. Elderly patients often prefer a lower intensity of care and care focused on comfort rather than undergoing invasive procedures [56] [57]. Recent evidence suggests that there are discrepancies between family preferences for end-of-life issues and actual care provided [58].

In the SUPPORT study, 85% of patients expressed specific wishes regarding do-not-resuscitate (DNR) orders; only 23% had discussed those wishes with their physician, and in half of these cases, the patient did not want to be resuscitated [58]. Fifty-eight percent did not want to discuss those wishes with their physician, and among these patients 25% did not want to be resuscitated. In 50% of cases, DNR orders were written by the physicians or requested by the families without the patients' consent.

Involvement of the patient and/or family in the decision-making process had a profound impact on ICU admission rate. The patient's relatives in most countries have no legal right to be involved in decision-making to limit LST. In the USA, the American College of Critical Care Medicine recommends that a family meeting should take place within 72 hours after admission of a patient to the ICU [59].

Strategies should be used to more consistently elicit, record, and harmonize documentation of patient preferences to attenuate confounding by unmeasured patient preferences and provide novel opportunities to improve the patient centeredness of medical care for serious illness [60].

23.7 How

At present, there is a strong consensus that age should not be considered as a sole decision-making criterion for limiting LST [61].

When an older patient has been admitted to the ICU, the most appropriate treatment should be given. However, this does not necessarily mean maximal treatment.

If, during the shared decision-making process, certain treatments such as invasive mechanical ventilation are thought to be disproportional to the chances of survival or certain treatments are refused by the patient, these treatments should not be forced upon the patient [56]. However, to give a patient a fair chance, all other treatments should be applied. The ethical climate has also been found to have an impact on treatment-limitation decisions and time until death [62] [63]. In a national, scenario-based, randomized trial, patient values had no effect on intensivists' decisions to discuss withdrawal of life support with family. However, requiring intensivists to record patients' estimated 3-month functional outcome substantially increased their intention to discuss withdrawal [64].

Apart from patient-related factors, other reasons to limit LSTs might play a role. Apparently, the ICU bed availability is associated with the timing of limitations of LSTs. Patients admitted in ICUs with a lower bed availability had a shorter time to do-not-resuscitate decisions, and patients who had do-not-resuscitate decisions had shorter time to death [65]. In the VIP1 study, there was no relation between the number of ICU beds and the percentage of LST limitations [48].

23.8 Treatment During the ICU Stay

LLST might be limited at ICU admission as reported by Rubio where most ICUs (94.8%) admitted patients with LLST, but only 7.8% patients had LLST on ICU admission [66]. A very restrictive admission policy will select out candidates for ICU treatment who are much less likely to fail a "trial of ICU" so that discussions regarding withholding/withdrawal of therapy are likely to be far less common than in ICU with liberal ICU policy. ICU survival might be better, but this relates to many potentially salvageable patients (especially the elderly) being denied ICU admission.

Older patients often receive a lower level of treatment intensity than their younger counterparts do. The prevalence of limitations of life-sustaining therapies increased with age in surgical population [67–69]. In addition, decisions to withhold LST were made earlier during the ICU stay in comparison to younger patients [42, 49]. In patients without improvement of their clinical situation, the therapeutic intensity level may no longer be in accordance with the patients' chances of long-term survival with acceptable quality of life, and a clinical decision might need to be made. In case of uncertainty or lack of information, the old critically ill patient might be admitted in ICU and the level of treatment reassessed after a few days. This pragmatic and sequential approach is often called time-limited trial (TLT).

23.9 Time-Limited Trial

The rationale of TLT is presented in ▶ Box 23.1. A TLT is an agreement between clinicians and a patient/family to use certain medical therapies over a defined period to see if the patient improves or deteriorates according to agreed-on clinical outcomes. If the patient improves, disease-directed therapy continues. If the patient deteriorates, the therapies involved in the trial are withdrawn, and goals frequently shift more purely curative to palliation. If significant clinical uncertainty remains, another TLT might be renegotiated. The different steps are presented in ▶ Box 23.2.

If accuracy of triage prior to the ICU at present is poorly evidence based, what is the alternative? The concept of an in-ICU-triage: a time-limited treatment trial (TLT) has emerged in the recent years and in particular in hemato-oncology and elderly ICU patients [70–73]. A TLT offers an admission to the ICU in order to observe if the patient profit from a full intensive care treatment [74]. A TLT is a formal process that must be discussed and agreed upon with the patient (if possible) or caregivers as well as medical stakeholders like referring physicians. After the time period, usually 2–4 days, a new evaluation is performed with the goal to document if there is objective improvement reflecting the effect of the treatment. This can be done in several ways, and objectively a serial measurement of organ dysfunction as with the sequential organ failure assessment (SOFA) score is important to document to avoid bias and subjective judgment. If organ function has improved, then the treatment is considered of value and continued; if organ dysfunction has increased, treatment may be considered futile and life-sustaining therapy withhold or withdrawn with a focus on palliative care. If situation is unaltered, a new TLT may or may be offered. A TLT must be explained and agreed on at ICU admission, so that these different trajectories can be described and discussed. The inclusion of a geriatrician will certainly add value to this process but remains to be demonstrated in a clinical trial.

A TLT begins with an assessment of the patient's current clinical status, preference, and prognosis with or without the treatment in question. In addition to disease-related factors, the patient's cognitive and functional status is generally relevant. This pragmatic approach is particularly relevant for old patient with short expected life and poor functional outcome. So given the uncertainty on short- but also long-term prognosis and the absence of complete information for the decision-making process of ICU admission, a trade-off could be to admit the old patient in ICU but with a formal reassessment a few days after admission in ICU. This could avoid futile treatment with consequences for the patient (suffering), for the family members (anxiety, grief, depression, and even economic impact in some countries), for the ICU team (burnout, grief, intention to quit), for other patients candidate for an ICU admission (distributive justice), and for the society (longer LOS translate into higher cost for the social security). These protocolized family support interventions reduce the ICU LOS without impacting mortality [75].

> **Box 23.1   Rationale for Time-Limited Trial**
> - Avoiding overutilization of ICU with potential detrimental effects for the patients, their relatives, and the ICU team and financial consequences for the society
> - Avoiding underutilization of ICU with critically ill old patient denied ICU admission (agism)
> - The main challenge is to identify who will benefit from admission to the intensive care unit when the chances of a meaningful outcome are unclear
> - In urgent situation, the estimation of ICU benefit (survival, HRQOL) is difficult to assess or predict; key information are often not available (advance directives, no relatives, etc.)

- For patients with uncertain prognosis and/or unclear preferences
- Requirement of comprehensive discussion with patient/family before and during ICU admission to facilitate an understanding of patient preferences and expectations
- Need to individualize the optimal duration of a trial of treatment but also the necessity for a fixed time for reevaluation

---

Box 23.2   Organization of Family Meetings (According to Quill) [73]

Preparation
- Select a senior ICU physician to involve
- Identify key family decision-maker(s)
- Seek consensus among medical teams
- Identify clear clinical markers of improvement or deterioration

Beginning of the family meeting
- Review purpose of meeting
- Solicit family members' views of patient's situation
- Reconcile clinicians' understanding with that of the patient or family

Propose key components of TLT
- If treatment is working, propose next steps
- If treatment is not working, next steps might include negotiating a different TLT or
- proposing a plan for treatment withdrawal
- In case of LST limitation, explain comfort care

Follow-up
- Discuss how progress will be measured and communicated
- Negotiate time frame for reevaluation
- Schedule a follow-up meeting
- Follow up at scheduled intervals depending on the TLT
- Regularly inform family about progress

23.10 Quality of Death

For patients with withholding or withdrawing of LST, an important goal is to achieve the most comfortable death [76]. Family members reported that the "patient be comfortable and suffer as little as possible" was their most important value and "the belief that life should be preserved at all costs" was their least important value considered in making treatment decisions [77]. Mobile palliative care team could be very useful to help in the decision process and even to propose admission in a palliative unit.

The care at the end of patients' lives—"end-of-life care" (EOLC)—has evolved into an important tool within the armamentarium of the modern critical care specialist, aided by palliative care specialists, if required and feasible [78, 79]. Despite widespread agreement as to the general need for adequate EOLC, there is considerable variation regarding its practice and implementation—not only between continents or countries but also within countries, regions, and even hospitals [8, 49, 80].

Arguably, the main proportion of the variation is attributable to the individual providers,

the reasons being, amongst others, schools of medical thinking, differences as to prognostication, hierarchy, ignorance, cultural norms, religion, and religiosity.

> **Take-Home Messages**
> Old patients have a higher risk of death during the ICU stay, in the hospital, and after discharge. When they survive, they may suffer from long-term sequel including loss of functional autonomy and poor quality of life, and they often represent a high burden for the caregivers. All these factors contribute to more frequent decisions to limit LST in old patients compared to younger patients. The work-up of the decision has an impact on the ICU team and the family members. Collegiality, timing, transparency, and objectivity are key to prevent conflict and complicated grief.

> **Clinical Protocol**
>
> Collection of objective information to decide to limit life-sustaining treatment (LST).
>
> To allow time for reassessment of the patient condition and response to previous treatment.
>
> In case of uncertainty or missing information, a time-limited trial can be proposed with definition of initial goal of treatment shared with the patient (if possible) and the caregivers with secondary decision to forgo LST or to continue treatment without any limitation.
>
> Limitation of LST is not synonym to end-of-life decision. This is particularly true for WH decision.

References

1. Guidet B, de Lange DW, Flaatten H. Should this elderly patient be admitted to the ICU? Intensive Care Med. 2018;44:1926–8.
2. Laake JH, Dybwik K, Flaatten HK, Fonneland I-L, Kvåle R, Strand K. Impact of the post-World War II generation on intensive care needs in Norway. Acta Anaesthesiol Scand. 2010;54:479–84.
3. Jones A, Toft-Petersen AP, Shankar-Hari M, Harrison DA, Rowan KM. Demographic shifts, case mix, activity, and outcome for elderly patients admitted to adult general ICUs in England, Wales, and Northern Ireland. Crit Care Med. 2020;48:466–74.
4. Angus D. Admitting elderly patients to the intensive care unit- is it the right decision? JAMA. 2017;318:1443–4.
5. Guidet B, Vallet H, Boddaert J, de Lange DW, Morandi A, Leblanc G, Artigas A, Flaatten H. Caring for the critically ill patients over 80: a narrative review. Ann Intensive Care. 2018;8:114.
6. Teno JM, Gozalo P, Trivedi AN, Bunker J, Lima J, Ogarek J, Mor V. Site of death, place of care, and health care transitions among US medicare beneficiaries, 2000-2015. JAMA. 2018;320:264–71.
7. Vallet H, Schwarz GL, Flaatten H, de Lange DW, Guidet B, Dechartres A. Mortality of older patients admitted to an intensive care unit a systematic review. Crit Care Med. 2021;49(2):324–34.
8. Mark NM, Rayner SG, Lee NJ, et al. Global variability in withholding and withdrawal of life-sustaining treatment in the intensive care unit: a systematic review. Intensive Care Med. 2015;41:1572–85.

9. Sprung CL, Woodcock T, Sjokvist P, et al. Reasons, considerations, difficulties and documentation of end-of-life decisions in European intensive care units: the ETHICUS Study. Intensive Care Med. 2008;34:271–7.
10. Sprung CL, Danis M, Iapichino G, Artigas A, Kesecioglu J, Moreno R, Lippert A, Curtis JR, Meale P, Cohen SL, Levy MM, Truog RD. Triage of intensive care patients: identifying agreement and controversy. Intensive Care Med. 2013;39:1916–24.
11. Quill CM, Ratcliffe SJ, Harhay MO, Halpern SD. Variation in decisions to forgo life-sustaining therapies in US ICUs. Chest. 2014;146(573–582):5.
12. Hart JL, Harhay MO, Gabler NB, Ratcliffe SJ, Quill CM, Halpern SD. Variability among US intensive care units in managing the care of patients admitted with preexisting limits on life-sustaining therapies. JAMA Intern Med. 2015;175:1019–26.
13. Barnato AE, Herndon MB, Anthony DL, Gallagher PM, Skinner JS, Bynum JP, Fisher ES. Are regional variations in end-of-life care intensity explained by patient preferences? A study of the US Medicare population. Med Care. 2007;45:386–93.
14. Oeyen S, Vermassen J, Piers R, et al. Critically ill octogenarians and nonagenarians: evaluation of long-term outcomes, posthospital trajectories and quality of life one year and seven years after ICU discharge. Minerva Anestesiol. 2017;83:598–609.
15. Sprung CL, Ricou B, Hartog CS, et al. Changes in end-of-life practices in European intensive care units from 1999 to 2016. JAMA. 2019;322(17):1–12.
16. Andersen FH, Flaatten H, Klepstad P, et al. Long-term outcomes after ICU admission triage in octogenarians. Crit Care Med. 2017;45:e363–71.
17. Ferrao C, Quintaneiro C, Camila C, et al. Evaluation of long-term outcomes of very old patients admitted to intensive care: survival, functional status, quality of life, and quality-adjusted life-years. J Crit Care. 2015;30(1150):e7–11.
18. Flaatten H, De Lange DW, Morandi A, et al. The impact of frailty on ICU and 30-day mortality and the level of care in very elderly patients (>/= 80 years). Intensive Care Med. 2017;43:1820–8.
19. Guidet B, de Lange DW, Boumendil A, et al. The contribution of frailty, cognition, activity of daily life and comorbidities on outcome in acutely admitted patients over 80 years in European ICUs: the VIP2 study. Intensive Care Med. 2020;46:57–69.
20. Le Borgne P, Maestraggi Q, Couraud S, et al. Critically ill elderly patients (>/= 90 years): clinical characteristics, outcome and financial implications. PLoS One. 2018;13:e0198360.
21. Le Maguet P, Roquilly A, Lasocki S, et al. Prevalence and impact of frailty on mortality in elderly ICU patients: a prospective, multicenter, observational study. Intensive Care Med. 2014;40:674–82.
22. Level C, Tellier E, Dezou P, et al. Outcome of older persons admitted to intensive care unit, mortality, prognosis factors, dependency scores and ability trajectory within 1 year: a prospective cohort study. Aging Clin Exp Res. 2018;30:1041–51.
23. Pietilainen L, Hastbacka J, Backlund M, et al. Premorbid functional status as a predictor of 1-year mortality and functional status in intensive care patients aged 80 years or older. Intensive Care Med. 2018;44:1221–9.
24. Roch A, Wiramus S, Pauly V, et al. Long-term outcome in medical patients aged 80 or over following admission to an intensive care unit. Crit Care. 2011;15:R36.
25. Rodríguez-Regañón I, Colomer I, Frutos-Vivar F, et al. Outcome of older critically ill patients: a matched cohort study. Gerontology. 2006;52:169–73.
26. Tabah A, Philippart F, Timsit JF, et al. Quality of life in patients aged 80 or over after ICU discharge. Crit Care. 2010;14:R2.
27. Fuchs L, Chronaki CE, Park S, et al. ICU admission characteristics and mortality rates among elderly and very elderly patients. Intensive Care Med. 2012;38:1654–61.
28. Heyland D, Cook D, Bagshaw SM, et al. The very elderly admitted to ICU: a quality finish? Crit Care Med. 2015;43:1352–60.
29. Pisani MA, Redlich CA, McNicoll L, et al. Short-term outcomes in older intensive care unit patients with dementia. Crit Care Med. 2005;33:1371–6.
30. Al-Dorzi HM, Tamim HM, Mundekkadan S, et al. Characteristics, management and outcomes of critically ill patients who are 80 years and older: a retrospective comparative cohort study. BMC Anesthesiol. 2014;14:126.
31. Kim J, Choi SM, Park YS, et al. Factors influencing the initiation of intensive care in elderly patients and their families: a retrospective cohort study. Palliat Med. 2016;30:789–99.
32. Lee SH, Lee TW, Ju S, et al. Outcomes of very elderly (>/= 80 years) critical-ill patients in a medical intensive care unit of a tertiary hospital in Korea. Korean J Intern Med. 2017;32:675–81.

33. Sim YS, Jung H, Shin TR, et al. Mortality and outcomes in very elderly patients 90 years of age or older admitted to the ICU. Respir Care. 2015;60:347–55.
34. Zampieri FG, Colombari F. The impact of performance status and comorbidities on the short-term prognosis of very elderly patients admitted to the ICU. BMC Anesthesiol. 2014;14:59.
35. Auclin E, Charles-Nelson A, Abbar B, et al. Outcomes in elderly patients admitted to the intensive care unit with solid tumors. Ann Intensive Care. 2017;7:26.
36. Seder DB, Patel N, McPherson J, et al. Geriatric experience following cardiac arrest at six interventional cardiology centers in the United States 2006-2011: interplay of age, do-not-resuscitate order, and outcomes. Crit Care Med. 2014;42:289–95.
37. Penasco Y, Gonzalez-Castro A, Rodriguez Borregan JC, et al. Limitation of life-sustaining treatment in severe trauma in the elderly after admission to an intensive care unit. Med Intensiva. 2017;41:394–400.
38. Azoulay E, Pochard F, Garrouste-Orgeas M, Moreau D, Montesino L, Adrie C, de Lassence A, Cohen Y, Timsit JF, Outcomerea Study Group. Decisions to forgo life-sustaining therapy in ICU patients independently predict hospital death. Intensive Care Med. 2003;29:1895–901.
39. Flaatten H, de Lange D, Jung C, Beil M, Guidet B. The impact of end of life care on ICU outcome. Intensive Care Med. 2021;47(5):624–25.
40. Gaudry S, Tubach F, Guillo S, Dreyfuss D, Hajage D, Ricard JD. Underreporting of end-of-life decisions in critical care trials: a call to modify the consolidated standards of reporting trials statement. Am J Respir Crit Care Med. 2018;197(2):263–6.
41. Guttman MP, Tillmann BW, Haas B, Nathens AB. Deaths following withdrawal of life-sustaining therapy: opportunities for quality improvement? J Trauma Acute Care Surg. 2020;89:743–51.
42. Azoulay E, Metnitz B, Sprung CL, Timsit JF, Lemaire F, Bauer P, Schlemmer B, Moreno R, Metnitz P, SAPS 3 investigators. End-of-life practices in 282 intensive care units: data from the SAPS 3 database. Intensive Care Med. 2009;35:623–30.
43. Guidet B, Hodgson E, Feldman C, Paruk F, Lipman J, Koh Y, Vincent JL, Azoulay E, Sprung C. The Durban World Congress Ethics Round Table conference report: II. Withholding or withdrawing of treatment in elderly patients admitted to the Intensive Care Unit. J Crit Care. 2014;29:896–901.
44. Hamel MB, Davis RB, Teno JM, et al. Older age, aggressiveness of care, and survival for seriously ill, hospitalized adults. SUPPORT investigators. Study to understand prognoses and preferences for outcomes and risks of treatments. Ann Intern Med. 1999;131:721–8.
45. Hakim RB, Teno JM, Harrell FE Jr, et al. Factors associated with do-not-resuscitate orders: patients' preferences, prognoses, and physicians' judgments. SUPPORT investigators. Study to understand prognoses and preferences for outcomes and risks of treatment. Ann Intern Med. 1996;125:284–93.
46. Bagshaw SM, Webb SA, Delaney A, et al. Very old patients admitted to intensive care in Australia and New Zealand: a multi-centre cohort analysis. Crit Care. 2009;13(2):R45.
47. Boumendil A, Aegerter P, Guidet B. Treatment intensity and outcome of patients aged 80 and over in intensive care unit. A multicenter matched-cohort study. J Am Geriatr Soc. 2005;53:88–93.
48. Guidet B, Flaatten H, Boumendil A, et al. VIP1 study group. Withholding or withdrawing of life-sustaining therapy in older adults (≥ 80 years) admitted to the intensive care unit. Intensive Care Med. 2018;44:1027–38.
49. Sprung CL, Truog RD, Curtis JR, et al. Seeking worldwide professional consensus on the principles of end-of-life care for the critically ill. The consensus for worldwide end-of-life practice for patients in intensive care units (WELPICUS) study. Am J Respir Crit Care Med. 2014;190(8):855–66.
50. Le Guen J, Boumendil A, Guidet B, Corval A, Saint-Jean O, Somme D. Are elderly patients' sought before admission to an intensive care unit? Results of the ICE-CUB study. Age Ageing. 2016;45:303–9.
51. Graw JA, Spies CD, Wernecke KD, Braun JP. Managing end of life decision making in intensive care medicine – a perspective from Charité Hospital, Germany. PLoS One. 2012;7:e46446.
52. Sprung CL, Cohen SL, Sjokvist P, et al.; Ethicus Study Group. End-of-life practices in European intensive care units: the Ethicus Study. JAMA. 2003;290(6):790–7.
53. Mullick A, Martin J, Sallnow L. An introduction to advance care planning in practice. BJM. 2013;347:f6064.
54. Prendergast TJ. Advance care planning : pitfalls, progress, promise. Crit Care Med. 2001;29(Suppl): N34–9.

55. Detering KM, Hancock AD, Reade MC, Silvester W. The impact of advance care planning on end of life care in elderly patients: randomised controlled trial. BMJ. 2010;340:c1345.

56. Philippart F, Vesin A, Bruel C, Kpodji A, Durand-Gasselin B, Garcon P, Levy-Soussan M, Jagot JL, Calvo-Verjat N, Timsit JF, Misset B, Garrouste-Orgeas M. The ETHICA study (part I): elderly's thoughts about intensive care unit admission for life-sustaining treatments. Intensive Care Med. 2013;39:1565–73.

57. Heyland DK, Dodek P, Mehta S, et al. Admission of the very elderly to the intensive care unit: family members' perspectives on clinical decision-making from a multicenter cohort study. Palliat Med. 2015;29:324–35.

58. Hofmann JC, Wenger NS, Davis RB, Teno J, Connors AF Jr, Desbiens N, Lynn J, Phillips RS. Patient preferences for communication with physicians about end-of-life decisions. SUPPORT investigators. Study to understand prognoses and preference for outcomes and risks of treatment. Ann Intern Med. 1997;127:1–12.

59. Truog RD, Campbell ML, Curtis JR, Haas CE, Luce JM, Rubenfeld GD, Rushton CH, Kaufman DC. Recommendations for end-of-life care in the intensive care unit: a consensus statement by the American College of Critical Care Medicine. Crit Care Med. 2008;36:953–63.

60. Walkey AJ, Barnato AE, Soylemez Wiener R, Nallamothu BK. Accounting for patient preferences regarding life-sustaining treatment in evaluations of medical effectiveness and quality. Am J Respir Crit Care Med. 2017;196:958–63.

61. Guidet B, De Lange DW, Christensen S, Moreno R, Fjølner J, Dumas G, Flaatten H. Attitudes of physicians towards the care of critically ill elderly patients - a European survey. Acta Anaesthesiol Scand. 2018;62(2):207–19.

62. Van den Bulcke B, Piers R, Jensen HI, Malmgren J, Metaxa V, Reyners AK, et al. Ethical decision-making climate in the ICU: theoretical framework and validation of a self-assessment tool. BMJ Qual Saf. 2018;27(10):781–9.

63. Benoit DD, Jensen HI, Malmgren J, Metaxa V, Reyners AK, Darmon M, et al. Outcome in patients perceived as receiving excessive care across different ethical climates: a prospective study in 68 intensive care units in Europe and the USA. Intensive Care Med. 2018;44(7):1039–49.

64. Turnbull AE, Hayes MM, Brower RG, Colantuoni E, Basyal PS, White DB, Curtis JR, Needham DM. Effect of documenting prognosis on the information provided to ICU proxies: a randomized trial. Crit Care Med. 2019;47(6):757–64.

65. Hua M, Halpern SD, Gabler NB, Wunsch H. Effect of ICU strain on timing of limitations in life-sustaining therapy and on death. Intensive Care Med. 2016;42(6):987–94.

66. Rubio O, Arnau A, Cano S, et al. Limitation of life support techniques at admission to the intensive care unit: a multicenter prospective cohort study. J Intensive Care. 2018;6:24.

67. Brandberg C, Blomqvist H, Jirwe M. What is the importance of age on treatment of the elderly in the intensive care unit? Acta Anaesthesiol Scand. 2013;57(6):698–703.

68. Hamel MB, Henderson WG, Khuri SF, Daley J. Surgical outcomes for patients aged 80 and older: morbidity and mortality from major noncardiac surgery. J Am Geriatr Soc. 2005;53(3):424–9.

69. Roger C, Morel J, Molinari N, Orban JC, Jung B, Futier E, et al. Practices of end-of-life decisions in 66 southern French ICUs 4 years after an official legal framework: a 1-day audit. Anaesth Crit Care Pain Med. 2015;34(2):73–7.

70. Lecuyer L, Chevret S, Thiery G, Darmon M, Schlemmer B, Azoulay E. The ICU trial: a new admission policy for cancer patients requiring mechanical ventilation. Crit Care Med. 2007;35(3):808–14.

71. Lee RY, Brumback LC, Sathitratanacheewin S, Lober WB, et al. Association of physician orders for life-sustaining treatment with ICU admission among patients hospitalized near the end of life. JAMA. 2020;323(10):950–60.

72. Shrime MG, Ferket BS, Scott DJ, et al. Time-limited trials of intensive care for critically ill Patients with cancer: how long is long enough? JAMA Oncol. 2016;2(1):76–83.

73. Quill TE, Holloway R. Time-limited trials near the end of life. JAMA. 2011;306:1483–4.

74. Vink EE, Azoulay E, Caplan A, Kompanje EJO, Bakker J. Time-limited trial of intensive care treatment: an overview of current literature. Intensive Care Med. 2018;44:1369–77.

75. Lee HW, Park Y, Jang EJ, Lee YJ. Intensive care unit length of stay is reduced by protocolized family support intervention: a systematic review and meta-analysis. Intensive Care Med. 2019;45(8):1072–81.

76. Lobo SM, De Simoni FHB, Jakob SM, Estella A, Vadi S, Bluethgen A, et al. Decision-making on withholding or withdrawing life support in the ICU: a worldwide perspective. Chest. 2017;152(2):321–9.

77. Heyland DK, Dodek P, Mehta S, Cook D, Garland A, Stelfox HT, et al. Admission of the very elderly to the intensive care unit: family members' perspectives on clinical decision-making from a multicenter cohort study. Palliat Med. 2015;29(4):324–35.
78. Baker M, Luce J, Bosslet GT, et al. Integration of palliative care services in the intensive care unit. A roadmap for overcoming barriers. Clin Chest Med. 2015;36:441–8.
79. Aslakson RA, Curtis JR, Nelson JE, et al. The changing role of palliative care in the ICU. Crit Care Med. 2014;42:2418–28.
80. Barnato AE, Tate JA, Rodriguez KL, et al. Norms of decision making in the ICU: a case study of two academic medical centers at the extremes of end-of-life treatment intensity. Intensive Care Med. 2012;38:1886–96.

Outcomes After Intensive Care

Contents

Outcomes After Intensive Care: Survival

Hans Flaatten

Contents

24

Learning Objectives

Probably the most frequently reported outcome in healthcare in general, and in intensive care in particular, is survival or its counterpart mortality. Obviously, other patient-centered outcomes are very often connected and even dependent on a patient that survives. It makes no meaning to talk about quality of life in patients not surviving the ICU stay, but for survivors post-hospital discharge, other issues than merely survival become more and more important.

Survival is reported in many ways, many of them then not directly comparable. The best is fixed time intervals, in particular to avoid hospital survival which is a very unprecise term since this may span from a week to months, also including or excluding transfer from one hospital to another. For this reason, the fixed time to report survival should be used whenever possible.

Crude survival with no or few other information of the patients is useless and cannot be used in any meaningful purpose. Often, we use survival to compare results between units, countries, or other studies. Then we need to have a lot of other information about the patient, like previous health and frailty, age and gender, severity of the acute disorder, and the limitation of life-sustaining therapy, to mention some important factors.

In this chapter I discuss several of these issues which are essential in order to understand mortality in general and within intensive care in particular.

24.1 Introduction

Controversies treating the very old in the ICU are not a new phenomenon. 40 years ago, a study was published in JAMA, *Medical Intensive Care for the elderly* [1], that evoked reactions. Although elderly in that paper was defined as ICU patients above 55 years, they also studied a subgroup of patients ≥75 years which is interesting in a historical perspective. In contrast with nowadays compared to those 55–64 years, the elderly more often was given "major interventions" like mechanical ventilation (32% compared to 22%). Today, this figure is reversed, and mechanical ventilation given to the very old usually occurs less often than in younger ICU patients. Of interest is that the absolute number of very old patients given mechanical ventilation is much higher today, being 51% in the VIP1 study [2].

Outcome in the group of very old was previously often reported to be poor, in particular if they were given mechanical ventilation. In a study from 1985 to 1987 in a single US ICU, 45 patients ≥80 years were followed, and only 10 patients survived to hospital discharge. If the sum of age and the number of ventilated days was >100, none survived to hospital discharge [3]. The message from these studies has followed us since, and in many situations most intensivists have probably been questioned about why elderly critical ill patients should be treated at all. Luckily, it is not very difficult to argue that today's octogenarians are different from 40–50 years ago, and our understanding of disease and treatment options is much improved, and survival has improved significantly!

24.2 Limitations of Crude Survival

Survival is probably the most used parameter to describe outcome after admission to an ICU, but it is difficult to really understand survival without putting it into a context.

Crude survival is just the number of survivors within a group, not necessarily further specified. An example is the ICU survival given for a given unit in the hospital, or in a registry, with no additional information. It is obvious that crude survival without any supplementary information is not meaningful in any form of comparison with other seemingly similar patient groups. Information mandatory to understand survival on group level is admission category, age, severity of disease, magnitude of organ dysfunction, pre-ICU condition (frailty-comorbidity-activity level, and cognition), and limitation of life-sustaining therapy (LST) during the ICU stay. All factors are seldom revealed together in outcome studies, which we recently have experienced during the COVID-19 pandemic, and this makes it hard to compare studies and also perform systematic review.

24.3 Survival After a Defined Procedure or Admission

This is a common way to report survival, and in our context both ICU survival and hospital survival fall into this group, where ICU can be seen both as a procedure and an admission. This use of survival is better than crude survival but still makes comparisons difficult. We know that mean admission time in an ICU typically vary between 1 and 10 days and hospital admission from 1 to 30(+) days.

Also, ICU admission is an ambiguous term. We can broadly dived ICU admissions as planned or unplanned. The former most often is a result of a major surgery and the latter after acute disease and trauma. The effect of this distinction was recently studied where it was found a huge 30-day survival difference between patients admitted after acute surgery (26%) or elective surgery (8%) [4], while the 30-day survival in the whole cohort including all medical admissions was 32.6%.

The mixture of acute and elective patients when reporting outcomes is probably one of the largest explanatory variables of differences in mortality. It is so profound that it should be mandatory to reveal this in any outcome study from the ICU.

24.4 Survival After a Fixed Period

This is most often used today since it makes comparisons fairer. Often 30 days/1 month is used for short time survival, 90 days/3 months for intermediate survival, and 6 months and above for long-term survival.

Previously ICU survival and hospital survival were the two most frequent reported survival outcomes and were also used in the development of our traditional scoring systems like APACHE and SAPS severity scores. But neither ICU stay nor hospital stay is a real-time variable and varies a lot in duration. In many countries hospital discharge can be difficult to reveal, since some ICU patients may be transferred to other hospitals before the final discharge home or elsewhere, and this may be difficult to find. Hence, this has been substituted with fixed time period reporting, often 30 days (short-term survival) and 3–6 months as intermediate-/long-term survival. This way to compare survival is obviously more robust, and cohorts are compared on equal terms. However, in particular post-hospital survival may be difficult for researchers to follow. In many countries with an easy access to a public people registry, where all births and deaths are registered, this information is easy to find. But such is not the case for most countries. For retrieving information about longer-term survival, one then has to use direct information from patients or caregivers, or information from primary care physicians, all more inconvenient to use, and hence compliance falls, and it is not often to get 100% of patients included in this follow-up.

24.5 Survival in Specific Cohorts

If one or more specific characteristics are connected to the cohort, this narrows the size, but increases the clinical use of survival analysis. Survival in patients ≥80 years admitted to an ICU is such an example. This cohort may then be further specified using subgroups like those admitted with sepsis [5]. Subgroups can also be specified using diagnostic codes. The problem then is that some groups will be very small since there are many relevant codes and may be impractical to use in comparisons. Another way to subdivide is to use admission categories. Both SAPS and APACHE severity scores use a simple three-item admission category with acute medical, acute surgical, and elective admissions. ◘ Table 24.1 reveals a more expanded admission group used in the VIP project. There is probably an overlap in how these categories are used, but the main principle for selection was to be specific (trauma, sepsis, surgery)

◘ **Table 24.1** Admission categories used in VIP1 and VIP2 studies [6]

Admission category	Explanation
Respiratory failure	Hypoxemic or hypercapnic ARF or combination
Circulatory failure	Any cause of circulatory failure/shock except sepsis
Respiratory and circulatory failure	Both signs of respiratory and circulatory failure found
Sepsis	According to sepsis 3 definition
Multitrauma without head injury	
Multitrauma with head injury	
Isolated head injury	
Non-trauma CNS cause	Other causes than trauma and intoxication
Intoxication	
Emergency surgery	Admission directly from the OT after acute surgery
Elective surgery	Planned admission after scheduled surgery
Other categories	

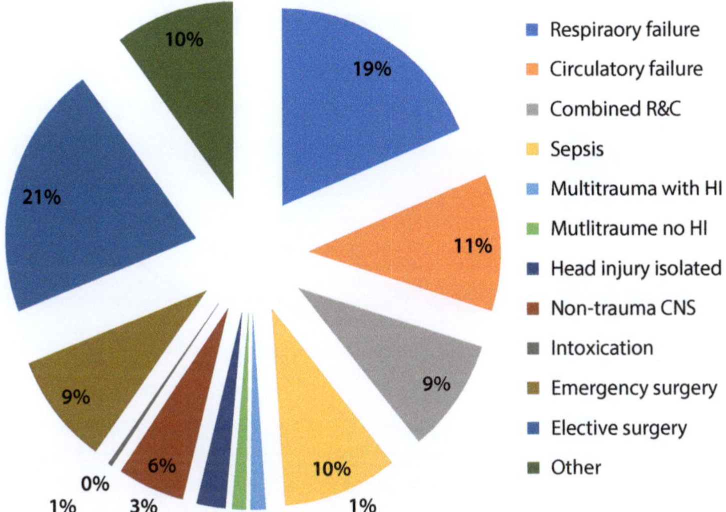

Fig. 24.1 Shows the distribution of admission categories for elderly ICU patients used in the VIP studies

if possible; if not use the first three categories even though other admissions could also qualify for respiratory and circulatory failure. As ◘ Fig. 24.1 reveals using this division makes it possible to divide patients into groups making comparisons easy, we also see there are two large (around 20%) groups – elective admission and respiratory failure – and four groups (around 10%): circulatory, combined respiratory and circulatory failure, sepsis, and emergency surgery.

The ◘ Fig. 24.1 shows the distribution of these categories in VIP1 study.

Obviously, combination of these ways to describe the cohort increases the understanding of survival as well as mortality, particularly in the very old intensive care patients. Knowledge of admission category can also be valuable in future prognostication.

In the further discussion of survival in very old intensive care patients, only experiences using survival put in a context will be included.

24.6   The Effect of Age

Some diverging reports have been found with regard to the effect of age in elderly ICU patients. It is well known that compared with young ICU patients (<65 years) the elderly group demonstrates an increased mortality. However, within a cohort of elderly patients, what are the effects of increasing age?

It seems to be a consistent finding that when studying a broader spectrum of elderly, like all above 65 years of age, and stratifying this group into smaller cohorts, there is still an influence of age. This has been demonstrated by Fuchs and coworkers [6]. In that retrospective study of 7265 emergency admitted ICU patients, they found significant differences in survival, most pronounced in post-hospital discharge and in the group >84 years (◘ Fig. 24.2).

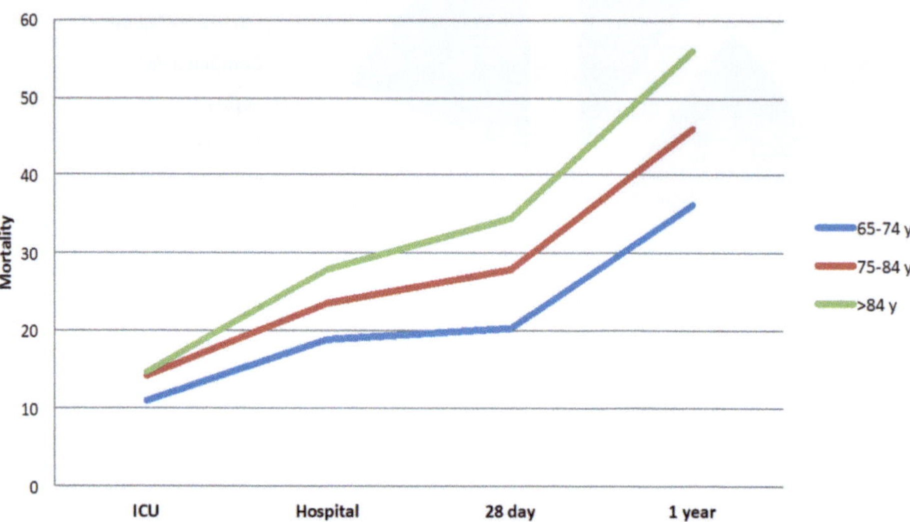

Fig. 24.2 Illustrates the develpment of mortality for three different age groups with time

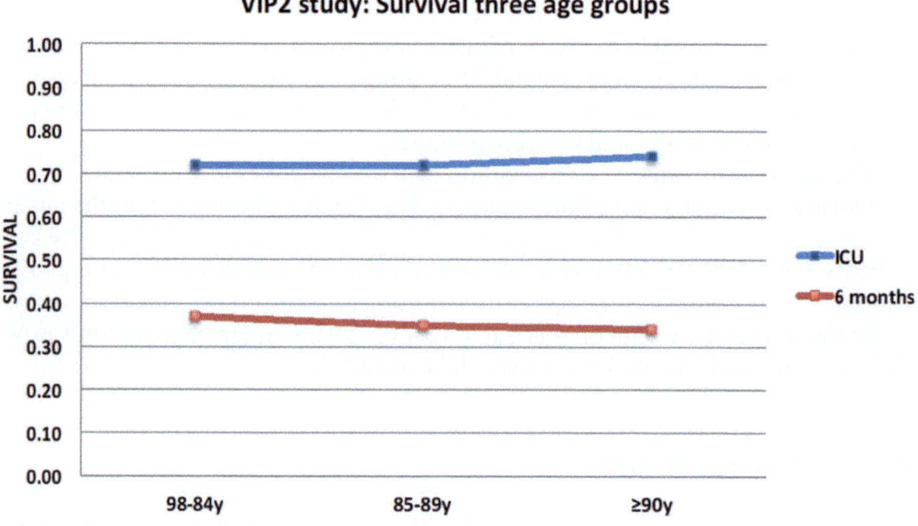

Fig. 24.3 Shows the ICU and 6 months mortality for three different age groups of very old ICU patients from the VIP studies

On the other hand, in a large prospective study of only acute ICU admissions including 3920 patients ≥80 years, there is a large difference in ICU versus 6 months survival going from 70% to 35% over 3 months [7]. However, no large differences could be found in the group 80–84 years compared with two older subgroups, although there is a small decrease in survival at 6 months in the two oldest subgroups (**Fig. 24.3**).

24.7 **The Effect of Gender**

There are not many studies of gender differences with regard to outcomes confined to the very old ICU patients. In general ICU patients, although only one third are females, there are usually no gender differences found with regard to survival [8]. In a recent study looking at gender differences in outcomes in a cohort of ICU patients ≥80 years, male sex was associated with increased 30-day mortality, but not ICU mortality [9].

24.8 **The Effect of Severity of Disease**

By tradition and experience, use of severity scores is the standard of care in intensive care, and the most frequently used scores are continuously improved by new versions. These scores are a mix of several sub-scores ranging from general patient specific items to values deviating from the normal in biochemistry or physiological measurements. To a certain degree, also items present pre-ICU are given weight like as they do in the SAPS-3 score.

Although not precise enough to warrant individual prognostications, most severity scores work well on group level, like in an ICU cohort from a single unit, often with an area under the receiver operating curve (AUROC) values around 0.7–0.8 which can be considered as acceptable but far from ideal [10].

All scores give extra points for increasing age, and age ≥80 years usually gives a high sub-score, often among the highest. The simplified acute physiology score (SAPS II) gives 18 points for age ≥80 years, only surpassed by GCS with 26 points for values <6. However, when analyzing the different age points given, most points are in fact given before the age of <70 (12 points) leaving only 6 points from 70 and onwards, so SAPS does not offer much extra points for being very old.

A problem worth mentioning is that we do in fact not know how many patients in the original publications of severity score that were very old, since such data are not easy to retrieve from the original publications, and mean age is around 60 years in most severity scores (see Table 2 in [11]).

Although not a severity score, organ failure score as the sequential organ failure assessment (SOFA) score may seem to be better suited to describe risk of dying in the ICU in the very old and has been found to be as good as traditional severity scores [12]. It has been used with frailty in order to improve mortality prediction with various success.

In a study specifically evaluating severity scores and their prediction in the elderly population, Minne et al. conducted a systematic review including seven studies with elderly cohorts [13]. They concluded: "none of them can be currently considered sufficiently credible or valid to be applicable in clinical practice for elderly patients." Only one study included additional information specific for the elderly population. This has led to a search for other factors than merely comorbidity and deranged physiology to be important prognostic factors. In particular frailty has been studied, mostly in smaller retrospective studies, but some large prospective studies are recently published. The so-called Very Old Intensive Care Patient (VIP) project within ESICM has focused on research in the very old intensive care patients ≥80 years. Also, a prognostic score was developed on the basis of VIP1 study data including frailty, and they found that an AUROC of 0.80 is better than traditional scores but still not good enough for individual use [14].

24.9 The Effect of Frailty

Frailty is described in more details in ▶ Chap. 12 and will just be mentioned briefly in the context of outcome.

It has been complicated to use crude age as selection criteria for medical treatment including intensive care and will today by many be considered ageism. The main reason that advanced age is associated with worse outcomes are probably better explained by other age-associated "syndromes," but these syndromes are far from confined to the elderly. Of interest here is comorbidity, cognitive decline, and sarcopenia, but frailty has probably attained most attention in the last 10 years since the ICU society was made aware of this phenomenon in 2011 [15]. There is a strong link between frailty and outcome, and in the very old several studies find frailty to outperform other factors in order to contribute to survival. In the VIP2 study where the interplay between age, frailty, cognition, comorbidity, and activity of daily life was investigated, frailty was found to be the best prognostic indicator [7] and had better discrimination in survival curves compared with the other geriatric syndromes. Recently frailty was found to be more important than age for survival in a group of ICU COVID-19 patients ≥70 years [16]. The effect of frailty in a general ICU population was recently described in retrospect from Alberta, Canada, in more the 15,000 ICU admissions (mean age 58 years) with assigned CFS. In their multivariate analysis, they found hospital mortality but not ICU mortality to be associated with increased CFS [17].

24.10 The Effect of Limitation of Care

It is not unusual in some multimorbid patients to withhold or even withdraw life-sustaining therapy (LST) after some time in the ICU. In a multinational study from Europe, this was overall found in more than one of four patients, most often as withholding LST (15%), but as many as 12% had treatment withdrawn [18]. There is a considerable variation within Europe with the northern parts more frequently using limitations of LST compared with eastern Europe particularly (◻ Table 24.2). Most usual are the decisions not to escalate treatment in patients where this is considered inappropriate, but also active withdrawing of ICU procedures occurs, like reducing vasoactive support or mechanical ventilation. Since such actions may influence the outcome and in particular ICU survival, this fraction is important to describe, also with separate outcome analysis. Without knowing the amount of this action, the mortality then can be claimed to be a self-fulfilling prophecy.

□ Table 24.2 The differences in end-of life care according to five European regions (from the VIP-1 study)

	Central	East	North	South	West	Test *p*-value
N	901	547	722	1702	1149	
Age, median (range) (IQR)	84 (range 80–99) (IQR 81-87)	83 (range 80–99) (IQR 81-86)	84 (range 80–98) (IQR 81-87)	84 (range 80–102) (IQR 82-86)	83 (range 80–99) (IQR 81-86)	0.001
Frailty	4 (range 1–9) (IQR 3-6)	5 (range 1–9) (IQR 4-6)	4 (range 1–9) (IQR 3-6)	4 (range 1–9) (IQR 3-6)	4 (range 1–9) (IQR 3-5)	<0.0001
Sofa score	6 (range 0–20) (IQR 3-9)	9 (range 0–24) (IQR 6-13)	7 (range 0–21) (IQR 4-9.75)	6 (range 0–22) (IQR 3-9)	8 (range 0–22) (IQR 4-11)	<0.0001
Frailty score						
Fit	286 (31.7%)	133 (24.3%)	241 (33.4%)	734 (43.1%)	499 (43.4%)	<0.0001
Vulnerable	174 (19.3%)	111 (20.3%)	131 (18.1%)	310 (18.2%)	246 (21.4%)	
Frail	441 (48.9%)	303 (55.4%)	350 (48.5%)	658 (38.7%)	404 (35.2%)	
Type of ICU admission						
Elective	241 (26.7%)	84 (15.4%)	40 (5.5%)	257 (15.1%)	284 (24.7%)	<0.0001
Acute	660 (73.3%)	463 (84.6%)	682 (94.5%)	1445 (84.9%)	865 (75.3%)	
Non invasive mechanical ventilation						
No	687 (76.2%)	466 (85.2%)	483 (66.9%)	1357 (79.7%)	879 (76.5%)	<0.0001
Yes	214 (23.8%)	81 (14.8%)	239 (33.1%)	345 (20.3%)	270 (23.5%)	
Invasive mechanical ventilation						
No	521 (57.8%)	108 (19.7%)	458 (63.4%)	679 (39.9%)	735 (64%)	<0.0001

(continued)

Table 24.2 (continued)

	Central	East	North	South	West	Test _p_-value
Yes	380 (42.2%)	439 (80.3%)	264 (36.6%)	1023 (60.1%)	414 (36%)	
Vasoactive drugs						
No	422 (46.8%)	157 (28.7%)	321 (44.5%)	969 (56.9%)	539 (46.9%)	<0.0001
Yes	479 (53.2%)	390 (71.3%)	401 (55.5%)	733 (43.1%)	610 (53.1%)	
Renal replacement therapy						
No	814 (90.3%)	452 (82.6%)	690 (95.6%)	1570 (92.2%)	1033 (89.9%)	<0.0001
Yes	87 (9.7%)	95 (17.4%)	32 (4.4%)	132 (7.8%)	116 (10.1%)	
None	580 (64.4%)	477 (87.2%)	396 (54.8%)	1268 (74.5%)	935 (81.4%)	<0.0001
withholding or withdrawing	321 (35.6%)	70 (12.8%)	326 (45.2%)	434 (25.5%)	214 (18.6%)	
None	580 (64.4%)	477 (87.2%)	396 (54.8%)	1268 (74.5%)	935 (81.4%)	<0.0001
Withholding alone	190 (21.1%)	40 (7.3%)	199 (27.6%)	218 (12.8%)	106 (9.2%)	
Withdrawing +/- withholding	131 (14.5%)	30 (5.5%)	127 (17.6%)	216 (12.7%)	108 (9.4%)	

24.11 What Is the Reported Mortality of Elderly ICU Patients?

As discussed above many important factors influence the reported mortality data; hence, comparison between studies is frequently impossible. A recent systematic review reveals that some of this diversity also is affected by study design [19]. In retrospective single-center studies, which also tend to be small, the reported ICU mortality varies from nearly 0 to 50%, while the larger (>1000 patients) prospective multicenter studies find a variation from 10 to 28%. According to this review, a substantial number of studies are very small, with <200 patients included in 25/45 studies among the single-center cohort.

24.12 The Future of Reporting Mortality

It is tempting to claim that since so many factors may influence mortality in the very old, it is important to use a checklist in order to include at least the most important confounding factors as per the following list:

> **Box**
> - Type of ICU admission: at least report outcomes seletcively in planned versus emergency admissions.
> - Age of the patients (mean and median): if age is ≥65 years, report results from the subgroup ≥80 years.
> - Frailty status, at least as frail-borderline-not frail.
> - Report organ dysfunctions at admission using a validated score.
> - Report mortality at fixed time after ICU discharge: 30 days-3 months-6 months.
> - Report the number of patients where limitation of life-sustaining therapy was decided, and apply this in multivariate analysis.

> **Take-Home Messages**
> - Mortality in the very old patients is much higher than that of its younger counterparts.
> - Usually, we can assume an ICU mortality of 25–30%, 30-day mortality around 40%, and 1-year mortality from 50 to 60%, but the numbers vary according to study design.
> - ICU mortality is first and foremost influenced by the type of ICU admission, planned or unplanned (acute), with mortality rates nearly four- to fivefold in acutely admitted patients.
> - Frailty seems to be a better predictor of death than crude age itself.
> - Obviously, a decision to forgo life-sustaining therapy like mechanical ventilation has a huge impact on survival.

References

1. Campion EW, Mulley AG, Goldstein RL, Barnett GO, Thibault GE. Medical intensive care for the elderly. A study of current use, costs, and outcomes. JAMA. 1981;246(18):2052–6.
2. Flaatten H, de Lange DW, Morandi A, et al. The impact of frailty on ICU and 30-day mortality and the level of care in very elderly patients (≥ 80 years). Intensive Care Med. 2017;43(12):1820–8.
3. Cohen IL, Lambrinos J, Fein IA. Mechanical ventilation for the elderly patient in intensive care. Incremental changes and benefits. JAMA. 1993;269(8):1025–9.
4. Jung C, Wernly B, Muessig JM, et al. A comparison of very old patients admitted to intensive care unit after acute versus elective surgery or intervention. J Crit Care. 2019;52:141–8.
5. Ibarz M, Boumendil A, Haas LEM, et al. Sepsis at ICU admission does not decrease 30-day survival in very old patients: a post-hoc analysis of the VIP1 multinational cohort study. Ann Intensive Care. 2020;10(1):56.

6. Fuchs L, Chronaki CE, Park S, et al. ICU admission characteristics and mortality rates among elderly and very elderly patients. Intensive Care Med. 2012;38(10):1654–61.
7. Guidet B, de Lange DW, Boumendil A, et al. The contribution of frailty, cognition, activity of daily life and comorbidities on outcome in acutely admitted patients over 80 years in European ICUs: the VIP2 study. Intensive Care Med. 2020;46(1):57-69. Hollinger A, Gayat E, Féliot E, et al. Gender and survival of critically ill patients: results from the FROG-ICU study. Ann Intensive Care. 2019;9(1):1–8.
8. Hollinger A, Gayat E, Féliot E, et al. Gender and survival of critically ill patients: results from the FROG-ICU study. Ann Intensive Care. 2019;9(1):1–8.
9. Wernly B, Bruno RR, Kelm M, et al. Sex-specific outcome disparities in very old patients admitted to intensive care medicine: a propensity matched analysis. Sci Rep. 2020;10(1):18671–9.
10. Moseson EM, Zhuo H, Chu J, et al. Intensive care unit scoring systems outperform emergency department scoring systems for mortality prediction in critically ill patients: a prospective cohort study. J Intensive Care. 2014;2(1):40–10.
11. Flaatten H, Lange DW, Artigas A, et al. The status of intensive care medicine research and a future agenda for very old patients in the ICU. Intensive Care Med. 2017;43(9):1–10.
12. Minne L, Abu-Hanna A, de Jonge E. Evaluation of SOFA-based models for predicting mortality in the ICU: a systematic review. Crit Care. 2008;12(6):R161. https://doi.org/10.1186/cc7160. Epub 2008 Dec 17
13. Minne L, Ludikhuize J, de Jonge E, de Rooij S, Abu-Hanna A. Prognostic models for predicting mortality in elderly ICU patients: a systematic review. Intensive Care Med. 2011;37(8):1258–68.
14. de Lange DW, Brinkman S, Flaatten H, et al. Cumulative prognostic score predicting mortality in patients older than 80 years admitted to the ICU. J Am Geriatr Soc. 2019;67:1263.
15. McDermid RC, Stelfox HT, Bagshaw SM Frailty in the critically ill: a novel concept. Crit Care (London, England) 2011;15:301.
16. Jung C. et al. The impact of frailty on survival in elderly intensive care patients with COVID-19: the COVIP study. Crit Care (London, England) 2021;25:149.
17. Montgomery CL, Zuege DJ, Rolfson DB, et al. Implementation of population-level screening for frailty among patients admitted to adult intensive care in Alberta, Canada. Can J Anaesth. 2019;66(11):1310–9.
18. Guidet B, Flaatten H, Boumendil A, et al. Withholding or withdrawing of life-sustaining therapy in older adults ($\geq$80 years) admitted to the intensive care unit. Intensive Care Med. 2018;43(1–11):1–12.
19. Vallet H, Schwarz GL, Flaatten H, de Lange DW, Guidet B, Dechartres A. Mortality of older patients admitted to an ICU: a systematic review. Crit Care Med. 2021;49(2):324–34.

Outcomes After Intensive Care: Functional Status

Sten M. Walther

Contents

> **Learning Objectives**
>
> In this chapter we will first describe functional status by applying models well known to other medical disciplines but not commonly used to understand functional outcome after critical illness in the very old. We will then discuss instruments to capture functional status, particularly in old and very old people, and finally summarise important contributions of functional outcome after critical illness as reported in the literature.

25.1 Introduction

Current accounts of patients' outcome after critical illness must look beyond saving lives to saving years with good functional status and perceived health. Functional status and health-related quality of life (HRQOL) have become fundamental endpoints of intensive care. The underlying assumption is that understanding relationships between functional status and HRQOL will inform and improve clinical care, rehabilitation and ultimately patient-centred outcomes. Ideally, every outcome should be evaluated with emphasis on capturing the patient's voice of her health and well-being.

Functional status is a wide-ranging concept that refers not only to physical function but also to cognitive, psychological and social functioning. While the relationship between functional status and perceived HRQOL may be multidirectional and complex, decline in functional status is the final common pathway of many chronic conditions and is an important foreshadow of poor HRQOL. Functioning decline in the elderly is highly predictive of loss of functional autonomy and mortality.

25.2 Framing Functional Status

Functional status and disability can best be understood and described by using the theoretical framework presented in the International Classification of Functioning, Disability and Health (ICF) published by the World Health Organization (WHO) in 2001 [1]. The ICF belongs to the family of international classifications with the aim to provide a unified framework and standard language for the description of health and health-related states. While the more familiar International Statistical Classification of Diseases and Related Health Problems (ICD) describes diseases, disorders and other health conditions, ICF enriches that description by classifying functioning and disability associated with health conditions. Together, information on diagnosis and functioning provide a fuller picture to describe patients' needs, develop interventions and prescribe appropriate rehabilitation care.

In order to integrate various perspectives of functioning, the ICF manual applies a bio-psycho-social model, advocated in a classical essay by George Engel [2]. This model considers not only the body-focused biological components of health but also the individual and societal contexts of patients' experience of health. The ICF contains six components of health linked by bidirectional relations, as illustrated in Fig. 25.1. There is a complex, dynamic and often unpredictable relationship among these components. To make simple linear inferences from one entity to another is incorrect, e.g. to infer overall disability from a diagnosis, activity limita-

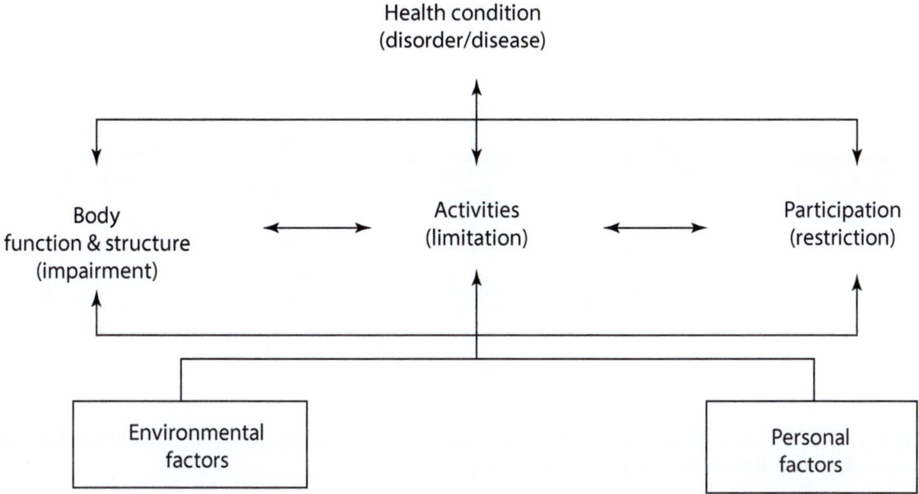

Fig. 25.1 Graphic representation of the six interactive components of the ICF. **Body functions** are physiological functions. **Body structures** refer to anatomical parts of the body. Diseases, illnesses and injuries cause **impairments** in body structures and functions. **Activities** are the execution of tasks or actions, and **activity limitations** are difficulties an individual encounter while performing tasks or actions. **Participation** is involvement in life situations, and **participation restrictions** are problems an individual faces when participating in life situations. The ICF also identifies contextual factors as components of a person's health. **Environmental factors** include the physical, social and attitudinal environment in which an individual lives and conducts his or her life. **Personal factors** include an individual's age, gender, coping style, education and work experience. Both environmental and personal factors can be either barriers or facilitators to participation in daily life

tions from one or more impairments or a participation restriction from one or more limitations.

The etiologically neutral framework of ICF provides a conceptual basis and standard language for description of health and health-related states. The hierarchical and high-resolution structure with roughly 1500 categories, each with one or more qualifier which denotes the presence and severity of the problem, supports a detailed analysis of functional status. This structure has been applied in various settings, including analysis of functional status and services provided to elderly people. However, one main challenge is the large number of domains, categories and qualifiers which, to be clinically helpful, need to be condensed to a more practical volume. For that purpose, a large number of ICF core sets have been developed to correspond to the needs of specific patient populations [3]. An early development of that kind was a comprehensive post-acute ICF core set for geriatric patients with 123 categories [4], which was reduced further to 39 and then to 29 categories in brief ICF core sets for geriatrics [5, 6] (▶ Box 25.1).

The resulting ICF profiles are impartial representations of functioning and health. They are not the patient's perception of health but still include factors of importance to the individual. The natural next step is to link the ICF taxonomy with a subjective person-centred perspective on health and well-being. The importance of person-centred assessments has been demonstrated repeatedly by showing that external observers are inaccurate judges of patients' perceived quality of life [7]. Self-rated HRQOL is about what patients feel about their state of health or its consequences.

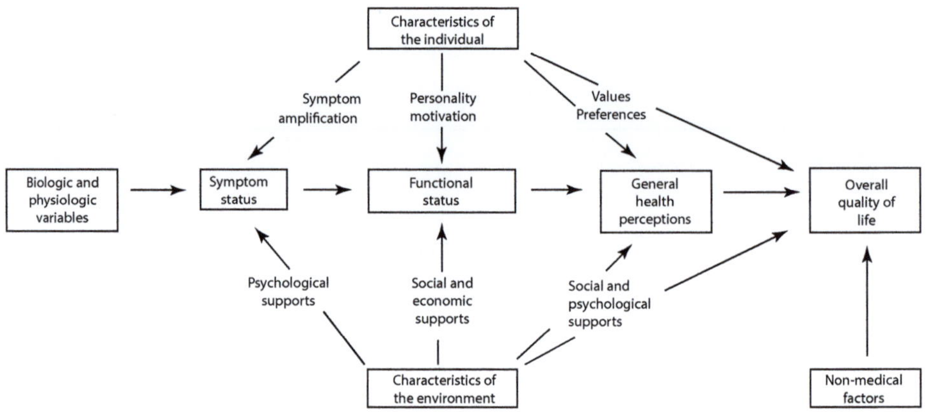

⬛ Fig. 25.2 Relationships among measures of patient outcome in a health-related quality of life conceptual model. (Reprinted with permission from [8])

A framework linking the traditional biomedical disease paradigm to HRQOL was proposed by Wilson and Cleary in the 1990s [8]. They identified the need to combine the breadth and relevance of the patient-centred HRQOL construct with the causal and mechanistic biomedical paradigm, providing conceptual links between specific clinical activities or processes and health outcomes that patients value. The Wilson-Cleary model focuses on five levels of patient outcomes, i.e. biologic and physiologic variables, symptoms, functioning, general health perceptions and overall quality of life. Extensions of the model propose mediating bidirectional relationships among these variables in addition to explanatory roles of several personal and environmental variables (⬛ Fig. 25.2). The relevance of this model has been shown in a variety of circumstances and patient populations, and its application to improve our understanding of outcomes after critical illness has also been suggested [9].

While the Wilson-Cleary model bridges the biomedical model of patient outcomes to the subjective patient-centred HRQOL construct, the systematic ICF model provides a common language to objectively describe impairments, limitations and restrictions. Together both models advance the understanding of how illness and disability constructions are causally linked to subjective health status outcomes.

> **Box 25.1   Brief Geriatric ICF Core Set with 29 Categories that Reflect the Most Relevant Health-Related Problems of Community-Living Older Adults Without Dementia**
>
> ICF category
>   Body functions
>   b144 Memory functions
>   b152 Emotional functions
>   b210 Seeing functions
>   b230 Hearing functions
>   b240 Sensations associated with hearing and vestibular function
>   b410 Heart functions
>   b420 Blood pressure functions

> b455 Exercise tolerance functions
> b525 Defecation functions
> b530 Weight maintenance functions
> b620 Urination functions
> b710 Mobility of joint functions
> b730 Muscle power functions
> b810 Protective functions of the skin
>
> Activities and participation
> d410 Changing basic body position
> d450 Walking
> d470 Using transportation
> d510 Washing oneself
> d520 Caring for body parts
> d530 Toileting
> d540 Dressing
> d550 Eating
> d560 Drinking
> d760 Family relationships
>
> Environmental factors
> e310 Immediate family
> e320 Friends
> e325 Acquaintances, peers, colleagues, neighbours and community members
> e570 Social security services, systems and policies
> e575 General social support services, systems and policies
> e580 Health services, systems and policies
>
> Reprinted with permission from [6]
>
> Each ICF code must be followed by a qualifier which specifies information about functioning status (i.e. magnitude of any problem: 0 no problem, 1 mild, 2 moderate, 3 severe, 4 complete, 8 not specified, 9 not applicable)

25.3 Instruments and Measures

Stimulated by the need to evaluate functioning in a standardised manner, clinicians and epidemiologists have developed a large array of measures to capture different domains of functional outcomes. The increasing acceptance of ICF as the universal language and framework to describe and classify functioning, health and disability has been instrumental for the development of objective measures of functional status. The ability of ICF to precisely describe the entire breadth of functional status of an individual, at a given time and at varying levels of resolution, opens the possibility to use the profile as a tool to track changes in the evolution of health and disability. An early proof of concept was shown by integrating clinical ratings of relevant ICF categories using the ICF qualifier in the development of instruments to capture musculoskeletal disabilities [10]. This was found to be a helpful approach and was followed by a number of initiatives based on relevant ICF core sets across medical disciplines (i.e. rheumatology, oncology, pulmonary medicine, rehabilitation medicine), specific patient populations (i.e. geriatrics [11], patients with cardiorespiratory diseases), settings (i.e. post-acute hospital care, community) and cultures. While not without problems [12], this approach provides a context-specific cross-cultural broad description of functional status.

A slightly different method was to link commonly employed tools for assessment of functional status to the ICF taxonomy. The ICF-linking rules [13] are an established method to identify the key concepts contained in any source of information, such as a data collection tool, and link it to the corresponding ICF category. An illustrative example was developed to evaluate activities of daily living in old people with a range of disability from healthy to Alzheimer's disease. The Katz index and Lawton scale were linked to ICF categories providing a detailed scoring system based on the ICF qualifiers resulting in an instrument with greater accuracy and discrimination than its progenitors [14].

In the same vein and more related to intensive care medicine, effective mapping of physical functioning outcome instruments to ICF subdomains was described [15]. While not primarily aimed to result in a composite instrument designed for the critically ill, it nevertheless demonstrated the utility of the ICF framework and common language as a scaffold in which clinicians can arrange and use outcome measures appropriate for different stages in the disease trajectory after critical illness.

25.4 Measuring Functional Status in the Old and Critically Ill

In old patients with chronic conditions the problems arising from focusing on single diseases (one at a time) were addressed many years back by the development of measures of functional status aimed to reflect the overall health of an individual [16, 17]. One of the ideas of these early measures of activities of daily living (ADL) was that they offered a means of making quantitative assessments of the overall effects of illness and treatment. This is supported by work showing that a broad set of components and categories of the ICF framework contribute to ADL [18]. However, a variety of instruments are currently used for assessment of functional status in geriatric patients with little agreement on the best set of tools [19–21]. Most commonly used instruments focus on basic and instrumental ADL and mobility, with few covering other functioning domains [20]. Furthermore, the original contents of instruments are used rarely, and score limits employed to identify functional decline vary, stressing a strong need for standardisation.

Critical care displays a similar proliferation of functional status outcome measures as geriatric medicine. A large array of diverse instruments applied to the critically ill was identified in a comprehensive review of studies published between 1970 and 1998 [22], with no apparent improvement when reviewed almost two decades later [23]. In addition to the large heterogeneity of instruments, there was a lack of information about measurement properties, which also did not improve over time [24]. For intensive care outcomes, a limited set of instruments was suggested early as remedy and to enable the building of a body of experience and knowledge around a few instruments and a core outcome set. While some evidence of consolidation around key instruments followed [23], there seems to be little agreement on which best to use. The absence of a formal needs' assessment in the field of intensive care outcomes research and the inexperience among caregivers and researchers on existing tools may have contributed to this lack of consensus.

In order to advance the state of affairs, it is obvious that agreement must be established about instruments to measure functional status in the old and critically ill. Progress in this field is impeded when we are unable to compare results across studies. The development of core outcome sets (COS) and core outcome measurement sets (COMS) is a systematic approach that may help resolve the confusion caused by heterogeneity in outcome measurements and instruments [25]. A large number of COS and corresponding COMS have been developed, primarily focusing on single diseases and conditions but none generic to geriatrics or intensive care medicine [26–28]. Reaching consensus on instruments and metrics in the elderly with multiple comorbidities may be particularly difficult, although feasible, as shown by published work on a standard set of health outcome measures for older persons [29].

Administrative data collected for other purposes may also provide important information of functional status. In the USA, information from the Outcome and Assessment Information Set (OASIS), which is a standardised assessment of physical, cognitive and mental health status, has been used to examine functional disability also after critical illness in the old [30].

Yet another way to capture the breadth of functional status is the Comprehensive Geriatric Assessment (CGA). This combines clinical evaluation and instruments to measure functional status, although there is currently no clear consensus about the contents. Several different CGA approaches have been developed; these are discussed in Chap. 14.

25.5 Functional Status in the Old After Intensive Care

Some past, but also current, studies which claim to examine functional status after intensive care have an overly simplistic definition and apply measures and instruments unable to capture the breadth of functioning [31, 32]. The label 'functional status' is occasionally used to refer to physical functioning only, although, as outlined in the ICF framework, it also encompasses cognitive, mental health, social and emotional functioning/well-being. Despite limitations with lack of conceptual framework to organise and capture relevant ICU outcomes with ensuant heterogeneity of measurements and instruments, there is important information in prior studies of ICU patients. Let us first consider research that captures a wide range of functioning measures and then turn to a few reports with more limited measurements. Studies on the cognitive aspects of functioning will not be considered since these are discussed in Chap. 14.

Many significant contributions to knowledge about functional status and disability trajectories in the old and very old have come from the Precipitating Events Project (the PEP Study). The PEP Study was established in 1998 to evaluate the epidemiology of disability in older persons and to elucidate the role of intervening illnesses and injuries (events) on the disabling process. Nondisabled persons, 70 years or older, living in greater New Haven on the American east-coast, were enrolled and followed with a comprehensive home-based assessment at 18-month intervals and monthly telephone interviews until death or dropout [33]. The comprehensive home-based assessments provided high-quality data on a core set of aging-relevant factors from multiple domains. The monthly assessments of functional status included 13 activities. Participants were asked about both difficulty and dependence (on another person) to complete each of the four basic activities (bathing, dressing, walking and transferring), five instrumental activities (shopping, housework, meal preparation, taking medications and managing finances) and four mobility activities (walking a quarter mile, climbing flight of stairs, lifting/carrying 10 pounds and driving).

Roughly 55% of those enrolled had at least one ICU admission through 2017, and their functional outcomes have been reported at the mean age of about 83 years in a series of detailed studies [34–39]. Many important findings from this rich data deserve to be highlighted, of which just a few will be listed here. First, more than 50% of the participants experienced functional decline or early death during the first year after ICU admission, underscoring the risks and complexity of ICU survivorship in this population. Second, among early survivors a majority showed some degree of recovery beginning at about 3 months after the ICU episode. Third, early survivors could be grouped into three distinct functional trajectories: a majority (51%) were severely disabled, while mild-to-moderate and minimal disability appeared in 28% and 21%, respectively. Fourth, a diverse set of potential targets for interventions to improve functional outcomes were identified. There was a strong independent association between the pre-ICU functional trajectories and functional outcome and death (◘ Fig. 25.3). Hearing and vision impairment and functional self-efficacy were also independent predictors of functional recovery. Precipitating events (illnesses/injuries) were common in the year after ICU admission, and these events were associated with a greater likelihood of subsequent functional decline than many traditional risk factors.

Additional valuable data about post-ICU functional status and recovery comes from the Canadian Critical Care Trials Group and the Canadian Researchers at the End of Life Network. These researchers enrolled critically ill patients aged

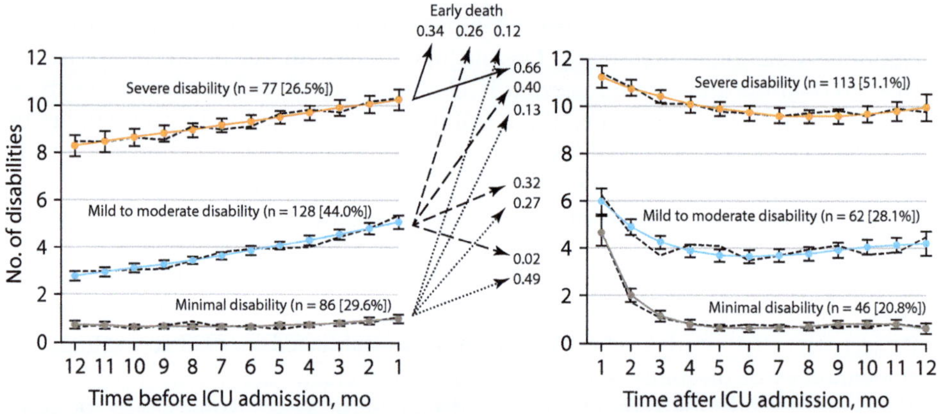

◘ **Fig. 25.3** Functional trajectories among older persons in the year before and after critical illness. Arrows and numbers indicate adjusted probabilities of transitioning from pre-ICU trajectories to early death (within 30 days of hospital admission) and post-ICU trajectories. The numbers of disabilities are expressed as least squares means (95% CIs); the possible number ranged from 0 to 13. (Modified from [34], published with permission)

80 years or older who spent at least 24 h in ICU from 2009 to 2013 [40, 41]. Functional status after hospitalisation was assessed 3, 6, 9 and 12 months after enrolment using the physical function domain and the summary physical component score of the Short Form 36 protocol in addition to the Palliative Performance Scale (PPS) version 2. About 33% of the patients died before hospital discharge, and 50% had died 1 year after ICU admission. At 1 year, only 26% had recovered back to, or near, their pre-hospital physical functioning. An extensive set of information was collected to reflect the patient's condition 2 weeks prior to hospitalisation. This data, which included variables related to both baseline function and acute illness, was used to build models to predict poor functional outcome. Measures related to the acute illness, chronic conditions and baseline health status (frailty, physical functioning and PPS score) were key determinants of functional status at 1 year.

Proportions and magnitude of disability among elderly ICU survivors have been reported with various durations and frequencies of follow-up from many other settings and circumstances [42–47]. Most show results at 1 year comparable to the PEP and Canadian network studies with about 50% survival. Roughly 25–30% of the studied populations recovered to functioning baseline at 1 year, and a significant proportion were considered to have good functional status at 2 years [43]. Not surprisingly, functional decline after critical illness was associated with worse quality of life and correlated with assessments of functional status before the ICU hospitalisation.

The findings indicate that assessment of baseline functional status could aid in prognostication and informed decision-making for very old critically ill patients. A logical consequence would be to start systematic collection and use of functioning measurements in all older patients who are admitted to ICU. This kind of systematic collection of functional status, though limited in extent, has been part of the basic dataset applied to patients older than 80 years in the Finnish Intensive Care Consortium since 2012. The combination of independence in ADL and ability to climb stairs was found to be a useful indicator of physiological reserves and ability to recover from critical illness in a large cohort of very old patients admitted to ICUs that were members of the Finnish consortium [48].

Few studies capture the entire breadth of functional status as pointed out earlier. Still, a couple of conclusions can be made though there is a lack of uniformity in instruments and inconsistent reporting of data that limit comparison of findings across studies. In general, when critically ill patients, 75 years or older, are admitted to ICU, about 30% of them die in hospital or within 30 days. A further 20% die within 1 year of ICU admission, with an overall 1-year survival of 50%. At 1 year roughly half of the survivors show complete or some degree of recovery of functional status. Many factors obvious for those familiar with intensive care may modify these numbers. The diagnosis leading to ICU admission, severity of illness on admission and duration of mechanical ventilation are some examples. The influence of other factors, i.e. impairment in hearing and vision, functional self-efficacy and frailty, have lately become apparent to clinicians. The influence of additional infrequently studied but possibly important factors, i.e. socio-economic status [49], remains to be determined.

25

> **Practical Implications**
>
> Lack of conceptual basis and generally accepted instruments to measure functional status in the old critically ill is a barrier to knowledge discovery and leads to preventable research waste.
>
> The International Classification of Functioning, Disability and Health provides a useful framework for understanding and describing functioning and disability.
>
> Systematic development of a core outcome set (an agreed, standardised collection of outcomes measured and reported in all trials) for the old and critically ill is a necessary way forward to identify and describe disability after critical illness in the elderly.
>
> Proper description of disability is essential for rehabilitation tailored to the patient's need. Functional status after critical illness in the old patient must be evaluated using standardised and widely accepted instruments that capture the entire breadth of functioning.

Conclusion

The ultimate goal in the old critically ill patient must be to maintain or improve functioning to achieve good perceived HRQOL, unless a shared decision to transit to palliative care exists. Functioning outcomes provide the linkage between the biomedical disease paradigm and the patient-centred HRQOL construct. The ICF classification provides a helpful framework so that we can understand, discuss and measure impairments, limitations and restrictions.

Inconsistencies in selection of functioning outcomes and metrics are important impediments to progress. Steps must be taken to reach consensus on a generic, multidimensional set of instruments that cover relevant domains of functional status in the old critically ill patient.

During the first year after critical illness, about one quarter of old patients who are admitted to ICU recover functioning completely or to some degree, one quarter encounter functional decline and two quarters decease. Prognostic factors represent potential targets for interventions to mitigate or prevent functional decline and death during or after critical illness.

Take-Home Messages

- Functional status provides a link between the biomedical disease paradigm and the patient-centred health-related quality of life construct.
- The International Classification of Functioning, Disability and Health offers a helpful framework so that we can measure, describe and discuss functioning impairments, limitations and restrictions.

References

1. World Health Organization. International classification of functioning, disability and health: ICF [Internet]. Geneva: WHO; 2001. Available from: https://www.who.int/standards/classifications/international-classification-of-functioning-disability-and-health.
2. Engel GL. The need for a new medical model: a challenge for biomedicine. Science. 1977;196(4286):129–36.

3. ICF Research Branch. Creation of an ICF-based documentation form [Internet]. Nottwil: ICF Research Branch; 2021. Available from: https://www.icf-core-sets.org/en/page0.php.

4. Grill E, Hermes R, Swoboda W, Uzarewicz C, Kostanjsek N, Stucki G. ICF Core Set for geriatric patients in early post-acute rehabilitation facilities. Disabil Rehabil. 2005;27(7/8):411–7.

5. Grill E, Müller M, Quittan M, Strobl R, Kostanjsek N, Stucki G. Brief ICF Core Set for patients in geriatric post-acute rehabilitation facilities. J Rehabil Med. 2011;43:139–44.

6. Spoorenberg SLW, Reijneveld SA, Middel B, Uittenbroek RJ, Kremer HPH, Wynia K. The Geriatric ICF Core Set reflecting health-related problems in community-living older adults aged 75 years and older without dementia: development and validation. Disabil Rehabil. 2015;37(25):2337–43. https://doi.org/10.3109/09638288.2015.1024337.

7. Albrecht GL, Devlieger PJ. The disability paradox: high quality of life against all odds. Soc Sci Med. 1999;48(8):977–88.

8. Wilson IB, Clearly PD. Linking clinical variables with health-related quality of life: a conceptual model of patient outcomes. JAMA. 1995;273:59–65.

9. Brummel NE. Measuring outcomes after critical illness. Crit Care Clin. 2018;34(4):515–26. https://doi.org/10.1016/j.ccc.2018.06.003.

10. Grill E, Stucki G. Scales could be developed based on simple clinical ratings of International Classification of Functioning, Disability and Health Core Set categories. J Clin Epidemiol. 2009;62:891–8.

11. de Vriendt P, Lambert M, Mets T. Integrating the International Classification of Functioning, Disability and Health (ICF) in the Geriatric Minimum Data Set-25 (GMDS-25) for intervention studies in older people. J Nutr Health Aging. 2009;13(2):128–34. https://doi.org/10.1007/s12603-009-0019-8.

12. Allguren B, Bostan C, Christensson L, Fridlund B, Cieza A. A multidisciplinary cross-cultural measurement of functioning after stroke: Rasch analysis of the Brief ICF Core Set for Stroke. Top Stroke Rehabil. 2011;18(Suppl 1):573–86.

13. Prodinger B, Tennant A, Stucki G. Standardized reporting of functioning information on ICF-based common metrics. Eur J Phys Rehabil Med. 2018;54:110–7. https://doi.org/10.23736/S1973-9087.17.04784-0.

14. Cornelis E, Gorus E, Beyer I, Bautmans I, De Vriendt P. Early diagnosis of mild cognitive impairment and mild dementia through basic and instrumental activities of daily living: development of a new evaluation tool. PLoS Med. 2017;14(3):e1002250. https://doi.org/10.1371/journal.pmed.1002250.

15. Parry SM, Huang M, Needham DM. Evaluating physical functioning in critical care: considerations for clinical practice and research. Crit Care. 2017;21:249. https://doi.org/10.1186/s13054-017-1827-6.

16. Katz S, Ford AB, Moskowitz RW, Jackson BA, Jaffe MW. Studies of illness in the aged. The index of ADL: a standardized measure of biological and psychological function. JAMA. 1963;185:914–9.

17. Mahoney FI, Barthel DW. Functional evaluation: the Barthel index. Md State Med J. 1965;14:61–5.

18. den Ouden ME, Schuurmans MJ, Mueller-Schotte S, Brand JS, van der Schouw YT. Domains contributing to disability in activities of daily living. J Am Med Dir Assoc. 2013;14(1):18–24. https://doi.org/10.1016/j.jamda.2012.08.014.

19. Demers L, Desrosiers J, Ska B, Wolfson N, Nikolova R, Pervieux I, et al. Assembling a toolkit to measure geriatric rehabilitation outcomes. Am J Phys Med Rehabil. 2005;84:460–72.

20. Buurman BM, van Munster BC, Korevaar JC, de Haan RJ, de Rooij SE. Variability in measuring (instrumental) activities of daily living functioning and functional decline in hospitalized older medical patients: a systematic review. J Clin Epidemiol. 2011;64(6):619–27. https://doi.org/10.1016/j.jclinepi.2010.07.005.

21. Wildiers H, Heeren P, Puts M, Topinkova E, Janssen-Heijnen MLG, Extermann M, et al. International Society of Geriatric Oncology consensus on geriatric assessment in older patients with cancer. J Clin Oncol. 2014;32(24):2595–603. https://doi.org/10.1200/JCO.2013.54.8347.

22. Hayes JA, Black NA, Jenkinson C, Young JD, Rowan KM, Daly K, et al. Outcome measures for adult critical care: a systematic review. Health Technol Assess. 2000;4:1e111.

23. Turnbull AE, Rabiee A, Davis WE, Nasser MF, Venna VR, Lolitha R, et al. Outcome measurement in ICU survivorship research from 1970 to 2013: a scoping review of 425 publications. Crit Care Med. 2016;44(7):1267–77.

24. Robinson KA, Davis WE, Dinglas VD, Mendez-Tellez PA, Rabiee A, Sukrithan V, et al. A systematic review finds limited data on measurement properties of instruments measuring outcomes in adult intensive care unit survivors. J Clin Epidemiol. 2017;82:37–46. https://doi.org/10.1016/j.jclinepi.2016.08.014.

25. Blackwood B, Marshall J, Rose L. Progress on core outcome sets for critical care research. Curr Opin Crit Care. 2015;21:439e44.

26. Dinglas VD, Cherukin SPS, Needham DM. Core outcomes sets for studies evaluating critical illness and patient recovery. Curr Opin Crit Care. 2020;26:489–99. https://doi.org/10.1097/MCC.0000000000000750.

27. The COMET initiative. Core outcome measures in effectiveness trials [Internet]. Liverpool: COMET; 2021. Available from: https://www.comet-initiative.org/.

28. Improving Long-Term Outcomes Research for Acute Respiratory Failure. Core outcome measurement set (COMS) [Internet]. US: Baltimore; 2021. https://www.improvelto.com/coms/.

29. Akpan A, Roberts C, Bandeen-Roche K, Batty B, Bausewein C, Bell D, et al. Standard set of health outcome measures for older persons. BMC Geriatr. 2018;18(1):36. https://doi.org/10.1186/s12877-017-0701-3.

30. Riegel B, Huang L, Mikkelsen ME, Kutney-Lee A, Hanlon AL, Murtaugh CM, et al. Early Post-Intensive Care Syndrome among older adult sepsis survivors receiving home care. J Am Geriatr Soc. 2019;67(3):520–6. https://doi.org/10.1111/jgs.15691.

31. Mahul P, Perrot D, Tempelhoff G, Gaussorgues P, Jospe R, Ducreux JC, et al. Short- and long-term prognosis, functional outcome following ICU for elderly. Intensive Care Med. 1991;17:7–10.

32. Ingraham NE, Vakayil V, Pendleton KM, Robbins AJ, Freese RL, Northrop EF, et al. National trends and variation of functional status deterioration in the medically critically ill. Crit Care Med. 2020;48(11):1556–64. https://doi.org/10.1097/CCM.0000000000004524.

33. Gill TM, Han L, Gahbauer EA, Leo-Summers L, Murphy TE. Cohort profile: the Precepitating Events Project (PEP Study). J Nutr Health Aging. 2020;24(4):438–44.

34. Ferrante LE, Pisani MA, Murphy TE, Gahbauer EA, Leo-Summers LS, Gill TM. Functional trajectories among older persons before and after critical illness. JAMA Intern Med. 2015;175(4):523–9. https://doi.org/10.1001/jamainternmed.2014.7889.

35. Ferrante LE, Pisani MA, Murphy TE, Gahbauer EA, Leo-Summers LS, Gill TM. Factors associated with functional recovery among older intensive care unit survivors. Am J Respir Crit Care Med. 2016;194(3):299–307.

36. Ferrante LE, Murphy TE, Gahbauer EA, Leo-Summers LS, Pisani MA, Gill TM. Pre–intensive care unit cognitive status, subsequent disability, and new nursing home admission among critically ill older adults. Ann Am Thorac Soc. 2018;15(5):622–9. https://doi.org/10.1513/AnnalsATS.201709-702OC.

37. Ferrante LE, Pisani MA, Murphy TE, Gahbauer EA, Leo-Summers LS, Gill TM. The association of frailty with post-ICU disability, nursing home admission, and mortality. A longitudinal study. Chest. 2018;153(6):1378–86. https://doi.org/10.1016/j.chest.2018.03.007.

38. Ferrante LE, Murphy TE, Gahbauer EA, Leo-Summers LS, Pisani MA, Gill TM. The combined effects of frailty and cognitive impairment on post-ICU disability among older ICU survivors. Am J Respir Crit Care Med. 2019;200(1):107–10. https://doi.org/10.1164/rccm.201806-1144LE.

39. Gill TM, Han L, Gahbauer EA, Leo-Summers L, Murphy TE, Ferrante LE. Functional effects of intervening illnesses and injuries after critical illness in older persons. Crit Care Med. 2021;49(6):956–66. https://doi.org/10.1097/CCM.0000000000004829.

40. Heyland DK, Garland A, Bagshaw SM, Cook D, Rockwood K, Stelfox HT. Recovery after critical illness in patients aged 80 years or older: a multi-center prospective observational cohort study. Intensive Care Med. 2015;41(11):1911–20. https://doi.org/10.1007/s00134-015-4028-2.

41. Heyland DK, Stelfox HT, Garland A, Cook D, Dodek P, Kutsogiannis J, et al. Predicting performance status 1 year after critical illness in patients 80 years or older: development of a multivariable clinical prediction model. Crit Care Med. 2016;44(9):1718–26. https://doi.org/10.1097/CCM.0000000000001762.

42. Broslawski GE, Elkins M, Algus M. Functional abilities of elderly survivors of intensive care. J Am Osteopath Assoc. 1995;95:712–7.

43. Boumendil A, Maury E, Reinhard I, Luquel L, Offenstadt G, Guidet B. Prognosis of patients aged 80 years and over admitted in medical intensive care unit. Intensive Care Med. 2004;30:647–54.

44. Daubin C, Chevalier S, Séguin A, Gaillard C, Valette X, Prévost F, et al. Predictors of mortality and short-term physical and cognitive dependence in critically ill persons 75 years and older: a prospective cohort study. Health Qual Life Outcomes. 2011;9:35.
45. Sacanella E, Pérez-Castejón JM, Nicolás JM, Masanés F, Navarro M, Castro P, López-Soto A. Functional status and quality of life 12 months after discharge from a medical ICU in healthy elderly patients: a prospective observational study. Crit Care. 2011;15:R105.
46. Demiselle J, Duval G, Hamel J-F, Renault A, Bodet-Contentin L, Martin-Lefèvre L, et al. Determinants of hospital and one-year mortality among older patients admitted to intensive care units: results from the multicentric SENIOREA cohort. Ann Intensive Care. 2021;11:35.
47. Hajeb M, Singh TD, Sakusic A, Graff-Radford J, Gajic O, Rabinstein AA. Functional outcome after critical illness in older patients: a population-based study. Neurol Res. 2021;43(2):103–9. https://doi.org/10.1080/01616412.2020.1831302.
48. Pietiläinen L, Hästbacka J, Bäcklund M, Parviainen I, Pettilä V, Reinikainen M. Premorbid functional status as a predictor of 1-year mortality and functional status in intensive care patients aged 80 years or older. Intensive Care Med. 2018;44:1221–9. https://doi.org/10.1007/s00134-018-5273-y.
49. Montuclard L, Garrouste-Orgeas M, Timsit J-F, Misset B, de Jonghe B, Carlet J. Outcome, functional autonomy, and quality of life of elderly patients with a long-term intensive care unit stay. Crit Care Med. 2000;28:3389–95.

Cognitive Disorders: Outcomes After Intensive Care

Marc Verny, Sandrine Greffard, and Sara Thietart

Contents

Learning Objectives
- In this chapter, we will first outline the epidemiology of neurocognitive disorders (NCD) in the oldest population and discuss the different concepts that will allow us to approach the complexity of diagnosis and prognosis in this population.
- Then we will briefly detail the epidemiology of delirium during ICU stay.
- In the third part, we will clarify the relationship between NCD and delirium.
- Finally, we will discuss the opportunities and perspectives for limiting the occurrence and the consequences of NCD.

26.1 Introduction

Throughout the world, the overall population is aging. In 2020, the worldwide population aged 65 years or over is estimated at 727 million. This number is projected to at least double by 2050, reaching over 1.5 billion persons [1]. This elderly population is characterized by increased multimorbidity, dependency, or risk of loss of functional ability. One of the significant risk factors of dependency and alteration of quality of life is the development of neurocognitive disorders (NCD). Prevalence of cognitive disorders increases in the course of aging.

Thus, all factors that increase the incidence of NCD must be identified in order to prevent (as best as possible) this unfavorable evolution. The Lancet Commission on Dementia Prevention, Intervention, and Care Report suggests that approximately one third of dementia cases might be preventable and suggests interventions to prevent this outcome [2].

On the other hand, the intensive care unit (ICU) admission rate of older patients is increasing dramatically. Older patients admitted in an ICU frequently present with delirium. Indeed, age is clearly identified as being one of the main risks of delirium during ICU stay. Many studies suggest an association between delirium and the risk of developing NCD after an ICU stay. It should be kept in mind that more than half of older critically ill patients recover their autonomy in the long term. Therefore, it is a compelling goal to develop care strategies to optimize the course of the older patients after their ICU stay.

26.2 Epidemiology and Generalities

As mentioned by the World Health Organization, worldwide prevalence of dementia (now designed by major NCD) is around 50 million people, with nearly ten million new cases every year. Alzheimer's disease is the most common form of major NCD and may contribute to 60–70% of cases [3]. More importantly, the older the patient is, the higher are the chances of developing major NCD (dementia). For example, the prevalence of major NCD in OCDE countries is over 2% in people aged 65–69 years but reaches 40% in people over 90 [4]. Thus, when admitting a patient over 80 years in an ICU, there is a high probability that he will have major NCD. NCD is even more frequent in this population when adding those with minor NCD.

26.2.1 The Different Stages of NCD

According to the *DSM-5*, NCD are composed of major neurocognitive disorder (previously called dementia) (▶ Box 26.1) and of minor neurocognitive disorder (previously called MCI). The diagnosis of minor NCD is made when there is modest impairment in one or more cognitive domains and the person is still fully independent notably for instrumental activities of daily living (IADL) [5]. Thus, the only significant difference between minor NCD and major NCD is the interference with independency in everyday activities. The concept of progression of neurodegenerative diseases as Alzheimer's disease (AD) distinguishes different stages of 10–15 years for each. As published by the National Institute on Aging – Alzheimer Association (NIA-AA) Work Group, the course of AD should now be considered as a continuum and can be diagnosed in its early stages, including asymptomatic (preclinical) subjects and those with minor NCD. The different stages are (1) preclinical without any cognitive disturbance, (2) minor NCD, and (3) major NCD. One can specify that Alzheimer's disease is the etiological process at the origin of NCD when one of these stages is combined with markers reflecting β-amyloid (Aβ) accumulation in the brain and indicating neuronal damage (neuronal death linked to hyperphosphorylated Tau) [6–8].

These conceptual advances have potential clinical implications: an asymptomatic cognitive patient entering an ICU may carry Alzheimer's pathological lesions! It can also be the case with patients presenting only minor NCD but unidentified by the family.

Different etiologies are responsible for NCD at different stages. Among older people, the first neurodegenerative cause of major NCD is AD, the second one being Lewy body dementia. Vascular dementia is also extremely prevalent in the older population [9].

Box 26.1 *DSM-5* **Criteria for Major Neurocognitive Disorder (Previously Called Dementia)**

A. Evidence of significant cognitive decline from a previous level of performance in one or more cognitive domains:
   - Learning and memory
   - Language
   - Executive function
   - Complex attention
   - Perceptual-motor
   - Social cognition

B. The cognitive deficits interfere with independence in everyday activities. At a minimum, assistance should be required with complex instrumental activities of daily living, such as paying bills or managing medications
C. The cognitive deficits do not occur exclusively in the context of a delirium
D. The cognitive deficits are not better explained by another mental disorder (e.g., major depressive disorder, schizophrenia)

26.2.2 Multiple Lesions Are Mainly Responsible for NCD in Older Patients

In fact, it is difficult to precisely determine the frequency of the different etiologies of NCD in older people because of the frequent association of different lesions. Follow-up of cohorts of patients older than 75 years with postmortem brain examination has demonstrated that a majority of patients presented an association of different types of lesions responsible for major NCD [10]. The most common combination is Alzheimer's lesions with vascular lesions, but it can also be Alzheimer's lesions with Lewy body, or Lewy body and vascular lesions, and so on. The more there are associations of lesions, the greater is the risk of developing major NCD [11]. Many studies suggest that the accumulation of different kinds of lesions does not have an additive effect, but a potentiating effect, with a potentially more severe clinical course. In clinical practice, the association of lesions makes etiological diagnosis more difficult.

26.2.3 Cognitive Reserve

The concept of cognitive reserve appeared many years ago. Indeed, the incidence of major NCD is significantly lower in subjects with a higher educational level than in the general population [12]. A longitudinal study showed that practicing leisure activities which demand planning (one part of executive functions), such as gardening, traveling, handiwork, and knitting, decreased the risk of major NCD [13]. In the "Nun Study" which took place in the global nun population, severity of cognitive impairment was significantly correlated with severity of AD neuropathology, as quantified in postmortem brains using Braak's staging. But in a small percentage of cases, this observation was wrong. These cases displayed Braak's stages V–VI (i.e., the most severe diffusion of lesions) with only minor cognitive impairment (minor NCD). For these nuns, the high density of AD lesion appears to be in advance with cognitive decline, suggesting that they were protected [14]. In fact, these people all had a high sociocultural status displaying the highest cognitive reserve [15]. Early and sustained practice of the most complex cognitive functions would build reserves against age-related cognitive declines due to pathological attacks. The cognitive reserve represents the capacity of individuals to resist neuropathological alterations. This concept has been further supported by an analysis of cognitive impairments among a population with AD, where individuals with higher reading levels remained cognitively intact despite the significant AD markers in brain pathology [16].

26.3 Delirium in ICU

Delirium is very frequently observed in older patients hospitalized in ICUs. The prevalence is around 70% in this population, age being one of the most important risk factors, with multimorbidity, cognitive status, and frailty [17, 18]. Diagnosis, risk factors, and scores will be discussed in the next chapter of this book and will not be detailed here. Delirium is associated with many adverse patient outcomes, notably increased ICU and hospital length of stay, reduced post-discharge quality of life, increased risk of functional disability in activities of daily living, and mortality rates. Delirium is also correlated with cognitive decline at 3, 6, and 12 months post-discharge [19, 20]. In these studies, global cognition, attentional processes, and executive functions were significantly impaired. While some patients showed reversible alterations, one third had persistent cognitive decline at 12 months. A longer duration of delirium during hospital stay was associated with worse cognition.

26.4 Relationship Between Cognitive Status Before ICU Stay, Delirium, and Post-ICU NCD

Delirium is more frequently observed in older patients with a medical or surgical condition. It is clearly linked with the slight cognitive decline which occurs with age (reduction of cognitive reserve), potentially associated with frequent cerebral lesions (neurodegenerative or vascular) responsible for minor or major NCD, and also with possible neurosensory impairment, multimorbidity, polypharmacy, and malnutrition. In this type of patients, delirium is usually provoked by an insult which is more or less severe, in regard to the level of vulnerability resulting from cognitive reserve and existence of cerebral lesions [21]. Clearly the ICU stay could be considered as a stressor. Many factors could be related to occurrence of delirium, such as the use of certain drugs, restrained movement, intubation, sleep disruptions, etc. But the main question is: could delirium influence incidence of NCD, or is it responsible for a greater deterioration of NCD than in the absence of delirium? Some studies with neuropathological correlations are in favor of a specific role of delirium. Davis et al. have studied the data of three population-based cohort studies where the mean age at death was 90 [22]. They demonstrated that patients with delirium had a greater slope of cognitive decline in comparison with matched patients without delirium. In the latter, density of neuropathological lesions responsible for NCD correlated with severity of cognitive impairment. However, this was not the case in patients with a history of delirium, suggesting that a specific type of alteration could be linked with delirium. They concluded that age-related cognitive decline has many contributors, and their findings support a role for delirium acting independently and multiplicatively on the pathological processes of classic dementia. Fong et al. reviewed some studies and underlined a strong interrelationship between delirium and major NCD, although they have distinct pathological mechanisms [23]. For example, a neuroimaging study demonstrated that longer duration of delirium was associated with greater brain atrophy and white matter disruption at discharge and 3 months after.

Many studies observed the role of inflammatory biomarkers and many cytokines such as insulin-like growth factor (IGF)-1, IL-1β, and IL-1 receptor antagonist (RA) which appear to be associated with delirium. Other biomarkers such as high levels of interferon (IFN-γ) with low levels of IGF-1 were associated with delirium severity [23]. Concerning cerebral spinal fluid biomarkers of AD (like Aβ40/Tau and Aβ42/Tau ratios), results are more conflicting but suggest a role of Aβ and Tau in the neuropathogenesis of postoperative delirium. On the other hand, in some cases, delirium may be the first sign of unknown NCD (subclinical dementia process) [23].

Thus, in patients with significant cognitive deterioration related to the "aggression" of intensive care practices, we can suggest different situations. The presence of post-ICU NCD in an older patient with reduced cognitive reserve could be due to the presence of previous NCD (known or unknown) which now appears evident or that has increased from minor to major NCD. But in some cases, it could be linked with the proper deleterious effect of delirium on a person with decreased cognitive reserve, without significant previous cerebral lesions.

Practical Implications: How to Reduce the Impact of ICU Stay on Post-ICU NCD?

All these studies are very important to propose methods to improve and prevent persistent NCD post-ICU stay.

1. A major step is to correctly select critically ill older patients for admission in ICUs. The more the patient presents major baseline NCD, the higher is the risk of having a negative impact on the cognition. This is probably also true if the patient has only minor NCD. It can be difficult in emergency settings to have all the elements to be formal on the presence of NCD. However, one can keep in mind that major NCD are present in 40% of population over 80 years and can at least check baseline autonomy (activities of daily living, i.e., ADL and IADL). From an ethical point of view, doubt must be in favor of the patient, and cognitive status is clearly not the only factor to consider when admitting an older patient in an ICU.
2. Once the patient is admitted in the ICU, it is necessary to control all the factors known to favor or major delirium. Many studies tried to determine the best way to prevent or treat delirium [18]. These include the use of neuroleptics (haloperidol or risperidone), cholinesterase inhibitor (donepezil, rivastigmine), and statins, but there is a lack of proven prophylactic agents to reduce delirium. Other methods such as the comparison of sedative treatment during mechanical ventilation (propofol, midazolam, dexmedetomidine) or nonpharmacological measures (cognitive stimulation and early mobilization) were explored.

Clinical Protocol

To date, there is no specific recommendation on management of delirium in older patients in ICUs.

A global management proposed in the ABCDEF model (► Box 26.2) recommended by the Society of Critical Care Medicine may be an interesting approach, but has not yet been evaluated in geriatric patients. However, the positive results of programs like these in medical wards can make one optimistic [24].

Box 26.2   The ABCDEF Building Blocks of ICU Delirium Management (► www.iculiberation.org)

A. Asses, prevent, and manage pain
B. Both spontaneous awakening and spontaneous breathing trials
C. Choice of sedation

D. Delirium monitoring and management
E. Early mobility and exercise
F. Family engagement and empowerment

Conclusions

Beyond these constatations and proposals, as suggested by Vallet et al., the creation of a genuine ICU-geriatric network appears essential [25]. The objectives of such a network could be to better determine the "good candidate" among older patients for ICU admission, to better evaluate our practices, to explore specific practices and protocols dedicated to older critically ill patients, and to propose special units in geriatric wards for immediate care post-ICU discharge. The role of these special geriatric units would be to pursue specialized care and to favor recovery of autonomy. Such a network needs a close collaboration between intensivists and geriatricians, as well as evaluation of procedures and organizations. This type of organization will be the best bastion against agism.

Take-Home Messages

- The presence of NCD is extremely prevalent in the older population (80 years and above) affecting 40% of this population.
- The presence of NCD post-ICU stay is one of the most important factors deteriorating quality of life.
- The evaluation of activities of daily living is important to help select patients for ICU admission.
- The occurrence and duration of delirium are determinant risk factors of appearance of NCD post-ICU stay. It seems possible to develop NCD post-ICU stay without any evidence of previous cognitive impairment.
- Prevention and management of delirium in ICUs are multifactorial as proposed in the ABCDEF building blocks.
- All these considerations should not be a pretext for refusing admission of an older patient in an ICU.

References

1. United Nations, Department of Economic and Social Affairs, Population Division (2019). World Population Ageing 2019: Highlights (ST/ESA/SER.A/430).
2. Livingston G, Sommerlad A, Orgeta V, Costafreda SG, Huntley J, Ames D, et al. Dementia prevention, intervention, and care. Lancet. 2017;390:2673–734. https://doi.org/10.1016/S0140-6736(17)31363-6.
3. Dementia prevalence. WHO; https://www.who.int/news-room/fact-sheets/detail/dementia.
4. OCDE. Prévalence de la démence. Health at a glance 2017: OECD indicators. Éditions OCDE, Paris; 2017. https://doi.org/10.1787/health_glance-2017-76-fr.
5. American Psychiatric Association. American Psychiatric Association. Diagnostic and statistical manual of mental disorders, 5th edn (DSM-5). Arlington; 2013.
6. Sperling RA, Aisen PS, Beckett LA, Bennett DA, Craft S, Fagan AM, et al. Toward defining the preclinical stages of Alzheimer's disease: recommendations from the National Institute on Aging-

Alzheimer's Association workgroups on diagnostic guidelines for Alzheimer's disease. Alzheimers Dement. 2011;7:280–92. https://doi.org/10.1016/j.jalz.2011.03.003.

7. Albert MS, DeKosky ST, Dickson D, Dubois B, Feldman HH, Fox NC, et al. The diagnosis of mild cognitive impairment due to Alzheimer's disease: recommendations from the National Institute on Aging-Alzheimer's Association workgroups on diagnostic guidelines for Alzheimer's disease. Alzheimers Dement. 2011;7:270–9. https://doi.org/10.1016/j.jalz.2011.03.008.

8. McKhann GM, Knopman DS, Chertkow H, Hyman BT, Jack CR, Kawas CH, et al. The diagnosis of dementia due to Alzheimer's disease: recommendations from the National Institute on Aging-Alzheimer's Association workgroups on diagnostic guidelines for Alzheimer's disease. Alzheimers Dement. 2011;7:263–9. https://doi.org/10.1016/j.jalz.2011.03.005.

9. Lopez OL, Kuller LH. Epidemiology of aging and associated cognitive disorders: prevalence and incidence of Alzheimer's disease and other dementias, Handbook of clinical neurology, vol. 167. Elsevier; 2019. p. 139–48. https://doi.org/10.1016/B978-0-12-804766-8.00009-1.

10. Yang Z, Slavin MJ, Sachdev PS. Dementia in the oldest old. Nat Rev Neurol. 2013;9:382–93. https://doi.org/10.1038/nrneurol.2013.105.

11. Kawas CH, Kim RC, Sonnen JA, Bullain SS, Trieu T, Corrada MM. Multiple pathologies are common and related to dementia in the oldest-old: the 90+ study. Neurology. 2015;85:535–42. https://doi.org/10.1212/WNL.0000000000001831.

12. Dartigues JF, Gagnon M, Barberger-Gateau P, Letenneur L, Commenges D, Sauvel C, et al. The Paquid epidemiological program on brain ageing. Neuroepidemiology. 1992;11(Suppl 1):14–8. https://doi.org/10.1159/000110955.

13. Fabrigoule C, Letenneur L, Dartigues JF, Zarrouk M, Commenges D, Barberger-Gateau P. Social and leisure activities and risk of dementia: a prospective longitudinal study. J Am Geriatr Soc. 1995;43:485–90. https://doi.org/10.1111/j.1532-5415.1995.tb06093.x.

14. Riley KP, Snowdon DA, Markesbery WR. Alzheimer's neurofibrillary pathology and the spectrum of cognitive function: findings from the Nun Study. Ann Neurol. 2002;51:567–77. https://doi.org/10.1002/ana.10161.

15. Riley KP, Snowdon DA, Desrosiers MF, Markesbery WR. Early life linguistic ability, late life cognitive function, and neuropathology: findings from the Nun Study. Neurobiol Aging. 2005;26:341–7. https://doi.org/10.1016/j.neurobiolaging.2004.06.019.

16. Negash S, Wilson RS, Leurgans SE, Wolk DA, Schneider JA, Buchman AS, et al. Resilient brain aging: characterization of discordance between Alzheimer's disease pathology and cognition. Curr Alzheimer Res. 2013;10:844–51. https://doi.org/10.2174/15672050113109990157.

17. Pisani MA, Murphy TE, Van Ness PH, Araujo KLB, Inouye SK. Characteristics associated with delirium in older patients in a medical intensive care unit. Arch Intern Med. 2007;167:1629–34. https://doi.org/10.1001/archinte.167.15.1629.

18. Hayhurst CJ, Pandharipande PP, Hughes CG. Intensive care unit delirium: a review of diagnosis, prevention, and treatment. Anesthesiology. 2016;125:1229–41. https://doi.org/10.1097/ALN.0000000000001378.

19. Pandharipande PP, Girard TD, Jackson JC, Morandi A, Thompson JL, Pun BT, et al. Long-term cognitive impairment after critical illness. N Engl J Med. 2013;369:1306–16. https://doi.org/10.1056/NEJMoa1301372.

20. Mitchell ML, Shum DHK, Mihala G, Murfield JE, Aitken LM. Long-term cognitive impairment and delirium in intensive care: a prospective cohort study. Aust Crit Care. 2018;31:204–11. https://doi.org/10.1016/j.aucc.2017.07.002.

21. Inouye SK, Westendorp RGJ, Saczynski JS. Delirium in elderly people. Lancet. 2014;383:911–22. https://doi.org/10.1016/S0140-6736(13)60688-1.

22. Davis DHJ, Muniz-Terrera G, Keage HAD, Stephan BCM, Fleming J, Ince PG, et al. Association of delirium with cognitive decline in late life: a Neuropathologic study of 3 population-based cohort studies. JAMA Psychiat. 2017;74:244–51. https://doi.org/10.1001/jamapsychiatry.2016.3423.

23. Fong TG, Davis D, Growdon ME, Albuquerque A, Inouye SK. The interface between delirium and dementia in elderly adults. Lancet Neurol. 2015;14:823–32. https://doi.org/10.1016/S1474-4422(15)00101-5.

24. Hshieh TT, Yang T, Gartaganis SL, Yue J, Inouye SK. Hospital elder life program: systematic review and meta-analysis of effectiveness. Am J Geriatr Psychiatry. 2018;26:1015–33. https://doi.org/10.1016/j.jagp.2018.06.007.

25. Vallet H, Riou B, Boddaert J. Elderly patients and intensive care: systematic review and geriatrician's point of view. Rev Med Interne. 2017;38:760–5. https://doi.org/10.1016/j.revmed.2017.01.014.

Rehabilitation

Jeremy M. Jacobs and Jochanan Stessman

Contents

> **ⓔ Learning Objectives**
> - Understand the general principles and particular challenges of geriatric rehabilitation in the critically ill very old patient.
> - Develop a personalized approach to assessment, focused upon the gap between individual capacity and optimal function.
> - Recognize the heterogeneity of aging, using measures of mobility, hearing, vision, frailty, resilience, mood, social function, and cognition to determine intrinsic capacity.
> - Explain the role of a multidisciplinary team, and outline rehabilitation interventions.
> - Acknowledge the unique challenges facing very old critically ill patients, and identify barriers to optimal rehabilitation.
> - Understand post-ICU care transitions of care.
> - Consider future directions in improving geriatric rehabilitation for critically ill older people.

27.1 Geriatric Rehabilitation: General Principles

Rehabilitation is the delivery of a set of interventions designed to meet the goal of optimal functioning and minimal disability among people with health conditions, in their interaction with the environment [1]. People aged over 65 years old are the fastest-growing population of rehabilitation patients, and the complex constellation of biological changes, which characterize the aging process, presents a unique set of rehabilitation challenges. Indeed, when viewed as vectors of change, aging and rehabilitation are frequently moving in different and opposite directions. It is the recognition and reconciliation of these divergent processes which define and delineate the subtle nuances characteristic of the art of geriatric rehabilitation. Previous models of rehabilitation dating from the 1960s [2] focused upon a causative model of events, whereby an active disease pathology leads to a structural impairment, resulting in a functional limitation and subsequent disability. This model of linear progression through a process of disablement and handicap was gradually replaced, and by 2001 the World Health Organization [3] adopted the International Classification of Functioning, Disability and Health (ICF). Emphasizing the multiplicity of different systems within which resides the concept of disability, the ICF recognizes that a person's activity or ability to execute a certain task reflects the interaction of their health status, body function, and participation, as well as personal and environmental factors. Distinct from the ICF model, the Ecological or Person-Environment Fit model of rehabilitation allows for a deeper understanding of the etiology of impaired function. Viewed as a mismatch between individual capacity and the task demands, optimal function and minimal disability require a highly personalized approach aimed at redressing the mismatch [4]. A shift in paradigm away from reacting to illness and preventing disability or impairments towards the promotion of healthy aging was recently adopted by the WHO *World Report on Ageing and Health* [5]. Rather than disability and disease, the report emphasizes optimal functioning and well-being in older age, which are considered expressions of the individual's intrinsic capacity, their environment, and the interaction between the two [6]. Understanding the optimal function of the aging person within this theoretical framework, it is proposed, may lead to a radical change in the principles of clinical practice and rehabilitation perspectives among older people. Moving away from screening for disease biomarkers and disease-oriented clinical care, this healthy aging approach would seek to promote individualized proactive interventions, aimed at enhancing intrinsic capacity and performance. Recent attempts to identify age-related correlates of intrinsic capacity, based upon a wide range of biogerontology and geroscience research into disability and function, consistently describe the following elemental domains: locomotion (including neuromuscular function), sensorium (including hearing and vision), physical vitality (e.g., homeostasis, frailty, resilience), psychology (mood and social function), and cognition [7–9]. Over and above the semantics within which to frame the language of disability, aging, and rehabilitation, it is these recurrent omnipresent core issues of geriatric medicine that are at the heart of rehabilitation of the older adult, irrespective of diagnostic categories, illness severity, intensity of treatment, or site of care.Geriatric rehabilitation, like all aspects of geriatric medicine, must inevitably account for the increasing heterogeneity which typifies the aging process. The interindividual variability in numerous biological systems observed between individuals of the same age group increases with advancing age, and the heterogeneity becomes even more pronounced across different age groups of older people [10]. Similarly, analyses of longitudinal data among very old people also confirm the increasing variability observed across different trajectories of health, disease, function, and survival [11, 12]. Recognizing the immense heterogeneity among very old people helps underline the importance of accurately differentiating between chronological and biological aging and is an important step towards an accurate and personalized assessment of the patient's specific rehabilitation potential and goals. Indeed, lack of awareness and appreciation among healthcare professionals of this critical difference is likely to result in critical decisions concerning triage and treatment to be made based upon chronological age alone.

There is a growing consensus concerning the important moderating influence of frailty within the rehabilitation process, and considerable evidence supports its usefulness as a prognostic factor among critically ill older people [13]. Numerous assessment tools to measure frailty exist reflecting the theoretical basis upon which frailty is derived: the model of phenotypic frailty, with its characteristic biological features closely related to muscle function and sarcopenia, alongside the stochastic "accumulation of impairments" Frailty Index [14–16]. These different yet complementary approaches respectively reflect a biological state of vulnerability and a gradual breakdown of complex networks. Irrespective of theoretical differences, when translated to clinically guided screening tools for frailty, all approaches have proven to be robust predictors of negative rehabilitation outcomes following intensive care [17–19]. In contrast to frailty, the notion of physical resilience is recently gaining growing attention as an additional moderating factor in the dynamics of recovery and rehabilitation from critical illness at the extremes of age [20–22].

It is within the microcosm of critical care for the very old patient that we are often witness to the entire spectrum of geriatric medicine. Critical illness within the ICU setting among the very old patient serves as both incubator and accelerator to highlight and intensify the core issues of geriatrics and rehabilitation. Provision of optimal care must first acknowledge, and subsequently address, the challenges of disability and functional decline; impaired neurocognitive, neuromuscular, and sensory function, set against a wide biological heterogeneity of comorbidities and frailty; resilience and intrinsic capacity; and unpredictable trajectories of health and disease progression.

27.2 Multidisciplinary Approach

A prerequisite for optimal geriatric rehabilitation is a fully functional, coordinated, and interactive multidisciplinary team, including a geriatric consultant specializing in rehabilitation, specialized geriatric nurses, physiotherapists, occupational and speech therapists, dietician, social worker, and, where appropriate, psychologist and specialized recreational therapists. Within the context of the critically ill very old patient in the intensive care setting, the importance of the multidisciplinary approach cannot be underestimated. Both as part of an initial assessment and also at regular multidisciplinary team meetings, decisions are continually updated concerning the patient's rehabilitation potential and their multimodal treatment plan, as well as an appraisal of both immediate-, short-, and long-term rehabilitation goals. Since rehabilitation involves multiple modalities of therapy, the involvement of all team members in joint decision-making is essential to assess progress, redefine goals, and if necessary consider the reduction or cessation of rehab therapy and a shift towards a more palliative orientated care. Rather than separate areas of therapy, the different modalities of rehabilitation care are widely overlapping, with interactive spheres of influence. Thus, for example, while physiotherapy for early mobilization is primarily aimed at improving locomotor and muscle function, nonetheless secondary effects include positive impact upon neurocognitive, affective and psychological, cardiovascular, hemodynamic, pulmonary, and metabolic function. Similarly, best standard nursing care might be aimed at optimal skin care and patient positioning, oral hygiene, sphincter control, preventing constipation, pain control, attention to sensory impairments by providing hearing and vision aids, reducing use of restraints and environmental stressors, and encouraging the engagement with family members. Nonetheless, secondary effects of these interventions are likely to also result in reduced levels of delirium and psychomotor agitation; improved sleep and mood; reduced degree of reactive depression, anxiety, and adjustment difficulties; and subsequently an improved degree of compliance and positive disposition towards early mobilization or other active rehabilitation treatment modalities.

27.3 Assessment of Rehabilitation Potential

Aims of rehabilitation assessment of the critically ill very old patient focus upon identifying potential reversible areas of functional deterioration, the determination of the patient's overall rehabilitation potential, and the initiation of early focused interventions. This being said, accurate predictions of subsequent rehabilitation potential and outcomes are notoriously difficult, and among very old people in particular, very little accurate evidence-based research exists. A growing body of literature exists, which repeatedly confirms the robust association between premorbid functional status, comorbid burden, and frailty with increased mortality as well as poor subsequent functional outcome in ICU survivors [13, 17–19, 23]. However, caution is needed in drawing conclusions from much of current data which is hampered by numerous methodological problems which include not only selection and survival bias but also fundamental issues such as lack of consensus concerning assessment tools [24] and the lack of standardization of rehabilitation treatment protocols among critically ill very old patients both within the ICU and post-ICU. Furthermore, there are wide disparities in both the availability of rehabilitation services and the degree of healthcare reimbursement provided by different healthcare systems.

That being said, medical assessment must include a determination of premorbidity, frailty, and level of disability, which, viewed through the rehabilitation paradigm, closely relates to the patient's prior level of activity, participation, and engagement with their environment. An assessment of neurocognitive status is essential, in order to identify the presence of agitation, delirium, and prior baseline cognitive state, as well as the patient's current degree of cognitive functioning and level of capacity for decision-making. Understanding the cognitive status is essential to help guide current interventions, to define treatment goals, with the aim of improving patient's insight, participation, and cooperation, as well promoting positive disposition and motivation towards rehabilitation therapy. Inadequate pain control presents a major barrier to rehabilitation efforts. Indeed, the close relationship between pain, agitation, delirium (PAD), and generalized impaired neurocognitive function was reinforced in the widely accepted 2013 PAD clinical practice guidelines [25]. Recognizing the importance of mobility and sleep, these guidelines were updated in the 2018 PADIS guideline to include pain, agitation, delirium, immobility (rehabilitation/ mobilization), and sleep (disruption) [26, 27]. Along similar lines, the additional importance of the family and caregiver involvement in critical care is included in the implementation of the ABCDEF Bundle (Assess/manage pain; Both spontaneous and awakening and breathing trials; Choice of analgesics and sedation; Delirium management; Early mobility and exercise; Family engagement and empowerment), which has been shown to have a significant and meaningful impact on numerous outcomes both during ICU and post-ICU [28].

Cardiovascular, pulmonary, and hemodynamic reserves are often rate limiting factors to the patient's tolerance, and are simultaneously often primary goals of rehabilitation, to be addressed alongside sarcopenia, ongoing infection, and inflammatory and catabolic status. The major sequelae of neuromuscular damage associated with critical illness among very old people are common and typically occur against a background of underlying current comorbidity, polypharmacy, immobility, and deep sedation, in addition to preexisting frailty, low levels of physical activity, sarcopenia, proinflammatory status, and poor nutritional status. Functional assessment of performance measures includes locomotion, gait, balance (static and dynamic), coordination, strength, and range of movement, in conjunction with determination of the patient's sensory integrity (vision, hearing, touch, proprioception, pain), autonomic and involuntary function, orthostatism, sphincter control, bowel function, and skin integrity. Nutritional screening and assessment of swallowing and oral hygiene are important, and where appropriate will be helpful to guide early intervention of speech therapy and assistive aids to help improve communication. Identifying the significant family members and caregivers is an important early step, aimed at facilitating their involvement and empowerment within the critical care environment. Furthermore, an understanding of the patient's social support and cultural background may contribute, indirectly, to improving the patient's disposition towards rehabilitation, as well as the early identification of potential barriers to future discharge and placement. Where possible the patient's advanced planning directives should be ascertained and surrogate decision-makers identified. The ultimate aim of assessment is to aid in determining the rehabilitation potential and help in "prognostication." While research over the last two decades has certainly identified risk factors associated with negative outcomes, nonetheless predicting longitudinal trajectories of change at the individual patient level remains notoriously unreliable. A body of literature now exists with evidence linking long-term post-ICU outcomes to the assessment at point of entry to ICU of the patient's degree of frailty, sarcopenia, premorbidity, and functional and cognitive status, as well as performance measures and illness severity [17–19, 23–25, 29]. Nonetheless, in addition to statistical models, algorithms, and heuristic approaches aimed at predicting outcomes and aiding in decision-making, there remains a highly significant role for clinical experience and judgment, and suggestions have been made for a time-limited trial of care rather than a single decision concerning triage for ICU [30].

27.4 Rehabilitation Interventions for the Critically Ill Very Old Patient

The sequelae of surviving critical illness are well documented, in both younger and older patients, and include, for example, sustained muscle weakness, cognitive impairment (memory and executive dysfunction), impaired pulmonary function, sustained weight loss, sarcopenia, frailty, functional decline as well as psychological symptoms (anxiety, depression, post trauma), and reduced levels of participation and engagement. In addition, the long-term negative impact of critical illness upon informal caregivers and the family unit is also recognized as a significant mental and physical health issue. Despite the frequent picture of negative outcomes, in the relatively little literature that exists among people age over 80, a wide variability is reported. Thus, for example, in a Canadian study of 610 patients aged >80 years old admitted to ICU, 25% of people had survived and returned to their baseline level of function at 12 months [31]. In contrast, a study from Finland among people aged over 80 years old admitted to ICU found that 62% were alive at 12 months, and 78% of these survivors had returned to a functional status comparable to their premorbid situation [23].

The fact that functional improvement is attainable among survivors of critical care, both young and old alike, is the driving reason behind the implementation of rehabilitation, and the initiation of rehabilitation early in the course of critical care is currently an accepted standard of care. For example, the National Institute for Health and Clinical Excellence (NICE) clinical guidelines for rehabilitation after critical illness in adults, which were published in 2009 and updated with quality standards in 2017 [32, 33], provide detailed outlines concerning minimal standards of rehabilitation. Interestingly, the guidelines are inclusive of patients of all ages. Although research efforts have primarily focused upon the examination of potential benefits of early rehabilitation interventions, particularly early mobilization and active exercise, nonetheless few have examined the very old ICU patients as a separate group. Despite the fact that numerous studies have shown benefits of both early mobilization and personalized exercise interventions among ICU patients of all ages, systematic reviews have repeatedly noted methodological difficulties and the lack of high-quality evidence [34–42]. Thus, conclusions are frequently limited in their scope, citing the lack of standardization of rehabilitation interventions, different criteria for patient inclusion, different timing and duration of treatment, and a variety of outcome measures, as well as a relative lack of very old patients included in the studies. That being said, a large number of individual research programs, upon which are based the numerous systematic reviews and meta-analyses, have found consistent evidence to support both early mobilization and exercise, which indeed appears to be persuasive. Among the large number of potential interventions, the positive effects of early mobilization and active exercise have been supported by existing evidence, primarily among ICU patients of all ages, of which the very old patients are included. Similarly, the safety of these interventions across a range of different patient populations has been shown [26, 27]. Recently the safety of exercise and early mobilization was also found to be beneficial among critically ill people aged over 80, recovering from acute cardiovascular disease in the cardiac critical care scenario [43].

The role of physiotherapy is perhaps the most common and dominant treatment modality, which is focused upon the restoration of muscle integrity: muscle strength, locomotor function, mobilization, and respiratory function, as well as improved and early weaning from ventilation. Aimed at improving muscle weakness and range of activities, techniques include passive and active assisted movements, postures, active limb exercises, peripheral muscle training, and respiratory muscle training, as well as neuromuscular stimulation. Specific respiratory techniques include manual hyperinflation, percussion, vibration, and in-exsufflation [44]. The increased use of in-bed cycling, among conscious ventilated patients in particular, is gaining interest, as is the early mobilization of ventilated patients [45].

Recognizing the importance of defining a key set of skills and interventions has led recent research to define a minimum set of standards for specialized physical therapists in the ICU setting. Like the majority of literature, little if any distinction is made concerning the often complex needs of very old people in the critical care setting, who by nature of preexisting mobility and neuromuscular impairments are likely to require specific and individualized care [46, 47].

Working in unison with physiotherapists, occupational therapists in critical care may aim at improving self-care skills, cognitive treatment, sensory input, optimal use of assistive technology, splints, and postural aids. Communication deficits, swallowing disorders, and optimal dietary considerations require close cooperation between both speech therapists and dieticians and nursing team. The rapidly developing area of virtual reality technology in rehabilitation is finding its way into the ICU, where its multiple uses in physical, exercise, communication, and cognitive therapy are likely to become established in the future. Recent reviews of available evidence remain inconclusive, and refrain from advising either for or against due to lack of evidence [26, 27]; however, current research is growing, including the niche relaxation and prevention of delirium – albeit among younger patients to date [48, 49].

27.5 Barriers to Early Rehabilitation

Among the critically old ill patient, it is likely that the patient-centered barriers to treatment (pain/fatigue/weakness/anxiety/fear/lack of motivation/confusion/restraints) may be even greater than their younger counterparts, and yet this area has been very poorly researched. Using qualitative, grounded theory to explore patient experiences of early rehabilitation in the ICU, reports of loss of sense of self, autonomy, and competence and dehumanization were repeatedly voiced, in conjunction with a gradual process of recalibration of the self-identity [50]. These common themes experienced by patients of all ages in the ICU are likely to resonate with pre-existing themes among the very old; however, to date it remains unknown if qualitative differences in the experience of ICU exist among the very old patients. Recent research from the USA suggest that among ICU patients of all ages, only 45% actually received early mobilization [51], and it is likely that among very old people, this lack of early rehab might be even higher. Numerous environmental barriers to early rehabilitation interventions in the ICU were identified in a review of 38 studies [52] and included not only an objective lack of dedicated and specialized therapists and lack of multidisciplinary regular rounds but also lack of positive perception of benefits from early rehabilitation by ICU staff members. Similar lack of adequate equipment, low staffing levels, and financial impediments were also commonly cited. The importance of the staff members' perception of the importance of early rehab and their appreciation of the potential benefits has been considered to be a critical aspect of the environmental barriers within the culture of the ICU department, with 63% of staff members reporting their underestimation of ICU weakness [53]. These findings were reinforced from a UK survey suggesting that less than one third of all ICU patients were offered appropriate rehabilitation care or follow-up, despite NICE guidelines [42].

27.6 Transitions Out of the ICU

As underlined by NICE guidelines, an important and necessary element in successful rehabilitation is the "seamless transition" of care following discharge from ICU, aimed at maintaining the continuity of an appropriate level of rehabilitation care. An accurate assessment of rehab potential prior to discharge remains challenging, and current efforts are directed at the development of a standardized assessment of core rehabilitation issues, according to which a tailored post-ICU rehab plan may be determined [54]. One such example is the Post-ICU Presentation Score (PICUPS), which is a screening and assessment tool aimed at improving the post-ICU care transition and continuity of rehabilitation care, at the decisive moment of "step-down" from ICU to continued care [55].

The range of rehabilitation services following ICU varies widely across different healthcare systems, and decisions concerning care are often a reflection of not only patient-dependent factors but also the availability of services, alongside the coverage provided within the healthcare system. Thus, the primary elements which must be considered concerning the most appropriate care setting will include the medical status, specific diagnosis for which rehabilitation is indicated, and medical stability; premorbid and current functional, neurocognitive, and neuromuscular status; motivational and psychological status; the tolerance and reserve necessary for sustained physical mobilization; the number of different therapeutic modalities required; psychosocial and family preferences; degree of health coverage provided; and local availability of services. Rehabilitation services providing intensive inpatient rehabilitation, often situated in a general hospital setting, will typically entail at least two or three modalities (physiotherapy, occupational therapy, and speech therapy), with a minimum of 3 h daily treatment, 5–6 times weekly. Geriatric rehabilitation (often referred to as subacute/post-acute/transitional care) is usually delivered in a step-down facility (geriatric medical center/skilled nursing facility) where, in addition to 24/7 nursing and geriatric care, patients will receive one to two modalities of therapy, often 1–2 h daily depending upon their reserve and tolerance. There is an increasing interest in the provision of home rehabilitation and home hospital services, with mounting evidence to support either non-inferiority or actual improved quality of care compared to inpatient rehabilitation, as well as improved patient and family satisfaction, and economic benefits for healthcare providers [56]. Multidisciplinary home care teams may provide long-term rehabilitation care for patients with an anticipated slow recovery, for whom the social support, informal caregivers, family, and home environment are deemed to be both willing and capable of providing adequate care in the community. As is the case for geriatric inpatient rehabilitation services, there is an even greater variability in the availability of home hospital and home care services in different healthcare systems [57].

The rapidly developing area of telemedicine is exploring numerous niches for both physio- and occupational therapy guided remotely, as well as the availability of virtual encounters with other healthcare professionals. Patients requiring long-term acute care, with poor or negligible rehabilitation potential, are also candidates for long-term provision of home hospital, as witnessed by the growing number of patients requiring prolonged mechanical or noninvasive ventilation, who are choosing home rather than hospital. One of the important drivers behind the emergence of home-based alternatives is the financial incentive. Thus, for example, a recent analysis of USA Medicare data concerning post-acute care at home versus long-term acute care or long-term skilled care among over 17 million patients discharged following an acute hospital-acquired deterioration found similar functional gain yet significantly reduced cost in favor of homecare [58]. Furthermore, evidence does exist to support the benefits associated with home-based rehabilitation specifically among post-ICU patients across a range of outcomes, including respiratory and locomotory function, quality of life, and patient safety [59]. Furthermore, when asked if they would choose again to undergo ventilation, a positive answer was given by over 80% of elderly survivors of ICU remaining on prolonged mechanical ventilation treated with home hospital, as well as those successfully weaned following a prolonged duration of ventilation [60–62].

27.7 Future Directions

Currently, there is a lack of high-quality, evidence-based research into rehabilitation of the critically ill very old patient. A central issue which must be addressed is the need to standardize the assessment of rehabilitation status, using a minimum set of core domains measured by accepted and validated tools. Improved assessment at numerous points along the transition of rehabilitation care is necessary to improve our understanding of initial triage, response to rehabilitation interventions, and decisions concerning post-ICU rehabilitation care. Similarly, a minimum standardized protocol of treatment, aimed particularly for early mobilization and exercise therapy, is essential in order to improve quality of care at the patient level, as well as determine the impact and potential benefits of treatment. A deeper understanding of patient-centered barriers is necessary, at numerous levels. Thus, for example, unravelling the interaction of sarcopenia, frailty, intrinsic capacity, and resilience with critical illness and rehabilitation will likely play a central role in translational research bridging the gap between assessment and prognostics. Environmental barriers to be addressed clearly involve educational advances aimed at the medical culture within the ICU. An important factor which is likely to help catalyze this change is the integration of geriatricians as an organic element within the ICU team [62]. The recent COVID-19 pandemic brought to the forefront the lack of rehabilitation services in general and among very old people in particular [63]. Addressing the need to integrate and promote rehabilitation with healthcare stems, at all points of care transition from ICU to home, will in all likelihood come about after the provision of hard evidence supporting the benefits of rehabilitation among critically ill very old people.

> **Take-Home Messages**
> - High-quality research into rehabilitation of critically ill very old patients is needed to improve assessment, interventions, and outcomes.
> - Always screen for agitation, delirium and dementia, pain, frailty, and locomotion and establish baseline premorbid level of function and advanced directives.
> - Multidisciplinary care, especially mobilization and exercise, can be safely delivered and should be started as soon as possible.
> - Successful transition from ICU to the optimal rehabilitation setting requires a tailored rehabilitation plan, using standardized assessment tools.
> - Barriers to rehabilitation include both patient-centered geriatric syndromes and environmental factors, including staff perception and education, as well as healthcare disparities.
> - Models of rehabilitation at home are increasingly common and for appropriate patients may provide the same level of functional gain as post-ICU hospital care but with substantially reduced costs and greater patient satisfaction.

References

1. World Health Organization. Rehabilitation: key for health in the 21st century. Geneva: World Health Organization; 2017.
2. Jette AM. Toward a common language for function, disability, and health. Phys Ther. 2006;86(5):726.
3. World Health Organization. The international classification of functioning, disability and health. Geneva: World Health Organization; 2001.
4. Lawton MP. Competence, environmental press, and the adaption of older people. In: Lawton MP, Windley PG, Byerts TO, editors. Aging and the environment. New York: Springer; 1982.
5. World Health Organization. World report on ageing and health. Geneva: World Health Organization; 2015.
6. Beard JR, Officer A, de Carvalho IA, et al. The world report on ageing and health: a policy framework for healthy ageing. Lancet. 2016;387:2145–54. https://doi.org/10.1016/S0140-6736(15)00516-4.
7. van der Vorst A, Zijlstra GA, Witte N, et al. D-SCOPE Consortium. Limitations in activities of daily living in community-dwelling people aged 75 and over: a systematic literature review of risk and protective factors. PLoS One. 2016;11(10):e0165127. https://doi.org/10.1371/journal.

pone.0165127. Erratum in: PLoS One. 2017 Jan 23;12 (1):e0170849. PMID: 27760234; PMCID: PMC5070862.

8. Cesari M, de Carvalho IA, Thiyagarajan JA, et al. Evidence for the domains supporting the construct of intrinsic capacity. J Gerontol A. 2018;73(12):1653–60. https://doi.org/10.1093/gerona/gly011.

9. Beard JR, Jotheeswaran AT, Cesari M, et al. The structure and predictive value of intrinsic capacity in a longitudinal study of ageing. BMJ Open. 2019;9(11):e026119. https://doi.org/10.1136/bmjopen-2018-026119. PMID: 31678933; PMCID: PMC6830681.

10. Mitnitski A, Howlett SE, Rockwood K. Heterogeneity of human aging and its assessment. J Gerontol A. 2017;72(7):877–84. https://doi.org/10.1093/gerona/glw089.

11. Cohen-Mansfield J, Skornick-Bouchbinder M, Brill S. Trajectories of end of life: a systematic review. J Gerontol B Psychol Sci Soc Sci. 2018;73(4):564–72. https://doi.org/10.1093/geronb/gbx093. PMID: 28977651.

12. Gerstorf D, Ram N. Inquiry into terminal decline: five objectives for future study. Gerontologist. 2013;53(5):727–37. https://doi.org/10.1093/geront/gnt046. Epub 2013 May 23. PMID: 23704220; PMCID: PMC3771675.

13. Brummel NE, Bell SP, Girard TD, et al. Frailty and subsequent disability and mortality among patients with critical illness. Am J Respir Crit Care Med. 2017;196(1):64–72. https://doi.org/10.1164/rccm.201605-0939OC. PMID: 27922747; PMCID: PMC5519959.F

14. Cesari M, Gambassi G, van Kan GA, Vellas B. The frailty phenotype and the frailty index: different instruments for different purposes. Age Ageing. 2014;43:10–2.

15. Mitnitski AB, Rutenberg AD, Farrell S, Rockwood K. Aging, frailty and complex networks. Biogerontology. 2017;18:433–46.

16. Clegg A, Young J, Iliffe S, Rikkert MO, Rockwood K. Frailty in elderly people. Lancet. 2013;381:752–62.

17. Flaatten H, De Lange DW, Morandi A, et al. VIP1 Study Group. The impact of frailty on ICU and 30-day mortality and the level of care in very elderly patients (≥ 80 years). Intensive Care Med. 2017;43(12):1820–8. https://doi.org/10.1007/s00134-017-4940-8. Epub 2017 Sept 21

18. Guidet B, de Lange DW, Boumendil A, et al. VIP2 Study Group. The contribution of frailty, cognition, activity of daily life and comorbidities on outcome in acutely admitted patients over 80 years in European ICUs: the VIP2 study. Intensive Care Med. 2020;46(1):57–69. https://doi.org/10.1007/s00134-019-05853-1. Epub 2019 Nov 29. PMID: 31784798; PMCID: PMC7223711.

19. Haas LEM, Boumendil A, Flaatten H, et al. VIP2 Study Group. Frailty is associated with long-term outcome in patients with sepsis who are over 80 years old: results from an observational study in 241 European ICUs. Age Ageing. 2021;50(5):1719–27. https://doi.org/10.1093/ageing/afab036. Epub ahead of print. PMID: 33744918.

20. Maley JH, Brewster I, Mayoral I, et al. Resilience in survivors of critical illness in the context of the survivors' experience and recovery. Ann Am Thorac Soc. 2016;13(8):1351–60. https://doi.org/10.1513/AnnalsATS.201511-782OC. PMID: 27159794; PMCID: PMC5021076.

21. Ferrante L, Stevens R. Functional loss and resilience in intensive care. Crit Care Med. 2020;48(11):1690–2. https://doi.org/10.1097/CCM.0000000000004603.

22. Varadhan R, Walston J, Bandeen-Roche K. Can physical resilience and frailty in older adults be linked by the study of dynamical systems? J Am Geriatr Soc. 2018;66(8):1455–8. https://doi.org/10.1111/jgs.15409.

23. Pietiläinen L, Hästbacka J, Bäcklund M, et al. Premorbid functional status as a predictor of 1-year mortality and functional status in intensive care patients aged 80 years or older. Intensive Care Med. 2018;44(8):1221–9. https://doi.org/10.1007/s00134-018-5273-y. Epub 2018 Jul 2. PMID: 29968013.

24. González-Seguel F, Corner EJ, Merino-Osorio C. International classification of functioning, disability, and health domains of 60 physical functioning measurement instruments used during the adult intensive care unit stay: a scoping review. Phys Ther. 2019;99(5):627–40. https://doi.org/10.1093/ptj/pzy158. PMID: 30590839; PMCID: PMC6517362.

25. Barr J, Fraser GL, Puntillo K, et al. Clinical practice guidelines for the management of pain, agitation, and delirium in adult patients in the intensive care unit. Crit Care Med. 2013;41(1):263–306. https://doi.org/10.1097/CCM.0b013e3182783b72. PMID: 23269131.

26. Devlin JW, Skrobik Y, Gélinas C, et al. Clinical practice guidelines for the prevention and management of pain, agitation/sedation, delirium, immobility, and sleep disruption in adult patients in the

ICU. Crit Care Med. 2018;46(9):e825–73. https://doi.org/10.1097/CCM.0000000000003299. PMID: 30113379.

27. Devlin JW, Skrobik Y, Gélinas C, et al. Executive summary: clinical practice guidelines for the prevention and management of pain, agitation/sedation, delirium, immobility, and sleep disruption in adult patients in the ICU. Crit Care Med. 2018;46(9):1532–48. https://doi.org/10.1097/CCM.0000000000003259. PMID: 30113371.

28. Pun BT, Balas MC, Barnes-Daly MA, et al. Caring for critically ill patients with the ABCDEF bundle: results of the ICU liberation collaborative in over 15,000 adults. Crit Care Med. 2019;47(1):3–14. https://doi.org/10.1097/CCM.0000000000003482. PMID: 30339549; PMCID: PMC6298815.

29. Villa P, Pintado MC, Luján J, et al. Functional status and quality of life in elderly intensive care unit survivors. J Am Geriatr Soc. 2016;64(3):536–42. https://doi.org/10.1111/jgs.14031. PMID: 27000326.

30. Beil M, Sviri S, Flaatten H, et al. On predictions in critical care: the individual prognostication fallacy in elderly patients. J Crit Care. 2021;61:34–8. https://doi.org/10.1016/j.jcrc.2020.10.006. Epub 2020 Oct 13. PMID: 33075607; PMCID: PMC7553132.

31. Heyland DK, Stelfox HT, Garland A, et al. Canadian critical Care Trials Group and the Canadian Researchers at the End of Life Network. Predicting performance status 1 year after critical illness in patients 80 years or older: development of a multivariable clinical prediction model. Crit Care Med. 2016;44(9):1718–26. https://doi.org/10.1097/CCM.0000000000001762. PMID: 27075141.

32. Centre for Clinical Practice at NICE (UK). Rehabilitation after critical illness [Internet]. London: National Institute for Health and Clinical Excellence; 2009. PMID: 20704055. https://www.nice.org.uk/guidance/cg83

33. Centre for Clinical Practice at NICE (UK). Rehabilitation after critical illness in adults. Quality standard [QS158]. Published: 7 September 2017. https://www.nice.org.uk/guidance/qs158

34. Calvo-Ayala E, Khan BA, Farber MO, et al. Interventions to improve the physical function of ICU survivors: a systematic review. Chest. 2013;144(5):1469–80. https://doi.org/10.1378/chest.13-0779. PMID: 23949645; PMCID: PMC3817929.

35. Sosnowski K, Lin F, Mitchell ML, White H. Early rehabilitation in the intensive care unit: an integrative literature review. Aust Crit Care. 2015;28(4):216–25. https://doi.org/10.1016/j.aucc.2015.05.002. Epub 2015 Jul 2. PMID: 26142542.

36. Doiron KA, Hoffmann TC, Beller EM. Early intervention (mobilization or active exercise) for critically ill adults in the intensive care unit. Cochrane Database Syst Rev. 2018;3(3):CD010754. https://doi.org/10.1002/14651858.CD010754.pub2. PMID: 29582429; PMCID: PMC6494211.

37. Connolly B, Salisbury L, O'Neill B, et al. Exercise rehabilitation following intensive care unit discharge for recovery from critical illness: executive summary of a Cochrane Collaboration systematic review. J Cachexia Sarcopenia Muscle. 2016;7(5):520–6. https://doi.org/10.1002/jcsm.12146. Epub 2016 Sep 16. PMID: 27891297; PMCID: PMC5114628.

38. Connolly B, Salisbury L, O'Neill B, et al. ERACIP Group. Exercise rehabilitation following intensive care unit discharge for recovery from critical illness. Cochrane Database Syst Rev. 2015;2015(6):CD008632. https://doi.org/10.1002/14651858.CD008632.pub2. PMID: 26098746; PMCID: PMC6517154.

39. Castro-Avila AC, Serón P, Fan E, Gaete M, Mickan S. Effect of early rehabilitation during intensive care unit stay on functional status: systematic review and meta-analysis. PLoS One. 2015;10(7):e0130722. https://doi.org/10.1371/journal.pone.0130722. PMID: 26132803; PMCID: PMC4488896.

40. Taito S, Yamauchi K, Tsujimoto Y, et al. Does enhanced physical rehabilitation following intensive care unit discharge improve outcomes in patients who received mechanical ventilation? A systematic review and meta-analysis. BMJ Open. 2019;9(6):e026075. https://doi.org/10.1136/bmjopen-2018-026075. PMID: 31182443; PMCID: PMC6561459.

41. Connolly B, O'Neill B, Salisbury L, Blackwood B, Enhanced Recovery After Critical Illness Programme Group. Physical rehabilitation interventions for adult patients during critical illness: an overview of systematic reviews. Thorax. 2016;71(10):881–90. https://doi.org/10.1136/thoraxjnl-2015-208273. Epub 2016 May 24. PMID: 27220357; PMCID: PMC5036250.

42. White C, Connolly B, Rowland MJ. Rehabilitation after critical illness. BMJ. 2021;373:n910. https://doi.org/10.1136/bmj.n910. PMID: 33858835.

43. Goldfarb M, Semsar-Kazerooni K, Morais JA, Dima D. Early mobilization in older adults with acute cardiovascular disease. Age Ageing. 2020;50(4):1166–72. https://doi.org/10.1093/ageing/afaa253. Epub ahead of print. PMID: 33247593.

44. Ambrosino N, Venturelli E, Vagheggini G, Clini E. Rehabilitation, weaning and physical therapy strategies in chronic critically ill patients. Eur Respir J. 2012;39(2):487–92. https://doi.org/10.1183/09031936.00094411. Epub 2011 Dec 1. PMID: 22135278.

45. Kho ME, Molloy AJ, Clarke FJ, et al. Canadian Critical Care Trials Group. TryCYCLE: a prospective study of the safety and feasibility of early in-bed cycling in mechanically ventilated patients. PLoS One. 2016;11(12):e0167561. https://doi.org/10.1371/journal.pone.0167561. PMID: 28030555; PMCID: PMC5193383.

46. Twose P, Jones U, Cornell G. Minimum standards of clinical practice for physiotherapists working in critical care settings in the United Kingdom: a modified Delphi technique. J Intensive Care Soc. 2019;20(2):118–31. https://doi.org/10.1177/1751143718807019. Epub 2018 Nov 20. PMID: 31037104; PMCID: PMC6475988.

47. Takahashi T, Kato M, Obata K, et al. Minimum standards of clinical practice for physical therapists working in intensive care units in Japan. Phys Ther Res. 2020;24(1):52–68. https://doi.org/10.1298/ptr.E10060. PMID: 33981528; PMCID: PMC8111421.

48. Gomes TT, Schujmann DS, Fu C. Rehabilitation through virtual reality: physical activity of patients admitted to the intensive care unit. Rev Bras Ter Intensiva. 2019;31(4):456–63. https://doi.org/10.5935/0103-507X.20190078. PMID: 31967219; PMCID: PMC7008986.

49. Naef AC, Jeitziner MM, Gerber SM, et al. Virtual reality stimulation to reduce the incidence of delirium in critically ill patients: study protocol for a randomized clinical trial. Trials. 2021;22(1):174. https://doi.org/10.1186/s13063-021-05090-2. PMID: 33648572; PMCID: PMC7923502.

50. Corner EJ, Murray EJ, Brett SJ. Qualitative, grounded theory exploration of patients' experience of early mobilisation, rehabilitation and recovery after critical illness. BMJ Open. 2019;9(2):e026348. https://doi.org/10.1136/bmjopen-2018-026348. PMID: 30804034; PMCID: PMC6443050.

51. Potter K, Miller S, Newman S. Patient-level barriers and facilitators to early mobilization and the relationship with physical disability post-intensive care: part 2 of an integrative review through the lens of the World Health Organization international classification of functioning, disability, and health. Dimens Crit Care Nurs. 2021;40(3):164–73. https://doi.org/10.1097/DCC.0000000000000470. PMID: 33792276.

52. Potter K, Miller S, Newman S. Environmental factors affecting early mobilization and physical disability post-intensive care: an integrative review through the lens of the World Health Organization international classification of functioning, disability, and health. Dimens Crit Care Nurs. 2021;40(2):92–117. https://doi.org/10.1097/DCC.0000000000000461. PMID: 33961378.

53. Koo KK, Choong K, Cook DJ, et al. Canadian Critical Care Trials Group. Early mobilization of critically ill adults: a survey of knowledge, perceptions and practices of Canadian physicians and physiotherapists. CMAJ Open. 2016;4(3):E448–54. https://doi.org/10.9778/cmajo.20160021. PMID: 27730109; PMCID: PMC5047804.

54. Connolly B, Denehy L, Hart N, et al. Physical Rehabilitation Core Outcomes in Critical Illness (PRACTICE): protocol for development of a core outcome set. Trials. 2018;19(1):294. https://doi.org/10.1186/s13063-018-2678-4. PMID: 29801508; PMCID: PMC5970518.

55. Turner-Stokes L, Corner EJ, Siegert RJ. The post-ICU presentation screen (PICUPS) and rehabilitation prescription (RP) for intensive care survivors part I: development and preliminary clinimetric evaluation. J Intensive Care Soc. 2021;0(0):1–11. https://doi.org/10.1177/1751143720988715.

56. Gearon E, O'Connor D, Wallis J, Han JX, Shepperd S, Mäkelä P, Buchbinder R. Factors influencing the implementation of early discharge hospital at home and admission avoidance hospital at home: a qualitative evidence synthesis. Cochrane Database Syst Rev. 2021;(3):CD014765. https://doi.org/10.1002/14651858.CD014765. Accessed 11 June 2021.

57. Falvey JR, Murphy TE, Gill TM, Stevens-Lapsley JE, Ferrante LE. Home health rehabilitation utilization among medicare beneficiaries following critical illness. J Am Geriatr Soc. 2020;68(7):1512–9. https://doi.org/10.1111/jgs.16412. Epub 2020 Mar 18. PMID: 32187664; PMCID: PMC7712590.

58. Werner RM, Coe NB, Qi M, Konetzka RT. Patient outcomes after hospital discharge to home with home health care vs to a skilled nursing facility. JAMA Intern Med. 2019;179(5):617–23. https://doi.org/10.1001/jamainternmed.2018.7998. PMID: 30855652; PMCID: PMC6503560.

59. Vitacca M, Barbano L, Vanoglio F, et al. Does 6-month home caregiver-supervised physiotherapy improve post-critical care outcomes?: a randomized controlled trial. Am J Phys Med Rehabil. 2016;95(8):571–9. https://doi.org/10.1097/PHM.0000000000000441. PMID: 26829083.
60. Jacobs JM, Marcus EL, Stessman J. Prolonged mechanical ventilation: symptomatology, well-being, and attitudes to life. J Am Med Dir Assoc. 2021;22(6):1242–7. https://doi.org/10.1016/j.jamda.2020.07.037. Epub 2020 Sep 6. PMID: 32907755; PMCID: PMC7474963.
61. Jubran A, Grant B, Duffner L, et al. Long-term outcome after prolonged mechanical ventilation. A long-term acute-care hospital study. Am J Respir Crit Care Med. 2019;199:1508–16. https://doi.org/10.1164/rccm.201806-1131oc.
62. De Biase S, Cook L, Skelton DA, et al. The COVID-19 rehabilitation pandemic. Age Ageing. 2020;49(5):696–700. https://doi.org/10.1093/ageing/afaa118. PMID: 32470131; PMCID: PMC7314277.
63. Brummel NE, Ferrante LE. Integrating geriatric principles into critical care medicine: the time is now. Ann Am Thorac Soc. 2018;15(5):518–22. https://doi.org/10.1513/AnnalsATS.201710-793IP. PMID: 29298089; PMCID: PMC5949609.

The Caregiver

J. Mellinghoff, M. van Mol, and N. Efstathiou

Contents

© The Author(s), under exclusive license to Springer Nature Switzerland AG 2022
H. Flaatten et al. (eds.), *The Very Old Critically Ill Patients*, Lessons from the ICU,
https://doi.org/10.1007/978-3-030-94133-8_28

Learning Objectives

By completing this chapter, the reader will be able to:

- Recognize and define the subject group of interest in the context of this book.
- Identify the individual roles caregivers fulfill.
- Relate the concept of caregiver burden to caregiving activities including post-intensive care syndrome (PICS-F).
- Describe individual consequences and effects of caregiving activities on the caregiver.
- Describe coping and support strategies that may be adopted to overcome negative aspects of caregiving.

28.1 Introduction

As life expectancy continues to increase and advances in medical technology bring many benefits to society, the provision of care within a healthcare system has taken central stage in health policy making. For example, Germany introduced long-term care insurance in 1995 which since has undergone several reforms taking account of population changes and increases in costs [1]. A shift from institutional care, such as hospitals or care homes, towards home care is believed to be of benefit to an individual's independence and reduces cost pressures on healthcare systems. However, these policy transformations also indicate a change in responsibility from the state as a provider of formal care activities to the informal sector which includes families, neighbors, and friends. In the UK, this informal sector is caring for 2 million adults and has been valued at £59.5 billion a year [2]. As such, informal caregivers form the backbone of care systems but seldom receive any recognition for their contribution and commitment.

Considering the impact that a critical care stay can have on a patient, it is not surprising that care will be required after discharge from hospital. In general, when we talk about the informal caregiver, we mean a relative, partner, child, family member, friend, or neighbor who has a significant personal relationship with the care recipient and provides a broad range of assistance without monetary gain. This role is dependent on its local context and often physically and emotionally demanding, particularly in cases where the carer has his/her own health-related morbidities, as it is common with the older aged population. The aim of this chapter is to provide an introduction into the role of the informal caregiver including a description of duties, its societal impact, consequences for the individual fulfilling this role, and relevant strategies that may be considered to support this important group. We also included a fictional scenario that we hope will highlight the practical implications of an ICU stay for the caregiver. For the purposes of this chapter, we will use the term caregiver (referring to the informal caregiver), while synonyms such as carer and caretaker have also been described in the English language.

Frances, a 76-year-old lady, collapsed at home and was found by her husband lying on the floor. She was unresponsive and brought to the specialist hospital by air ambulance presenting with hypothermia, hypotension, and impaired consciousness. She required mechanical ventilation and was transferred to the intensive care unit (ICU) with a diagnosis of new-onset atrial fibrillation that subsequently had led to a stroke with a left-sided weakness and aspiration pneumonia.

Frances stayed in the ICU for 3 weeks and required a tracheostomy. Naturally, she was going to have a long recovery but was supported by her husband Harry and their two children who visited frequently. After completing her neuro recovery and rehabilitation, she was discharged home after 8 weeks in hospital. There, she was supported by her older spouse and nearby living children. For the initial period, primary care services were involved who came daily to ensure she settled back into her normal life. She continued to be affected by some long-term disabilities due to the not completely resolved left-sided weakness.

28.2 Definitions and Roles of Caregivers

Before taking a closer look at the specific roles that caregivers adopt, it is imperative to recognize who these individuals are, who have been defined to provide most of the financial, emotional, and physical support to a patient on an unpaid basis [1]. Data from 21 OECD countries suggest that between 9 and 21% of older adults (age $\geq$ 50 years) undertake caring activities at least on a weekly basis, and the distribution among sexes is skewed towards women in most countries except for Sweden [3]. While this instance is not surprising due to women's increased life expectancy, analysis from the UK suggests that women are also more likely to be employed while being a caregiver, affecting their other life commitments more than in men. The age distribution increasingly affects older workers in society with the greatest number being between the age of 60 and 69 years [3]. Similar data is reported by the USA demonstrating a global trend in the developed world [4].

Overall, there is great uncertainty about the roles caregivers adopt. Anyone who finds themselves in that position goes through a period of experiential autodidactic learning with little formalized training. In 2008, the Institute of Medicine acknowledged that the definition of "healthcare workforce" must be expanded to include informal caregivers who need to be equipped with knowledge, tools, and training to provide high-quality care [5]. More than 10 years on, the reality paints a different picture, namely, a disconnect between formal and informal care provision [6]. Especially in the later stages of convalescence of a patient's recovery process, a clear distinction between what is formal and informal care would be helpful in assigning responsibilities. In order to explore the roles of the caregiver in more detail, Tramm's model (2017) is a useful tool to explore different functions that caregivers perform individually or in parallel [7]. This "carousel of roles" (■ Fig. 28.1) includes the decision-maker, carer, manager, and recorder with some fluency between these different roles.

◘ Fig. 28.1 Carousel of roles

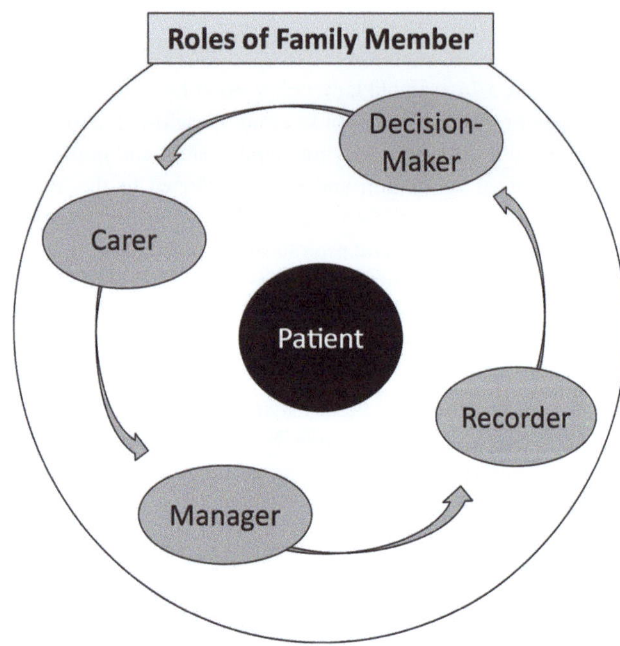

28.2.1 The Recorder

Over the last 10 years, a wealth of evidence has recognized that cognitive decline of patients recovering from critical illness affects both younger and older patients [8, 9]. Dependent on the cognitive impairments experienced by the affected individual, caregivers have to compensate for these including activities such as communicating with healthcare professionals and organizations and interpreting information received from healthcare providers as well as record keeping. The latter activity is of particular importance when dealing with multiple specialties and agencies. Taking different healthcare contexts into account, the provision of a functional model of care which is based on the needs of the care recipient and incorporates the concerns of the caregiver, should ensure that all services are coordinated and complement each other [10]. The administrative burden that arises with this task may be overwhelming, notably for the more complex cases, but certain existing services may provide support to caregivers with its completion. For example, the gatekeeping role of general practitioners may help the caregiver to communicate across professional care services and share information [11].

28.2.2 The Manager

Managing one's own life is difficult enough at the best of time, and usually an individual balances one's own needs against those in the immediate surroundings. During a critical illness and its aftermath, this balance is tilted towards the care recipient because their affairs require organization. Consequently, more time and effort are necessary in order to secure a person's health or well-being. Managerial activities in the acute disease stage include relocation to somewhere near to the hospital to be present and provide support for the acutely unwell patient [12]. In the latter stages, travel is more focused on medical or rehabilitation appointments and the organization of schedules [7]. Other aspects to be managed are the financial affairs of either the caregiver, care recipient, or both. Although this is dependent on the relationship between the two, it may not be a skill the caregiver is familiar with. In such circumstances, support by family and friends in the immediate surroundings is detrimental but not always available. Financial loss due to reduction in employment and out-of-pocket expenses may be the consequence [13]. There is acknowledgment that due to the time constraints of these activities, caregivers forego other undertakings including their own employment [2].

28.2.3 The Decision-Maker

Decision-making responsibilities commonly start early for anyone affected by a serious illness of a close relative or friend. Patients admitted to ICU are incapacitated for at least some of the time, and the caregiver in conjunction with other members of a patient's close circle makes decisions on their behalf [7]. If a relationship between the patient and caregiver is formally documented prior to the illness, this concept is referred to as "power of attorney." For the early period of illness, this includes providing consent/assent to medical investigations and procedures, comprehending and processing complex treatment information all the way to decision-making about end-of-life care or continuous therapeutic options and where such treatments may take place [5]. Stepping up to this role, caregivers provide leadership and advocacy for the patient looking after their medical affairs. But clearly all the other issues of normal life continue, such as making decisions on applying for assistance through official support services and accessing rehabilitation and long-term care institutions if services are not provided in the patient's own home. Thus, caregivers take a lot of responsibility for the patients' situation, continuously making decisions in the best interest of the care recipient and subsequently navigating through the labyrinth of a complex healthcare system.

Considerations for Practice – A Case Scenario

While Frances was in the hospital, Harry, Frances's husband, stayed in a local bed and breakfast to be able to visit and support his wife on a continuous basis. He only occasionally went home as he had stopped driving 2 years ago. He was talking to the health-care professionals daily in order to receive information on his wife's progress and participated in decision-making, providing important information about her normal life. He was writing down information so he could keep his children up to date because they could not come every day due to work and childcare commitments.

When Frances moved onto the rehabilitation ward of the hospital, Harry started to get more involved in her personal care aspects, being supervised by the nurses and allied health professionals. While he continued to be in hospital most of the time, the children looked after their personal affairs and investigated local care provision by contacting the GP, community nurses, and rehabilitation center in preparation for her return to home.

28.2.4 The Carer

Tramm's model of caregiving activities includes both the physical and psychological dimension [7]. In low- and middle-income countries caregiver involvement is much more common due to the unavailability of professionally trained staff [14]. In contrast, in high income countries contributing to care in the hospital setting is mostly left to the healthcare professional but some participation by caregivers may include the support of activities of daily living for example oral feeding or personal care. In view of the psychological dimension, a growing body of evidence suggests that caregivers have a role to play in the prevention and treatment of delirium by their participation in reorientation and rehabilitation exercises [15, 16]. Clearly, in the later stages of rehabilitation, for example in the home setting, the role of the caregiver becomes more prominent. In these cases, the question arises if there is any oversight of the quality of care provided and who is taking responsibility for it, in case of neglect – is it the healthcare system i.e., by proxy the general practitioner? Complex activities and technical tasks, such as suctioning of tracheostomised patients, changing settings of ventilation equipment, all the way to the provision of emotional welfare, require training and expertise to be transferred from the healthcare professional to the caregiver. The inherent difficulties manifesting themselves include the possibility of an imbalance between the care provided and the care needed, as well as the willingness of the caregiver to provide these tasks [17].

28.3 Caregiver Burden and Measurements

The concept of caregiver burden has been described as a multi-dimensional construct by Zarit et al. (1980): "the extent to which caregivers perceive the adverse effect that caregiving has on their emotional, social, financial, and physical functioning" [18]. While the word burden as such has a negative connotation, caregiving should not only be seen in the light of undesirable consequences for the person providing care [19]. Indeed, a study among older caregivers suggests the opposite, with caregiving resulting in a greater sense of self-fulfillment and a positive impact on people's lives [20]. Still, caregivers are often not adequately prepared for their role and may become overwhelmed [21]. Care activities vary from supporting discharged ICU patients while adjusting and returning to their previous physical and psychological state to supporting and caring for survivors who will experience long-term disabilities. Caregiver burden in the older population has been described related to Alzheimer's disease and other advance illnesses such as cancer and obstructive pulmonary disease [22] with more than one third suffering from mild to severe burden 6 months after critical illness. Adelman et al. (2014) stated that spousal caregivers, as compared with adult children that take caregiving roles for their parents, face greater challenges because they are more likely to live with the care recipient, have little choice in taking on the caregiving role, are less aware of the toll that caregiving is taking on them, and are more vulnerable because of their older age and associated morbidities [23]. The burden in caregivers is associated with the severity of illness, loss of functional autonomy, and the need for help in daily activities [24, 25]. The burden for caregivers of patients admitted to the ICU has not been studied extensively; however, it seems to be underestimated [26].

28.3.1 Post-Intensive Care Syndrome-Family (PICS-F)

As generally known, an ICU admission is a stressful moment for both the patient and its family members. As a result, family members of ICU patients are at risk of developing several psychological impairments, such as post-traumatic stress disorder (PTSD), anxiety, depression, and complicated grief in the unfortunate event of a patients dying during ICU treatment. These impairments are collectively referred to as the post-intensive care syndrome-family (PICS-F) [27–29]. A literature review revealed that anxiety, depression, and symptoms of PTSD are evident to a large number of caregivers 6 months after ICU discharge [30]. Additionally, loss of employment, financial burden, lifestyle interference, and a decreased health-related quality of life were frequently reported [30]. Development of PICS-F might exacerbate through unexpected illness of the ICU patient, the level of communication of the ICU staff, and inadequate information [31, 32].

Relatives of deceased ICU patients may develop complicated grief because of the unpredictable and burdensome situation of losing their loved one. Therefore, complicated grief has been included in the PICS-F framework [27, 28]. Demographic variables, such as gender, relationship status, and cultural background, might be associated with complicated grief [33, 34]. In addition, factors related to quality of dying and death, communication of staff, and bereavement care might impact the process of grieving for ICU relatives [35, 36]. Providing bereavement care to relatives in the ICU is an important part of high-quality ICU care [37].

28.3.2 Relationship Between Caregiver and Care Recipient After ICU Admission

A conceptual framework describing the long-term mental and social health-related outcomes of ICU survivors' relatives is based on a model of post-intensive care syndrome (PICS) created at an international stakeholder conference [28], ongoing scientific work [27, 38–41], and an extension to pediatrics [42]. It integrates the importance of physical, cognitive, emotional, and social health as a result of critical illness (◘ Fig. 28.2).

Emotional distress or the psychological domain includes symptoms of depression, anxiety, and post-traumatic stress reactions. Beyond doubt, emotional distress due to critical illness, resilience, and social outcomes are intricately intertwined. The domain of social health acknowledges an increasing focus on persons' social functioning. This means participating in activities related to family and friends, reintegration with work, and continuing in economic fundamentals of life.

Additionally, this framework recognizes that the interrelationship between the ICU survivor and their relatives is central to the trajectory of recovery. The impact of critical illness on relatives may also be profound, as they can experience emotional and social consequences due to the critical illness of their loved one [29]. Post-

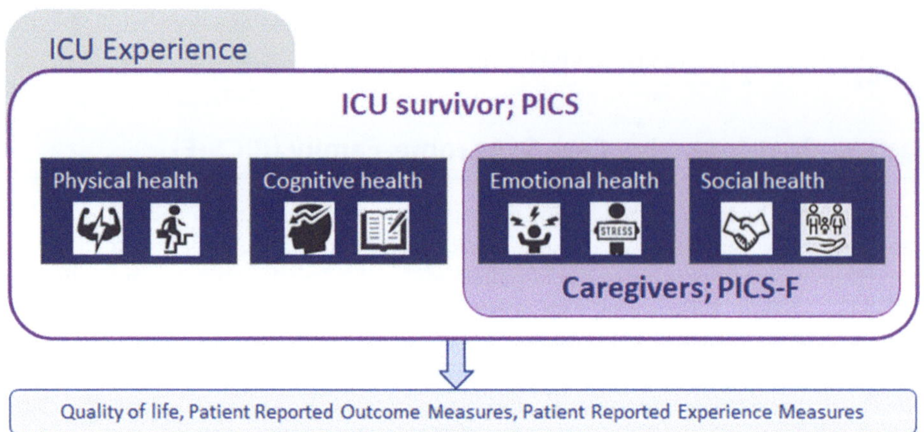

Fig. 28.2 Conceptual framework on PICS/PICS-F. (©van Mol – den Ouden Management)

traumatic stress reactions may remain from their ICU experiences. In their role as a caregiver, after hospital discharge, the new situation may lead to worries, anxiety, and symptoms of depression. Additionally, caregivers may reduce social activities [30], which further increases the risk of PICS-F. These health-related outcomes, in turn, influence the outcomes of ICU survivors following critical illness. Support of relatives contributes both to their own psychological health and to the recovery of the patient.

28.3.3 Psychological Effects

After discharge of a patient from the ICU, family members gain caregiver responsibilities that can create anxiety and stress. These feelings tend to be due to the unpredictability related to the patient's condition following discharge from ICU and changes in roles and responsibilities [43].

Researchers have investigated the prevalence of depression, anxiety, and PTSD among caregivers of ICU survivors, although not always exploring the specific factors that have contributed to developing psychological symptoms. A systematic review reported prevalence of depression that had an increasing trend from 3 months to 12 months after the patient's discharge (range between 12.2% and 26.2% at 3 months, 4.7% and 36.4% at 6 months, and 22.8% and 44% at 12 months) [30]. Anxiety tended to be higher at 3 months after discharge and reduced at 6 months (range between 24.4% and 62.5% at 3 months and 15% and 24% at 6 months). PTSD increased considerably in months following ICU discharge (between 29.8% and 42% at 3 months, 35% and 57.1% at 6 months, and 31.7% and 80% at 12 months). Similar findings are reported in an integrative review in which the included studies indicated a prevalence of moderate to severe depressive symptoms (20–43% of respondents) 2–3 months after ICU discharge [44]. In addition, 15–57% of relatives reported the presence of PTSD symptoms at up to 6 months after the patients' discharge from ICU. Up to one third of caregivers reported taking anxiolytics or antidepressants at 90 days that they had not required prior to the patient's admission to ICU [45, 46]. Interestingly, in a study of 280 caregivers, psychological outcomes did not appear to be related to patient demographics, clinical characteristics, and changes in patient functional and psychological outcomes over time; however, it was identified that younger caregivers were more likely to have worse psychological outcomes [47].

28.3.4 Physical Effects

Apart from psychological effects, the role of caregiving has also physical consequences. In a study of caregivers of ICU survivors, physical health among caregivers was low [47]. Older caregivers providing more assistance and having less sense of control had lower physical health scores.

There is some evidence to suggest that sleep is also affected among caregivers. This is quite significant as the caregiving ability of relatives can be affected by sleep deprivation. Van den Born (2016) suggests that the quality of sleep is continuously disrupted 3 months after discharge from critical care as around 40% of relatives reported sleeping difficulties in their study. Anxiety and strain because of the caregiving role appear to be major causes of insomnia [48]. Other factors such as support required by discharged patients or concerns about the physical status of the discharged patient during the night can also have an impact on sleeping patterns. Frivold et al. (2016, p. 397) described how carers were worried about their relative's vital functions such as "stopping breathing during the night."

28.3.5 Socioeconomic Effects

Adopting a caregiving role can have immense socioeconomic effects [30]. A caregiver-related systematic review reported that employment is reduced around 2 months after discharge, and two studies reported that almost 50% of caregivers, who had been employed at enrolment, reduced their work hours, quit their job, or were fired in order to provide informal care. Similarly, an integrative review inferred that after adopting a caregiving role, 25–48% of relatives reported a reduction in employment; they reduced their working hours, quit, or were fired [44]. In another study, one quarter of 94 caregivers had reduced their hours of gainful employment prior to ICU admission, and 2% had completely stopped working [21].

The social life of caregivers can also be affected. Choi and colleagues report that 75% of 69 caregivers in their study reported moderate or greater restrictions in visiting friends at 1 month after ICU discharge. Moderate or greater restrictions in participating in hobbies and recreation were reported by 48% of caregivers, but these subsided at 6 months. However, in the subgroup of patients who never regained their pre-ICU functional abilities, caregivers' lifestyle restrictions and distress were high and unchanged over 6 months' period [49].

28.3.6 Measurements

Caregiver burden has not been recognized in the International Classification of Diseases, Ninth Revision (ICD-9) or ICD-10, although the severity of this strain of caring might overshadow joy in life [23]. A range of instruments have been developed to measure caregivers' burden. They have been developed either for caregivers in general or for a specific condition. An example of a general caregiver instrument is the Carer Strain Index (CSI) which measures strain related to care provision from the caregivers' perspective including seven elements related to emotional adjustment, social issues, and physical and financial strain [50]. Each question is given one point. A score of 7 or higher is the generally accepted cutoff point indicating a high level of stress. Other validated general measurement tools include the Caregiver Well-Being Scale (CWBS) for which a short form has been devised [51, 52] and the Caregiver Burden Inventory (CBI) [53] or Caregiver Burden Scale (CBS) [54].

In comparison with general instruments, the Zarit Burden Interview (ZBI) is a 22-item questionnaire that was developed specifically for dementia patients in which caregivers self-assess their level of burden [18]. More recently it has also been validated for other neurological conditions. Each item of the questionnaire is a statement which the caregiver is asked to endorse using a 5-point scale. Response categories vary from 0 (Never) to 4 (Nearly Always). The total score ranges from 0 to 88 with interpretation as following: from 0 to 20, there is no or a low burden; from 21 to 40, the burden is mild to moderate; from 41 to 60, the burden is moderate to severe; and above 61 the burden is severe. As with other validated long questionnaires, a short form of the measurement tool has also been devised and tested in different diseases [55]. A few other disease specific tools exist in the measurement of caregiver burden such as the Caregiver Burden Questionnaire for Heart Failure (CBQ-HF) [56].

> **Consideration for Practice – A Case Scenario**
>
> Since Frances was discharged home, Harry has become her main caregiver. Although he had some training while being with his wife in hospital, he found the transition to home caring difficult, felt stressed, and started suffering with insomnia – "It is this sense of responsibility that I had to get used to as I was feeling a bit depressed. I obviously didn't want anything to happen to her under my supervision." Their son, who is self-employed, was initially able to reduce his working hours to support them but found the whole situation unmanageable and was considering the possibility of a nursing home. Harry categorically said no to that option, "obviously, our life has changed completely, and I need to help Frances in the morning with some of her personal care which I find physically hard to do – but I don't mind! I now feel physically fitter than I was before she became sick."

28.3.7 Coping Strategies

As alluded to in the introduction of this subchapter, the negative meaning of the word burden is not giving a realistic picture of what the provision of care means to individuals who deliver it on a day-to-day basis. Indeed, if we think in what context we discuss caregivers, we might recognize a subjective feeling of sorrow for someone who fulfills this role with a lot of pride. According to Lin et al. (2012), "negative and positive caregiving experiences are affected by caregivers' demographic characteristics, care recipients' problem behavior and dependency, caregivers' involvement, reciprocal help from care recipients, and social support available" [57]. Leading on from this, we need to consider the question of coping strategies that caregivers can use or intrinsically have to mitigate risks of negative consequences to their emotional and physical health and well-being, something also referred to as resilience [58].

According to Pearlin et al. (1990), coping together with social support forms part of the mediating conditions that influence how stress is being experienced by caregivers [59]. The thought that one can experience positive emotions during stressful times may also have a physiological explanation, for example, due to the release of endorphins and other immune responses. However, even during times of chronic stress, some evidence points to the fact that positive emotions can counterbalance the negative ones [60]. Folkman and Moskowitz (2000) refer to the process of positive reappraisal, which means a negative view of a situation is changed in such a way that it can be seen with a positive perspective in mind [61]. The intrinsic processes that are involved in this reappraisal are related to the value system of each individual which also explains why in the experimental setting people react differently to stressful situations even though the stressor is the same [62]. Relating this to the caregiver, older female family caregivers have been found to be more resilient than younger ones and cope better with higher mastery and self-esteem [63].

A systematic review of older caregivers investigating coping strategies identified four themes of coping mechanisms including problem-focused coping, emotion-focused coping, approach coping, and avoidance coping [64]. The problem-focused and emotion-focused coping framework was first recognized as the main scheme individuals may be able to deal with stressors [65]. Lazarus and Folkman concluded that if a source of a problem or a stressor can be identified, it can be managed or possibly removed. One such tool that can help to accomplish this is the S.M.A.R.T. mnemonic acronym goals approach (Specific, Measurable, Achievable, Realistic, Time-related), a mechanism widely used in project management, performance management, and personal development planning. In case the stressor cannot be managed, the emotion-focused mechanism might be utilized to deal with the stressor. Focusing on breathing, mindfulness, relaxation exercises, or distraction with pleasurable activities might help to prevent stress escalation. Since Lazarus and Folkman, other conceptual frameworks have been developed such as approach coping and avoidance coping [66]. The former relates to any emotional, cognitive, or behavioral activity directed towards the stressor in order to problem solve, while the latter is concerned with its denial or withdrawal.

28.4 Interventions to Support Caregivers

As critical illness of a loved one has enormous effects on family members during and after the ICU admission, we need to consider the interventions available to support these caregivers. Interventions during an ICU stay that are associated with improved family satisfaction include communication strategies, more liberal visiting policies, hiring support coordinators, direct involvement of family members in their relative's care, and patient- and family-friendly changes to the ICU structural environment [67–69]. Notably, the use of diaries has been promoted with varying significant effects on outcomes such as anxiety and post-traumatic stress in former ICU patients or their caregivers [70–73]. Practice guidelines about family-centered care are developing but are not well evidenced since research in this area is generally of low quality [74, 75]. Nevertheless, ICUs should provide families with leaflets that give information about the ICU setting to reduce anxiety and stress. As far as is known, no specific interventions for older caregivers have been introduced in ICU, as data from this specific group are scarce [22].

Overall, ICU professionals and management will need to decide which interventions are most suitable in current daily practice and how these should be implemented. Clear information and leaflets can provide a solid foundation for evidence-based family-centered care policy. Because of limited effectiveness of a single intervention, multifaceted and/or multidisciplinary sets of interventions are recommended [76].

28.4.1 Communication Strategies

Caregivers have an important role in the physical and psychosocial recovery process of the ICU patient [77, 78]. They can support their beloved ones in an emotional, cognitive, and practical way, provided that they themselves are able to cope with the stressful situation. They also might enhance the trust into the support network of the patient, a significant aid in the recovery process [79], and act as surrogate decision-makers [80]. This complex interaction of role requires a careful information and communication process that starts immediately after hospitalization.

Providing information to family members can mitigate insecurity and anxiety. It should include general or basic information on procedures, rules, and practices common in the ICU, for example, contact details, visiting hours, hygiene and isolation, monitoring, sounds, general treatment, and team composition. This could be presented in leaflets [81], although information via tablets [82] and web-based technologies [83] have shown promising possibilities. Moving from information to communication, by allowing family members to ask questions and voice their concerns on medical treatment and prognosis, will establish a high-quality relationship supportive to consensus regarding the goals of care [84]. It is crucial to take time for family conferences and monitor needs and non-verbal signals as well as the informational processes.

Communication between professionals and families is a key factor in experiences and satisfaction with care. Families appreciate conferences with ICU professionals which are routinely scheduled, having time set aside in a dedicated room, and where they felt listened to [85]. Conversations with families should be clear, honest, supportive, and comprehensive. In addition, detecting good and bad feelings, as well as anticipating requests, will build a relationship of trust, which is a requirement for shared decision-making.

Most studies on communication with caregivers in the ICU have found insufficient effectiveness of interventions tested. Difficulties to measure the effectiveness might be no specific directions of communication, an individualistic approach and outcome measures not sensitive enough to important changes [86]. The PARTNER (Pairing Re-engineered ICU Teams with Nurse-Driven Emotional Support and Relationship-Building) trial, which studied the effect of nurses who were specially trained on supporting the families daily according to a family-support pathway, did not significantly affect the family members' burden of psychological symptoms [87]. However, the families rated the quality of communication and the patient and family centeredness of care higher in the intervention group than the group with usual care. Another multicomponent intervention, including among others a family facilitator and several family meetings, found preliminary positive results with a reduction of depressive symptoms in bereaved family members at 6 months after death of the patient [88]. The results of this study suggested that early decision-making about withdrawing life support through a diligent communication process might reduce psychological burden in caregivers.

28.4.2 Digital Means

The COVID-19 pandemic influenced, among others, the visiting policies and communication with family members in the ICU. Due to the necessary quarantine measures, restricted presence at the bedside had his toll on levels of stress in relatives [89]. Therefore, existing or innovative digital means to enhance possibilities to interact were developed in fast-track processes. Videoconferencing from different digital platforms was employed across the globe as a method to communicate, both between the family members and their loved one and between the family members and the professional team. Although appreciated by all stakeholders, privacy, network, and functionality considerations limited the utility of commercially available video communication tools [90]. Newly created communication platforms, especially adapted to enable virtual family visits in a safe hospital setting, have been implemented as a response. It is encouraging that ICU teams are embracing and developing these new virtual communication techniques.

Some precaution should be considered in regard to elderly family members. The digital world is not as familiar or accessible to them as to younger people. Extra effort, for example, through clear and user-friendly instructions, is essential to support the use of digital communication tools. Offering digital devices such as tablets during the ICU admission of their loved one could also enable practical help in virtual connecting.

28.4.3 Use of Diaries

Diaries in ICUs have been used in several ways, mostly in the form of paper journal, hard- or softcover, including a short introduction and blank lines to make notes. In some settings, ICU nurses write in lay language the events and successive recovery processes [91], while in other ICUs the families are invited to participate or own the filling of the diary [92, 93]. In either way, the effect of a diary on PICS-F symptoms was found inconclusive. A block-randomized, single-blinded, controlled trial conducted at four medical-surgical ICUs has shown diaries to reduce symptoms of post-traumatic stress in relatives, although no effect was found on anxiety and depression [93]. Another study in 35 French ICUs did not support the use of diaries for preventing symptoms of post-traumatic stress [94]. Studies exploring the effectiveness of ICU diaries in reducing symptoms of PICS-F have often been conducted with small numbers of participants [95], various outcome measures, and length of follow-up

[96]. Other methodological challenges include lack of blinding and incomplete knowledge about the outcome measure of significance. Yet it is broadly accepted that a diary intervention has benefits for processing emotions for those relatives who have affinity with keeping notes for themselves or put effort in extensive journaling for future reading by their loved one.

Writing in a diary might be useful during the ICU stay by helping family members to assimilate and understand medical information [97]. In addition, they start doing a valuable activity, having a focus and hope for the future when their loved one is recovering. The diary supports the urge to discuss the ICU period in the aftermath of critical illness, which could be beneficial for both the former ICU patient and the family member. Thus, writing a diary might contribute to their perceived quality of life.

28.4.4 Bereavement Support

Highly valued aspects of care in the relatives' perspective, particularly during the dying and death process of the patient, are effective communication with ICU professionals, professionals' empathic attitudes, and personalized interactions [98]. When a patient is approaching death in the ICU, relatives need to make a rapid transition from focusing on the recovery of their beloved one to preparing for their unavoidable death. Supporting this bereavement process of relatives has been incorporated into the daily care offerings of professionals worldwide [99]. A multicenter randomized clinical trial to determine the effect of informational and emotional support meetings for caregivers of patients with chronic critical illness led by palliative care specialists reported no effects in clinical outcomes such as anxiety and depression [100, 101]. Therefore, other potential interventions should be taken into account. In today's society and culture, talking about death is not always taken for granted. Therefore, the added value of research projects in this domain is to improve psychosocial care for family members during and after the death of their loved one, thus reducing long-term grieving and disruption in personal life.

28.4.5 Discharge Support

Discharge from the ICU might provoke relocation stress in patients due to less monitoring and reduced number of professionals [102]. Despite a big step forward in the recovery process of the patient, this transfer to a general ward might also be accompanied with insecurity among family members. An informational package guiding the discharge from the ICU seemed a promising intervention to prepare both the patients and their caregivers on upcoming physical rehabilitation and emotional distress [103]. In contrast, the preparation and guidance of discharge from the ICU by a liaison nurse were not effective in reducing family members' anxiety [104]. To support the family members after discharge, general practitioners have ongoing opportunities to assess, monitor, and manage the health of those who are in mental distress. However, usually general practitioner contact has to be initiated by the caregivers themselves [105].

Follow-up programs, including ICU outpatient clinics, should be tailored to caregivers' needs and health status. However, in most countries caregivers still do not receive the attention and recognition they deserve. A practical drawback is the lack of a formal treatment agreement with the ICU team, and consequently support services have hardly focused on this group.

> **Consideration for Practice – A Case Scenario**
>
> While Harry was residing near the hospital for most of Frances' stay, they both developed relationships with some of the hospital staff. Once home, the occupational therapist and ICU follow-up team contacted them a couple of times to ascertain if they required any further support. They also made an appointment with the ICU consultant for a visit of the intensive care unit, on which occasion the liaison nurse handed them a patient diary which had been completed during Frances's admission. Overall, both were happy with the support they had received throughout their hospital stay but also acknowledged that communication with all the different people was challenging. Harry said, "I initially felt overwhelmed with all the professionals there and did not know who was doing what. It took me a considerable amount of time to get used to that situation." The liaison nurse got them in touch with the local peer support group which met every 3 months.
>
> At home, with the support from neighbors, carers, and children the situation had improved, and a daily routine was established. Frances made progress gaining back some of her strength and it seemed that both reassured their children that they were able to cope at their own home.

28.4.6 Peer Support

Peer support is acknowledged as a method; individuals can face, accept, and overcome the challenges arising from a stressful event [106]. In peer support groups, participating people share experiences, talk with each other, recognize emotions, and provide and receive informal support. They help each other to learn how to manage feelings and situations, which might lead to acceptance of the person they are right at the moment. Peer support is hypothesized to act by building social relationships that have a reciprocal influence on health and well-being, as shown in patients with cancer and depression [107]. Through peer support both former ICU patients and the family members realize that they are not alone and that others understand what they are going through.

One of the first critical care peer support groups was set up by the patient charity ICU steps, who continue to run several groups in the UK [108]. Variance in the design of these groups exists in frequency and location of the meetings; leading committee such as patient experts, ICU nurses, or other healthcare professionals; the number of attendances; and funding [106]. Among the Society of Critical Care Medicine Thrive Peer Support Collaborative, with 17 sites from the USA, UK, and Australia, six general models of peer support were identified: community-based, psychologist-led outpatient, models based within ICU follow-up clinics, online, groups based within ICU, and peer mentor models [107].

Few studies have investigated peer support interventions in critical care cohorts. Although of generally low quality, the existing studies indicate that peer support has potential to reduce psychological morbidity and increase social support [109]. The most common barriers to implementation were recruitment to groups, personnel input and training, sustainability and funding, risk management, and measuring success.

As Groves et al. (2020) advised from the perspectives of former ICU patients and their family members, peer support should be offered in a standard way to support dealing with the psychological distress after an ICU admission [106].

Conclusion

Becoming a caregiver is a common occurrence within our society, and individual healthcare systems have developed policy recommendations to support the informal caregiving sector with varied success. Most recent policy proposals are geared towards the assistance of those who need care in their own homes, moving them away from the institutional long-term care sector. This narrative has a significant impact on caregivers and is further exacerbated by the more complex caring needs of an aging population. An ever-growing body of evidence points towards increased responsibilities on behalf of caregivers which result in burden, psychological morbidity, and an impact on their socioeconomic status. Less studied in the scientific debate is the positive impact that caregiving may hold for those fulfilling this role.

In this chapter, we outlined the main themes impacting caregivers in the transition into this important role and how they can be supported. While they fulfill many different functions willingly and without protest, their impact on the wider society is not fully appreciated, particularly when taking into account their economic benefit. As such, family-centered care is important by using interventions that will prepare and support caregivers during and after a hospital stay. The lack of strong evidence on interventions does not allow us to recommend a specific one. However, the use of diaries and peer support appear to be helpful. In addition, technology (digital means) can offer some solutions but will have to be simple. More research is needed to identify older caregivers' needs and how to address them as they are more likely to have comorbidities and problems in accessing support services. Therefore, taking care of the caregivers involved, and supporting their adaptation to the new situation, is essential to deliver high-quality care.

Take-Home Messages

- Caregivers provide an invaluable service to society that is only going to increase in an aging population.
- Policymakers should ensure that there is societal recognition of the unpaid services that caregivers provide.
- Policy solutions should focus on the recognition of the complexity of care required by patients and the development of associated services.
- More evidence on interventions is required to make clear recommendations on which work best to support caregivers.

References

1. Theobald H. Combining welfare mix and new public management: the case of long-term care insurance in Germany. Int J Soc Welf. 2012;21:S61–74.
2. Office for National Statistics. Living longer: caring in later working life. 2021. Retrieved from https://www.ons.gov.uk/peoplepopulationandcommunity/birthsdeathsandmarriages/ageing/articles/livinglongerhowourpopulationischangingandwhyitmatters/2019-03-15.
3. OECD Informal carers. 2017. https://doi.org/10.1787/health_glance-2017-78-en.
4. AARP 2020. Caregiving in the US. 2020. Retrieved from https://www.aarp.org/content/dam/aarp/ppi/2020/05/full-report-caregiving-in-the-united-states.doi.10.26419-2Fppi.00103.001.pdf.
5. Institute of Medicine (US) Committee on the Future Health Care Workforce for Older Americans. Retooling for an aging America: building the health care workforce. Washington (DC): National Academies Press (US); 2008.
6. Lilleheie I, et al. The tension between carrying a burden and feeling like a burden: a qualitative study of informal caregivers' and care recipients' experiences after patient discharge from hospital. Int J Qual Stud Health Well Being. 2021;16(1):1855751.
7. Tramm R, et al. Experience and needs of family members of patients treated with extracorporeal membrane oxygenation. J Clin Nurs. 2017;26(11–12):1657–68.
8. Pandharipande PP, et al. Long-term cognitive impairment after critical illness. N Engl J Med. 2013;369(14):1306–16.
9. Rengel KF, et al. Long-term cognitive and functional impairments after critical illness. Anesth Analg. 2019;128(4):772–80.
10. Sullivan AB, Miller D. Who is taking care of the caregiver? J Patient Exp. 2015;2(1):7–12.
11. van Beusekom I, et al. Dutch ICU survivors have more consultations with general practitioners before and after ICU admission compared to a matched control group from the general population. PLoS One. 2019;14(5):e0217225.
12. Kulnik ST, Wulf A-K, Brunker C. Experiences of long-distance visitors to intensive care units at a regional major trauma centre in the United Kingdom: a cross-sectional survey. Intensive Crit Care Nurs. 2019;55:102754.
13. Keating NC, et al. A taxonomy of the economic costs of family care to adults. J Econ Ageing. 2014;3:11–20.
14. Lambert SD, et al. Impact of informal caregiving on older adults' physical and mental health in low-income and middle-income countries: a cross-sectional, secondary analysis based on the WHO's Study on global AGEing and adult health (SAGE). BMJ Open. 2017;7(11):e017236.
15. Mitchell ML, et al. A family intervention to reduce delirium in hospitalised ICU patients: a feasibility randomised controlled trial. Intensive Crit Care Nurs. 2017;40:77–84.
16. Martínez F, et al. Implementing a multicomponent intervention to prevent delirium among critically ill patients. Crit Care Nurse. 2017;37(6):36–46.
17. Teixeira M, et al. Understanding family caregivers' needs to support relatives with advanced disease at home: an ethnographic study in rural Portugal. BMC Palliat Care. 2020;19:73.
18. Zarit SH, Reever KE, Bach-Peterson J. Relatives of the impaired elderly: correlates of feelings of burden. The Gerontologist. 1980;20(6):649–55.
19. Choi J, Son Y-J, Tate JA. Exploring positive aspects of caregiving in family caregivers of adult ICU survivors from ICU to four months post-ICU discharge. Heart Lung. 2019;48(6):553–9.
20. Potier F, et al. A high sense of coherence protects from the burden of caregiving in older spousal caregivers. Arch Gerontol Geriatr. 2018;75:76–82.
21. van den Born-van Zanten S, et al. Caregiver strain and posttraumatic stress symptoms of informal caregivers of intensive care unit survivors. Rehabil Psychol. 2016;61(2):173.
22. Vallet H, et al. Acute critically ill elderly patients: what about long term caregiver burden? J Crit Care. 2019;54:180–4.
23. Adelman RD, et al. Caregiver burden: a clinical review. JAMA. 2014;311(10):1052–60.
24. Kamiya M, et al. Factors associated with increased caregivers' burden in several cognitive stages of A lzheimer's disease. Geriatr Gerontol Int. 2014;14:45–55.
25. Garlo K, et al. Burden in caregivers of older adults with advanced illness. J Am Geriatr Soc. 2010;58(12):2315–22.

26. Douglas SL, et al. Impact of a disease management program upon caregivers of chronically critically ill patients. Chest. 2005;128(6):3925–36.

27. Harvey MA, Davidson JE. Postintensive care syndrome: right care, right now… and later. Crit Care Med. 2016;44(2):381–5.

28. Needham DM, et al. Improving long-term outcomes after discharge from intensive care unit: report from a stakeholders' conference. Crit Care Med. 2012;40(2):502–9.

29. Davidson JE, Jones C, Bienvenu OJ. Family response to critical illness: postintensive care syndrome–family. Crit Care Med. 2012;40(2):618–24.

30. van Beusekom I, et al. Reported burden on informal caregivers of ICU survivors: a literature review. Crit Care. 2015;20(1):1–8.

31. Siegel MD, et al. Psychiatric illness in the next of kin of patients who die in the intensive care unit. Crit Care Med. 2008;36(6):1722–8.

32. Azoulay É, Kentish-Barnes N, Pochard F. Health-related quality of life: an outcome variable in critical care survivors. Chest. 2008;133(2):339–41.

33. Kentish-Barnes N, et al. Complicated grief after death of a relative in the intensive care unit. Eur Respir J. 2015;45(5):1341–52.

34. Savelkoul C, et al. Culturally sensitive communication in end-of-life care: the care for Muslim patients as an example. Ned Tijdschr Geneeskd. 2017;161:–D1410.

35. Lautrette A, et al. A communication strategy and brochure for relatives of patients dying in the ICU. N Engl J Med. 2007;356(5):469–78.

36. Kentish-Barnes N, et al. Effect of a condolence letter on grief symptoms among relatives of patients who died in the ICU: a randomized clinical trial. Intensive Care Med. 2017;43(4):473–84.

37. van Mol MM, et al. Developing and testing a nurse-led intervention to support bereavement in relatives in the intensive care (BRIC study): a protocol of a pre-post intervention study. BMC Palliat Care. 2020;19(1):1–10.

38. Inoue S, et al. Post-intensive care syndrome: its pathophysiology, prevention, and future directions. Acute Med Surg. 2019;6(3):233–46.

39. Geense WW, et al. New physical, mental, and cognitive problems 1-year post-ICU: a prospective multicenter study. Am J Respir Crit Care Med. 2021;203(12):1512–21.

40. Fuke R, et al. Early rehabilitation to prevent postintensive care syndrome in patients with critical illness: a systematic review and meta-analysis. BMJ Open. 2018;8(5):e019998.

41. Lee M, Kang J, Jeong YJ. Risk factors for post–intensive care syndrome: a systematic review and meta-analysis. Aust Crit Care. 2020;33(3):287–94.

42. Manning JC, et al. Conceptualizing post intensive care syndrome in children—the PICS-p framework. Pediatr Crit Care Med. 2018;19(4):298–300.

43. Frivold G, Slettebø Å, Dale B. Family members' lived experiences of everyday life after intensive care treatment of a loved one: a phenomenological hermeneutical study. J Clin Nurs. 2016;25(3–4):392–402.

44. Stayt LC, Venes TJ. Outcomes and experiences of relatives of patients discharged home after critical illness: a systematic integrative review. Nurs Crit Care. 2019;24(3):162–75.

45. Lemiale V, et al. Health-related quality of life in family members of intensive care unit patients. J Palliat Med. 2010;13(9):1131–7.

46. De Miranda S, et al. Postintensive care unit psychological burden in patients with chronic obstructive pulmonary disease and informal caregivers: a multicenter study. Crit Care Med. 2011;39(1):112–8.

47. Cameron JI, et al. One-year outcomes in caregivers of critically ill patients. N Engl J Med. 2016;374(19):1831–41.

48. McPeake J, et al. Caregiver strain following critical care discharge: an exploratory evaluation. J Crit Care. 2016;35:180–4.

49. Choi J, et al. Caregivers of the chronically critically ill after discharge from the intensive care unit: six months' experience. Am J Crit Care. 2011;20(1):12–23.

50. Robinson BC. Validation of a caregiver strain index. J Gerontol. 1983;38(3):344–8.

51. Berg-Weger M, Rubio DM, Tebb SS. The caregiver well-being scale revisited. Health Soc Work. 2000;25(4):255–63.

52. Tebb SS, Berg-Weger M, Rubio DM. The caregiver well-being scale: developing a short-form rapid assessment instrument. Health Soc Work. 2013;38(4):222–30.

53. Novak M, Guest C. Application of a multidimensional caregiver burden inventory. The Gerontologist. 1989;29(6):798–803.
54. Fukahori H, et al. Psychometric properties of the caregiving burden scale for family caregivers with relatives in nursing homes: scale development. Jpn J Nurs Sci. 2010;7(2):136–47.
55. Higginson IJ, et al. Short-form Zarit caregiver burden interviews were valid in advanced conditions. J Clin Epidemiol. 2010;63(5):535–42.
56. Humphrey L, et al. The caregiver burden questionnaire for heart failure (CBQ-HF): face and content validity. Health Qual Life Outcomes. 2013;11(1):1–12.
57. Lin IF, Fee HR, Wu HS. Negative and positive caregiving experiences: a closer look at the intersection of gender and relationship. Fam Relat. 2012;61(2):343–58.
58. Folkman S. The Oxford handbook of stress, health, and coping. Oxford: Oxford University Press; 2011.
59. Pearlin LI, et al. Caregiving and the stress process: an overview of concepts and their measures. The Gerontologist. 1990;30(5):583–94.
60. Folkman S, et al. Caregiver burden in HIV-positive and HIV-negative partners of men with AIDS. J Consult Clin Psychol. 1994;62(4):746.
61. Folkman S, Moskowitz JT. Stress, positive emotion, and coping. Curr Dir Psychol Sci. 2000;9(4):115–8.
62. Schneiderman N, Ironson G, Siegel SD. Stress and health: psychological, behavioral, and biological determinants. Annu Rev Clin Psychol. 2005;1:607–28.
63. Carter JH, et al. Does age make a difference in caregiver strain? Comparison of young versus older caregivers in early-stage Parkinson's disease. Mov Disord. 2010;25(6):724–30.
64. del Pino Casado R, et al. Coping and subjective burden in caregivers of older relatives: a quantitative systematic review. J Adv Nurs. 2011;67(11):2311–22.
65. Lazarus RS, Folkman S. Stress, appraisal, and coping. New York: Springer; 1984.
66. Roth S, Cohen LJ. Approach, avoidance, and coping with stress. Am Psychol. 1986;41(7):813.
67. Goldfarb MJ, et al. Outcomes of patient-and family-centered care interventions in the ICU: a systematic review and meta-analysis. Crit Care Med. 2017;45(10):1751–61.
68. Junior APN, et al. Flexible versus restrictive visiting policies in ICUs: a systematic review and meta-analysis. Crit Care Med. 2018;46(7):1175–80.
69. Scheunemann LP, et al. Randomized, controlled trials of interventions to improve communication in intensive care: a systematic review. Chest. 2011;139(3):543–54.
70. Barreto BB, et al. The impact of intensive care unit diaries on patients' and relatives' outcomes: a systematic review and meta-analysis. Crit Care. 2019;23(1):411.
71. McIlroy PA, et al. The effect of ICU diaries on psychological outcomes and quality of life of survivors of critical illness and their relatives: a systematic review and meta-analysis. Crit Care Med. 2019;47(2):273–9.
72. Ullman AJ, et al. Intensive care diaries to promote recovery for patients and families after critical illness: a Cochrane systematic review. Int J Nurs Stud. 2015;52(7):1243–53.
73. Nielsen AH, Angel S. How diaries written for critically ill influence the relatives: a systematic review of the literature. Nurs Crit Care. 2016;21(2):88–96.
74. Davidson JE, et al. Guidelines for family-centered care in the neonatal, pediatric, and adult ICU. Crit Care Med. 2017;45(1):103–28.
75. Gerritsen RT, Hartog CS, Curtis JR. New developments in the provision of family-centered care in the intensive care unit. Intensive Care Med. 2017;43(4):550–3.
76. Zante B, Camenisch SA, Schefold JC. Interventions in post-intensive care syndrome-family: a systematic literature review. Crit Care Med. 2020;48(9):e835–40.
77. Verhaeghe STL, et al. The focus of family members' functioning in the acute phase of traumatic coma part two: protecting from suffering and protecting what remains to rebuild life. J Clin Nurs. 2010;19(3–4):583–9.
78. Bailey JJ, et al. Supporting families in the ICU: a descriptive correlational study of informational support, anxiety, and satisfaction with care. Intensive Crit Care Nurs. 2010;26(2):114–22.
79. Thüm S, et al. The association between psychosocial care by physicians and patients' trust: a retrospective analysis of severely injured patients in surgical intensive care units. Psycho-Social-Medicine. 2012;9:Doc04.
80. van Mol M, et al. Relatives' perspectives on the quality of care in an intensive care unit: the theoretical concept of a new tool. Patient Educ Couns. 2014;95(3):406–13.

81. Kleinpell R, et al. Patient and family engagement in the ICU: report from the task force of the World Federation of Societies of Intensive and Critical Care Medicine. J Crit Care. 2018;48:251–6.

82. Chiang VCL, et al. Fulfilling the psychological and information need of the family members of critically ill patients using interactive mobile technology: a randomised controlled trial. Intensive Crit Care Nurs. 2017;41:77–83.

83. Nguyen Y-L. Dealing with internet-based information obtained by families of critically ill patients. Intensive Care Med. 2019;45(8):1119–22.

84. Azoulay E, et al. Questions to improve family–staff communication in the ICU: a randomized controlled trial. Intensive Care Med. 2018;44(11):1879–87.

85. Garrouste-Orgeas M, et al. Impact of proactive nurse participation in ICU family conferences: a mixed-method study. Crit Care Med. 2016;44(6):1116–28.

86. Curtis JR, et al. Development and evaluation of an interprofessional communication intervention to improve family outcomes in the ICU. Contemp Clin Trials. 2012;33(6):1245–54.

87. White DB, et al. A randomized trial of a family-support intervention in intensive care units. N Engl J Med. 2018;378(25):2365–75.

88. Curtis JR, et al. Randomized trial of communication facilitators to reduce family distress and intensity of end-of-life care. Am J Respir Crit Care Med. 2016;193(2):154–62.

89. Azoulay E, Kentish-Barnes N. A 5-point strategy for improved connection with relatives of critically ill patients with COVID-19. Lancet Respir Med. 2020;8(6):E52.

90. Montauk TR, Kuhl EA. COVID-related family separation and trauma in the intensive care unit. Psychol Trauma Theory Res Pract Policy. 2020;12(S1):S96–7.

91. Gjengedal E, et al. An act of caring - patient diaries in Norwegian intensive care units. Nurs Crit Care. 2010;15(4):176–84.

92. Engström Å, Grip K, Hamrén M. Experiences of intensive care unit diaries: 'touching a tender wound'. Nurs Crit Care. 2009;14(2):61–7.

93. Nielsen AH, et al. The effect of family-authored diaries on posttraumatic stress disorder in intensive care unit patients and their relatives: a randomised controlled trial (DRIP-study). Aust Crit Care. 2020;33(2):123–9.

94. Garrouste-Orgeas M, et al. Effect of an ICU diary on posttraumatic stress disorder symptoms among patients receiving mechanical ventilation: a randomized clinical trial. JAMA. 2019;322(3):229–39.

95. Knowles RE, Tarrier N. Evaluation of the effect of prospective patient diaries on emotional Well-being in intensive care unit survivors: a randomized controlled trial. Crit Care Med. 2009;37(1):184–91.

96. Garrouste-Orgeas M, et al. Impact of an intensive care unit diary on psychological distress in patients and relatives. Crit Care Med. 2012;40(7):2033–40.

97. Garrouste-Orgeas M, et al. Writing in and reading ICU diaries: qualitative study of families' experience in the ICU. PLoS One. 2014;9(10):e110146.

98. Kentish-Barnes N, Chevret S, Azoulay E. Guiding intensive care physicians' communication and behavior towards bereaved relatives: study protocol for a cluster randomized controlled trial (COSMIC-EOL). Trials. 2018;19(1):698.

99. Aslakson R, Spronk P. Tasking the tailor to cut the coat: how to optimize individualized ICU-based palliative care? Intensive Care Med. 2016;42(1):119–21, Springer.

100. Carson SS, et al. Effect of palliative care–led meetings for families of patients with chronic critical illness: a randomized clinical trial. JAMA. 2016;316(1):51–62.

101. Efstathiou N, et al. The state of bereavement support in adult intensive care: a systematic review and narrative synthesis. J Crit Care. 2019;50:177–87.

102. Bench S, Day T. The user experience of critical care discharge: a meta-synthesis of qualitative research. Int J Nurs Stud. 2010;47(4):487–99.

103. Bench S, et al. Evaluating the feasibility and effectiveness of a critical care discharge information pack for patients and their families: a pilot cluster randomised controlled trial. BMJ Open. 2015;5(11):e006852.

104. Chaboyer W, et al. The effect of an ICU liaison nurse on patients and family's anxiety prior to transfer to the ward: an intervention study. Intensive Crit Care Nurs. 2007;23(6):362–9.

105. van Sleeuwen D, et al. Health problems among family caregivers of former intensive care unit (ICU) patients: an interview study. BJGP Open. 2020;4(4):bjgpopen20X101061.

106. Groves J, et al. Patient support groups: a survey of United Kingdom practice, purpose and performance. J Intensive Care Soc. 2020;22(4):300–4.

107. McPeake J, et al. Models of peer support to remediate post-intensive care syndrome: a report developed by the SCCM thrive international peer support collaborative. Crit Care Med. 2019;47(1):e21.
108. Peskett M, Gibb P. Developing and setting up a patient and relatives intensive care support group. Nurs Crit Care. 2009;14(1):4–10.
109. Haines KJ, et al. Peer support in critical care: a systematic review. Crit Care Med. 2018;46(9):1522–31.

Specific Diseases and Conditions

Contents

Acute Respiratory Failure

Marta Lorente-Ros, Antonio Artigas, and José A. Lorente

Contents

Learning Objectives

In this chapter the reader will learn the basics of age-related changes in respiratory physiology and in inflammatory response and immune function pertaining to acute respiratory failure. The different clinical manifestation, susceptibility to acute lung injury, response to treatments of acute respiratory failure (ARF), and physiology of weaning that characterize the elderly, as compared to younger patients, will also be reviewed here.

Practical Implications

In the elderly, loss of elastic tissue surrounding the alveoli and alveolar ducts, increased anteroposterior diameter, and decreased elastance are associated with lung collapse at the lung bases (where intrapleural pressure is less negative), ventilation/perfusion mismatch, decreased muscle strength and decreased vital capacity, forced expiratory volume in 1 second (FEV1), and FEV1/forced vital capacity.

Aging is associated with low-grade inflammation and immune dysfunction (inflammaging and immunosenescence).

In the elderly, the presenting signs and symptoms of ARF are often not respiratory. The incidence of acute lung injury increases markedly with age.

29.1 Introduction

ARF requiring mechanical ventilation has some specific peculiarities with pathophysiological, treatment, and prognostic implications. These peculiarities include age-dependent changes in respiratory physiology, increased susceptibility to respiratory failure after a given insult, longer intensive care unit (ICU) length of stay, increased ICU cost, and increased healthcare cost after ICU discharge [1–4].

Advanced age is associated with less aggressive ICU treatment, more frequent ICU admission refusal, and more frequent withholding of mechanical ventilation, as compared with younger patients [5–7]. Determining the causes of these differences and whether they are associated with different outcomes as compared to the younger patient population need to be studied.

The effectiveness of therapies commonly used in patients with ARF may differ in the elderly. Physiological changes in respiratory system mechanics and immune function could determine different responses to specific therapies in the elderly as compared to younger patients. Thus, efforts to prove specifically in the aged population the effectiveness of therapies commonly used in patients with ARF, including infection prevention measures, sedation protocols, and transfusion practices, as well as advanced treatments for refractory hypoxemia, are warranted.

29.2 Changes in Respiratory Physiology Associated with Aging

The most important physiological changes in respiratory physiology are (i) loss of elastic tissue surrounding the alveoli and alveolar ducts; (ii) increased anteroposterior diameter of the chest; and (iii) decreased muscle strength (▶ Box 29.1).

Morphological changes include increased size of the trachea, large bronchi, and alveolar ducts. The alveolar sacs thicken, and the alveoli become dilated. Intra-alveolar fenestration decreases alveolar surface area [8]. Associated functional changes include smaller and more collapsible distal airways and decreased gas exchange surface. Unlike in emphysema, there is no septal destruction, but decreased elastic tissue and increased collagen associated with aging. The mechanism underlying the loss of elastic tissue is probably a low-grade inflammation and increased oxidative stress. There is also increased neutrophil count in the bronchoalveolar lavage (BAL) fluid and neutrophil elastase, whose relative role in the loss of elastic tissue is not known [9].

Aging is associated with decreased outward chest wall force and decreased inward elastic recoil (elastance); therefore, total lung capacity remains unchanged. But because elastance decreases more than chest wall recoil, there is an age-related increase in residual volume with a stable total lung capacity, resulting in decreased vital capacity [10]. Vital capacity is related to the probability of death and to the risk of myocardial infarction, indicating that the decline in vital capacity is a reflection of the general state of health.

The decrease in elastance also leads to a decrease in maximal expiratory flow rates measured as a decline in forced expiratory volume in 1 second (FEV1) and FEV1/forced vital capacity (FVC) ratio [11]. Since maximal expiratory flow rates decrease and residual volume increases, increases in minute ventilation requirements are met by an increased respiratory rate rather than by an increased tidal volume.

As closing volume approaches functional residual capacity, small airways tend to close during expiration, when intrapleural pressure becomes less negative. Areas of lung collapse appear at the lung bases (where intrapleural pressure is less negative than in the apex), and ventilation decreases in the dependent lung regions, leading to V/Q mismatch, increased alveolar-arterial oxygen tension difference, and hypoxemia. PaO_2 can increase during deep breaths, minimizing early airway closure [9–11].

Changes in shape and function of the chest wall in the elderly are related to osteoporosis, kyphosis, and costovertebral joint changes and are associated with decreased chest wall compliance and increased anteroposterior diameter of the thorax. The resulting flattening of the diaphragm and decreased radius of the diaphragm lead to decreased maximum pressure generated. Although the response of the respiratory system to physical exertion seems to be preserved, the response to hypoxia and hypercapnia is less vigorous in older adults [12].

Box 29.1   Specific Considerations on Acute Respiratory Failure in Elderly Patients

- **Demographic and clinical factors**
  - Increased proportion of elderly patients in the ICU
  - Increased risk of acute respiratory failure
  - Unknown response to therapies shown to be effective in other age groups
  - Possible increased susceptibility to ventilator-induced lung injury
- **Physiological changes**
  - Loss of elastic recoil
  - Increased closing volume

- Decreased chest wall compliance
- Increased lung compliance
- Increased residual volume
- Collapse of the dependent lung regions
- FEV1 and FEV1/FVC decline
- Forced vital capacity decreases
- Decreased response to hypoxia or hypercapnia
- Increased anteroposterior diameter of the thorax
- Flattening of the diaphragm
- **Prognostic factors**
  - Age
  - Comorbidities
  - Frailty
  - Cognition decline
  - Activity of daily life
  - Severity of acute illness

29.3   Changes in Cardiovascular Physiology and ARF

Cardiovascular changes related to aging are pertinent for a better understanding of ARF in the elderly. Aging is associated with a decreased myocyte number, maximal heart rate, myocardial contractility, coronary flow reserve, ventricular compliance and beta-adrenoceptor-mediated inotropism, and increased myocardial collagen content [9, 13]. Elderly patients present an increased prevalence of hypertension as a result of decreased arterial distensibility which leads to increased afterload. Subsequently, compensatory myocyte hypertrophy, left ventricular hypertrophy, and decreased left ventricular ejection fraction ensue.

The elderly is characterized by reduced sympathetic responsiveness, and during periods of stress, an inappropriate increase in heart rate may lead to inadequate cardiac output. Given the high prevalence of diastolic dysfunction, older patients are more susceptible to hypovolemia, and a normal preload is critical to maintain cardiac output. In the context of diastolic dysfunction and ventricular hypertrophy, ventricular relaxation is altered and may become more apparent during episodes of hypoxemia, resulting in heart failure (HF). Given the diminished functional reserve, rate-related ischemia may develop in conditions of increased metabolic demand or sepsis. Older patients often have atypical symptoms of HF including fatigue, failure to thrive, somnolence, weakness, and altered mental status as well as symptoms of volume overload [9, 13].

Age-related changes in the pulmonary circulation include intimal fibrosis, loss of capillaries, and decreased pulmonary artery distensibility. Pulmonary artery pressure is normal at rest but increases excessively during exercise [9, 13]. Because of the decreased number of capillaries, diffusing capacity declines over time.

The relationship between cardiac and respiratory changes should be underlined. For instance, an episode of respiratory infection may precipitate HF, and low cardiac output may lead to diaphragmatic hypoperfusion, alveolar hypoventilation, and cardiac arrest in a patient with reduced respiratory reserve.

Sedation, analgesic treatment, and tracheal intubation may make the diagnosis of acute myocardial infarction (AMI) difficult. Elevation of troponin can be due to many causes other than myocardial ischemia due to coronary artery thrombus formation. In a single-center study of medical ICU patients [14], among 93 patients with at least 1 electrocardiogram (ECG) and 1 troponin measurement, 44 (47.3%) had at least 1 elevated troponin, and 24 (25.8%) had AMI. Worsening clinical status or difficulty weaning from mechanical ventilation should prompt inquiry into the possibility of myocardial ischemia in the ICU.

29.4 Inflammatory Response and Immune Function in ARF

The incidence and mortality of acute respiratory distress syndrome (ARDS) increase with age [15–17]. This worse outcome in the elderly seems to be independent of comorbidities [18–20] suggesting that ARDS in young adults and in the elderly may not obey the same pathophysiology. Well-described changes in the function of the immune system, in the inflammatory response, and in the biological pathways involved in the host response to injurious pulmonary and non-pulmonary insults in the different age groups may play roles in the observed clinical differences.

Aged individuals exhibit a persistent low-grade innate immune activation generating a constitutive proinflammatory environment (inflammaging) as well as a gradual deterioration of the immune system (immunosenescence) [21, 22]. Differences in neonates and adults in the immune and inflammatory response include less absolute number of neutrophils, immaturity of the proliferative pool, lower expression of adhesion molecules, less production of chemotactic mediators by resident inflammatory cells, and reduced responsiveness and diminished extravasation of white cells [23]. Increasing age is associated with increased endothelial-epithelial permeability, altered function of alveolar macrophages, increased influx of neutrophils, exaggerated inflammatory mediator response, and increased oxidative stress [24].

Other aging-associated alterations in the inflammatory response include dysfunctional immune cells, senescent cells that secrete proinflammatory cytokines, and deficient autophagy [22]. Recent evidence indicates that neutrophils from humans of advanced age show untargeted tissue migration with increased primary granule release and neutrophil elastase activity leading to more tissue inflammation [25]. This may in part explain the marked inflammatory cell recruitment and extensive alveolar damage found in elderly animals with lung injury. In addition, aging in general is associated with changes in intracellular signaling pathways involved in inflammation and cell integrity and overactivation of nuclear factor-kB pathway.

There are age-related differences in proteolytic activity of sheddases [26, 27] which is important as P-selectin and intercellular adhesion molecule (ICAM)-1 are known to be cleaved by different enzymes, and levels of adhesion molecules in BAL fluid are the result of both protein expression and proteolytic activity of sheddases [28].

With increasing age, the balance between the two main enzymes of the pulmonary renin-angiotensin system (RAS), angiotensin-converting enzyme (ACE) and its natural counteracting enzyme ACE2, shifts toward the lung injurious axis (i.e., ACE), an imbalance that has been associated with aggravating inflammation and increased lung injury [24, 29–31].

Mesenchymal stem cells (MSCs) possess the ability to protect the endothelium and the alveolar epithelium through multiple paracrine mechanisms. Young bone marrow MSCs (B-MSCs) exert protective effect in animal models of LPS-induced injury [32–36]. Thus, a role of MSC in age-related increased susceptibility to lung injury has been proposed. Aged B-MSCs exhibit reduced migration and expression of soluble factors compared with young B-MSCs. Gene expression of several cytokine and chemokine receptors such as tumor necrosis factor receptor (TNFR), IFN-gamma receptor (IFNGR), and CCR7 decreases in aged B-MSCs. In in vivo experiments, it was shown by adoptive transfer of aged B-MSCs to young mice treated with LPS that aged cells lacked the anti-inflammatory protective effect of young B-MSCs and that aged B-MSCs have lower migration rates in a classical parabiosis model independently of the age of the injured animal. Aged B-MSCs were associated with increased severity of lung injury [32]. In summary, the decreased expression of cytokine and chemokine receptors in aged B-MSCs compromises their protective role by impairing their activation and migration to the site of injury.

In a recent systematic review [37], Schouten et al. analyzed 51 studies in animal models in which at least 2 age groups were compared. Studies showed that, in response to a pulmonary insult, increasing age is associated with more marked neutrophil infiltration, pulmonary inflammation, edema and alveolar damage, and a higher mortality. In addition, results indicate the existence of age-dependent changes in key components of the intracellular signaling pathways involved in the inflammatory response. The results of this meta-analysis [37] indicate that care should be taken when extrapolating results from preclinical models (generally in young adult animals) [37–39] to adult clinical practice.

Schouten et al. [40] conducted the first clinical study in which the pulmonary host response in ARDS was compared between patients of different age groups. The authors studied 20 neonates (<28 days), 29 children (28 days–18 years), 26 adults (18–65 years), and 17 older adults (>65 years of age). They found that BAL fluid levels of myeloperoxidase, IL-6, IL-10, and P-selectin were higher with increasing age, whereas ICAM-1 followed the opposite pattern (higher in neonates). The reported age-dependent differences in proteolytic activity of sheddases [26, 27] might account for the discrepancy found between P-selectin and ICAM-1 levels. No differences in activity of ACE and ACE2 were seen between the four age groups. This discrepancy could be due, among other reasons, to the wide variability on the levels of ACE and ACE2 [40]. It is also possible that the pulmonary RAS is not the most prominent inflammatory pathway in human ARDS, as inflammatory biomarkers showed only a weak correlation with ACE and ACE2 activities and no correlation with ACE2/ACE ratio.

The findings reported by Schouten et al. [40] of higher levels of markers involved in the neutrophil response with increasing age are in line with the findings from the above-cited preclinical studies of greater pulmonary edema, neutrophil infiltration, and alveolar damage after identical insults in older than in younger animals [37, 41–46].

29.5   Diagnosis of ARF

When discussing ARF in the elderly, two considerations are important. First, the presenting signs and symptoms may not be primarily respiratory. Delirium may be often the presenting sign of respiratory failure. Second, inappropriate diagnosis is related to mortality, highlighting the importance of an early correct diagnosis [47].

There is an age-related decreased sensitivity of respiratory centers to hypoxemia and hypercapnia, and the perception of dyspnea and the capacity to perceive resistive loads are diminished [48]. Thus, the ventilatory response to the different causes of ARF is decreased in the elderly. Increased heart rate in response to hypoxemia may be absent because of blunted autonomic drive. Finally, cognitive impairment reduces the ability of elderly patients to communicate their symptoms. All those age-related changes may result in delay in the diagnosis.

29.6   Causes of ARF

In one study, common causes of ARF in patients older than 80 years of age presenting to the emergency department included HF (43%), pneumonia (35%), chronic obstructive pulmonary disease (COPD) exacerbation (32%), and pulmonary embolism (PE) (18%). Less frequent causes (<5%) were pneumothorax, lung cancer, sepsis, and acute asthma. The definitive diagnosis was delayed by more than 72 h in 62% of patients [47].

HF may present as peripheral edema, confusion, or wheezing. The ECG (indicating arrhythmias, ischemic heart disease, or left ventricular hypertrophy), chest X-ray (showing signs of pulmonary edema), spirometry (showing a preserved peak expiratory flow rate), and echocardiography (showing signs of systolic or diastolic ventricular dysfunction) may aid in the diagnosis of HF in the elderly.

The risk of **pneumonia** is increased due to poor nutrition, decreased T-cell function, decreased mucociliary function, impaired airway secretion due to muscle weakness, decreased secretory immunoglobulin (Ig) A, and increased upper airway bacterial colonization. Other predisposing factors include the increased prevalence of cerebrovascular disease, COPD, renal failure, and dysphagia (in the context of, for instance, cerebrovascular accident or Parkinson's disease) predisposing to aspiration of gastric contents.

General symptoms (confusion, agitation) rather than respiratory symptoms (cough, dyspnea) often dominate the clinical picture. Typical signs and symptoms of pneumonia, such as dyspnea, cough, and fever, were observed in combination in only one third of patients with community-acquired pneumonia [49, 50].

COPD is a chronic, progressive disease, in which the pathologic process accelerates the age-related impairment in respiratory function. Clinical symptoms during an exacerbation episode resemble those of asthma. COPD is rarely diagnosed before the age of 40 years. Pathophysiologically, two distinct forms are defined: **Chronic bronchitis**, characterized by mucous gland hyperplasia in the large airways, goblet cell hyperplasia, chronic inflammation, and mucous plugging in the small airways. These changes lead to ventilation/perfusion mismatching, resulting in hypoxemia and hypercapnia. **Emphysema** is characterized by abnormal enlargement of the airway distal to the terminal bronchiole and destruction of the alveolar wall, leading to loss of elastic recoil and increased airway resistance. The capillaries are destroyed along with alveolar walls, so that ventilation/perfusion matching is better preserved than in chronic bronchitis, resulting in only mild hypoxemia and normocapnia. The increased lung volume results in flattening of the diaphragm, leading to decreased force of contraction. The normal 65% contribution of the diaphragm to ventilation decreases to 35%, resulting in increased work of breathing. In the elderly population, these pure forms are rarely diagnosed, and they most often present together.

COPD is often diagnosed to explain the complaint of dyspnea and signs and symptoms resembling emphysema (herein the term "senile emphysema"). However, the symptoms are often simply explained by the increased anteroposterior diameter of the chest and alveoli dilatation that accompany aging.

Aspiration pneumonia is common in the elderly. Healthy elderly subjects do not seem to have increased risk of aspiration. However, conditions more prevalent in the elderly population are associated with an increased risk of aspiration. The risk of aspiration is increased due to cerebrovascular disease, Parkinson's disease, or recent endotracheal intubation. Aspiration of gastric contents manifests as respiratory distress 2–12 h after a vomiting episode in a patient with decreased level of consciousness or glottic dysfunction from any cause (neurological disease, drug overdose, use of a nasogastric tube) or esophageal dysfunction. Bacterial pneumonia may result from repeated aspirations of colonized gastric contents.

Asthma is relatively common in the elderly, affecting 5% of this population. Asthma is characterized by paroxysmal dyspnea, wheezing, and coughing, with no respiratory distress between episodes, except in long-standing disease. It may have been present for several years, may be a recurrence of an attack at a younger age, or even may occur for the first time in patients older than 65 years.

It is important to identify the cause. As atopy decreases with age, it is less likely in the elderly to find a specific antigen, and viral infections or nonspecific irritants are more likely to be the precipitating factor.

The risk of **pulmonary embolism** increases with age [51]. ECG, chest X-ray, and a ventilation-perfusion lung scan may aid in the diagnosis, but the most common diagnostic test used is a high-resolution CT. Elevation of D-dimer concentration is sensitive, but its specificity is low as it is increased in many other disease conditions. Its specificity for the diagnosis of PE is higher if other causes of D-dimer elevation are ruled out.

29.7 Susceptibility of the Elderly to ARDS

Acute respiratory distress syndrome (ARDS) is an important precipitating cause of ARF in the ICU. In adult ICUs 26% of cases with ARF result from ARDS [15, 52]. According to the previous definition of acute lung injury (ALI) and ARDS (acute hypoxemic respiratory failure with bilateral pulmonary infiltrates that is associated with both pulmonary and non-pulmonary risk factors and that is not primarily due to left atrial hypertension) [53], the reported incidences in the USA are 78.9×10^5 person-years for ALI ($200 < PaO_2/FiO_2 \leq 300$) and 58.7×105 person-years for ARDS ($PaO_2/FiO_2 \leq 200$) [17].

The incidence of ALI increases markedly with age, from 16×10^5 person-years for the 15–19 years of age group to 306×10^5 person-years for the 74–85 years of age group [15]. This age-related change may be determined to a great extent by the higher incidence of sepsis, the major risk factor for ALI, among older patients [54].

In another study, patients older than 70 years of age, as compared to younger patients, developed more often ARDS, as well as renal failure, ventilator-associated pneumonia, sepsis, shock, and liver failure [55]. Likewise, in a cohort study of 100 ICU patients older than 75 compared to 100 patients younger than 75, matched for severity of illness as measured by the APACHE II score, older patients developed more often ARF than younger ones (67% vs. 32%) [56].

However, other studies have indicated that age by itself is not a risk factor for the development of ALI. For instance, Gajic et al. [57] validated a lung injury prediction score (LIPS) that predicts the development of ALI in patients with predefined risk factors, such as sepsis, shock, pancreatitis, pneumonia, aspiration, high-risk trauma, or high-risk surgery. Predisposing conditions and risk modifiers were included in the LIPS according to logistic regression analysis, but age was not part of the model. Thus, according to these results, age by itself does not determine a higher susceptibility for the development of ALI in patients with a risk factor.

29.8 Treatments of ARDS in the Elderly

Different clinical trials have tested the efficacy of a number of interventions in patients with ARDS, but elderly patients as well as those with chronic pulmonary conditions seem to be underrepresented in those studies, limiting the applicability of the results to certain patient populations. For instance, the ARDS Network trial compared low (6 ml/kg IBW) with high (12 ml/kg IBW) V_T ventilation [58]. The same group also tested the efficacy of other interventions, such as the addition of high positive end-expiratory pressure (PEEP) to a low V_T strategy [59], and a liberal versus restrictive fluid management strategy in selected hemodynamically stable patients with ARDS [60]. These studies included patients with a mean age in the early 50s. Exclusion criteria were significant COPD, FEV1 < 20 ml/kg IBW, signs of hyperinflation in the chest X-ray, and PaO2 < 55 mm Hg on room air. Thus, generalizability of the results of these trials to the elderly population is questionable.

On the other hand, the strategies used for ventilation in these trials use V_T and plateau pressure as surrogates for alveolar volume, assuming the same pulmonary response across all age groups. However, this assumption may not hold true, as the elderly experience higher lung compliance and lower chest wall compliance as compared to younger patients.

The same concern about applicability across the different age groups applies to other trials testing different therapies for ARDS, such as high-frequency oscillation (HFO), airway pressure release ventilation (APRV), or corticosteroids. For instance, it is not known whether the increased necessity for sedation associated with the use of HFO, and the subsequent increased risk for delirium in the elderly, negates any beneficial effect associated with this particular ventilatory mode or if the physiological benefits of APRV and the decreased need for sedation are associated with decreased incidence of delirium and dementia and therefore a decreased mortality in elderly patients. In a similar way, the effects of corticosteroids in elderly patients, in whom the treatment-induced muscle weakness may be related to a higher ventilator dependency, are not known.

29.9 Weaning the Elderly Patient from the Ventilator After ARF

The study showing superiority of the spontaneous breathing trial (SBT) to other weaning methods [61] studied a population whose average age was 58 years. The generalizability of these findings to older patients is questionable, as age-related changes in respiratory physiology may impact how patients respond to spontaneous breathing. In addition, of the 546 patients studied [61], only 319 (58%) had acute lung injury (others had other causes of respiratory failure, such as COPD or neurologic diagnoses), and only 23 cases (4%) had ARDS.

In addition, commonly used signs to assess the tolerability to an SBT include the appearance of rapid shallow breathing (or a high f/V_T ratio) and the identification of signs of increased sympathetic tone (hypertension, tachycardia). However, elderly patients tend to have under normal conditions a pattern of rapid shallow breathing [10] so that the observation of this ventilatory pattern may not necessarily indicate failure of the SBT.

On the other hand, older patients have a decreased ventilatory response to hypoxemia and hypercapnia [12]. Thus, the patient may appear to be breathing normally when in fact hypoxemia and hypercapnia may be developing. These observations suggest that routine use of arterial blood gases might have greater utility in the older adult population to detect weaning failure in a patient who seems to be comfortable on a SBT.

The need to assess different weaning methods in the elderly is also suggested by the results of El Solh et al. [62], who observed that patients over the age of 70, as compared with a younger matched cohort, were much more likely to fail extubation because of the inability to handle secretions, and those who failed had a higher risk of developing nosocomial pneumonia. In addition, although older persons achieved physiologic recovery from ALI in equal proportion to younger patients, their ICU length of stay and duration of mechanical ventilation were increased because of a higher reintubation rate [18].

29.10 Outcome of ARF in the Elderly

An increasing number of very old (aged 80 or older) patients are being admitted to ICUs [63, 64], mostly for ARF and requirement of ventilatory support. Survival of elderly patients is poor. In a large study on 2709 ICU patients, long-term mortality at 3 years was 57% and 40% (for patients ≥65 years of age versus <65 years of age, respectively) [65]. In a smaller study of 233 patients aged ≥80 years, mortality at 3 years was 71% [66].

ICU admission refusal by the physician of elderly patients with ARF is frequently based on the estimation of potential benefit of ICU admission, the consideration of advanced age as a poor prognostic factor, the estimation of their long-term survival, and the quality of life as assessed by family members. However, the presence of comorbidities and the severity of acute physiological disturbances are more related to adverse outcomes in acutely ill patients than age itself [67]. In addition, the validity of the assessment of patients' quality of life by proxies or physicians has been questioned [68].

It is generally admitted that **ICU admission improves prognosis of elderly patients**. Observational studies generally report lower crude mortality rates for patients admitted to the ICU than in patients whose ICU admission was refused [69]. However, studies of very old patients find similar crude mortality rates [70]. A large study of 2646 patients >80 years of age visiting the emergency department with a condition potentially warranting ICU admission showed an adjusted decrease in survival for patients admitted to the ICU compared with those not admitted. Thus, benefit of ICU admission for very old patients could not be appreciated [71].

Several studies have shown that **age is independently associated with mortality** in patients requiring mechanical ventilation. Heuser et al. found in a large series of 3050 patients with respiratory disease, whether or not receiving mechanical ventilation, that age was independently associated with mortality [72]. In another prospective study of mechanically ventilated elderly patients [73], Zilberberg et al. compared 31 patients >65 years of age with 76 patients ≤65 years of age. After multivariable analysis to adjust for confounding variables, it was found that older age was an independent predictor of death.

In a large international cohort of mechanically ventilated patients including 5183 patients, taking patients with age < 40 years as the reference, age was independently associated with mortality for patients 40–70 years of age (odds ratio [OR] = 1.58, 95% confidence interval [CI] 1.27–1.98]) and more strongly for patients >70 years of age (OR = 2.18 [95% CI 1.71–2.76]) [74]. In a subanalysis of 467 patients with the diagnosis of ARDS [75], the adjusted mortality risk factors included age (in addition to early and late renal failure, SAPS II score, and low PEEP).

Ely et al., using the ARDSNet database [18], analyzed retrospectively 902 patients and found that age 70 or older was a strong predictor of hospital death (hazard ratio 2.5, 95% CI [2.0, 3.2]). Age was also associated with longer duration of mechanical ventilation (median of 19 days vs. 10 days), ICU length of stay (21 days vs. 16 days), and 28-day mortality (50% vs. 25%). Interestingly the proportion of survivors achieving physiological recovery landmarks did not differ in the older and younger patient age groups, and the median time to pass a spontaneous breathing trial was similar (4 days vs. 5 days). However, after passing a spontaneous breathing trial, it took older patients 1 more day as compared to younger patients to achieve unassisted breathing and 3 more days to be discharged from the ICU. This is likely related to the decreased respiratory reserve and the age-related increased incidence of other conditions such as delirium.

In a cohort study of 100 ICU patients older than 75 years of age compared to 100 patients younger than 75 years matched for severity of illness as assessed by the APACHE II score, a non-significant trend toward a higher mortality (26% versus 19%, $p = 0.23$) and longer duration of mechanical ventilation (7 days [IQR 3–15] versus 3 days [IQR 2–8]) and ICU length of stay (8 days [IQR 3–17] versus 5 days [IQR 3–9]) was reported [56]. Do-not-resuscitate orders were written more often in the elderly group than in the younger group (9% vs. 3%, $p = 0.07$). Considering only those patients under mechanical ventilation, mortality was higher, not reaching statistical significance, in the older age group (30% vs. 23%). Thus, there was a strong trend in this study for a higher mortality and worse outcomes in older patients, not reaching statistical significance probably due to lack of statistical power.

In a retrospective analysis from three multicenter clinical studies, a model combining age and cardiorespiratory function on day 3 predicted a combined outcome of mortality and ventilator dependence [76]. In a multicenter retrospective study of adult ICU patients receiving at least 24 hours of mechanical ventilation, Ma et al. analyzed 853 patients, of whom 61.5% were $\geq$ 65 years of age and 26.0% were $\geq$ 80 years of age [77]. Advanced age was significantly associated with total duration of mechanical ventilation, ICU length of stay, and ICU costs, but not with hospital length of stay and hospital costs. Mortality rates in the ICU, hospital, and at 60 days significantly increased with age and for patients $\geq$80 years were 47.7%, 49.5%, and 50.0%, respectively. Age, APACHE II score, PaO2/FiO2, total duration of mechanical ventilation, ICU length of stay, and the decision to withhold/withdraw life-sustaining treatments were independent risk factors for mortality.

In the VIP2, a very large prospective multicentric observational study [78], conducted using the European Very elderly Intensive Patient (VIP) network, ICU and 30-day survival of 3920 ICU patients $\geq$80 years were, respectively, 72.5% and 61.2%, and age was independently associated with mortality.

On the other hand, there are studies providing evidence that **age by itself is not related to mortality** after adjusting for other risk factors and that the association between mortality and age becomes non-significant in adjusted analysis [47, 50]. For instance, one study compared 130 ICU patients older than 75 years of age with a cohort of patients aged 55–65 years with the same severity of illness [79]. Hospital mortality was significantly greater in the older age group (51% vs. 39%) with a crude relative risk of 1.32 (95% CI 1.01–1.73). However, after adjusting for other variables (APACHE II, whether the patient had a private attending physician, primary admitting diagnosis, or presence of cancer), older patients did not have a significantly greater risk of dying (adjusted relative risk, 1.05 [95% CI 0.97–1.12]).

Ely et al. [80] analyzed prospectively collected data on mechanically ventilated patients using a multivariable analysis and adjustment for ethnicity, sex, and severity of illness, to evaluate the independent effect of age on different outcomes. Patients $\geq$75 years of age spent similar lengths of time on mechanical ventilation, had a lower cost of care, and presented similar in-hospital mortality rates (38% compared with 39%, $p < 0.2$).

The discrepancies between studies [73, 80] might be explained by the different patient sample, the ICU referral criteria, and the underlying comorbidity. For example, patients in the study by Zilberberg and Epstein [73] had a high mortality, and two thirds of the patients had cancer, cirrhosis, HIV disease, or transplant-associated illnesses, whereas patients in the study by Ely et al. [80] had a lower overall mortality, and these diagnoses accounted for less than 10% of the comorbid conditions.

Finally, a recent retrospective study in Turkey [81] evaluated the risk factors for mortality in a medical ICU. They studied 693 patients, of whom 414 (59.7%) were $\geq$ 65 years of age. Median age of the young and elderly groups was significantly different (55 and 77 years, respectively), and median age was similar in survivors and non-survivors (69 versus 68 years). Different risk factors (ICU stay, hospital stay before ICU, APACHE II and Charlson Comorbidity Index scores, pneumonia, acute hepatic failure/coma, malignancy, acute hemodialysis, need for vasopressors, and invasive mechanical ventilation), but not age, were independent predictors of ICU mortality. Mortality was comparable in the young (<65 years) and elderly (≥65 years) groups (58.8% versus 58.5%, respectively). The authors concluded that in developing countries, age should not be a determining factor for ICU triage.

In an interesting analysis, Farfel et al. [82] reported in 840 ICU patients older than 55 years of age that in-hospital mortality was independently associated with age only in patients requiring mechanical ventilation (in paimpact of frailty on survitients receiving mechanical ventilation, OR = 1.60 [95% CI 1.01–2.54] for 65–74 years old, OR = 2.68 [95% CI 1.58–4.56] for ≥75 years old; in patients not receiving mechanical ventilation, OR = 2.28 [95% CI 0.99–5.25] for 65–74 years old, OR = 1.95 [95% CI = 0.82–4.62] for ≥75 years old). In our view, the conclusion is not quite supported by their results, as the point estimate of the mortality risk for patients not receiving mechanical ventilation was still greater than 1, and the confidence interval was not significant probably because of lack of power, as the low number of events in these groups suggest. Indeed, the number of deaths in patients receiving mechanical ventilation was only 14, 18, and 16 in the three age groups, respectively.

The nonagenarian patient population with ARF was studied by Becker et al. in a single-center retrospective observational study. 372 ICU patients ≥90 years of age were studied [83], of whom 40% of patients required mechanical ventilation (30% of survivors and 84% of non-survivors). ICU, hospital, and 1-year after hospital discharge mortalities were, respectively, 18.3%, 30.9%, and 65.1%. Independent risk factors for 28-day mortality were creatinine, bilirubin, age, and requirement of catecholamines. Thus, even though mortality of the nonagenarian population is of course high, these results suggest that admission should not be uniformly refused based on age.

Unlike the previous study [83], another study in nonagenarian did not find age to be an independent risk factor for mortality [84]. Le Borgne et al., in a retrospective single-center study of 317 ICU patients ≥90 years [84], reported that the main admission diagnosis was ARF in 52.4% of cases, and 49.2% required mechanical ventilation (more often non-survivors than survivors: 81.4% and 31.4%, respectively). Median age was 92 years, both in the survivors and in the non-survivors group, and ICU and hospital mortality rates were 35.7% and 42.6%, respectively. Mechanical ventilation (OR = 4.83, 95% CI 1.59–15.82) was an independent predictor of ICU mortality, whereas age was not (OR = 0.88, 95% CI 95% 0.72–1.08). Thus, these results suggest that among critically ill elderly patients aged ≥90 years, chronological age was not an independent factor of ICU mortality. In addition, the reported mortality of patients ≥90 years of age allows the contention that chronological age by itself would not be an exclusion criterion for ICU admission (▶ Box 29.1).

Of great importance when assessing prognosis of elderly ICU patients is the consideration and measurement of frailty. The VIP2 study [78] showed that frailty assessment using the clinical frail scale is able to predict short-term mortality in elderly patients admitted to the ICU, and other geriatric syndromes do not add improvement to the prediction model. A more in-depth discussion on the importance of frailty in the treatment and prognostication of critically ill patients is discussed elsewhere in this work.

29.11   Outcome of ARF in Elderly Patients with COVID-19

COVID-19 merits particular attention in the discussion of ARF in the elderly. Old patients admitted to the ICU with COVID-19 are at increased risk of death [85], and the decision of ICU admission can be challenging [86]. The case fatality rates observed in ARDS-related SARS-CoV-2 are close to 30–40% [87–89] but can reach 70% in the older patients [90–92].

Some studies have reported the management and prognosis of elderly patients in the context of SARS-CoV-2 lower respiratory tract infection [93, 94], and some have focused on a population admitted to the ICU. In a large German study enrolling 10,021 patients, 923 (9%) patients over 70 years old received ventilatory support. In-hospital mortality reached 63% for patients 70–79 years of age [89]. This result concurred with the poor prognosis reported in previous studies focused on elderly patients with ARDS not related to SARS-CoV-2 infection [95].

In an ancillary analysis of the COVID-ICU study of 1199 old patients (>70 years) admitted to the ICU with the diagnosis of COVID-19 [96], overall day-90 mortality was 46% and reached 67% among the 193 patients over 80 years old. In multivariable analysis, clinical frailty scale, diabetes mellitus, a shorter time from the first symptom to ICU admission, cardiovascular dysfunction, admission early in the pandemic, and the PaO2/FiO2 ratio, but not age, were associated with day-90 mortality.

A large multicenter transnational study described the characteristics and outcomes of 4244 patients admitted to the ICU with laboratory-confirmed COVID-19 during the first wave of the pandemic and post-ICU admission status available [97]. Patient age (median [IQR]) for all patients, survivors and non-survivors, was, respectively, 63 [54–71], 61 [52–69], and 68 [59–74] years. On ICU admission, standard oxygen therapy, high-flow oxygen therapy, noninvasive ventilation, and invasive mechanical ventilation were used, respectively, in 29%, 19%, 6%, and 63% of patients (more than one therapy could be used in one patients), and 80% received invasive mechanical ventilation at some point during their ICU stay. Considering patients on invasive mechanical ventilation or noninvasive ventilation within the first 24 h in ICU, pulmonary embolism and ventilator-associated pneumonia were diagnosed in 207 (9%) and 1209 (58%) cases, respectively, and different advanced therapies were used on day 1 of mechanical ventilation, including paralyzing agents (88%), prone position (70%), inhaled NO (19%), and ECMO (11%). Mortality at day 90 was 31%, increasing with the severity of ARDS at ICU admission (30%, 34%, and 50% for mild, moderate, and severe ARDS, respectively), and decreased from 42% to 25% over the study period. Early independent predictors of 90-day mortality were older age, immunosuppression, severe obesity, diabetes, higher renal and cardiovascular SOFA score components, lower PaO2/FiO2, and a shorter time between the first symptom and ICU admission.

In a recent meta-analysis [98], studies reporting the case fatality rate (CFR) for patients with confirmed COVID-19 requiring IMV were analyzed. In the 69 studies included, overall reported CFR of 57,420 adult patients was estimated at 45% (95%

CI 39–52%). Among studies in which age-stratified CFR was available, pooled CFR estimates ranged from 47.9% (95% CI 46.4–49.4%) in younger patients (age ≤ 40 years) to 84.4% (95% CI 83.3–85.4%) in older patients (age > 80 yr). CFR was also higher early in the pandemic.

After the identification of age and comorbidity as prognostic factor in patients with ARF in the context of COVID-19 [99–101], frailty was soon recognized as a mortality risk factor in these patients [102, 103], and the clinical frailty scale (CFS) was included in critical care escalation guidelines [104, 105]. However, studies on the relationship between frailty and mortality in COVID-19 have yielded positive [94] and negative [106, 107] results. In a recent large multicenter international cohort study of 5711 adult patients hospitalized with COVID-19 [108] (median age 74), it was found that the risk of death increased independently with increasing age (>80 versus 18–49: hazard ratio 3.57 [95% CI 2.54–5.02]), frailty (CFS 8 versus 1–3: hazard ratio 3.03 [95% CI 2.29–4.00]), inflammation, renal disease, cardiovascular disease, and cancer.

The COVIP study [109], a prospective multicentric study of COVID-19 ICU patients ≥70 years of age, included 1346 patients (median age of 75 years [IQR 72–78], 16.3% > 80 years), of whom 21% were frail and 72% were under MV at 10 days. The overall survival at 30 days was 59% and was dependent on frailty status (66% in fit, 53% in vulnerable, 41% in frail patients). In frail patients, there was no difference in 30-day survival between different age categories, and frailty was independently associated with lower survival [109]. Thus, in elderly patients with COVID-19, frailty provides relevant prognostic information in addition to age and comorbidities.

In summary, the largest studies show that age, comorbidities, and frailty are independently related to outcome in patients with ARF and COVID-19. However, reporting methods between studies are variable, and mortality of these patients is changing over time. Thus, although prognosis of elderly patients with ARF in the context of COVID-19 is certainly poor, individual case assessment is recommended when the decision whether to admit an elderly patient with COVID-19 to the ICU is faced.

Conclusion

ARF in the elderly presents specific characteristics that should be taken into consideration for the diagnosis, treatment, and prognostication of these patients in the ICU.

Elderly patients are at increased risk of ARF after a given insult. Their response to interventions used for the treatment of ARF may differ as compared to other age groups.

Prognosis should be assessed when an elderly patient requires invasive treatment in the ICU for ARF. Age interplays with other factors to determine mortality. These factors include the presence of comorbidities, previous functional status, and diminished functional reserve, as well as the risk for the development of complications known to be associated with outcome (i.e., delirium). Thus, age should not be used alone to determine treatment decisions. The concept of physiological age, rather than chronologic age, reflecting the underlying level of disease, may be a more important determinant of outcome.

> **Take Home Message**
> - Elderly patients as well as those with chronic pulmonary conditions seem to be underrepresented in large clinical trials on protective ventilation in ARDS, limiting the applicability of the results to certain patient populations.
> - Strategies used for ventilation in clinical trials on the role of protective ventilation strategies use V_T and plateau pressure as surrogates for alveolar volume, assuming the same pulmonary response across all age groups. However, this assumption may not hold true, as the elderly experience higher lung compliance and lower chest wall compliance as compared to younger patients.
> - Age interplays with other factors to determine mortality, such as the presence of comorbidities, previous functional status, and diminished functional reserve. The concept of physiological age, rather than chronologic age, may be a more important determinant of outcome.

References

1. Milbrandt EB, Eldadah B, Nayfield S, Hadley E, Angus DC. Toward an integrated research agenda for critical illness in aging. Am J Respir Crit Care Med. 2010;182(8):995–1003.
2. Angus DC, Kelley MA, Schmitz RJ, White A, Popovich J Jr. Committee on Manpower for Pulmonary and Critical Care Societies (COMPACCS). Caring for the critically ill patient. Current and projected workforce requirements for care of the critically ill and patients with pulmonary disease: can we meet the requirements of an aging population? JAMA. 2000;284(21):2762–70.
3. Nin N, Lorente JA, De Paula M, et al. Aging increases the susceptibility to injurious mechanical ventilation. Intensive Care Med. 2008;34(5):923–31.
4. Wunsch H, Linde-Zwirble WT, Angus DC, Hartman ME, Milbrandt EB, Kahn JM. The epidemiology of mechanical ventilation use in the United States. Crit Care Med. 2010;38(10):1947–53.
5. Boumendil A, Aegerter P, Guidet B, CUB-Rea Network. Treatment intensity and outcome of patients aged 80 and older in intensive care units: a multicenter matched-cohort study. J Am Geriatr Soc. 2005;53(1):88–93.
6. Hamel MB, Teno JM, Goldman L, et al. Patient age and decisions to withhold life-sustaining treatments from seriously ill, hospitalized adults. SUPPORT investigators. Study to understand prognoses and preferences for outcomes and risks of treatment. Ann Intern Med. 1999;130(2):116–25.
7. Giugliano RP, Camargo CA Jr, Lloyd-Jones DM, et al. Elderly patients receive less aggressive medical and invasive management of unstable angina: potential impact of practice guidelines. Arch Intern Med. 1998;158(10):1113–20.
8. Aghasafari P, Heise RL, Reynolds A, Pidaparti RM. Aging effects on alveolar sacs under mechanical ventilation. J Gerontol A Biol Sci Med Sci. 2019;74(2):139–46.
9. Pisani MA. Considerations in caring for the critically ill older patient. J Intensive Care Med. 2009;24(2):83–95.
10. Sprung J, Gajic O, Warner DO. Review article: age related alterations in respiratory function: anesthetic considerations [Article de synthese: les modifications de fonction respiratoire liees a l'age - considerations anesthesiques]. Can J Anaesth. 2006;53(12):1244–57. [in French]
11. Knudson RJ, Slatin RC, Lebowitz MD, et al. The maximal expiratory flow-volume curve: normal standards, variability, and effects of age. Am Rev Respir Dis. 1976;113(5):587–600.
12. Peterson DD, Pack AI, Silage DA, et al. Effects of aging on ventilatory and occlusion pressure responses to hypoxia and hypercapnia. Am Rev Respir Dis. 1981;124(4):387–91.
13. Crispell KA. Common cardiovascular issues encountered in geriatric critical care. Crit Care Clin. 2003;19(4):677–91.
14. Lim W, Qushmaq I, Cook DJ, Crowther MA, Heels- Ansdell D, Devereaux PJ. Elevated troponin and myocardial infarction in the intensive care unit: a prospective study. Crit Care. 2005;9:R636–44.

15. Rubenfeld GD, Caldwell E, Peabody E, et al. Incidence and outcomes of acute lung injury. N Engl J Med. 2005;353(16):1685–93.
16. Phua J, Badia JR, Adhikari NK, et al. Has mortality from acute respiratory distress syndrome decreased over time?: a systematic review. Am J Respir Crit Care Med. 2009;179(3):220–7.
17. Zimmerman JJ, Akhtar SR, Caldwell E, Rubenfeld GD. Incidence and outcomes of pediatric acute lung injury. Pediatrics. 2009;124(1):87–95.
18. Ely EW, Wheeler AP, Thompson BT, Ancukiewicz M, Steinberg KP, Bernard GR. Recovery rate and prognosis in older persons who develop acute lung injury and the acute respiratory distress syndrome. Ann Intern Med. 2002;136(1):25–36.
19. Wood JH, Partrick DA, Johnston RB Jr. The inflammatory response to injury in children. Curr Opin Pediatr. 2010;22(3):315–20.
20. Johnston CJ, Rubenfeld GD, Hudson LD. Effect of age on the development of ARDS in trauma patients. Chest. 2003;124(2):653–9.
21. Brubaker AL, Palmer JL, Kovacs EJ. Age-related dysregulation of inflammation and innate immunity: lessons learned from rodent models. Aging Dis. 2011;2(5):346–60.
22. López-Otín C, Blasco MA, Partridge L, Serrano M, Kroemer G. The hallmarks of aging. Cell. 2013;153(6):1194–217.
23. Lawrence SM, Corriden R, Nizet V. Age-appropriate functions and dysfunctions of the neonatal neutrophil. Front Pediatr. 2017;5:23. https://doi.org/10.3389/fped.2017.00023. PMID: 28293548; PMCID: PMC5329040
24. Schouten LR, Helmerhorst HJ, Wagenaar GT, et al. Age-dependent changes in the pulmonary renin-angiotensin system are associated with severity of lung injury in a model of acute lung injury in rats. Crit Care Med. 2016 Dec;44(12):e1226–35. https://doi.org/10.1097/CCM.0000000000002008.
25. Sapey E, Greenwood H, Walton G, et al. Phosphoinositide 3-kinase inhibition restores neutrophil accuracy in the elderly: toward targeted treatments for immunosenescence. Blood. 2014;123(2):239–48.
26. Bonnema DD, Webb CS, Pennington WR, et al. Effects of age on plasma matrix metalloproteinases (MMPs) and tissue inhibitor of metalloproteinases (TIMPs). J Card Fail. 2007;13(7):530–40.
27. Tayebjee MH, Lip GY, Blann AD, Macfadyen RJ. Effects of age, gender, ethnicity, diurnal variation and exercise on circulating levels of matrix metalloproteinases (MMP)-2 and −9, and their inhibitors, tissue inhibitors of matrix metalloproteinases (TIMP)-1 and −2. Thromb Res. 2005;115(3):205–10.
28. Zonneveld R, Martinelli R, Shapiro NI, Kuijpers TW, Plötz FB, Carman CV. Soluble adhesion molecules as markers for sepsis and the potential pathophysiological discrepancy in neonates, children and adults. Crit Care. 2014;18(2):204.
29. Xie X, Chen J, Wang X, Zhang F, Liu Y. Age- and gender-related difference of ACE2 expression in rat lung. Life Sci. 2006;78(19):2166–71.
30. Kuba K, Imai Y, Rao S, Jiang C, Penninger JM. Lessons from SARS: control of acute lung failure by the SARS receptor ACE2. J Mol Med (Berl). 2006;84(10):814–20.
31. Imai Y, Kuba K, Rao S, et al. Angiotensin-converting enzyme 2 protects from severe acute lung failure. Nature. 2005;436(7047):112–6.
32. Bustos ML, Huleihel L, Kapetanaki MG, et al. Aging mesenchymal stem cells fail to protect because of impaired migration and antiinflammatory response. Am J Respir Crit Care Med. 2014;189(7):787–98.
33. Xu J, Woods CR, Mora AL, Joodi R, Brigham KL, Iyer S, Rojas M. Prevention of endotoxin-induced systemic response by bone marrow-derived mesenchymal stem cells in mice. Am J Physiol Lung Cell Mol Physiol. 2007 Jul;293(1):L131–41.
34. Matthay MA, Goolaerts A, Howard JP, Lee JW. Mesenchymal stem cells for acute lung injury: preclinical evidence. Crit Care Med. 2010;38(10 Suppl):S569–73.
35. Zhu YG, Feng XM, Abbott J, et al. Human mesenchymal stem cell microvesicles for treatment of Escherichia coli endotoxin-induced acute lung injury in mice. Stem Cells. 2014;32(1):116–25.
36. Martínez-González I, Roca O, Masclans JR, et al. Human mesenchymal stem cells overexpressing the IL-33 antagonist soluble IL-1 receptor-like-1 attenuate endotoxin-induced acute lung injury. Am J Respir Cell Mol Biol. 2013;49(4):552–62.
37. Schouten LR, Schultz MJ, van Kaam AH, Juffermans NP, Bos AP, Wösten-van Asperen RM. Association between maturation and aging and pulmonary responses in animal models of lung injury: a systematic review. Anesthesiology. 2015;123(2):389–408.

38. Matute-Bello G, Downey G, Moore BB, et al. Acute Lung Injury in Animals Study Group. An official American Thoracic Society workshop report: features and measurements of experimental acute lung injury in animals. Am J Respir Cell Mol Biol. 2011;44(5):725–38.

39. Matute-Bello G, Frevert CW, Martin TR. Animal models of acute lung injury. Am J Physiol Lung Cell Mol Physiol. 2008;295(3):L379–99.

40. Schouten LR, van Kaam AH, Kohse F, et al. MARS consortium. Age-dependent differences in pulmonary host responses in ARDS: a prospective observational cohort study. Ann Intensive Care. 2019;9(1):55. https://doi.org/10.1186/s13613-019-0529-4. PMID: 31089908; PMCID: PMC6517452

41. Kling KM, Lopez-Rodriguez E, Pfarrer C, Mühlfeld C, Brandenberger C. Aging exacerbates acute lung injury-induced changes of the air-blood barrier, lung function, and inflammation in the mouse. Am J Physiol Lung Cell Mol Physiol. 2017;312(1):L1–L12.

42. Ito Y, Betsuyaku T, Nagai K, Nasuhara Y, Nishimura M. Expression of pulmonary VEGF family declines with age and is further down-regulated in lipopolysaccharide (LPS)-induced lung injury. Exp Gerontol. 2005;40(4):315–23.

43. Smith LS, Gharib SA, Frevert CW, Martin TR. Effects of age on the synergistic interactions between lipopolysaccharide and mechanical ventilation in mice. Am J Respir Cell Mol Biol. 2010;43(4):475–86.

44. Martin TR, Ruzinski JT, Wilson CB, Skerrett SJ. Effects of endotoxin in the lungs of neonatal rats: age-dependent impairment of the inflammatory response. J Infect Dis. 1995;171(1):134–44.

45. Sordelli DO, Djafari M, García VE, Fontán PA, Döring G. Age-dependent pulmonary clearance of Pseudomonas aeruginosa in a mouse model: diminished migration of polymorphonuclear leukocytes to N-formyl-methionyl-leucyl-phenylalanine. Infect Immun. 1992;60(4):1724–7.

46. Smith LS, Zimmerman JJ, Martin TR. Mechanisms of acute respiratory distress syndrome in children and adults: a review and suggestions for future research. Pediatr Crit Care Med. 2013;14(6):631–43.

47. Ray P, Birolleau S, Lefort Y, et al. Acute respiratory failure in the elderly: etiology, emergency diagnosis and prognosis. Crit Care. 2006;10(3):R82. https://doi.org/10.1186/cc4926. Epub 2006 May 24. PMID: 16723034; PMCID: PMC1550946

48. Connolly MJ, Crowley JJ, Charan NB, Nielson CP, Vestal RE. Reduced subjective awareness of bronchoconstriction provoked by methacholine in elderly asthmatic and normal subjects as measured on a simple awareness scale. Thorax. 1992;47(6):410–3.

49. Marrie TJ. Community-acquired pneumonia in the elderly. Clin Infect Dis. 2000;31(4):1066–78.

50. Riquelme OR, Riquelme OM, Rioseco ZML, Gómez MV, Cárdenas G, Torres C. Neumonía adquirida en la comunidad en el anciano hospitalizado: Aspectos clínicos y nutricionales [Community-acquired pneumonia in the elderly: clinical and nutritional aspects]. Rev Med Chil. 2008;136(5):587–93.

51. Yernault JC. Dyspnoea in the elderly: a clinical approach to diagnosis. Drugs Aging. 2001;18(3):177–87.

52. Roupie E, Lepage E, Wysocki M, et al. Prevalence, etiologies and outcome of the acute respiratory distress syndrome among hypoxemic ventilated patients. SRLF Collaborative Group on Mechanical Ventilation. Société de Réanimation de langue Française. Intensive Care Med. 1999;25(9):920–9.

53. Ware LB, Matthay MA. The acute respiratory distress syndrome. N Engl J Med. 2000;342(18):1334–49.

54. Angus DC, Linde-Zwirble WT, Lidicker J, Clermont G, Carcillo J, Pinsky MR. Epidemiology of severe sepsis in the United States: analysis of incidence, outcome, and associated costs of care. Crit Care Med. 2001;29(7):1303–10.

55. Esteban A, Anzueto A, Frutos-Vivar F, et al. Mechanical Ventilation International Study Group. Outcome of older patients receiving mechanical ventilation. Intensive Care Med. 2004;30(4):639–46.

56. Rodríguez-Regañón I, Colomer I, Frutos-Vivar F, Manzarbeitia J, Rodríguez-Mañas L, Esteban A. Outcome of older critically ill patients: a matched cohort study. Gerontology. 2006;52(3):169–73.

57. Gajic O, Dabbagh O, Park PK, et al. U.S. Critical Illness and Injury Trials Group: Lung Injury Prevention Study Investigators (USCIITG-LIPS). Early identification of patients at risk of acute lung injury: evaluation of lung injury prediction score in a multicenter cohort study. Am J Respir Crit Care Med. 2011;183(4):462–70.

58. Acute Respiratory Distress Syndrome Network, Brower RG, Matthay MA, Morris A, Schoenfeld D, Thompson BT, Wheeler A. Ventilation with lower tidal volumes as compared with traditional

tidal volumes for acute lung injury and the acute respiratory distress syndrome. N Engl J Med. 2000;342(18):1301–8.

59. Brower RG, Lanken PN, MacIntyre N, et al. National Heart, Lung, and Blood Institute ARDS Clinical Trials Network. Higher versus lower positive end-expiratory pressures in patients with the acute respiratory distress syndrome. N Engl J Med. 2004;351(4):327–36.

60. National Heart, Lung, and Blood Institute Acute Respiratory Distress Syndrome (ARDS) Clinical Trials Network, Wiedemann HP, Wheeler AP, Bernard GR, et al. Comparison of two fluid-management strategies in acute lung injury. N Engl J Med. 2006;354(24):2564–75.

61. Esteban A, Frutos F, Tobin MJ, et al. A comparison of four methods of weaning patients from mechanical ventilation. Spanish Lung Failure Collaborative Group. N Engl J Med. 1995;332(6):345–50.

62. El Solh AA, Bhat A, Gunen H, et al. Extubation failure in the elderly. Respir Med. 2004;98(7):661–8.

63. Wunsch H, Linde-Zwirble WT, Harrison DA, Barnato AE, Rowan KM, Angus DC. Use of intensive care services during terminal hospitalizations in England and the United States. Am J Respir Crit Care Med. 2009;180(9):875–80.

64. Bagshaw SM, Webb SA, Delaney A, et al. Very old patients admitted to intensive care in Australia and New Zealand: a multi-centre cohort analysis. Crit Care. 2009;13(2):R45.

65. Kaarlola A, Tallgren M, Pettilä V. Long-term survival, quality of life, and quality-adjusted life-years among critically ill elderly patients. Crit Care Med. 2006;34(8):2120–6.

66. Boumendil A, Maury E, Reinhard I, Luquel L, Offenstadt G, Guidet B. Prognosis of patients aged 80 years and over admitted in medical intensive care unit. Intensive Care Med. 2004;30(4):647–54.

67. Marik PE. Management of the critically ill geriatric patient. Crit Care Med. 2006;34(9 Suppl):S176–82.

68. Lum TY, Lin WC, Kane RL. Use of proxy respondents and accuracy of minimum data set assessments of activities of daily living. J Gerontol A Biol Sci Med Sci. 2005;60(5):654–9.

69. Sinuff T, Kahnamoui K, Cook DJ, Luce JM, Levy MM. Values Ethics and Rationing in Critical Care Task Force. Rationing critical care beds: a systematic review. Crit Care Med. 2004;32(7):1588–97.

70. Garrouste-Orgeas M, Boumendil A, Pateron D, et al. ICE-CUB Group. Selection of intensive care unit admission criteria for patients aged 80 years and over and compliance of emergency and intensive care unit physicians with the selected criteria: an observational, multicenter, prospective study. Crit Care Med. 2009;37(11):2919–28.

71. Boumendil A, Latouche A, Guidet B. ICE-CUB Study Group. On the benefit of intensive care for very old patients. Arch Intern Med. 2011;171(12):1116–7.

72. Heuser MD, Case LD, Ettinger WH. Mortality in intensive care patients with respiratory disease. Is age important? Arch Intern Med. 1992;152(8):1683–8.

73. Zilberberg MD, Epstein SK. Acute lung injury in the medical ICU: comorbid conditions, age, etiology, and hospital outcome. Am J Respir Crit Care Med. 1998;157(4 Pt 1):1159–64.

74. Esteban A, Anzueto A, Frutos F, et al. Mechanical Ventilation International Study Group. Characteristics and outcomes in adult patients receiving mechanical ventilation: a 28-day international study. JAMA. 2002;287(3):345–55.

75. Ferguson ND, Frutos-Vivar F, Esteban A, et al. Mechanical Ventilation International Study Group. Airway pressures, tidal volumes, and mortality in patients with acute respiratory distress syndrome. Crit Care Med. 2005;33(1):21–30.

76. Gajic O, Afessa B, Thompson BT, et al. Second International Study of Mechanical Ventilation and ARDS-net Investigators. Prediction of death and prolonged mechanical ventilation in acute lung injury. Crit Care. 2007;11(3):R53.

77. Ma JG, Zhu B, Jiang L, Jiang Q, Xi XM. Clinical characteristics and outcomes of mechanically ventilated elderly patients in intensive care units: a Chinese multicentre retrospective study. J Thorac Dis. 2021;13(4):2148–59.

78. Guidet B, de Lange DW, Boumendil A, et al. VIP2 study group. The contribution of frailty, cognition, activity of daily life and comorbidities on outcome in acutely admitted patients over 80 years in European ICUs: the VIP2 study. Intensive Care Med. 2020;46(1):57–69.

79. Wu AW, Rubin HR, Rosen MJ. Are elderly people less responsive to intensive care? J Am Geriatr Soc. 1990;38(6):621–7.

80. Ely EW, Evans GW, Haponik EF. Mechanical ventilation in a cohort of elderly patients admitted to an intensive care unit. Ann Intern Med. 1999;131(2):96–104.

81. Kır S, Bahçeci BK, Ayrancı E, et al. Age is not a risk factor in survival of severely ill patients with co-morbidities in a medical intensive care unit. Ir J Med Sci. 2021;190(1):317–24.

82. Farfel JM, Franca SA, Sitta Mdo C, Filho WJ, Carvalho CR. Age, invasive ventilatory support and outcomes in elderly patients admitted to intensive care units. Age Ageing. 2009;38(5):515–20.

83. Becker S, Müller J, de Heer G, Braune S, Fuhrmann V, Kluge S. Clinical characteristics and outcome of very elderly patients ≥90 years in intensive care: a retrospective observational study. Ann Intensive Care. 2015;5(1):53. https://doi.org/10.1186/s13613-015-0097-1. Epub 2015 Dec 21. PMID: 26690798; PMCID: PMC4686461

84. Le Borgne P, Maestraggi Q, Couraud S, et al. Critically ill elderly patients (≥ 90 years): clinical characteristics, outcome and financial implications. PLoS One. 2018;13(6):e0198360. https://doi.org/10.1371/journal.pone.0198360. PMID: 29856809; PMCID: PMC5983531

85. Richardson S, Hirsch JS, Narasimhan M, et al. Presenting characteristics, comorbidities, and outcomes among 5700 patients hospitalized with COVID-19 in the New York City area. JAMA. 2020;323(20):2052–9.

86. Haas LEM, de Lange DW, van Dijk D, van Delden JJM. Should we deny ICU admission to the elderly? Ethical considerations in times of COVID-19. Crit Care. 2020;24(1):321. https://doi.org/10.1186/s13054-020-03050-x. PMID: 32517776; PMCID: PMC7282209

87. Wang Y, Lu X, Li Y, et al. Course and outcomes of 344 intensive care patients with COVID-19. Am J Respir Crit Care Med. 2020;201(11):1430–4.

88. Grasselli G, Zangrillo A, Zanella A, et al. COVID-19 Lombardy ICU Network. Baseline characteristics and outcomes of 1591 patients infected with SARS-CoV-2 admitted to ICUs of the Lombardy Region, Italy. JAMA. 2020;323(16):1574–81.

89. Karagiannidis C, Mostert C, Hentschker C, et al. Case characteristics, resource use, and outcomes of 10 021 patients with COVID-19 admitted to 920 German hospitals: an observational study. Lancet Respir Med. 2020;8(9):853–62.

90. Jiménez E, Fontán-Vela M, Valencia J, et al. COVID@HUIL Working Group. Characteristics, complications and outcomes among 1549 patients hospitalised with COVID-19 in a secondary hospital in Madrid, Spain: a retrospective case series study. BMJ Open. 2020;10(11):e042398. https://doi.org/10.1136/bmjopen-2020-042398. PMID: 33172949; PMCID: PMC7656887

91. Nijman G, Wientjes M, Ramjith J, et al. Risk factors for in-hospital mortality in laboratory-confirmed COVID-19 patients in the Netherlands: a competing risk survival analysis. PLoS One. 2021;16:e0249231.

92. Grasselli G, Greco M, Zanella A, et al. COVID-19 Lombardy ICU Network. Risk factors associated with mortality among patients with COVID-19 in intensive care units in Lombardy, Italy. JAMA Intern Med. 2020;180(10):1345–55.

93. Ma Y, Hou L, Yang X, et al. The association between frailty and severe disease among COVID-19 patients aged over 60 years in China: a prospective cohort study. BMC Med. 2020;18(1):274. https://doi.org/10.1186/s12916-020-01761-0. PMID: 32892742; PMCID: PMC7474968

94. Hewitt J, Carter B, Vilches-Moraga A, et al. COPE Study Collaborators. The effect of frailty on survival in patients with COVID-19 (COPE): a multicentre, European, observational cohort study. Lancet Public Health. 2020;5(8):e444–51. https://doi.org/10.1016/S2468-2667(20)30146-8. Epub 2020 Jun 30. PMID: 32619408; PMCID: PMC7326416

95. Milberg JA, Davis DR, Steinberg KP, Hudson LD. Improved survival of patients with acute respiratory distress syndrome (ARDS): 1983-1993. JAMA. 1995;273(4):306–9.

96. Dres M, Hajage D, Lebbah S, et al. COVID-ICU investigators. Characteristics, management, and prognosis of elderly patients with COVID-19 admitted in the ICU during the first wave: insights from the COVID-ICU study : Prognosis of COVID-19 elderly critically ill patients in the ICU. Ann Intensive Care. 2021;11(1):77. https://doi.org/10.1186/s13613-021-00861-1. PMID: 33988767; PMCID: PMC8120254

97. COVID-ICU Group on behalf of the REVA Network and the COVID-ICU Investigators. Clinical characteristics and day-90 outcomes of 4244 critically ill adults with COVID-19: a prospective cohort study. Intensive Care Med. 2021;47(1):60–73.

98. Lim ZJ, Subramaniam A, Ponnapa Reddy M, et al. Case fatality rates for patients with COVID-19 requiring invasive mechanical ventilation. A meta-analysis. Am J Respir Crit Care Med. 2021;203(1):54–66.

99. Onder G, Rezza G, Brusaferro S. Case-fatality rate and characteristics of patients dying in relation to COVID-19 in Italy. JAMA. 2020;323(18):1775–6.

100. Guan WJ, Ni ZY, Hu Y, et al. China Medical Treatment Expert Group for COVID-19. Clinical characteristics of coronavirus disease 2019 in China. N Engl J Med. 2020;382(18):1708–20.

101. Atkins JL, Masoli JAH, Delgado J, et al. Preexisting comorbidities predicting COVID-19 and mortality in the UK biobank community cohort. J Gerontol A Biol Sci Med Sci. 2020 Oct 15;75(11):2224–30.

102. Vallet H, Schwarz GL, Flaatten H, de Lange DW, Guidet B, Dechartres A. Mortality of older patients admitted to an ICU: a systematic review. Crit Care Med. 2021;49(2):324–34.

103. Pulok MH, Theou O, van der Valk AM, Rockwood K. The role of illness acuity on the association between frailty and mortality in emergency department patients referred to internal medicine. Age Ageing. 2020;49(6):1071–9.

104. National Institute for Health and Care Excellence. COVID- 19 rapid guideline: critical care in adults. In: National Institute for Health and Care Excellence, 2020. Available online at: https://www.nice.org.uk/guidance/ng159. Accessed 15 Sept 2021.

105. Azoulay É, Beloucif S, Guidet B, Pateron D, Vivien B, Le Dorze M. Admission decisions to intensive care units in the context of the major COVID-19 outbreak: local guidance from the COVID-19 Paris-region area. Crit Care. 2020;24(1):293. https://doi.org/10.1186/s13054-020-03021-2. PMID: 32503593; PMCID: PMC7274070

106. Owen RK, Conroy SP, Taub N, et al. Comparing associations between frailty and mortality in hospitalised older adults with or without COVID-19 infection: a retrospective observational study using electronic health records. Age Ageing. 2021;50(2):307–16.

107. Miles A, Webb TE, Mcloughlin BC, et al. Outcomes from COVID-19 across the range of frailty: excess mortality in fitter older people. Eur Geriatr Med. 2020;11(5):851–5.

108. Geriatric Medicine Research Collaborative, Covid Collaborative, Welch C. Age and frailty are independently associated with increased COVID-19 mortality and increased care needs in survivors: results of an international multi-centre study. Age Ageing. 2021;50(3):617–30.

109. Jung C, Flaatten H, Fjølner J, et al. COVIP study group. The impact of frailty on survival in elderly intensive care patients with COVID-19: the COVIP study. Crit Care. 2021;25(1):149.

Sepsis in Older Adults

Lenneke van Lelyveld-Haas, Dylan de Lange, and I. Martin-Loeches

Contents

🏠 Learning Objectives

- The sepsis 3.0 criteria:
  - Sepsis is defined as life-threatening organ dysfunction caused by a dysregulated host response to infection [1, 2]. Organ dysfunction is defined as an increase of two or more points in the sequential (sepsis-related) organ failure assessment (SOFA) score (appendix I).
  - Septic shock is defined as sepsis with circulatory, cellular, and metabolic abnormalities, associated with a greater mortality risk. These patients require vasopressors to maintain a mean arterial pressure (MAP) $\geq$65 mmHg and have a lactate >2 mmol/L (>18 mg/dL), despite adequate fluid resuscitation.
- Sepsis risks and incidences increase with age.
- Immunosenescence, additional comorbidities (including diabetes and chronic kidney disease and other risk factors including malnutrition), and inflammaging lead to increased risk of infection in older adults.
- Sepsis can be more difficult to diagnose in elderly, who frequently present with nonspecific signs and symptoms.
- Overall treatment of sepsis in the elderly should be according SSC guidelines. However, some points require special attention in this vulnerable patient population, including the following:
  - Fluid resuscitation should be done carefully, since very old patients are at higher risk for both under- and over-resuscitation.
  - Vasopressors may be needed in order to help achieve appropriate MAP levels; however, appropriate MAP levels in older adults have not been specified, nor have the appropriate vasopressors for older adults been identified.
  - Older adults are at increased risk of having infections with drug-resistant pathogens and additional gram-negative bacteria.
  - Drug selection can be challenging in this patient population due to multiple pharmacokinetic and pharmacodynamics changes related to aging.
- Older adults are at higher risk of developing ICU delirium, and clinicians need to perform routine delirium assessments, adequate pain control, prevention of constipation, and avoidance of benzodiazepines, anticholinergic agents, and other deliriogenic medications.
- Mortality rates of very old patients with sepsis are quite high. Age, severity of disease (SOFA), and frailty are important independent risk factors for mortality. Sepsis at admission is, however, not independently associated with 30-day or 6-month mortality.
- Special care should be taken when decisions need to be made about ICU treatment of these patients, since the ethical principles of avoiding (net) harm and respect for patients' autonomy are easily violated in very old patients with sepsis. Physicians are obliged not to provide treatment that is not for the patient's good, especially if that treatment is burdensome. First do no harm. Clinicians should discuss goals of care and prognosis with patients and families, incorporate those goals into treatment, and end of life care planning. A framework to decide on withholding intensive care in older patients, based on explicit estimations of baseline physical and cognitive status, subjective quality of life, the likelihood of long-term survival and acceptable functional performance, individual preferences, and the burden of treatment might be helpful.

30.1 Introduction to the Chapter

Sepsis is a major worldwide healthcare problem. It has been estimated that sepsis affects almost 50 million people per year and causes approximately 11 million deaths worldwide and accounts billions in healthcare costs annually [1]. The WHO estimated that sepsis causes 20% of deaths worldwide. The patients that do survive often suffer long-term physical, psychological, and cognitive disability.

In Europe, sepsis is responsible for about a quarter of all ICU admissions, and although sepsis occurs at all ages, incidences increase with age, and most sepsis episodes are seen in elderly patients (age ≥ 65 years) [2–4].

Since sepsis disproportionally affects older adults, elderly patients are responsible for the majority of all episodes of sepsis, with incidences that are still increasing [5, 6]. Sepsis is one of the leading causes of morbidity and mortality in the very elderly patients, and understanding and knowledge of recognition, treatment, and outcome are of utmost importance.

30.2 Definition

Sepsis is described as a variable, nonspecific, acute syndrome caused by an infection. It is not a specific illness, but rather a syndrome which is defined by consensus. The definition of sepsis has undergone three major revisions since 1991 [7–9]. This latest sepsis 3.0 definition defines sepsis as life-threatening organ dysfunction caused by overwhelming, dysregulated host response to infection [2, 10]. This new definition accentuates the dysregulated and maladaptive host response to infection. Organ dysfunction is defined as an acute increase of two or more points in the Sequential Organ Failure Assessment (SOFA) score [11]. What was previously called severe sepsis is now the new definition of sepsis. Septic shock is a subset of sepsis in which there is circulatory, cellular, and metabolic dysfunction. Septic shock is defined as persisting hypotension requiring vasopressors to maintain a mean arterial pressure (MAP) of 65 mmHg or higher and a serum lactate level greater than 2 mmol/L (18 mg/dL) despite adequate volume resuscitation.

30.3 Epidemiology

Elderly are, compared with younger patients, more susceptible to sepsis. They have less physiologic reserve to tolerate the insult from infection and are more likely to have underlying diseases. As a consequence, sepsis is a frequent cause of morbidity and mortality in elderly patients and appears to be a very common reason for very elderly patients to be admitted to the ICU. Very elderly patients are responsible for the majority of all episodes of sepsis. Incidences of sepsis increased last decades and are still increasing, and these increases are particularly seen in elderly patients [5, 6, 12–14]. The severity of disease increased also last years. At present, most sepsis episodes are observed in patients older than 60 years, with a sharp increase of the incidence in people older than 80 years. More than 60% of sepsis diagnoses are made in adults aged ≥65 years and approximately 64% of elderly patients with a mean age of 75 years admitted to an ICU met the definition of sepsis [4, 15]. Older adults are more likely to develop infections because of several reasons (see below, paragraph about immunity and pathophysiology).

30.4 Diagnosis

Sepsis is a syndrome defined by consensus and cannot be diagnosed by a "gold standard" clinical or laboratory tests. Diagnosing sepsis is still mainly clinical. However, since older adults with infection often present atypically, diagnosing sepsis in elderly patients can be challenging [16]. Since the body's immune response to infection is reduced with aging, sepsis in elderly often presents more atypically. Signs and symptoms may be more obscure in the elderly patients, and although the definition is the same in the elderly, you may need more diagnostic techniques, like CT scans or other ancillary tests. For example, fever, the most recognized clinical feature of infection, is absent in approximately 30–50% of the elderly patients with infection [17]. And in addition, typical localizing symptoms might be absent, or symptoms may be masked by concomitant use of drugs such as beta-blockers (no increase of heart rate) [18, 19]. The physiologic reserve of very elderly is diminished, and they are more likely to have underlying diseases.

30.5 Pathogen Detection in Elderly

Positive blood cultures are found in only 30% of patients with sepsis [20]. Molecular techniques, such as polymerase chain reaction/electrospray ionization-mass spectrometry (PCR-ESI-MS), have demonstrated higher rates of pathogen identification than standard blood culture and can provide results within 6 hours, but these assays require broader clinical evaluation and are frequently too expensive for many institutions [21]. A diagnostic blood culture is too slow and may be falsely negative and is thus inappropriate for early identification of sepsis.

Causative pathogens differ depending on the source and site of infection (community acquired or nosocomial sepsis). Respiratory tract and genitourinary tract infections are the most common infectious sources of sepsis in the elderly, and infections are more frequent than in younger adults caused by gram-negative organisms [6]. Elderly have higher risk for multiple drug resistance due to antibiotic pressure. *Escherichia coli* is the predominant cause (50%) of urinary tract infections (UTI) both in younger and older adults, but older adults are at increased risk for infection from other gram-negative bacteria, such as *Proteus* spp., *Klebsiella* spp., and *Pseudomonas* spp. Common gram-positive organisms in older adults with bloodstream infections include *Staphylococcus aureus*, *Enterococcus* spp., and *Streptococcus* spp. [22]. For the most frequent sources, the following pathogens are frequently found in elderly patients: urinary tract, *Escherichia coli*, *Proteus mirabilis*, *Klebsiella* species *(spp.)*, and *Enterobacter* spp.; lung (non-aspiration pneumonia), *Streptococcus pneumoniae*, *Enterobacteriaceae*, *Staphylococcus aureus, and*

Pseudomonas aeruginosa; in the case of aspiration pneumonia: *Streptococcus pneumoniae, Staphylococcus aureus, Fusobacterium* spp., *Prevotella* spp., and *Peptostreptococcus* spp.; and in the case of skin and soft tissue infections: *Streptococcus* spp., *Staphylococcus* spp., and *Pseudomonas aeruginosa* (diabetic foot infections) [23].

Traditional biomarkers of sepsis (like the total white cell count, neutrophil count, and C-reactive protein) lack the specificity to discriminate sepsis from inflammation due to noninfectious causes (e.g., pancreatitis, burns, and trauma). Newer biomarkers, such as procalcitonin (PCT) and sTREM-1 (soluble triggering receptor expressed on myeloid cells-1), do not have enough sensitivity or specificity and have not yet been sufficiently validated in the very elderly patients with sepsis. Consequently, at present, biomarkers unfortunately are not helpful in the diagnosis, or exclusion, of sepsis in VIPs.

30.6 Immunity

Elderly are, compared with younger patients, more susceptible to sepsis. First, because of immunosenescence, there is a gradual decline of the immune system with aging. The adaptive immune system is affected more than the innate immune system [24]. Elderly patients have a considerable decrease in both cell-mediated immune function and reduced humoral immune function [25]. Hallmarks of immunosenescence are "inflammaging" (the lingering level of low-grade inflammation), the reduced ability to respond to new antigens, and the accumulation of memory T cells [26, 27]. It is a multifactorial condition, resulting from several age-dependent biological changes of the immune system, contributing to enhanced susceptibility of elderly patients to sepsis [25, 28, 29] (see also the separate ▶ Chap. 6).

Second, elderly are more prone to infections due to their diminished functional status, frailty, and malnutrition. Third, many common comorbid diseases, including decreased cardiac and pulmonary reserves, malignancies, diabetes mellitus, and chronic liver failure, increase the risk sepsis and are all frequently seen in older patients [30]. Fourth, other factors which are quite common in elderly (e.g., an altered vaginal flora due to declining estrogen levels, urinary retention and stasis due to prostatic hypertrophy, poor skin integrity due to age-associated changes, immobility, swallowing difficulty, diminished cough reflex, and inadequate oral care) all increase the risk for infections [18, 31–35]. In addition, decreases in circulating thyroid hormone and endogenous corticosteroids make elderly more prone for infection. Fifth, institutionalization and instrumentation (e.g., urinary catheters) are all associated with sepsis. Nursing home residents were seven times more likely to be diagnosed with severe sepsis compared with non-nursing home residents, and rates of ICU admissions were twice as high [36]. Cognitive impairment is another risk factor for severe infection. After controlling for multiple factors, including age, sex, and comorbidities, dementia showed to be associated with a 50% higher risk of severe sepsis [37].

30.7 **Pathophysiology**

The pathophysiology of sepsis and septic shock is not precisely understood, but is considered to involve a complex interaction between the pathogen and the host's immune system. In health, humans live in a state of symbiosis with microorganisms, but in sepsis, microorganisms invade normally sterile host tissues and become a threat to the host. The normal physiologic response to (localized) infection includes activation of host defense mechanisms that result in the influx of activated neutrophils and monocytes, release of inflammatory mediators, local vasodilation, increased endothelial permeability, and activation of coagulation pathways. Sepsis, however, results from an exaggerated systemic inflammatory response induced by infecting organisms, leading to secondary organ system failure. A profoundly deranged host-microbial homeostasis with early activation of both pro- and anti-inflammatory responses occurs, along with major alterations in non-immunologic pathways such as the cardiovascular, neuronal, hormonal, metabolic, and coagulation systems. Inflammatory mediators are the key players in the pathogenesis of sepsis, but other factors such as the causative pathogen, initial site of infection, comorbidities, and iatrogenic interventions also affect the host response [38]. Genetic defects have also been identified to play in role in sepsis development.

Several biochemical processes occur and are responsible for the clinical manifestation of sepsis [39, 40]. The first process is vasodilatation, caused by a number of cytokines and involving small arterioles and nutrient vessels. Expression of inducible nitric oxide synthase (iNOS) in vascular endothelial cells is induced and nitric oxide generated, which is a potent smooth muscle relaxing agent that causes local vasodilatation. Due to the vasodilatation, the vascular resistance is reduced, and relative hypovolemia and decreased effective blood pressure occur. The diminished capacity of the heart to cope with hypovolemia and low blood pressure is described in the chapter on vasoactive drugs of this book. The loss of normal microvasculature resistance results in accelerated passage of blood through capillary beds, reducing the time available for the passive unloading of oxygen from saturated erythrocytes. The second is loss of endothelial barrier function. Disruption of the endothelial tight junctions and loss of endothelial cells result in the loss of proteins and fluid into the interstitium, which further decreases the effective intravascular volume. The resulting edema aggravates cellular hypoxia by increasing the distance between the erythrocyte in the capillary and the adjacent cells. The third biochemical process is occlusion of capillaries by thrombi, activated leukocytes, and aggregates of erythrocytes, impairing perfusion. Oxygenated blood will bypass the occluded capillaries, resulting in an increase in the local tissue oxygen deficit. The fourth is impaired myocardial contractility that occurs as a consequence of poorly characterized myocardial depressant factors. However, its significance is uncertain, since the cardiac output is characteristically increased in sepsis. Finally, mitochondrial dysfunction occurs in sepsis. Mitochondria are affected in several ways, including insufficient oxygen at the mitochondrial level to allow function; the generation of excess amounts of multiple reactive oxygen species (e.g., NO, CO, H2S), causing direct damage to mitochondrial structures; hormone-induced alterations in function and efficiency; and the downregulation of mitochondrial gene transcription proteins. These processes lead to a bioenergetic-metabolic shutdown, similar to a state of hibernation. An association between the degree of mitochondrial impairment and either clinical severity, organ dysfunction, or poor outcomes has been demonstrated. However, whether this is a causal pathway to organ damage, death is unclear. It may also represent a mechanism through which eventual survival is enhanced.

30.8 Treatment of Sepsis in Elderly

Treatment of very elderly patients with sepsis should follow the Surviving Sepsis Campaign (SSC) guidelines in general, the same as for younger adults, although there are some important considerations when managing very old patients. Therefore, we will present the general SSC guidelines and highlight and discuss where more attention or another approach is required in very old patients. Nevertheless, robust evidence about sepsis treatment of very old patients is scarce. Older adults often were excluded or underrepresented in sepsis trials. And when they were included, no subgroup analyses were performed, so specific recommendations for treatment of older adults could be made.

In 2002, the SSC was initiated [41]. The SSC campaign had the aim to reduce mortality from sepsis worldwide through the development of guidelines for diagnosis and treatment. After 2002, the campaign progressed in several phases, with publication of four editions (every 4 years) of evidence-based guidelines, implementation of a performance improvement program, and analysis and publication of multiple studies from around the world [42–45]. The SSC have strongly influenced our clinical practice regarding the septic patient the past decades. In 2018, the SSC published a revision to the bundle based on the 2016 guidelines. The bundle changed from 3 hours and 6 hours to an Hour-1 bundle to encourage more rapid interventions for adult patients with sepsis and septic shock, which is crucial. The four items of this 1-hour bundle are: measurement of lactate level (and remeasure if elevated (i.e. >2 mmol/L), obtaining cultures, (including blood cultures), administration of broad-spectrum antibiotics, rapid fluid administration in case of hypotension or lactate level $\geq$ 4 mmol/L, and vasopressors if hypotension persist during or after fluid resuscitation to maintain MAP $\geq$65 mm Hg [46].

30.8.1 Fluid Resuscitation

Fluid resuscitation is important in all patients with sepsis and serves to optimize cardiac preload and improve or preserve organ perfusion pressure. All patients with sepsis who are hypotensive require fluid resuscitation; however, in VIPs with sepsis, fluid resuscitation requires special attention and should be done carefully. The SSC recommends fluid resuscitation to maintain or achieve MAP $\geq$65 mm Hg, but it is questioned if higher MAP goals (80–85 mm Hg) are required in VIPs with sepsis, due to their additional comorbidities, although clinical trials nor the SSC support this goal elevation (see the ▶ Chap. 19). Elderly patients more often are known with chronic arterial hypertension, which results in a rightward shift of the autoregulatory pressure-organ perfusion curve [47]. Therefore, higher MAP targets may be needed to prevent acute kidney injury (AKI). It seems essential to carefully define an individualized target MAP for the resuscitation phase goals by considering the patient's pre-admission MAP in elderly patients with sepsis and septic shock. Although no difference in 28-day mortality rates was found between the patients (with septic shock) with high (80–85 mmHg) or low (65–70 mmHg) MAP targets, the subset of patients with chronic arterial hypertension indeed had a lower incidence of serum creatinine doubling and required less renal replacement therapy when randomized to the high MAP target group. However, the higher MAP target group also had a higher incidence of atrial fibrillation [48]. Another study demonstrated a relation between the incidence of AKI and the difference between pre- and post-resuscitation MAP values in patients with severe sepsis or septic shock. The MAP differences were demonstrated as a risk factor for sepsis-associated (SA)-AKI, with significantly lower incidence of AKI in the patients with MAP differences (pre-admission MAP minus post-resuscitation MAP) values in the lowest quartile (i.e., patients with post-resuscitation MAP mostly higher than their pre-admission MAP). Analysis of the subgroup of patients with hypertension showed the same relationship [49]. Though these VIPs might be at greater risk of under-resuscitation, some caution should be taken to avoid excessive resuscitation, particularly in patients with known heart failure or significant renal impairment. It is also important to timely start de-resuscitation with diuretics. Very old patients more often suffer systolic and also diastolic dysfunction. Diastolic dysfunction is associated with age and other comorbidities that are more frequent in elderly, like hypertension, diabetes mellitus, and ischemic heart disease (IHD). In addition, diastolic dysfunction is common during severe sepsis and septic shock in patients of all ages. It was demonstrated that diastolic dysfunction is a strong independent predictor of mortality [50, 51]. Fluid challenge assessment techniques, like transthoracic echocardiogram (TTE), pulse pressure variation (PPV), cardiac output (CO), and/or end-diastolic volume (EDV) measurements (e.g., with Pulse Contour Cardiac Output (PICCO) method), may be helpful to identify VIPs who require further fluid resuscitation during severe sepsis and septic shock.

The SSC recommends an initial fluid challenge of 30 mL/kg IV in all patients, followed by additional fluid therapy until the patient no longer demonstrates hemodynamic improvement (strong recommendation, low quality of evidence). A fluid challenge technique should be applied, and fluid administration is continued as long as hemodynamic factors continue to improve [45, 52–57].

Crystalloids are the fluid of choice and preferred over colloids, both for initial resuscitation as for subsequent intravascular volume replacement (strong recommendation, moderate quality of evidence). Either balanced crystalloids (e.g., Ringer's lactate or Plasmalyte®) or saline is suggested for fluid resuscitation. Irrespective of the crystalloid solution selected, hyperchloremia should be avoided [58, 59]. Hydroxyethyl starch (HES) should not be used (due to higher rates of mortality and RRT as compared to crystalloid). The place of human albumin is still a matter of debate. Human albumin could eventually be considered for intravascular volume replacement in addition to crystalloids for patients with low albumin and requiring substantial amounts of crystalloids (albumin concentration target of 3 g/dL) (weak recommendation, low quality of evidence). Although the general guidelines recommend against transfusing to hemoglobin levels >9 g/dL (strong recommendation, high quality of evidence), the optimal transfusion threshold in VIPs with sepsis is not exactly defined.

30.8.2 Vasopressors (See Also ▶ Chap. 19)

Vasopressors may be needed in order to help achieve appropriate MAP levels and to improve and preserve sepsis-induced end-organ perfusion for elderly patients exhibiting hypotension despite adequate fluid resuscitation (septic shock). The SSC guidelines strongly recommend to target an initial goal MAP ≥65 mm Hg, but as discussed above higher goals may be beneficial in patients with hypertension or atherosclerosis, which are common comorbidities in older patients, since it is demonstrated that a target MAP of 80–85 mm Hg resulted in improved renal function when compared to standard targets in patients with a history of arterial hypertension. However, no differences in mortality were seen, and patients in the high target group had a greater incidence of atrial fibrillation (AF). Individualized assessments of regional and global perfusion, such as lactate concentration, mental status, and diuresis, might be more important monitoring and treatment targets.

Norepinephrine is the first choice for patients in general. However, as discussed above, appropriate MAP levels in VIPs have not been specified, nor have the appropriate vasopressors for VIPs with sepsis. Vasoactive agents can be classified as vasopressors, inotropes, or vasodilators. The receptor pharmacology of each vasoactive agent ultimately determines the physiologic properties and impacts on various hemodynamic parameters in terms of both important beneficial and adverse effects. The selection of a specific agent is largely guided by balancing the beneficial hemodynamic effects and unwanted adverse effects. Safety concerns may be amplified in older adults, particularly those with multiple comorbid disease states.

30.8.3 Antibiotics

Timely administration of appropriate and effective antimicrobial therapy is a cornerstone of sepsis management, because poor outcomes are associated with inadequate therapy across all ages (strong recommendation, moderate quality of evidence) [60]. The SSC recommend starting broad-spectrum intravenous antibiotics within 1 h of sepsis recognition (strong recommendation, moderate quality of evidence).

Empiric regimens should be determined by several factors, including epidemiological risk factors, the likely source of infection based on presenting signs and symptoms comorbidities, severity of illness, and local epidemiology. Empiric therapy should be tailored to definitive regimens and/or stopped if the balance of evidence is that infection is unlikely [61, 62]. When starting broad-spectrum antibiotics in VIPs with sepsis, special considerations to the selection and dosing of the antimicrobials should be given, since VIPs are at higher risk, compared with younger adults, for having an infection with a multidrug-resistant organism (MDRO), because of multiple reasons, including comorbid conditions like COPD, renal failure, and diabetes mellitus; recent hospitalizations; recent exposure to antibiotics; residing in a long-term care facility; foreign bodies (urinary catheter, vascular access devices); and prior colonization with an MDRO.

Dosing receives special attention, because of alterations in pharmacokinetics and pharmacodynamics that occur with aging, due to physiologic changes. Several antibiotics require dosage adjustment to prevent toxicity, and using standard adult dosing nomograms is often not appropriate.

30.8.4 Sedation

As in general, continuous or intermittent sedation should be minimized in VIPs with sepsis. Specific titration endpoints should be targeted, to reduce duration of mechanical ventilation and support earlier mobilization. Limiting the use of sedatives, regardless of the used drug, is associated with a reduction of the duration of mechanical ventilation, ICU, and hospital length of stay (LOS). Targeting prespecified sedation levels (like Ramsay Sedation Scale, Richmond Agitation Sedation Scale (RASS), or Riker Sedation-Agitation Scale (SAS)) eventually with daily interruptions and/or the use of short acting drugs both may all contribute to faster weaning from mechanical ventilation, shorter ICU LOS, and improved outcomes of VIPs with sepsis [63–65]. Due to the aforementioned alterations in pharmacokinetics and pharmacodynamics of drugs in older patients, the life span of sedatives may be prolonged. Therefore, dosing of sedatives also should be done carefully, and the use of short acting drugs and individualized sedation protocols may be useful.

Due to underlying cognitive changes, VIPs have higher delirium risks. Delirium itself is associated with increased mortality in VIPs [66]. Nonpharmacologic approaches to the management of pain, agitation, and delirium should be explored, and use of benzodiazepines should be minimized [67].

30.8.5 Corticosteroids

The use of steroids in sepsis is controversial, and up till now, evidence for a mortality benefit is contradictory [68–72]. The SSC guidelines suggest hydrocortisone administration at 200 mg/day if the restoration of hemodynamics cannot be achieved and in patients with known prior steroid therapy or suspected impaired adrenal function. Critical illness-related corticosteroid insufficiency (CIRCI) might be more frequent in elderly patients, but data are scarce. Blockage of adrenal cortisol production by etomidate (by inhibition of 11-β-hydroxylase) is prolonged in elderly patients. ACTH or random cortisol testing is not recommended. Corticosteroid therapy can be tapered when there is no longer a need for vasopressor support [68, 69, 73].

We believe the same recommendations can be given for very old patients with sepsis. Normal aging results in subtle changes both in ACTH and cortisol secretion. Daily cortisol levels are increased in the elderly, without a noteworthy alteration in the normal circadian rhythm pattern [74]. Hyperglycemia and hypernatremia may develop during therapy with steroids, and since type 2 diabetes is already more frequent in elderly, blood glucose levels should be monitored carefully and insulin therapy started if necessary.

30.8.6 Glucose Control

For patients with sepsis in general, insulin therapy should be started after two blood glucose levels >180 mg/dL (10 mmol/l). Blood glucose levels should be monitored every 1–2 hours until stabilization and every 4 hours thereafter if the patient receives an insulin infusion and targeted ≤180 mg/dL (10 mmol/l). In addition, diabetes mellitus is more frequent in elderly. Therefore, glucose control should be done in every elderly patient with sepsis. However, it is not determined if the same or other glucose levels should be targeted in the very old patients with sepsis.

30.8.7 Thromboembolic Prophylaxis

Pharmacologic prophylaxis with LMWH is recommended in general for patients with sepsis, in the absence of any contraindications, to prevent deep vein thrombosis (DVT) and pulmonary embolism (PE). Elderly patients are more prone to DVT and PE, and incidences rise with age. Aging is one of the strongest and most prevalent risk factor for venous thrombosis [75, 76]. Age-specific risk factors of thrombosis, that is, endothelial dysfunction and frailty, may be important in the explanation of the increased incidence of VT in the elderly. Other risk factors for venous thromboembolism in elderly are immobilization, comorbidities (including congestive heart failure, chronic obstructive pulmonary disease, diabetes mellitus, altered hormone hemostasis, and malignancy), and increased levels of coagulation factors.

Since elderly are more prone to DVT and PE, pharmacologic prophylaxis with LMWH is of utmost importance. In VIPs with impaired renal function, it might be necessary to reduce the LMWH dose, since LMWH is renally excreted. It is recommended to monitor anti-Xa levels in VIPs with a creatinine clearance of <30 ml/minute and subsequently adjust LMWH doses according to the measured anti-Xa levels.

Nevertheless, older patients also have increased bleeding risks. These increased thromboembolic and bleeding risks should be evaluated individually. If pharmacologic prophylaxis is contraindicated, mechanical thromboembolism prophylaxis is recommended [77].

30.8.8 Stress Ulcer Prophylaxis (SUP)

Patients with sepsis or septic shock should in general receive SUP, with either histamine-2 receptor antagonists (H2RAs) or proton pump inhibitors (PPIs). Since very old patients with sepsis are at risk for gastrointestinal (GI) stress ulcers with clinically significant bleeding, the need for SUP should be evaluated in every elderly patient with sepsis, with attention to the presence of risk factors for hemorrhage [78, 79].

30.9 Medication: Pharmacokinetics and Pharmacodynamics (See Also ▶ Chap. 7)

Pharmacokinetics (PK) and pharmacodynamics (PD) are different in very old patients, and this should be taken into consideration when medication, including antibiotics, is prescribed for these patients [23, 80, 81].

Age is a well-documented risk factor for the development of both liver and kidney insufficiency, and dose adjustments may be necessary. In addition, older adults with multiple comorbidities are susceptible to polypharmacy, which may pose additional risks of adverse drug reactions. A number of changes are seen in the absorption, distribution, metabolism, and elimination of drugs in older patients (see also the separate ▶ Chap. 7).

Absorption of medications may decline in older adults, due to atrophy of the gastric parietal cells with increased gastric pH, delayed emptying time and a decreased intestinal surface area, and decreased abdominal blood flow [80, 82].

Distribution can be different due to the altered body composition of very old patients, a decreased lean muscle mass, increased body fat, and decreased total body water. This leads to a decreased volume of distribution for hydrophilic medications and an increased volume of distribution for lipophilic medications. In addition, VIPs have decreased serum albumin leading to an increased concentration of free fraction of drugs which are normally highly protein bound [19].

Metabolism and elimination of drugs are often also altered in very old patients. Due to age-related decline in hepatic blood flow and impairment in hepatic enzymes (including P450 system activity), first-pass effects decrease, and half-lives of hepatically cleared medications increase. Renal function is difficult to estimate in VIPs due to an age-related decrease in muscle mass and decreased renal filtration capacity due to age-related damage to glomeruli. Clearance of renally cleared medications may be decreased.

Very old patients mostly have decreased systemic perfusion as a result of atherosclerosis and increased peripheral vascular resistance, and this effect may be further enhanced in cases of sepsis. As a consequence, medications have decreased penetration into tissue with sub-therapeutic concentrations and lead to a higher incidence of treatment failure. Alternatively, due to decreased perfusion to the liver and kidneys, metabolism and elimination of antimicrobials may be decreased leading to increased risks of various toxicities.

30.10 Outcomes: Mortality, Predictive Values of Scoring Systems, Functional Outcome, and Quality of Life

Advanced age is associated with worse outcomes of sepsis [6]. Although several recent studies repeatedly demonstrated that age is one of the important independent risk factors for mortality in very elderly patients with sepsis, many other factors, including frailty, severity of organ failure, and comorbidities, play also an important role [83, 84]. Sepsis as admission diagnosis, however, was not independently associated with 30-day or 6-month mortality, after adjusting for organ dysfunction [85, 86].

Although advances in diagnosis and management have led to significant improvements in outcomes of ICU patients overall and across all ages, mortality rates of very old patients with sepsis remain quite high [4, 5, 84, 87–89]. In a large prospective multicenter trial, the 28-day and hospital mortality rates of very old patients with sepsis were, respectively, 46.8% and 54.2% ($p = 0.02$) [84]. A systematic review describing the outcome of very old patients with sepsis documented ICU-, hospital-, and 1-year mortality rates of respectively 43%, 47%, and 68% [89]. Mortality rates of the very old patients admitted with sepsis were higher compared with very elderly admitted to the ICU for another reason than sepsis. Older adult non-survivors tend to die earlier during hospitalization. In the VIP-1 study, a large European multicenter study, the ICU- and 30-day mortality rates of the patients aged ≥80 years admitted with sepsis were respectively 31.2% and 44.6% [90]. ICU- and 6-month mortality rates of the patients aged ≥80 years admitted with sepsis in the VIP-2 study were 31.4% and 53.8% [83].

The predictive value for mortality of the different scoring systems, including APACHE IV, SOFA, SAPS, MPM, in elderly patients is lower, compared to younger patients. Age provides a high weight into the variables for prognostication, along with the presence of comorbidities. The prognostic model of SAPS 3 was not found to be accurate in predicting mortality in geriatric patients requiring ICU admission [91]. Alternative modeling approaches might be needed to customize the model coefficients to the elderly population for more accurate probabilities or to develop specialized models for the elderly patients. Since the use of the SOFA score requires laboratory values that may not be readily available at the bedside, the qSOFA was developed [10]. The qSOFA is an easy to use risk stratification tool for non-ICU settings to recognize sepsis at an early stage. It can be obtained without laboratory testing and contains the following three components: systolic blood pressure ≤ 100 mm Hg, respiratory rate ≥ 22 breaths per minute, and altered mentation. However, in very elderly admitted to Dutch ICUs with sepsis, the discriminative performance of qSOFA for in-hospital mortality was poor (AUC 0.596) and lower than that of SOFA, APACHE IV, and SAPS II (0.704, 0.722, and 0.780, respectively). A qSOFA model extended with several other characteristics (AUC 0.643) was non-inferior to the full SOFA but still inferior to APACHE IV and SAPS II, for all age groups [92].

Many very old patients who survive their hospitalization because of sepsis suffer from significant functional disability and cognitive decline and cannot be discharged home. They frequently require skilled nursing or rehabilitation after hospitalization. They suffer from long-term impairments; cognitive, psychological, and physical impairments; and complaints like muscle weakness, fatigue, poor memory, difficulty concentrating, cloudy thinking, difficulty sleeping, sadness, anxiety, and difficulty swallowing, known as post-intensive care syndrome (PICS) [93, 94]. PICS is more likely to affect VIPs and has become an increasingly important phenomenon in very elderly for several reasons. First, the number of VIPs increases as the population ages, and patients 85 and over make up the fastest growing age group for ICU admissions. Second, a majority of VIPs develop delirium, which is a major risk factor for developing ICU-acquired cognitive impairment. Third, cognitive and functional impairment before an ICU hospitalization increases the likelihood of cognitive and functional decline afterward [93].

Severe sepsis was found to be associated with a threefold higher rate of progression from moderate to severe cognitive impairment. Sepsis has also been associated with decreased quality of life (QoL) [95, 96]. However, several studies have demonstrated that elderly ICU survivors might accept their disabilities and accommodate to a degree of physical disability quite well, consider their QoL to be good or satisfactory, and report good emotional and social well-being after hospital discharge [97].

30.11 Triage and Medical Ethics

The decision whether to admit a very old patient with sepsis to the ICU can be difficult. Since elderly patients have a higher risk of death and of functional decline than younger patients, discussions about proportionality of ICU care may arise.

In medical ethics, there are four leading principles to guide treatment decisions: non-maleficence, beneficence, respect for the patient's autonomy, and distributive justice [98]. For very old patients admitted because of sepsis, these four principles may be in conflict with each other. Most ICU treatments are not without side effects and have high costs. For example, the principle of non-maleficence is usually violated by invasive treatments such as intubation and central venous catheterization. Violating this principle is usually justified, since the intended benefit of these measures is expected to outweigh the harm. However, this balance might be different in very old patients with sepsis. The harm (suffering) caused by the ICU treatment may be similar to that in younger ICU patients, but the benefit of the ICU treatment is often much smaller.

With regard to the principle of patient autonomy, it is important to know that it is not obvious that all very old patients with sepsis would like to be admitted to the ICU. Some of them might prefer care focused on "quality of dying" and relieving pain and discomfort over life-extending treatment [99, 100]. The assessment of a tolerable degree of suffering and acceptable outcome of ICU treatment should be in the eye of the patient, rather than that of the treating team. Medical treatment has to be justified by the autonomous wish of the patient and the benefit of treatment for that unique patient. Therefore, goals of care should be discussed in all very old patients with sepsis. This carefully balancing of pros and cons of ICU treatment should not only be done before ICU admission but also during a (prolonged) ICU admission. All decisions on starting, continuing, or foregoing life-sustaining treatments (LST) should be justified by serving the well-being of that particular patient, aligned with his or her wishes. A framework to decide on withholding intensive care in older patients, based on explicit estimations of baseline physical and cognitive status, subjective quality of life, the likelihood of long-term survival and acceptable functional performance, individual preferences, and the burden of treatment has been proposed [101].

30.12 Cost Burden of Very Old Patients with Sepsis

As a consequence of the aging of the population and the high rate of sepsis among the older population, sepsis has a significant burden on our society and important implications for our healthcare system [102–104]. Sepsis is the most expensive condition treated in hospitals in the United States [105]. The annual cost of sepsis treatment in 2017 was almost $40 billion (38.2 billion), representing 8.8% of aggregate hospital costs and with more than 50% of these costs attributed to the care of individuals over the age of 65 years. Readmission after sepsis is more frequent and more expensive than readmissions for other medical conditions, like COPD, pneumonia, and heart failure [106].

For very old patients in general, it has been demonstrated that they consume more healthcare resources in the year before, the year of, and the year after ICU admission, compared to younger ICU patients and a very elderly control population [107]. Although this study was not exclusively about very old patients admitted with sepsis, high costs can also be expected after hospital discharge for the very elderly admitted with sepsis, since the majority of the very old patients who survive their hospitalization because of sepsis suffer from significant functional disability and cognitive decline, requiring skilled nursing or rehabilitation after hospitalization.

> **Conclusion**
>
> Sepsis is a major worldwide healthcare problem. Older patients are, compared with younger patients, more susceptible to sepsis and responsible for the majority of all episodes of sepsis, with incidences that are still increasing. Elderly frequently present with nonspecific signs and symptoms, and diagnosing sepsis may be more challenging. Overall treatment of sepsis in the elderly should be according SSC guidelines. However, as discussed, some points require special attention in this vulnerable patient population. Although treatment modalities improved, mortality rates of older patients with sepsis still are quite high.

30

> **Take Home Message**
> - Sepsis is a major worldwide healthcare problem. Elderly patients are, due to several reasons, more susceptible to infection and as a consequence responsible for the majority of all episodes of sepsis, with incidences that are still increasing.
> - Sepsis can be more difficult to diagnose in elderly, who frequently present with nonspecific signs and symptoms.
> - The sepsis 3.0 definition defines sepsis as life-threatening organ dysfunction caused by overwhelming, dysregulated host response to infection.
> - Overall treatment of sepsis in the elderly should be according SSC guidelines. However, several aspects (e.g., fluid resuscitation, vasopressors, choice of antibiotics, sedation, and drug selection) require special attention in this vulnerable patient population.
> - Mortality rates of very old patients with sepsis are quite high. Age, severity of disease (SOFA), and frailty are important independent risk factors for mortality.
> - Special care should be taken when decisions need to be made about ICU treatment of these patients, since the ethical principles of avoiding (net) harm and respect for patients' autonomy are easily violated in very old patients with sepsis. Physicians are obliged not to provide treatment that is not for the patient's good, especially if that treatment is burdensome. First do no harm.
> - Clinicians should discuss goals of care and prognosis with patients and families. A framework to decide on withholding intensive care in older patients based on explicit estimations of baseline physical and cognitive status, subjective quality of life, the likelihood of long-term survival and acceptable functional performance, individual preferences, and the burden of treatment might be helpful.

References

1. Organization WH. Global report on the epidemiology and burden of sepsis: current evidence, identifying gaps and future directions. Geneva: World Health Organization; 2020. Licence: CC BY-NC-SA 3.0 IGO ISBN: 978 92 4 001078 9.
2. Singer M, Deutschman CS, Seymour CW, Shankar-Hari M, Annane D, Bauer M, et al. The third international consensus definitions for sepsis and septic shock (sepsis-3). JAMA [Internet]. 2016 [cited 2019 Jan 23];315(8):801–10. Available from: http://jama.jamanetwork.com/article.aspx?doi=10.1001/jama.2016.0287.
3. Vincent J-L, Sakr Y, Singer M, Martin-Loeches I, Machado FR, Marshall JC, et al. Prevalence and outcomes of infection among patients in intensive care units in 2017. JAMA. 2020;323(15):1478–87.
4. Kaukonen K-M, Bailey M, Suzuki S, Pilcher D, Bellomo R. Mortality related to severe sepsis and septic shock among critically ill patients in Australia and New Zealand, 2000–2012. JAMA [Internet]. 2014 [cited 2019 Jan 23];311(13):1308–16. Available from: http://jama.jamanetwork.com/article.aspx?doi=10.1001/jama.2014.2637
5. Angus DC, Linde-Zwirble WT, Lidicker J, Clermont G, Carcillo J, Pinsky MR. Epidemiology of severe sepsis in the United States: analysis of incidence, outcome, and associated costs of care. Crit Care Med [Internet]. 2001 [cited 2019 Jan 23];29(7):1303–10. Available from: http://www.ncbi.nlm.nih.gov/pubmed/11445675.
6. Martin GS, Mannino DM, Moss M. The effect of age on the development and outcome of adult sepsis. Crit Care Med [Internet]. 2006 [cited 2019 Jan 23];34(1):15–21. Available from: http://www.ncbi.nlm.nih.gov/pubmed/16374151.
7. Bone RC, Balk RA, Cerra FB, Dellinger RP, Fein AM, Knaus WA, et al. Definitions for sepsis and organ failure and guidelines for the use of innovative therapies in sepsis. The ACCP/SCCM Consensus Conference Committee. American College of Chest Physicians/Society of Critical Care Medicine. Chest [Internet]. 1992 [cited 2019 Jan 23];101(6):1644–55. Available from: http://www.ncbi.nlm.nih.gov/pubmed/1303622.
8. Levy MM, Fink MP, Marshall JC, Abraham E, Angus D, Cook D, et al. 2001 SCCM/ESICM/ACCP/ATS/SIS international sepsis definitions conference. Crit Care Med [Internet]. 2003 [cited 2019 Jan 23];31(4):1250–6. Available from: http://www.ncbi.nlm.nih.gov/pubmed/12682500.
9. Kaukonen K-M, Bailey M, Pilcher D, Cooper DJ, Bellomo R. Systemic inflammatory response syndrome criteria in defining severe sepsis. N Engl J Med [Internet]. 2015 [cited 2019 Jan 23];372(17):1629–38. Available from: http://www.nejm.org/doi/10.1056/NEJMoa1415236.
10. Seymour CW, Liu VX, Iwashyna TJ, Brunkhorst FM, Rea TD, Scherag A, et al. Assessment of clinical criteria for sepsis: for the third international consensus definitions for sepsis and septic shock (sepsis-3). JAMA [Internet]. 2016 [cited 2019 Jan 23];315(8):762–74. Available from: http://jama.jamanetwork.com/article.aspx?doi=10.1001/jama.2016.0288
11. Vincent JL, Moreno R, Takala J, Willatts S, De Mendonça A, Bruining H, et al. The SOFA (Sepsis-related Organ Failure Assessment) score to describe organ dysfunction/failure. On behalf of the Working Group on Sepsis-Related Problems of the European Society of Intensive Care Medicine. Intensive Care Med [Internet]. 1996 [cited 2019 Jan 23];22(7):707–10. Available from: http://www.ncbi.nlm.nih.gov/pubmed/8844239.
12. Gavazzi G, Krause K-H. Ageing and infection. Lancet Infect Dis. 2002;2(11):659–66.
13. Pawelec G, Solana R, Remarque E, Mariani E. Impact of aging on innate immunity. J Leukoc Biol. 1998;64(6):703–12.
14. Martin GS, Mannino DM, Eaton S, Moss M. The epidemiology of sepsis in the United States from 1979 through 2000. N Engl J Med. 2003;348(16):1546–54.
15. Rowe T, KLB A, Van Ness PH, Pisani MA, Juthani-Mehta M. Outcomes of older adults with sepsis at admission to an intensive care unit. Open forum Infect Dis. 2016;3(1):ofw010.
16. Ginaldi L, Loreto MF, Corsi MP, Modesti M, De Martinis M. Immunosenescence and infectious diseases. Microbes Infect. 2001;3(10):851–7.
17. Norman DC. Fever in the elderly. Clin Infect Dis an Off Publ Infect Dis Soc Am. 2000;31(1):148–51.
18. van Duin D. Diagnostic challenges and opportunities in older adults with infectious diseases. Clin Infect Dis an Off Publ Infect Dis Soc Am. 2012;54(7):973–8.

19. Bellmann-Weiler R, Weiss G. Pitfalls in the diagnosis and therapy of infections in elderly patients--a mini-review. Gerontology. 2009;55(3):241–9.
20. Calandra T, Cohen J. The international sepsis forum consensus conference on definitions of infection in the intensive care unit. Crit Care Med. 2005;33(7):1538–48.
21. Vincent J-L, Brealey D, Libert N, Abidi NE, O'Dwyer M, Zacharowski K, et al. Rapid diagnosis of infection in the critically ill, a multicenter study of molecular detection in bloodstream infections, pneumonia, and sterile site infections. Crit Care Med. 2015;43(11):2283–91.
22. Blot S, Cankurtaran M, Petrovic M, Vandijck D, Lizy C, Decruyenaere J, et al. Epidemiology and outcome of nosocomial bloodstream infection in elderly critically ill patients: a comparison between middle-aged, old, and very old patients. Crit Care Med. 2009;37(5):1634–41.
23. Clifford KM, Dy-Boarman EA, Haase KK, Maxvill K, Pass SE, Alvarez CA. Challenges with diagnosing and managing sepsis in older adults. Expert Rev Anti-Infect Ther. 2016;14(2):231–41.
24. Pangrazzi L, Weinberger B. T cells, aging and senescence. Exp Gerontol. 2020;134:110887.
25. Opal SM, Girard TD, Ely EW. The immunopathogenesis of sepsis in elderly patients. Clin Infect Dis an Off Publ Infect Dis Soc Am. 2005;41(Suppl 7):S504–12.
26. Aiello A, Farzaneh F, Candore G, Caruso C, Davinelli S, Gambino CM, et al. Immunosenescence and its hallmarks: how to oppose aging strategically? A review of potential options for therapeutic intervention. Front Immunol. 2019;10:2247.
27. Soysal P, Stubbs B, Lucato P, Luchini C, Solmi M, Peluso R, et al. Inflammation and frailty in the elderly: a systematic review and meta-analysis. Ageing Res Rev. 2016;31:1–8.
28. Castle SC, Uyemura K, Fulop T, Makinodan T. Host resistance and immune responses in advanced age. Clin Geriatr Med. 2007;23(3):463–79. v
29. Norman DC. Clinical features of infection in older adults. Clin Geriatr Med. 2016;32(3):433–41.
30. Esper AM, Moss M, Lewis CA, Nisbet R, Mannino DM, Martin GS. The role of infection and comorbidity: factors that influence disparities in sepsis. Crit Care Med. 2006;34(10):2576–82.
31. Raz R, Gennesin Y, Wasser J, Stoler Z, Rosenfeld S, Rottensterich E, et al. Recurrent urinary tract infections in postmenopausal women. Clin Infect Dis an Off Publ Infect Dis Soc Am. 2000;30(1):152–6.
32. Jackson SL, Boyko EJ, Scholes D, Abraham L, Gupta K, Fihn SD. Predictors of urinary tract infection after menopause: a prospective study. Am J Med. 2004;117(12):903–11.
33. Rowe TA, Juthani-Mehta M. Diagnosis and management of urinary tract infection in older adults. Infect Dis Clin N Am. 2014;28(1):75–89.
34. Quagliarello V, Ginter S, Han L, Van Ness P, Allore H, Tinetti M. Modifiable risk factors for nursing home-acquired pneumonia. Clin Infect Dis an Off Publ Infect Dis Soc Am. 2005;40(1):1–6.
35. Juthani-Mehta M, De Rekeneire N, Allore H, Chen S, O'Leary JR, Bauer DC, et al. Modifiable risk factors for pneumonia requiring hospitalization of community-dwelling older adults: the Health, Aging, and Body Composition Study. J Am Geriatr Soc. 2013;61(7):1111–8.
36. Ginde AA, Moss M, Shapiro NI, Schwartz RS. Impact of older age and nursing home residence on clinical outcomes of US emergency department visits for severe sepsis. J Crit Care. 2013;28(5):606–11.
37. Shen H-N, Lu C-L, Li C-Y. Dementia increases the risks of acute organ dysfunction, severe sepsis and mortality in hospitalized older patients: a national population-based study. PLoS One. 2012;7(8):e42751.
38. Cinel I, Opal SM. Molecular biology of inflammation and sepsis: a primer. Crit Care Med. 2009;37(1):291–304.
39. De Backer D, Creteur J, Preiser J-C, Dubois M-J, Vincent J-L. Microvascular blood flow is altered in patients with sepsis. Am J Respir Crit Care Med. 2002;166(1):98–104.
40. Singer M. The role of mitochondrial dysfunction in sepsis-induced multi-organ failure. Virulence. 2014;5(1):66–72.
41. SSC declaration.
42. Dellinger RP, Carlet JM, Masur H, Gerlach H, Calandra T, Cohen J, et al. Surviving sepsis campaign guidelines for management of severe sepsis and septic shock. Crit Care Med. 2004;32(3):858–73.
43. Dellinger RP, Levy MM, Carlet JM, Bion J, Parker MM, Jaeschke R, et al. Surviving sepsis campaign: international guidelines for management of severe sepsis and septic shock: 2008. Crit Care Med. 2008;36(1):296–327.
44. Dellinger RP, Levy MM, Rhodes A, Annane D, Gerlach H, Opal SM, et al. Surviving sepsis campaign: international guidelines for management of severe sepsis and septic shock: 2012. Crit Care Med. 2013;41(2):580–637.

45. Rhodes A, Evans LE, Alhazzani W, Levy MM, Antonelli M, Ferrer R, et al. Surviving sepsis campaign: international guidelines for management of sepsis and septic shock: 2016. Intensive Care Med. 2017;43(3):304–77.
46. Levy MM, Evans LE, Rhodes A. The surviving sepsis campaign bundle: 2018 update. Intensive Care Med. United States. 2018;44:925–8.
47. Hill JV, Findon G, Appelhoff RJ, Endre ZH. Renal autoregulation and passive pressure-flow relationships in diabetes and hypertension. Am J Physiol Renal Physiol. 2010;299(4):F837–44.
48. Asfar P, Meziani F, Hamel J-F, Grelon F, Megarbane B, Anguel N, et al. High versus low blood-pressure target in patients with septic shock. N Engl J Med. 2014;370(17):1583–93.
49. Moman RN, Ostby SA, Akhoundi A, Kashyap R, Kashani K. Impact of individualized target mean arterial pressure for septic shock resuscitation on the incidence of acute kidney injury: a retrospective cohort study. Ann Intensive Care. 2018;8(1):124.
50. Landesberg G, Gilon D, Meroz Y, Georgieva M, Levin PD, Goodman S, et al. Diastolic dysfunction and mortality in severe sepsis and septic shock. Eur Heart J. 2012;33(7):895–903.
51. Brown SM, Pittman JE, Hirshberg EL, Jones JP, Lanspa MJ, Kuttler KG, et al. Diastolic dysfunction and mortality in early severe sepsis and septic shock: a prospective, observational echocardiography study. Crit Ultrasound J. 2012;4(1):8.
52. Self WH, Semler MW, Bellomo R, Brown SM, DeBoisblanc BP, Exline MC, et al. Liberal versus restrictive intravenous fluid therapy for early septic shock: rationale for a randomized trial. Ann Emerg Med. 2018;72(4):457–66.
53. Serpa Neto A, Martin Loeches I, Klanderman RB, Freitas Silva R, Gama de Abreu M, Pelosi P, et al. Balanced versus isotonic saline resuscitation-a systematic review and meta-analysis of randomized controlled trials in operation rooms and intensive care units. Ann Transl Med. 2017;5(16):323.
54. Caironi P, Tognoni G, Masson S, Fumagalli R, Pesenti A, Romero M, et al. Albumin replacement in patients with severe sepsis or septic shock. N Engl J Med. 2014;370(15):1412–21.
55. Finfer S, Bellomo R, Boyce N, French J, Myburgh J, Norton R. A comparison of albumin and saline for fluid resuscitation in the intensive care unit. N Engl J Med. 2004;350(22):2247–56.
56. Holst LB, Haase N, Wetterslev J, Wernerman J, Guttormsen AB, Karlsson S, et al. Lower versus higher hemoglobin threshold for transfusion in septic shock. N Engl J Med. 2014;371(15):1381–91.
57. Hjortrup PB, Haase N, Bundgaard H, Thomsen SL, Winding R, Pettilä V, et al. Restricting volumes of resuscitation fluid in adults with septic shock after initial management: the CLASSIC randomised, parallel-group, multicentre feasibility trial. Intensive Care Med. 2016;42(11):1695–705.
58. Self WH, Semler MW, Wanderer JP, Wang L, Byrne DW, Collins SP, et al. Balanced crystalloids versus saline in noncritically ill adults. N Engl J Med. 2018;378(9):819–28.
59. Semler MW, Self WH, Wanderer JP, Ehrenfeld JM, Wang L, Byrne DW, et al. Balanced crystalloids versus saline in critically ill adults. N Engl J Med. 2018;378(9):829–39.
60. Kumar A, Roberts D, Wood KE, Light B, Parrillo JE, Sharma S, et al. Duration of hypotension before initiation of effective antimicrobial therapy is the critical determinant of survival in human septic shock. Crit Care Med. 2006;34(6):1589–96.
61. Prescott HC, Iwashyna TJ. Improving sepsis treatment by embracing diagnostic uncertainty. Ann Am Thorac Soc. 2019;16(4):426–9.
62. Strich JR, Heil EL, Masur H. Considerations for empiric antimicrobial therapy in sepsis and septic shock in an era of antimicrobial resistance. J Infect Dis. 2020;222(Supplement_2):S119–31.
63. Shehabi Y, Bellomo R, Reade MC, Bailey M, Bass F, Howe B, et al. Early intensive care sedation predicts long-term mortality in ventilated critically ill patients. Am J Respir Crit Care Med. 2012;186(8):724–31.
64. Kress JP, Pohlman AS, O'Connor MF, Hall JB. Daily interruption of sedative infusions in critically ill patients undergoing mechanical ventilation. N Engl J Med. 2000;342(20):1471–7.
65. Fraser GL, Devlin JW, Worby CP, Alhazzani W, Barr J, Dasta JF, et al. Benzodiazepine versus nonbenzodiazepine-based sedation for mechanically ventilated, critically ill adults: a systematic review and meta-analysis of randomized trials. Crit Care Med. 2013;41(9 Suppl 1):S30–8.
66. Pisani MA, Kong SYJ, Kasl SV, Murphy TE, Araujo KLB, Van Ness PH. Days of delirium are associated with 1-year mortality in an older intensive care unit population. Am J Respir Crit Care Med. 2009;180(11):1092–7.
67. Barr J, Fraser GL, Puntillo K, Ely EW, Gélinas C, Dasta JF, et al. Clinical practice guidelines for the management of pain, agitation, and delirium in adult patients in the intensive care unit. Crit Care Med. 2013;41(1):263–306.

68. Sprung CL, Annane D, Keh D, Moreno R, Singer M, Freivogel K, et al. Hydrocortisone therapy for patients with septic shock. N Engl J Med. 2008;358(2):111–24.

69. Annane D, Bellissant E, Bollaert P-E, Briegel J, Confalonieri M, De Gaudio R, et al. Corticosteroids in the treatment of severe sepsis and septic shock in adults: a systematic review. JAMA. 2009;301(22):2362–75.

70. Kalil AC, Sun J. Low-dose steroids for septic shock and severe sepsis: the use of Bayesian statistics to resolve clinical trial controversies. Intensive Care Med. 2011;37(3):420–9.

71. Annane D, Bellissant E, Bollaert PE, Briegel J, Keh D, Kupfer Y, et al. Corticosteroids for treating sepsis in children and adults. Cochrane Database Syst Rev. 2019;12(12):CD002243.

72. Batzofin BM, Sprung CL, Weiss YG. The use of steroids in the treatment of severe sepsis and septic shock. Best Pract Res Clin Endocrinol Metab. 2011;25(5):735–43.

73. Keh D, Trips E, Marx G, Wirtz SP, Abduljawwad E, Bercker S, et al. Effect of hydrocortisone on development of shock among patients with severe sepsis: the HYPRESS randomized clinical trial. JAMA. 2016;316(17):1775–85.

74. Yiallouris A, Tsioutis C, Agapidaki E, Zafeiri M, Agouridis AP, Ntourakis D, et al. Adrenal aging and its implications on stress responsiveness in humans. Front Endocrinol (Lausanne). 2019;10:54.

75. Righini M, Le Gal G, Perrier A, Bounameaux H. The challenge of diagnosing pulmonary embolism in elderly patients: influence of age on commonly used diagnostic tests and strategies. J Am Geriatr Soc. 2005;53(6):1039–45.

76. Weberová D, Weber P, Kubesová H, Meluzínová H, Polcarová V, Ambrosová P, et al. Occurrence of pulmonary embolism among 260 in-patients of acute geriatric department aged 65+ years in 2005–2010. Adv Gerontol = Uspekhi Gerontol. 2012;25(3):506–12.

77. Alhazzani W, Lim W, Jaeschke RZ, Murad MH, Cade J, Cook DJ. Heparin thromboprophylaxis in medical-surgical critically ill patients: a systematic review and meta-analysis of randomized trials. Crit Care Med. 2013;41(9):2088–98.

78. Young PJ, Bagshaw SM, Forbes AB, Nichol AD, Wright SE, Bailey M, et al. Effect of stress ulcer prophylaxis with proton pump inhibitors vs histamine-2 receptor blockers on in-hospital mortality among ICU patients receiving invasive mechanical ventilation: the PEPTIC randomized clinical trial. JAMA. 2020;323(7):616–26.

79. Krag M, Perner A, Wetterslev J, Wise MP, Hylander MM. Stress ulcer prophylaxis versus placebo or no prophylaxis in critically ill patients. A systematic review of randomised clinical trials with meta-analysis and trial sequential analysis. Intensive Care Med. 2014;40(1):11–22.

80. Weber S, Mawdsley E, Kaye D. Antibacterial agents in the elderly. Infect Dis Clin N Am. 2009;23(4):881–98, viii

81. Noreddin AM, El-Khatib W, Haynes V. Optimal dosing design for antibiotic therapy in the elderly: a pharmacokinetic and pharmacodynamic perspective. Recent Pat Antiinfect Drug Discov. 2008;3(1):45–52.

82. Herring AR, Williamson JC. Principles of antimicrobial use in older adults. Clin Geriatr Med. 2007;23(3):481–97. v

83. Guidet B, de Lange DW, Boumendil A, Leaver S, Watson X, Boulanger C, et al. The contribution of frailty, cognition, activity of daily life and comorbidities on outcome in acutely admitted patients over 80 years in European ICUs: the VIP2 study. Intensive Care Med. 2020;46(1):57–69.

84. Martin-Loeches I, Guia MC, Vallecoccia MS, Suarez D, Ibarz M, Irazabal M, et al. Risk factors for mortality in elderly and very elderly critically ill patients with sepsis: a prospective, observational, multicenter cohort study. Ann Intensive Care. 2019;9(1):26.

85. Ibarz M, Boumendil A, Haas LEM, Irazabal M, Flaatten H, de Lange DW, et al. Sepsis at ICU admission does not decrease 30-day survival in very old patients: a post-hoc analysis of the VIP1 multinational cohort study. Ann Intensive Care. 2020;10(1):56.

86. Haas LEM, Boumendil A, Flaatten H, Guidet B, Ibarz M, Jung C, et al. Frailty is associated with long-term outcome in patients with sepsis who are over 80 years old: results from an observational study in 241 European ICUs. Age Ageing. 2021;50(5):1719–27.

87. Karakus A, Haas LEM, Brinkman S, de Lange DW, de Keizer NF. Trends in short-term and 1-year mortality in very elderly intensive care patients in the Netherlands: a retrospective study from 2008 to 2014. Intensive Care Med. 2017;43(10):1476–84.

88. Nasa P, Juneja D, Singh O. Severe sepsis and septic shock in the elderly: an overview. World J Crit care Med [Internet]. 2012 [cited 2019 Jan 23];1(1):23–30. Available from: http://www.ncbi.nlm.nih.gov/pubmed/24701398.

89. Haas LEM, van Dillen LS, de Lange DW, van Dijk D, Hamaker ME. Outcome of very old patients admitted to the ICU for sepsis: a systematic review. Eur Geriatr Med [Internet]. 2017 [cited 2019 Jan 23];8(5–6):446–53. Available from: https://linkinghub.elsevier.com/retrieve/pii/S1878764917301602.

90. Flaatten H, De Lange DW, Morandi A, Andersen FH, Artigas A, Bertolini G, et al. The impact of frailty on ICU and 30-day mortality and the level of care in very elderly patients (≥ 80 years). Intensive Care Med [Internet]. 2017 [cited 2019 Jan 23];43(12):1820–8. Available from: http://link.springer.com/10.1007/s00134-017-4940-8.

91. Sánchez-Hurtado LA, Ángeles-Veléz A, Tejeda-Huezo BC, García-Cruz JC, Juárez-Cedillo T. Validation of a prognostic score for mortality in elderly patients admitted to intensive care unit. Indian J Crit care Med peer-reviewed, Off Publ Indian Soc Crit Care Med. 2016;20(12):695–700.

92. Haas LEM, Termorshuizen F, de Lange DW, van Dijk D, de Keizer NF. Performance of the quick SOFA in very old ICU patients admitted with sepsis. Acta Anaesthesiol Scand. 2020;64(4):508–16.

93. Wang S, Allen D, Kheir YN, Campbell N, Khan B. Aging and post-intensive care syndrome: a critical need for geriatric psychiatry. Am J Geriatr Psychiatry Off J Am Assoc Geriatr Psychiatry. 2018;26(2):212–21.

94. Lee M, Kang J, Jeong YJ. Risk factors for post-intensive care syndrome: a systematic review and meta-analysis. Aust Crit care Off J Confed Aust Crit Care Nurses. 2020;33(3):287–94.

95. Winters BD, Eberlein M, Leung J, Needham DM, Pronovost PJ, Sevransky JE. Long-term mortality and quality of life in sepsis: a systematic review. Crit Care Med. 2010;38(5):1276–83.

96. Iwashyna TJ, Ely EW, Smith DM, Langa KM. Long-term cognitive impairment and functional disability among survivors of severe sepsis. JAMA [Internet]. 2010 [cited 2019 Jan 23];304(16):1787. Available from: http://jama.jamanetwork.com/article.aspx?doi=10.1001/jama.2010.1553.

97. Kaarlola A, Tallgren M, Pettila V. Long-term survival, quality of life, and quality-adjusted life-years among critically ill elderly patients. Crit Care Med. 2006;34(8):2120–6.

98. Beauchamp TL, Childress JF. Principles of biomedical ethics. 7th ed. Oxford: Oxford University Press; 2013.

99. Fried TR, Bradley EH, Towle VR, Allore H. Understanding the treatment preferences of seriously ill patients. N Engl J Med. 2002;346(14):1061–6.

100. Philippart F, Vesin A, Bruel C, Kpodji A, Durand-Gasselin B, Garcon P, et al. The ETHICA study (part I): elderly's thoughts about intensive care unit admission for life-sustaining treatments. Intensive Care Med. 2013;39(9):1565–73.

101. de Jonge E, Mooijaart S. Framework to decide on withholding intensive care in older patients. Netherlands J Crit Care. 2019;27:150–4.

102. Lagu T, Rothberg MB, Shieh M-S, Pekow PS, Steingrub JS, Lindenauer PK. Hospitalizations, costs, and outcomes of severe sepsis in the United States 2003 to 2007. Crit Care Med. 2012;40(3):754–61.

103. Kumar G, Kumar N, Taneja A, Kaleekal T, Tarima S, McGinley E, et al. Nationwide trends of severe sepsis in the 21st century (2000-2007). Chest. 2011;140(5):1223–31.

104. Stoller J, Halpin L, Weis M, Aplin B, Qu W, Georgescu C, et al. Epidemiology of severe sepsis: 2008-2012. J Crit Care. 2016;31(1):58–62.

105. Liang L, Moore B, Soni A. National inpatient hospital costs: the most expensive conditions by Payer, 2017. Healthcare cost and utilization project Statistical Brief #261. Agency for Healthcare Research and Quality, Rockville, MD. [Internet]. 2020. [cited 2020 Aug 26]. Available from: https://www.hcup-us.ahrq.gov/reports/statbriefs/sb261-Most-Expensive-Hospital-Conditions-2017.jsp.

106. Mayr FB, Talisa VB, Balakumar V, Chang C-CH, Fine M, Yende S. Proportion and cost of unplanned 30-day readmissions after sepsis compared with other medical conditions. JAMA, United States. 2017;317:530–1.

107. van Beusekom I, Bakhshi-Raiez F, de Keizer NF, van der Schaaf M, Busschers WB, Dongelmans DA. Healthcare costs of ICU survivors are higher before and after ICU admission compared to a population based control group: a descriptive study combining healthcare insurance data and data from a Dutch national quality registry. J Crit Care. 2017;44:345–51.

Acute Kidney Injury

*Carmen A. Pfortmueller, Patrick Zuercher,
and Joerg C. Schefold*

Contents

© The Author(s), under exclusive license to Springer Nature Switzerland AG 2022
H. Flaatten et al. (eds.), *The Very Old Critically Ill Patients*, Lessons from the ICU,
https://doi.org/10.1007/978-3-030-94133-8_31

🏠 Learning Objectives

Aging is associated with a decline in glomerular filtration rate (GFR) resulting in diminished both renal function and renal reserve ("renal aging"). Elderly patients thus have increased chronic kidney disease (CKD) prevalence and, in cases of critical illness (e.g., sepsis/systemic inflammation, acute heart failure/cardiorenal interactions, need for surgical interventions, and/or multiple organ dysfunction), an increased likelihood of acute-on-chronic renal dysfunction. Further, significant (e.g., cardiovascular) comorbidity and polypharmacy are often present in ICU patients. The presence of age-related comorbidities (such as cardiovascular disease and/or heart failure) contributes significantly to frailty and implies a key independent risk factor for unfavorable clinical outcomes from AKI in aged ICU populations.

In the future, and with an overall aging population, this will become even more evident against the background of an increased incidence of age-associated comorbidities and an expected continuous rise in AKI incidence.

Practical Implications

AKI is characterized by a rapid loss in renal function resulting in increased systemic levels of nitrogen products as well as electrolyte, acid-base, hormonal, and fluid dysbalance. In aged patients with critical illness, the prevention of loss in renal function seems of paramount importance.

In respective elderly patients, AKI is associated with high incidence of development of end-stage renal disease (ESRD) and high in-hospital mortality rates. Prevention of AKI should be considered pivotal on intensive care units (ICUs), which imply, for example, avoidance of both nephrotoxic medication (including limiting the use of contrast media) and/or hyperglycemia as well as adequate therapy of hemodynamics. This includes the therapy for eventual right heart failure and/or avoidance of fluid overload which may result in renal venous congestion. Despite respective clinical efforts, causal therapeutic approaches, that is, interventions, for AKI are currently unavailable.

31.1 Introduction

Acute kidney injury (AKI) is a global health concern, and the prognosis of affected aged patients is poor. In respective aged ICU populations, AKI mostly presents as acute-on-chronic AKI, as aging itself is associated with a decline in glomerular filtration rates (GFR). Thus, in aged populations, renal reserve is diminished and typically impedes AKI recovery.

Increased numbers of aged ICU patients initially have AKI, later followed by accelerated chronic kidney disease (CKD) and/or end-stage renal disease (ESRD). Importantly, a number of critical illness including sepsis/ shock, acute heart failure, and/or multiple organ dysfunction prone respective patients to AKI development. However, risk profiling identifies age-related comorbidities, in particular cardiovascular disease, as a key AKI risk factor. In the light of aging populations worldwide, this will become even more evident against the background of an associated increased incidence of age-associated comorbidities. Here we summarize definitions, epidemiology, risk, (patho)physiology, diagnosis, and potential therapy for AKI in this vulnerable adult patient group. Finally, available biomarkers and current and future therapeutic approaches will be discussed.

31.2 AKI Definitions

Acute kidney injury (AKI), less precise earlier referred to as "acute renal failure," is defined as an acute (within 7 days) loss in kidney function. In 2012, the Kidney Disease Improving Global Outcomes (KDIGO [1], ◘ Table 31.1 initiative) proposed specific diagnostic AKI criteria. These definitions include increased (A) serum creatinine ≥0.3 mg/dl (≥26.5 µmol/l) within 48 h: or (B) increased serum creatinine to

◘ **Table 31.1** AKI categories: KDIGO, AKIN, RIFLE grading system

AKI staging criteria	KDIGO[a]	AKIN[b]	RIFLE[c]
Stage 1 (KDIGO/AKIN), risk (RIFLE)	+ SCr ≥ 0.3 mg/dl or 1.5–1.9 × baseline OR urine output <0.5 ml/kg/h for 6–12 h	+ SCr ≥ 0.3 mg/dl or 150–200% baseline OR urine output <0.5 ml/kg/h for 6–12 h	+ SCr ≥ 1.5 × baseline OR GFR decrease >25% OR urine output <0.5 ml/kg/h for 6 h
Stage 2 (KDIGO/AKIN), injury (RIFLE)	+ SCr ≥ 2.0–2.9 × baseline OR urine output <0.5 ml/kg/h for 12–24 h	+ SCr ≥ 200–300% baseline OR urine output <0.5 ml/kg/h for 12–24 h	+ SCr ≥ 2 × baseline OR GFR decrease > 50% OR urine output <0.5 ml/kg/h for 12 h
Stage 3 (KDIGO/AKIN), failure (RIFLE)	+ SCr ≥ 3.0 × baseline OR + SCr ≥ 0.3 mg/dl to ≥4.0 mg/dl OR urine output <0.3 ml/kg/h for ≥24 h OR anuria for ≥12 h OR start of RRT	+ SCr > 300% baseline OR + SCr > 0.5 mg/dl to ≥4.0 mg/dl OR urine output <0.3 ml/kg/h for >24 h OR anuria for >12 h OR start of RRT	+ SCr ≥ 3 × baseline OR GFR decrease >75% OR + SCr > 0.5 mg/dl (acute) to >4.0 mg/dl OR urine output <0.3 ml/kg/h for 24 h OR anuria for 12 h OR start of RRT
Loss (RIFLE)			Need for RRT for >4 weeks
End stage (RIFLE)			Need for RRT for >3 months

[a]KDIGO Clinical Practice Guideline for Acute Kidney Injury [1]
[b]Mehta et al. [2]
[c]Bellomo et al. [3]

≥1.5 times baseline, which has occurred within the prior 7 days: or (C) reduced urine volumes (<0.5 ml/kg/h for >6 h). Prior to classification, the KDIGO criteria allow for volume status correction and obstructive causes of AKI.

The Acute Kidney Injury Network (AKIN) [2] stated that these criteria should be applied in the context of clinical presentation and (where applicable) after adequate fluid resuscitation. Further, use of urine output (UO) criteria alone would require exclusion of obstruction AKI etiology and/or other reversible causes of reduced UO.

In addition, the RIFLE (Risk, Injury, Failure, Loss of kidney function, End-stage kidney disease) grading system was proposed by the Acute Dialysis Quality Initiative (ADQI) [3]: (risk) 1.5-fold increase in the serum creatinine, or GFR decrease by 25%, or urine output <0.5 mL/kg/h for 6 h; (injury) twofold increase in serum creatinine, or GFR decrease by 50%, or urine output <0.5 mL/kg/h for 12 h; (failure) threefold increase in serum creatinine, or GFR decrease by 75%, or urine output of <0.3 mL/kg/h for 24 h, or anuria for 12 h; (loss) complete loss of kidney function (e.g., need for renal replacement therapy) for more than 4 weeks; and (ESRD): complete loss of kidney function (e.g., need for renal replacement therapy) for more than 3 months.

31.3 AKI Epidemiology

In light of partly differing AKI definitions and variations in populations between geographic areas, exact numbers on AKI incidence in aged ICU populations are missing. AKI incidence in hospitalized patients was described as less than 10%, whereas in the ICU population, incidences rise from 20% to 40% [4]. Among critically ill patients, those presenting with AKI seem significantly older [5]. Another report observed an incidence ranging from 28.5% to 35.5%, with 25% of ICU patients with AKI being 75 years old or above [6]. Age-related yearly AKI incidence in adults was reported to increase from 17 per million aged (<50 years) up to 949 per million in the 80–89-year-old age group [7]. The incidence of renal replacement therapy (RRT)-treated AKI in a large representative data set (decade of recording) from a nationwide US inpatient sample showed an association with age, with an absolute AKI incidence highest in elderly individuals [8].

31.4 Risk Factors for AKI in Elderly ICU Patients

Factors that render elderly ICU patients more susceptible for AKI can likely be categorized into four groups:
(a) Structural and/or functional changes due to renal aging
(b) Comorbidities
(c) Acute medical conditions directly and/or or indirectly affecting the kidneys
(d) Medical diagnostic and/or therapeutic interventions

Renal aging, that is, age-related structural and functional changes, leads to a decrease in kidney weight, number of functioning nephrons, and overall kidney function. The medulla remains relatively unaltered, whereas the loss is primarily cortical [9, 10].

Interestingly, evidence demonstrates that the observed loss of kidney mass is not accompanied by a concurrent volume reduction with imaging studies showing that parenchymal kidney volume in aged kidney remains relatively unaltered [11–13]. Compensatory mechanisms in response to this loss may be an explanation, with an increase in size of the unaffected, remaining glomeruli due to hypertrophy [14, 15]. Tubulointerstitial changes, thickening of the glomerular basement membrane, and glomerulosclerosis are age-related histologic alterations, often referred to as nephrosclerosis [16, 17]. More precisely, nephrosclerosis is present whenever two or more of the following histologic features are apparent: tubular atrophy, any global glomerulosclerosis, interstitial fibrosis (>5%), and any arteriosclerosis. Despite a known correlation between nephrosclerosis, aging, mild hypertension, and healthy living donor kidneys [18], its impact on functional changes in aging is not fully explored [19, 20]. Further, morphological and anatomical changes seen in senile kidneys embrace mesangium expansion, decrease of tubules (number, size, and length), atherosclerosis, growth of the internal elastic lamina leading to fibro-intimal hyperplasia, and luminar hyalinization with an impact of lumen diameters, potentially causing stenosis [21–24].

Another functional change in the aging kidney is that active transports by the tubule can be impaired, due to reduced mitochondrial energy production leading to altered reabsorption and/or secretion [21]. With a reduction in functional nephrons, sodium retention is impaired which impacts on urine concentration ability and hence volume depletion with a consecutively increased risk of dehydration [21]. Another physiological process is impaired in the aging kidney, which is urine acidification, especially during stress, leading to systemic metabolic acidosis. A decreased production of renal 1-alpha-hydroxylase (located mainly in the proximal tubules) induces direct changes in vitamin D and calcium metabolism and possibly triggers renal osteoporosis. With an increased apoptosis rate and a concomitant reduced amount of growth factors, the senile kidney shows a slower regeneration rate in response to injury [22, 23]. This may impede the aging kidney to complete recovery. Further, animal models show an age-related decrease in podocyte density (i.e., glomerular volume per podocyte increased) which was associated with podocyte hypertrophic stress and failure leading to glomerulosclerosis [25]. Results from different models reported that glomerular enlargement alone causes glomerulosclerosis, in a podocyte-dependent manner [26]. These experimental results show that reduced podocyte density and podocyte stress can trigger age-related glomerulosclerosis [25]. More recent research analyzing human kidneys [27] (i.e., from living and deceased donors and nephrectomy samples) support a hypothesis that a gradual decline in podocyte density over the human lifespan cause hypertrophic podocyte stress in some glomeruli. Over time, this may result in glomerular tuft collapse and glomerulosclerosis (i.e., focal global glomerulosclerosis), which may present a significant etiology of ESRD in aged kidneys.

Comorbidities may lead to pre-, intra-, and/ or post-renal conditions. According to the majority of data, chronic medical conditions such as diabetes mellitus (DM), arterial hypertension (AHT), heart disease/congestive heart failure (HD/CHF), and chronic kidney disease (CKD) are considered the most common comorbidities in the elderly, proning for development of AKI [28]. Approximately 20–30% of the elderly are affected by DM and are thus at risk for diabetic nephropathy consisting in particular of glomerular and microvascular changes. Increased blood glucose levels may induce microvascular injury and, secondary to its direct toxic effect, microinfarcts, which further decrease the number of functional nephrons (thus limiting renal functional reserve). In addition, changes in the production of extracellular matrix components, triggered by metabolites of nonenzymatic glycation induced by diabetic hyperglycemia, can lead to glomerular obstruction/occlusion. Furthermore, sorbitol, a metabolite of the pathway of polyols, can directly cause cellular damage via hyperosmotic stress [29, 30].

In AHT, hypertension stresses the vessel wall chronically, causing endothelial damage. Loss of elasticity of the tunica intima by hyalinization and stenosis of the lumen as well as proliferating of the internal elastic lamina, subsequently reducing renal blood flow and rising the risk for pre-renal AKI [21, 23, 30]. Atheromatous plaques may further decrease vessel lumen, therefore reducing renal blood flow even more and hence impacting on the renin-angiotensin-aldosterone system (RAAS), impairing its regulatory function. Its activity can be altered by up to 50% in elderly people when compared to a younger population [21]. Importantly, functioning feedback loops are depending on elastic afferent and efferent vessels in order to adequately respond to ischemic insults, and this may not be the case in aged kidneys.

In addition, acute and/or chronic systemic disorders can impact both on heart and on renal function. An acute and/or chronic dysfunction of one of the two organs can induce an acute and/or chronic dysfunction in the other organ [31]. Such interactions were previously referred to as cardiorenal syndromes (CRS), of which five types were classified [32] (please see below). Comorbidities proning to post-renal AKI are medical conditions associated with mass or infiltrating processes causing obstruction of the urinary tract (e.g., benign prostate hyperplasia, neoplasia, kidney stones, and/or bleeding conditions).

Acute medical conditions, for example, urinary tract infections, may lead to urinary sepsis with the risk of deterioration into septic shock with consecutive septic AKI.

Medical diagnostic and/or therapeutic interventions incl. Polypharmacy: In light of a limited drug excretion capacity, the aging kidney of polymorbid ICU patients is especially prone for "iatrogenic" AKI when contrast media and/or nephrotoxic drugs are applied [21–24, 29, 30, 33–36]. Iodinated contrast agents may cause direct tubular injury with an additional impact on intra-renal hemodynamics [28]. Commonly prescribed drugs in the elderly, such as anti-inflammatory nonsteroidals and/or antihypertensive agents such as angiotensin-converting enzyme inhibitors, may impair renal autoregulation and contribute to ATN development. Additionally, when prescribing potentially harmful nephrotoxic drugs for elderly ICU patients, one should not (over)estimate a given patients' renal function in the presence of (near to) normal serum creatinine levels. In ICU patients, this may be of particular importance in cases of presence of, for example, cachexia, sarcopenia, critical illness-induced muscular weakness (ICU-acquired weakness) [37–40], and/or other related (neuro)muscular conditions [37, 39, 41] that can typically be observed in aged ICU patients.

31.5 Pathophysiology of AKI

With advancing age, the kidneys undergo specific structural and functional changes (◘ Fig. 31.1) resulting in a decrease in kidney weight, the number of functioning nephrons, and baseline kidney function [22, 42, 43]. The loss of renal mass mainly affects the renal cortex, especially the proximal tubules [44], while the medulla does

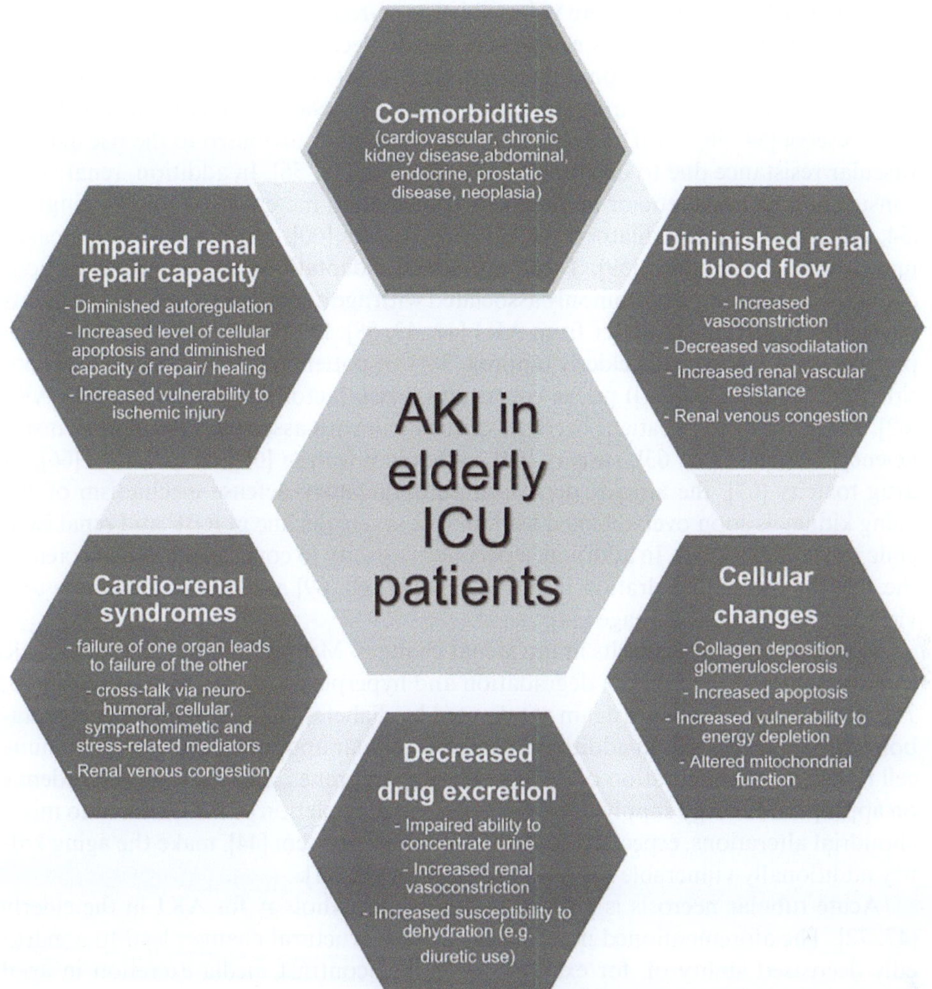

Fig. 31.1 Risk factors and pathophysiology of AKI in the elderly

change relatively little in aged individuals [10]. Aging however affects not only the number of nephrons but also proper glomerular function [22]. Data show that the number of sclerotic glomeruli reaches 10–30% by the age of 80 [45]. All of these factors result in a significant decline in renal function (eGFR) and renal autoregulatory capacity in aged individuals [22, 43]. While the extent of age-related reduction of renal function is individual and depends on several factors (e.g., gender, race, or genetic predisposition) [46], age-related renal functional decline together with important comorbidities (such as chronic heart failure, abdominal, or chronic inflammatory disease) makes, as discussed above, the kidney of elderly ICU patients particular susceptible to AKI [47, 48]. In addition, as mentioned, the repair capacity of the aging kidney is also impaired [49–51], leading to a transition to chronic kidney disease in 20–30% of elderly patients suffering from AKI [42, 52].

Pre-renal AKI is considered the most common cause of AKI in the elderly, accounting for about 40–60% of cases [42, 53, 54]. Several age-related factors that make elderly ICU patients more vulnerable to pre-renal AKI were identified. One of the key underlying changes is a relatively steady decline in renal blood flow (RBF) with advancing age [54], amounting to a loss of about 10% per decade of life [55]. As touched above, another important factor is the age-related reduction in functional renal reserve [54, 56, 57]. The decrease in RBF might be attributed to the rise in renal vascular resistance due to decrease NO production [55, 56]. In addition, renal vaso-constriction (sympathetic or angiotensin-II mediated) increases with advancing age [54, 58, 59], while vasodilatory mechanisms decline [60], resulting in an increased renal vascular resistance [59]. These age-related adaptations are enhanced by con-comitant comorbidities commonly associated with age and make elderly ICU patients particular vulnerable to suffer from AKI [42, 43, 58]. In addition, the relatively high prevalence of CKD in the elderly (approx. 38% of patients >65 years of age are con-sidered to be affected [61]) per se constitutes a risk factor for development of AKI [62]. When the elderly patient becomes critically ill with associated circulatory insuf-ficiency/ ischemia [42, 63], surgery [64], systemic infection [65], dehydration [66], or drug toxicity [67], the already decreased autoregulatory defense mechanism of the aging kidney is soon overwhelmed leading to a severe decline in RBF and renal isch-emic injury [22, 63, 67]. In addition, a declined capacity to concentrate urine increases the risk for severe dehydration in the elderly [22, 68, 69] and might contribute to a vicious cycle of renal damage [54].

Advancing age also results in intrarenal changes. Morphological changes include increased interstitial collagen degradation and hyperplasia of fibrotic tissues [67, 70, 71]. Respective changes are again accelerated by diabetes mellitus and/or other meta-bolic disorders [22, 42]. In addition, increased cellular apoptosis, changes in immune cell functions, disintegration of cellular basal membranes, and the high dependency on appropriate energy supply due to an accelerated depletion of ATP related to mito-chondrial alterations, especially in proximal tubular system [44], make the aging kid-ney additionally vulnerable for AKI progression [52, 71].

Acute tubular necrosis is a typical underlying pathology for AKI in the elderly [47, 72]. The aforementioned morphological and structural changes lead to a mark-edly decreased ability of, for example, drug and contrast media excretion in aged kidneys, which in turn increases the risk for additional kidney injury [47, 67]. The use of diuretics, which are commonly prescribed in elderly patients (e.g., for treatment of systemic arterial hypertension), may accelerate drug toxicity by impairing the kid-neys ability to concentrate urine and thus facilitate dehydration [52]. Further, advancing age is associated with increased levels of neurohumoral mediators that result in renal vasoconstriction, which make the kidney susceptible to nephrotoxic agents [52]. This may be especially problematic in cases of nonsteroidal anti-inflammatory drug use which not only leads to dehydration but also inhibits prosta-glandin-mediated renal vasodilatation [73].

While post-renal causes account for only about 2–4% of AKI cases in the criti-cally ill [54], the prevalence increases with age [22, 74, 75]. For example, high preva-lence of prostatic disease increases the risk of the elderly male patient to suffer from post-renal AKI by up to 35% [76]. Further, other post-renal diseases such as kidney stones, malignancies, and/or dysfunctional bladder diseases increase the vulnerability of elderly patients to develop post-renal AKI [42].

A further important mechanism associated with AKI is cardiorenal syndromes [77, 78]. The cardiorenal syndrome is pathophysiological disorder of the heart and kidney in which the organs "cross talk" with dysfunction of one organ resulting in acute or chronic dysfunction of the other organ [31, 77]. Pathophysiologically, there are several underlying mechanisms involved. First, altered hemodynamics such as low cardiac output and diminished venous return may affect both organs [31]. Second, neurohumoral dysregulation (especially of the RAAS system), inflammatory, cellular immune-mediated, and stress-related mechanisms may play a key role [31]. Third, cardiovascular disease-related factors such as cachexia/malnutrition-associated clinical problems, mineral bone disease, and/ or anemia may play a role [31]. Given the rather high incidence of cardiovascular disease in the elderly, the cardiorenal syndromes are an entity for AKI that warrants recognition in the elderly [22].

Another potential contributor to increased rates of AKI in the critically ill, especially in the elderly ICU population, is the occurrence of renal venous hypertension resulting in renal venous congestion [31]. It is thought to mainly occur in cases of acute or chronic heart failure with increased backward pressure to venous return, diminished efferent renal blood flow, and resulting increased intra-glomerular hydrostatic pressure [31]. Neurohumoral, inflammatory, hyperhydration, and sympathomimetically mediated factors are considered to be important also [31]. Renal venous hypertension may induce decreased arterial RBF, increase plasma renin activity, and increase aldosterone levels, which may ultimately result in diminished glomerular filtration rates [79, 80]. Morphologically, tubular hypertrophy, tubulointerstitial renal fibrosis, and intra-glomerular sclerosis were observed [81]. It thus seems that renal venous congestion could accelerate the natural aging process of the kidney and thus progression to chronic kidney disease.

31.6 Diagnosis of AKI in Aged ICU Patients

Serum creatinine (SCr) likely is the most commonly used biomarker to assess renal function despite obvious limitations of the marker. When renal filtration capacity declines, SCr levels typically rise not immediately, but in a delayed fashion. Therefore, SCr levels may not adequately reflect "real-time" renal function. When a SCr increase is documented, however, loss of renal function has occurred.

Further, SCr levels depend on production, removal rates, and volumes of distribution, all of which are typically impaired in the elderly population [55]. Among the many variables influencing SCr levels, age may be somewhat neglected. With loss of muscle mass due to aging, baseline SCr levels in the elderly may be lower than expected and should likely be adjusted. Kidney injury with an expected rise in SCr levels may be masked and a diagnosis of AKI therefore missed or delayed. In addition, low protein intake and/or altered protein metabolism is another factor for a low baseline SCr levels [21, 22, 24]. Thus, SCr does not constitute an ideal marker for AKI diagnosis in the elderly [82]. Novel AKI markers that are currently under investigation include cystatin C, neutrophil gelatin-associated lipocalin (NGAL), kidney injury molecule-1, kidney injury molecule 1 (KIM-1), L-type fatty acid-binding protein (L-FABP), netrin 1, N-acetyl-beta-D-glucosaminidase (NAG), alfa1-macroglobulin, or interleukin-18 [23, 24, 29, 35]. Some were investigated and validated in multiple studies as predictors of AKI in specific patient cohorts, both in adults and children, but none of these studies specifically analyzed elderly ICU populations [22, 29, 33, 35, 36]. Of the respective markers, it appears that only cystatin C was thoroughly validated and could be considered a reliable alternative biomarker for AKI, especially when used in combination with SCr [83–88]. Among the additional markers, NGAL was tested extensively. An increase in urinary NGAL may indicate unfavorable outcome in septic patients with AKI or in ICU patients [89, 90]. In elderly patients with CKD, serum NGAL reflects renal impairment and was found associated with cystatin C, urea, SCr, and eGFR. In a recent study among elderly CKD patients (mean age 75.3 +/− 12.1 years), increasing NGAL levels correlate with an increased 2- and 5-year risk of ESRD [91].

31.7 Treatment of AKI in the Elderly

No targeted, that is, specific, treatment for AKI in the elderly population is currently available. In association with a considerably increased mortality rate in this patient population, the focus of clinical management lies on preventive measures. Elderly ICU patients have to be monitored closely with regard to clinical course: fluid balance, electrolytes, hemodynamics, addressing hypovolemia, and hypotension, together aiming for an optimal volume status with preserved macro- and microcirculation (and organ perfusion). Respective clinical parameters should especially be remembered when operations and/or invasive interventions are performed.

Drug-induced AKI, iatrogenic, either via direct (dose-independent) or indirect (dose-dependent) nephrotoxicity, poses another key element, necessitating vigilant patient monitoring. Drugs that should be used with caution include drugs that impact on renal/intrarenal hemodynamics (e.g., anti-inflammatory substances), diuretics, and angiotensin-converting enzyme inhibitors. Medication should ideally be individualized and tailored based on GFR [23]. Whenever imaging studies become necessary, it is recommended to prefer studies that would not require contrast media. However, when indicated and unavoidable, iso-osmotic nonionic low osmolar contrast media should be applied in the lowest volumes possible. Protocols to prevent contrast media-induced AKI should be adhered to and be present on all ICUs.

Globally, rising attention of health-care professionals for the particular renal vulnerability will be important in the future. Key in management of respective patients at risk may be careful monitoring of the elderly ICU patient, with the overall aim to prevent AKI or limit respective complications.

> **Take-Home Messages**
> - Elderly ICU patients are at risk for AKI due to a number of reasons including (a) renal aging, (b) presence of age-related comorbidities, and (c) polypharmacy and/or application of potentially nephrotoxic agents.
> - Assessment of urinary output and repeat assessment of, for example, 6-h SCr-clearance may best allow to monitor individual renal (dys)function.
> - No causative therapy for AKI is currently available which places the clinical management focus on effective AKI prevention.
> - With an overall aging society, the incidence of AKI on intensive care units will likely increase, rendering AKI a major concern of global health-care systems.

Conflict of Interest Statement (Full Departmental Disclosure)   The Dept. of Intensive Care Medicine received research and/or development grants from Orion Pharma, Abbott Nutrition International, B. Braun Medical AG, CSEM AG, Edwards Lifesciences Services GmbH, Kenta Biotech Ltd., Maquet Critical Care AB, Omnicare Clinical Research AG, Nestle, Pierre Fabre Pharma AG, Pfizer, Bard Medica S.A., Abbott AG, Anandic Medical Systems, Pan Gas AG Healthcare, Bracco, Hamilton Medical AG, Fresenius Kabi, Getinge Group Maquet AG, Dräger AG, Teleflex Medical GmbH, Glaxo Smith Kline, Merck Sharp and Dohme AG, Eli Lilly and Company, Baxter, Astellas, Astra Zeneca, CSL Behring, Novartis, Covidien, Phagenesis Ltd., Philips Medical, Prolong Pharmaceuticals and Nycomed outside of the submitted work. The money went into departmental funds. No personal financial gain applied.

References

1. KDIGO. KDIGO Clinical practice guideline for acute kidney injury. Kidney Int Suppl. 2012;2:1–141.
2. Mehta RL, Kellum JA, Shah SV, Molitoris BA, Ronco C, Warnock DG, Levin A, Acute Kidney Injury Network. Acute kidney injury network: report of an initiative to improve outcomes in acute kidney injury. Crit Care. 2007;11(2):R31.
3. Bellomo R, Ronco C, Kellum JA, Mehta RL, Palevsky P, Acute Dialysis Quality Initiative Workgroup. Acute renal failure – definition, outcome measures, animal models, fluid therapy and information technology needs: the Second International Consensus Conference of the Acute Dialysis Quality Initiative (ADQI) Group. Crit Care. 2004;8(4):R204–12.
4. Nash K, Hafeez A, Hou S. Hospital-acquired renal insufficiency. Am J Kidney Dis. 2002;39(5):930–6.
5. Santos ER. RIFLE: association with mortality and length of stay in critically ill acute kidney injury patients. Rev Bras Ter Intensiva. 2009;21(4):359–68.
6. Joannidis M, Metnitz B, Bauer P, Schusterschitz N, Moreno R, Druml W, Metnitz PG. Acute kidney injury in critically ill patients classified by AKIN versus RIFLE using the SAPS 3 database. Intensive Care Med. 2009;35(10):1692–702.
7. Groeneveld AB, Tran DD, van der Meulen J, Nauta JJ, Thijs LG. Acute renal failure in the medical intensive care unit: predisposing, complicating factors and outcome. Nephron. 1991;59(4):602–10.
8. Hsu RK, McCulloch CE, Dudley RA, Lo LJ, Hsu CY. Temporal changes in incidence of dialysis-requiring AKI. J Am Soc Nephrol. 2013;24(1):37–42.
9. Zhou XJ, Saxena R, Liu Z, Vaziri ND, Silva FG. Renal senescence in 2008: progress and challenges. Int Urol Nephrol. 2008;40(3):823–39.
10. Tauchi H, Tsuboi K, Okutomi J. Age changes in the human kidney of the different races. Gerontologia. 1971;17(2):87–97.
11. Herts BR, Sharma N, Lieber M, Freire M, Goldfarb DA, Poggio ED. Estimating glomerular filtration rate in kidney donors: a model constructed with renal volume measurements from donor CT scans. Radiology. 2009;252(1):109–16.
12. Jeon HG, Lee SR, Joo DJ, Oh YT, Kim MS, Kim YS, Yang SC, Han WK. Predictors of kidney volume change and delayed kidney function recovery after donor nephrectomy. J Urol. 2010;184(3):1057–63.
13. Johnson S, Rishi R, Andone A, Khawandi W, Al-Said J, Gletsu-Miller N, Lin E, Baumgarten DA, O'Neill WC. Determinants and functional significance of renal parenchymal volume in adults. Clin J Am Soc Nephrol. 2011;6(1):70–6.
14. Goyal VK. Changes with age in the human kidney. Exp Gerontol. 1982;17(5):321–31.
15. Hoy WE, Douglas-Denton RN, Hughson MD, Cass A, Johnson K, Bertram JF. A stereological study of glomerular number and volume: preliminary findings in a multiracial study of kidneys at autopsy. Kidney Int Suppl. 2003;83:S31–7.

16. Newbold KM, Sandison A, Howie AJ. Comparison of size of juxtamedullary and outer cortical glomeruli in normal adult kidney. Virchows Arch A Pathol Anat Histopathol. 1992;420(2):127–9.

17. Nyengaard JR, Bendtsen TF. Glomerular number and size in relation to age, kidney weight, and body surface in normal man. Anat Rec. 1992;232(2):194–201.

18. Denic A, Alexander MP, Kaushik V, Lerman LO, Lieske JC, Stegall MD, Larson JJ, Kremers WK, Vrtiska TJ, Chakkera HA, et al. Detection and clinical patterns of nephron hypertrophy and Nephrosclerosis among apparently healthy adults. Am J Kidney Dis. 2016;68(1):58–67.

19. Meyrier A. Nephrosclerosis: a term in quest of a disease. Nephron. 2015;129(4):276–82.

20. Meyrier A. Nephrosclerosis: update on a centenarian. Nephrol Dial Transplant. 2015;30(11):1833–41.

21. Chronopoulos A, Cruz DN, Ronco C. Hospital-acquired acute kidney injury in the elderly. Nat Rev Nephrol. 2010;6(3):141–9.

22. Chronopoulos A, Rosner MH, Cruz DN, Ronco C. Acute kidney injury in elderly intensive care patients: a review. Intensive Care Med. 2010;36(9):1454–64.

23. Coca SG. Acute kidney injury in elderly persons. Am J Kidney Dis. 2010;56(1):122–31.

24. Schinstock CA, Semret MH, Wagner SJ, Borland TM, Bryant SC, Kashani KB, Larson TS, Lieske JC. Urinalysis is more specific and urinary neutrophil gelatinase-associated lipocalin is more sensitive for early detection of acute kidney injury. Nephrol Dial Transplant. 2013;28(5):1175–85.

25. Wiggins JE, Goyal M, Sanden SK, Wharram BL, Shedden KA, Misek DE, Kuick RD, Wiggins RC. Podocyte hypertrophy, "adaptation," and "decompensation" associated with glomerular enlargement and glomerulosclerosis in the aging rat: prevention by calorie restriction. J Am Soc Nephrol. 2005;16(10):2953–66.

26. Fukuda A, Chowdhury MA, Venkatareddy MP, Wang SQ, Nishizono R, Suzuki T, Wickman LT, Wiggins JE, Muchayi T, Fingar D, et al. Growth-dependent podocyte failure causes glomerulosclerosis. J Am Soc Nephrol. 2012;23(8):1351–63.

27. Hodgin JB, Bitzer M, Wickman L, Afshinnia F, Wang SQ, O'Connor C, Yang Y, Meadowbrooke C, Chowdhury M, Kikuchi M, et al. Glomerular aging and focal global glomerulosclerosis: a podometric perspective. J Am Soc Nephrol. 2015;26(12):3162–78.

28. Yokota LG, Sampaio BM, Rocha EP, Balbi AL, Sousa Prado IR, Ponce D. Acute kidney injury in elderly patients: narrative review on incidence, risk factors, and mortality. Int J Nephrol Renov Dis. 2018;11:217–24.

29. Anderson S, Eldadah B, Halter JB, Hazzard WR, Himmelfarb J, Horne FM, Kimmel PL, Molitoris BA, Murthy M, O'Hare AM, et al. Acute kidney injury in older adults. J Am Soc Nephrol. 2011;22(1):28–38.

30. Silveira Santos CGD, Romani RF, Benvenutti R, Ribas Zahdi JO, Riella MC, do Nascimento MM. Acute kidney injury in elderly population: a prospective observational study. Nephron. 2018;138(2):104–12.

31. Schefold JC, Filippatos G, Hasenfuss G, Anker SD, von Haehling S. Heart failure and kidney dysfunction: epidemiology, mechanisms and management. Nat Rev Nephrol. 2016;12(10):610–23.

32. Ronco C, Haapio M, House AA, Anavekar N, Bellomo R. Cardiorenal syndrome. J Am Coll Cardiol. 2008;52(19):1527–39.

33. Funk I, Seibert E, Markau S, Girndt M. Clinical course of acute kidney injury in elderly individuals above 80 years. Kidney Blood Press Res. 2016;41(6):947–55.

34. Hsu RK, Siew ED. The growth of AKI: half empty or half full, it's the size of the glass that matters. Kidney Int. 2017;92(3):550–3.

35. Martensson J, Bell M, Oldner A, Xu S, Venge P, Martling CR. Neutrophil gelatinase-associated lipocalin in adult septic patients with and without acute kidney injury. Intensive Care Med. 2010;36(8):1333–40.

36. Petronijevic Z, Selim G, Petkovska L, Georgievska-Ismail L, Spasovski G, Tozija L. The effect of treatment on short-term outcomes in elderly patients with acute kidney injury. Open Access Maced J Med Sci. 2017;5(5):635–40.

37. Schefold JC, Wollersheim T, Grunow JJ, Luedi MM, Z'Graggen WJ, Weber-Carstens S. Muscular weakness and muscle wasting in the critically ill. J Cachexia Sarcopenia Muscle. 2020;11(6):1399–412.

38. Schefold JC, Bierbrauer J, Weber-Carstens S. Intensive care unit-acquired weakness (ICUAW) and muscle wasting in critically ill patients with severe sepsis and septic shock. J Cachexia Sarcopenia Muscle. 2010;1(2):147–57.

39. Berger D, Bloechlinger S, von Haehling S, Doehner W, Takala J, Z'Graggen WJ, Schefold JC. Dysfunction of respiratory muscles in critically ill patients on the intensive care unit. J Cachexia Sarcopenia Muscle. 2016;7(4):403–12.
40. Vanhorebeek I, Latronico N, Van den Berghe G. ICU-acquired weakness. Intensive Care Med. 2020;46(4):637–53.
41. Zuercher P, Moret CS, Dziewas R, Schefold JC. Dysphagia in the intensive care unit: epidemiology, mechanisms, and clinical management. Crit Care. 2019;23(1):103.
42. Rosner MH. Acute kidney injury in the elderly. Clin Geriatr Med. 2013;29(3):565–78.
43. Haase M, Story DA, Haase-Fielitz A. Renal injury in the elderly: diagnosis, biomarkers and prevention. Best Pract Res Clin Anaesthesiol. 2011;25(3):401–12.
44. Sato Y, Takahashi M, Yanagita M. Pathophysiology of AKI to CKD progression. Semin Nephrol. 2020;40(2):206–15.
45. Kappel B, Olsen S. Cortical interstitial tissue and sclerosed glomeruli in the normal human kidney, related to age and sex. A quantitative study. Virchows Arch A Pathol Anat Histol. 1980;387(3):271–7.
46. Epstein M. Aging and the kidney. J Am Soc Nephrol. 1996;7(8):1106–22.
47. Cheung CM, Ponnusamy A, Anderton JG. Management of acute renal failure in the elderly patient: a clinician's guide. Drugs Aging. 2008;25(6):455–76.
48. Pascual J, Liaño F, Ortuño J. The elderly patient with acute renal failure. J Am Soc Nephrol. 1995;6(2):144–53.
49. Macedo E, Bouchard J, Mehta RL. Renal recovery following acute kidney injury. Curr Opin Crit Care. 2008;14(6):660–5.
50. Wald R, Quinn RR, Luo J, Li P, Scales DC, Mamdani MM, Ray JG. Chronic dialysis and death among survivors of acute kidney injury requiring dialysis. JAMA. 2009;302(11):1179–85.
51. Harel Z, Bell CM, Dixon SN, McArthur E, James MT, Garg AX, Harel S, Silver S, Wald R. Predictors of progression to chronic dialysis in survivors of severe acute kidney injury: a competing risk study. BMC Nephrol. 2014;15:114.
52. Schmitt R, Cantley LG. The impact of aging on kidney repair. Am J Physiol Renal Physiol. 2008;294(6):F1265–72.
53. Liu JQ, Cai GY, Liang S, Wang WL, Wang SY, Zhu FL, Nie SS, Feng Z, Chen XM. Characteristics of and risk factors for death in elderly patients with acute kidney injury: a multicentre retrospective study in China. Postgrad Med J. 2018;94(1111):249–53.
54. Infante B, Franzin R, Madio D, Calvaruso M, Maiorano A, Sangregorio F, Netti GS, Ranieri E, Gesualdo L, Castellano G, et al. Molecular mechanisms of AKI in the elderly: from animal models to therapeutic intervention. J Clin Med. 2020;9(8):2574.
55. Fliser D. Ren sanus in corpore sano: the myth of the inexorable decline of renal function with senescence. Nephrol Dial Transplant. 2005;20(3):482–5.
56. Fliser D, Zeier M, Nowack R, Ritz E. Renal functional reserve in healthy elderly subjects. J Am Soc Nephrol. 1993;3(7):1371–7.
57. Fliser D, Ritz E, Franek E. Renal reserve in the elderly. Semin Nephrol. 1995;15(5):463–7.
58. Lakatta EG. Cardiovascular regulatory mechanisms in advanced age. Physiol Rev. 1993;73(2):413–67.
59. Zhang XZ, Qiu C, Baylis C. Sensitivity of the segmental renal arterioles to angiotensin II in the aging rat. Mech Ageing Dev. 1997;97(2):183–92.
60. Baylis C, Fredericks M, Wilson C, Munger K, Collins R. Renal vasodilatory response to intravenous glycine in the aging rat kidney. Am J Kidney Dis. 1990;15(3):244–51.
61. Coresh J, Selvin E, Stevens LA, Manzi J, Kusek JW, Eggers P, Van Lente F, Levey AS. Prevalence of chronic kidney disease in the United States. JAMA. 2007;298(17):2038–47.
62. Stevens LA, Li S, Wang C, Huang C, Becker BN, Bomback AS, Brown WW, Burrows NR, Jurkovitz CT, McFarlane SI, et al. Prevalence of CKD and comorbid illness in elderly patients in the United States: results from the Kidney Early Evaluation Program (KEEP). Am J Kidney Dis. 2010;55(3 Suppl 2):S23–33.
63. Gong Y, Zhang F, Ding F, Gu Y. Elderly patients with acute kidney injury (AKI): clinical features and risk factors for mortality. Arch Gerontol Geriatr. 2012;54(2):e47–51.
64. Mangano CM, Diamondstone LS, Ramsay JG, Aggarwal A, Herskowitz A, Mangano DT, The Multicenter Study of Perioperative Ischemia Research Group. Renal dysfunction after myocardial

revascularization: risk factors, adverse outcomes, and hospital resource utilization. Ann Intern Med. 1998;128(3):194–203.

65. Bagshaw SM, Uchino S, Bellomo R, Morimatsu H, Morgera S, Schetz M, Tan I, Bouman C, Macedo E, Gibney N, et al. Septic acute kidney injury in critically ill patients: clinical characteristics and outcomes. Clin J Am Soc Nephrol. 2007;2(3):431–9.

66. Brennan M, O'Keeffe ST, Mulkerrin EC. Dehydration and renal failure in older persons during heatwaves-predictable, hard to identify but preventable? Age Ageing. 2019;48(5):615–8.

67. Aymanns C, Keller F, Maus S, Hartmann B, Czock D. Review on pharmacokinetics and pharmacodynamics and the aging kidney. Clin J Am Soc Nephrol. 2010;5(2):314–27.

68. Epstein M, Hollenberg NK. Age as a determinant of renal sodium conservation in normal man. J Lab Clin Med. 1976;87(3):411–7.

69. Mimran A, Ribstein J, Jover B. Aging and sodium homeostasis. Kidney Int Suppl. 1992;37:S107–13.

70. Martin JE, Sheaff MT. Renal ageing. J Pathol. 2007;211(2):198–205.

71. O'Sullivan ED, Hughes J, Ferenbach DA. Renal aging: causes and consequences. J Am Soc Nephrol. 2017;28(2):407–20.

72. Lameire N, Hoste E, Van Loo A, Dhondt A, Bernaert P, Vanholder R. Pathophysiology, causes, and prognosis of acute renal failure in the elderly. Ren Fail. 1996;18(3):333–46.

73. Jerkić M, Vojvodić S, López-Novoa JM. The mechanism of increased renal susceptibility to toxic substances in the elderly. Part I. the role of increased vasoconstriction. Int Urol Nephrol. 2001;32(4):539–47.

74. Macías-Núñez JF, López-Novoa JM, Martínez-Maldonado M. Acute renal failure in the aged. Semin Nephrol. 1996;16(4):330–8.

75. Pascual J, Liaño F, Madrid Acute Renal Failure Study Group. Causes and prognosis of acute renal failure in the very old. J Am Geriatr Soc. 1998;46(6):721–5.

76. Feest TG, Round A, Hamad S. Incidence of severe acute renal failure in adults: results of a community based study. BMJ. 1993;306(6876):481–3.

77. Ronco C, Bellasi A, Di Lullo L. Cardiorenal syndrome: an overview. Adv Chronic Kidney Dis. 2018;25(5):382–90.

78. Ronco C, Chionh CY, Haapio M, Anavekar NS, House A, Bellomo R. The cardiorenal syndrome. Blood Purif. 2009;27(1):114–26.

79. Doty JM, Saggi BH, Sugerman HJ, Blocher CR, Pin R, Fakhry I, Gehr TW, Sica DA. Effect of increased renal venous pressure on renal function. J Trauma. 1999;47(6):1000–3.

80. Doty JM, Saggi BH, Blocher CR, Fakhry I, Gehr T, Sica D, Sugerman HJ. Effects of increased renal parenchymal pressure on renal function. J Trauma. 2000;48(5):874–7.

81. Cops J, Mullens W, Verbrugge FH, Swennen Q, De Moor B, Reynders C, Penders J, Achten R, Driessen A, Dendooven A, et al. Selective abdominal venous congestion induces adverse renal and hepatic morphological and functional alterations despite a preserved cardiac function. Sci Rep. 2018;8(1):17757.

82. Chao CT, Lin YF, Tsai HB, Wu VC, Ko WJ. Acute kidney injury network staging in geriatric postoperative acute kidney injury patients: shortcomings and improvements. J Am Coll Surg. 2013;217(2):240–50.

83. Han WK, Wagener G, Zhu Y, Wang S, Lee HT. Urinary biomarkers in the early detection of acute kidney injury after cardiac surgery. Clin J Am Soc Nephrol. 2009;4(5):873–82.

84. Parikh CR, Abraham E, Ancukiewicz M, Edelstein CL. Urine IL-18 is an early diagnostic marker for acute kidney injury and predicts mortality in the intensive care unit. J Am Soc Nephrol. 2005;16(10):3046–52.

85. Shlipak MG, Sarnak MJ, Katz R, Fried LF, Seliger SL, Newman AB, Siscovick DS, Stehman-Breen C. Cystatin C and the risk of death and cardiovascular events among elderly persons. N Engl J Med. 2005;352(20):2049–60.

86. Siew ED, Ware LB, Gebretsadik T, Shintani A, Moons KG, Wickersham N, Bossert F, Ikizler TA. Urine neutrophil gelatinase-associated lipocalin moderately predicts acute kidney injury in critically ill adults. J Am Soc Nephrol. 2009;20(8):1823–32.

87. Soni SS, Cruz D, Bobek I, Chionh CY, Nalesso F, Lentini P, de Cal M, Corradi V, Virzi G, Ronco C. NGAL: a biomarker of acute kidney injury and other systemic conditions. Int Urol Nephrol. 2010;42(1):141–50.

88. Lopes MB, Araujo LQ, Passos MT, Nishida SK, Kirsztajn GM, Cendoroglo MS, Sesso RC. Estimation of glomerular filtration rate from serum creatinine and cystatin C in octogenarians and nonagenarians. BMC Nephrol. 2013;14:265.
89. Haase M, Bellomo R, Devarajan P, Schlattmann P, Haase-Fielitz A, Group NM-aI. Accuracy of neutrophil gelatinase-associated lipocalin (NGAL) in diagnosis and prognosis in acute kidney injury: a systematic review and meta-analysis. Am J Kidney Dis. 2009;54(6):1012–24.
90. Park HS, Kim JW, Lee KR, Hong DY, Park SO, Kim SY, Kim JY, Han SK. Urinary neutrophil gelatinase-associated lipocalin as a biomarker of acute kidney injury in sepsis patients in the emergency department. Clin Chim Acta. 2019;495:552–5.
91. Guo L, Zhu B, Yuan H, Zhao W. Evaluation of serum neutrophil gelatinase-associated lipocalin in older patients with chronic kidney disease. Aging Med. 2020;3(1):32–9.

The Very Old Critically Ill Patient Neurointensive Care

Louis Morisson and Benjamin G. Chousterman

Contents

> **Learning Objectives**
>
> The proportion of elderly patients admitted to neurointensive care is increasing. Appropriate care of this specific subgroup of patient necessitates a good understanding of the changes of brain physiology with age, the therapeutic specificities of elderly patients, and the outcome of these patients when admitted for neurological conditions.
>
> In this chapter, we will review the latest epidemiologic data on neurointensive care for elderly patients, we will present the physiology of the aging central nervous system and the therapeutics peculiarities of aging patients, and we will discuss what can be the expected outcomes and the related ethical considerations when taking care of an old patient admitted to neurointensive care.

32.1 Introduction

The increase in life expectancy has been accompanied by an increase in the proportion of people living in old age and in relatively good health. On one hand, the resulting aging of the population is accompanied by medical issues that present peculiarities in their pathophysiology and etiology. On the other hand, this leads to consider treatments that were previously reserved for younger subjects.

When caring for elderly subjects in neurological intensive care units, clinicians must keep in mind the specificities related to the physiology of aging as well as the relevant elements of the neurological prognosis assessment.

This chapter presents the main acute neurological conditions that can lead to the management of the elderly patient in intensive care with adapted therapeutic objectives. The notion of functional prognosis will be addressed, as it may or may not ultimately justify the intensity of treatment of these patients.

32.2 Epidemiology

The proportion of elderly critically ill patients is rapidly increasing in developed countries, and epidemiological data concerning neurocritical care of these patients are emerging. In 2010, Chibbaro et al. showed a significant increase in the proportion of patients aged 70 and over admitted to a monocentric neurosurgical unit: from 11% in 1983 to 25% in 2007 [1]. When looking at very old patients, the overall incidence of neurological causes of admission in intensive care unit (ICU) is about 8.6% in a recent European cohort with 3.7% concerning head injury [2] and 8.5% in Australia and New Zealand [3].

Neurological causes of admission are varied and depend on the care facility. In a UK neurosurgical center, it seems that main causes of neurosurgical admissions are degenerative spine disease and traumatic brain injury (Table 32.1) [4]. Concerning the causes for nonsurgical neurological admissions, they seem to be relatively similar in elderly subjects as those reported in younger subjects: ischemic stroke (31%), intracranial hemorrhage (ICH) (26%), subarachnoid hemorrhage (SAH) (5%), epileptic seizures (12%), meningoencephalitis (6%), and Guillain-Barré syndrome and myasthenia gravies (3%) [5].

□ Table 32.1 Causes of neurosurgical admission

Diagnostic category	Elective admissions	Emergency admissions	Total
Degenerative spine disease	36.1%	5.2%	41.2%
Traumatism (including spinal fracture)	0.9%	35.7%	36.6%
Tumor	5%	5.6%	10.6%
SAH	0	4.9%	4.9%
Disorders of CSF flow	1.8%	0.6%	2.5%
Hemorrhagic cerebrovascular event	0	1.7%	1.7%
Ischemic cerebrovascular event	0	0.2%	0.2%
Infection	0.1%	1.3%	1.4%
Other	0.3%	0.3%	0.6%
Total	**44.4%**	**55.6%**	**100%**

SAH subarachnoid hemorrhage, *CSF* cerebrospinal fluid
From Whitehouse et al. [4]

32.2.1 Traumatic Brain Injury

Traumatic brain injury (TBI) is a leading cause of death and disability worldwide. In the United States, the highest incidence of TBI occurs in older adults (incidence 2000 in 100,000) [6]. From 2007 to 2013, TBI-related hospitalizations increased more than 25%. This increasing incidence of TBI hospitalizations (and deaths) among older adults in the United States has also been confirmed in European countries [7–9]. The majority of TBI in the elderly are attributed to falls (>50% after 65 years old and 75% after 75 years old) [10]. This is clinically important since fall-related TBIs more frequently result in mass lesions (e.g., subdural hemorrhage), while motor vehicle accident-related TBIs more frequently result in diffuse axonal injury. The proportion of women who experience a TBI increases with age, reaching over 75% after age 85 [11]. Another particularity of TBI in the elderly is that preexisting conditions are extremely common. Preexisting conditions including past history of TBI, dementia, diabetes, and cardiovascular disease are risk factors of TBI and are associated with worse outcomes [9, 12].

32.2.2 Stroke

Each year in the United States, about 795,000 people experience a stroke. In 2017, stroke accounted for about one of every 19 deaths. Stroke risk increased with age, and 66% of people hospitalized for stroke were more than 65 years old in 2009. Of all strokes, 87% are acute ischemic stroke (AIS), 10% are intracerebral hemorrhage (ICH), and 3% are subarachnoid hemorrhage (SAH) [13]. Incidences rates are 1.5 times higher in men than in women [14]. This is particularly marked in people aged 55–75 years, whereas an inverse trend has been reported in older people [15]. Most of the population-based registries have reported stable or decreasing incidence rates. But because of aging of the population, the absolute annual number of new strokes has risen over the last 20 years (from 10.1 to 16.9 million in high-income countries) [14].

32.2.3 Epilepsy

Like stroke, epilepsy is a pathology whose incidence increases with age [16]. It represents the third most common neurological disorder in older people after stroke and dementia. Incidence increases steadily after 50 years old, from about 50 cases per 100,000 to more than 150 per 100,000 after 75 years of age. While the main etiologies of seizures in the young are genetic or constitutive, epilepsy in the elderly is mostly secondary. The most common cause of seizures and epilepsy in older people is cerebrovascular disease which account for more than 50%. Other causes of epilepsy in older people are neoplasms, Alzheimer's disease, and metabolic and iatrogenic causes. In addition to the numerous treatments and their polypathology, elderly subjects present a lowering of the epileptogenic threshold which explains in part the increase in incidence with age. The diagnosis of epilepsy in older people can be more challenging than in younger people. For the latter, there is a preponderance of temporal lobe seizures, while most seizures in older people are of extra-temporal onset and diverse in semiology. Convulsions are relatively rare and may occur at night, and one ictus out of four is manifested by a predominantly cognitive symptomatology. Finally, in older subjects, there are a lot of differential diagnoses for a potential seizure. Differentiating between syncope, fluctuating cognitive impairment, delirium, transient ischemic attack, or impairment of cerebral circulation due to seizures can be difficult.

32.2.4 Brain Tumors

The incidence rate of brain cancer is relatively stable over the years and is about six per 100,000 people for the overall population, but this incidence rate rises to 56 per 100,000 persons after 65 years old [17]. The aging of the population and the expansion of surgical indications have led to an increase in the proportion of elderly subjects undergoing neurosurgery. The experience of the neurosurgical department of Lariboisière Hospital in Paris shows that over a period of 25 years, this proportion has increased from 10 to 24%. At the same time, the proportion of surgical interventions performed in emergency decreased from 46 to 26% during the same period, suggesting that the increase in surgical procedures in elderly subjects is essentially related to elective interventions [1].

32.3 Physiology of the Aging Central Nervous System

32.3.1 Structural Modifications

32.3.1.1 Neurons

During aging, there is a progressive cerebral atrophy associated with neuronal loss. Progressive decline in brain weight begins at 50 years of age and reaches its lowest values after 85 years (the mean brain weight has decreased by about 11% relative to the maximum brain weight) [18]. Cerebral atrophy is mainly observed in the hippocampal region, in the prefrontal and temporal associative neocortex, in the cerebellum, and in the brain stem nuclei. The cell bodies concerned are essentially the large pyramidal cells. These are notably the cells on which neurofibrillary degeneration is observed in Alzheimer's disease.

Apart from cell atrophy, the loss of mass of the brain during aging can be explained by a quantitative neuronal loss, particularly in the gray matter. Gray matter loss is most pronounced for orbital and inferior frontal, cingulate, insular, inferior parietal, and to a lesser extent mesial temporal region as shown in longitudinal magnetic resonance imaging studies [19, 20]. The changes in the white matter are widespread. It should be noted that these neuronal structural changes correspond to normal brain aging and differ from those observed in Alzheimer's disease [21]. The overall neuronal loss is about 10% with more than 15% difference between males and females favoring females [19]. This is probably due to protective effect of estrogens on neurons and intracerebral vessels. Another notably structural change, which has a direct impact of intracerebral lesions' constitution, is the phenomenon of increased adhesion of the dura mater to the underlying bone over time. It trends to fix the dura mater to the cranial vault.

32.3.1.2 Vessels

Morphological structure and biomechanical properties of intracranial vessels are affected by aging. These modifications concern macro-vessels and intraparenchymal micro-vessels.

From an anatomical point of view, atherosclerosis is first observed in the vessels of the Willis circle [22, 23] particularly at the level of the bifurcations and the birth of the collateral branches. While vessels appear to maintain a constant diameter, there is thickening of the media as a result of the deposition of type IV collagen. It leads to a decrease in their internal diameter through a phenomenon of concentric hypertrophy [24–27].

Biomechanical properties of intracranial arteries are also altered. Indeed, aging is responsible of major elasticity loss with a direct negative impact of cerebral blood flow (CBF) autoregulation. Arterial stiffness is partly explained by elastin fibers modification. During the aging process, there is no decrease in the number of fibers but a reorganization of their positioning and a fragmentation of the fibers. Normally organized in a circumferential manner, perpendicular to the blood flow, the elastin fibers are oriented in the direction of the flow in the elderly. This phenomenon is leading to a loss of arterial elastic deformability [25, 28, 29].

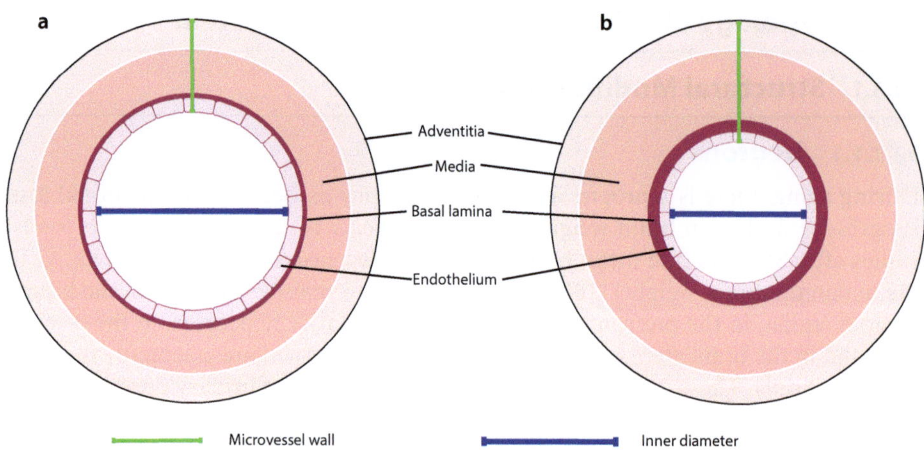

◘ Fig. 32.1 Analysis of the thickness of the vessel wall and the inner diameter of the vessel lumen in young and old patients. **a** young patient, **b** old patient. (From Uspenskaia et al. [24])

The thickening of the basal membrane and media together with endothelial volume decrease are responsible of microcirculation alteration (◘ Fig. 32.1) [24, 30]. Histological sections of micro-vessels show a decrease in endothelium thickness, and functional assays attest to the lack of intrinsic regulation of vasomotor tone in response to sympathetic nervous system activation or in response to flow. The damage to the micro-vessels, particularly the perforating arteries, is due to lipohyalinosis following fibrinoid necrosis leading to the disappearance of the smooth muscle cells of the small arteries [28, 29]. In addition to lipohyalinosis, these vessels are subject to a fibrotic phenomenon by collagen deposition. These lesions are aggravated by arterial hypertension and are associated with other cardiovascular risk factors. These very peripheral vascular lesions are at the origin of intracerebral lacunar lesions.

These lesions are also at the origin of blood-brain barrier alteration which is weakened [31]. In pathological situation, this may represent a risk factor of cerebral edema constitution. Finally, intracranial arterial aneurysms, responsible for, among others, SAH, are twice as frequent in the elderly [32, 33].

From a functional point of view, the question of cerebral autoregulation alteration in aging is still not answered. Cerebral autoregulation consists of diameter adaptation of intracerebral vessels in response to mean arterial pressure variations in order to provide a constant CBF over a large scale [34]. Current hypotheses suggest that preservation of cerebral autoregulation with aging serves as a "reserve" to compensate for impairment of other systems [35]. But if age is not directly responsible for an alteration of cerebral autoregulation, it is reasonable to think that comorbidities and cardiotropic treatments have an adverse effect on cerebral autoregulation in the elderly subject (◘ Fig. 32.2). Moreover, in basal state, cerebral metabolic rate and CBF are decreased of about 15% [36]. These physiological observations are confirmed by transcranial dopplers (TCD) which showed a decrease in intracranial arteries' velocities of 10–20%. Together with intern caliber reduction, this leads to a decrease in CBF.

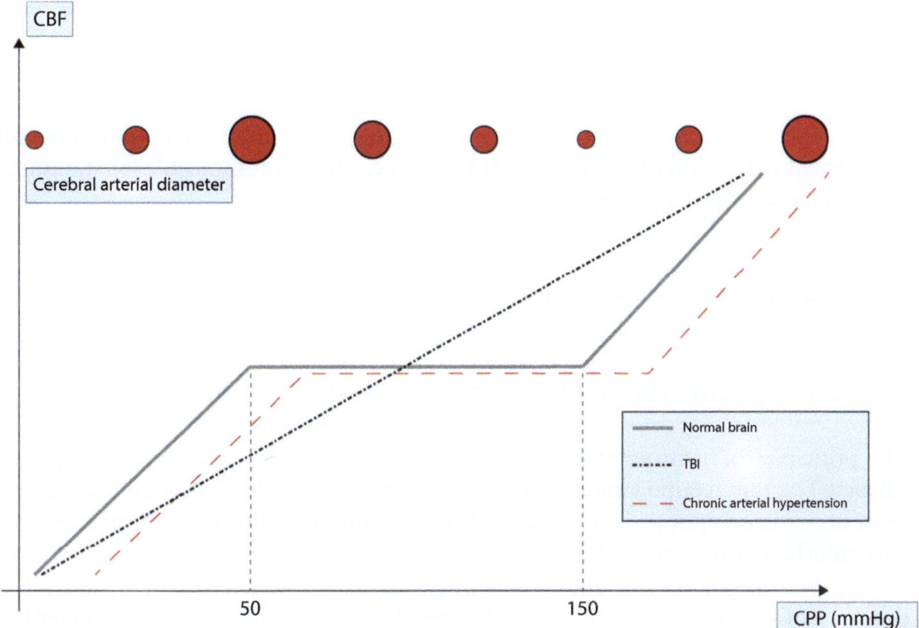

■ **Fig. 32.2** Cerebral autoregulation. Cerebral autoregulation curve is shifted on the right in chronic hypertension patients. TBI traumatic brain injury, CPP cerebral perfusion pressure, CBF cerebral blood flow

A study investigated the relationship between age and cerebral autoregulation (evaluated with intracranial pressure (ICP) and TCD) after traumatic brain injury. On the one hand, the authors report a link between initial ICP and age, older subjects having lowest ICP values and TCD didn't seem to be affected by age. On the other hand, cerebral autoregulation was notably altered in older subjects. This was associated with a relative deterioration in outcome despite better initial Glasgow Coma Scale (GCS) [37].

32.3.2 Functional Modifications

Aging is responsible of neuronal physiology modification which is linked not only to structural changes of the neurons, vessels, and the connective tissue but also to qualitative change in nervous cells. Several mechanisms are involved in the disruption of nerve conduction. At the cellular level, the long-term consequences of oxidative stress can be observed as the endogenous regulatory systems become defective [38–40]. Oxygen-free radicals and lipid peroxidation weaken and modify the ability of the cellular membrane to assume its barrier and nervous signal transmission functions.

Neurotransmitters and neurotransmitters receptors are also diminished in the elderly subject together with post-synaptic enzymatic degradation increase [41]. Acetylcholine and dopamine synthesis decrease are mainly observed in the frontal and cingulate cortex, respectively [42–45]. Certain conditions or disease can amplify this phenomenon. For example, Alzheimer's disease is characterized by an increase of cholinesterase expression, while Parkinson's disease is characterized by a decrease in dopamine synthesis in neurons of *locus niger*. Inflammatory infections also play a role in neurotransmission's alteration by decreasing neurotransmitter receptor's number (e.g., NMDA receptor) [46].

DNA repair mechanisms degrade during aging [47]. Thus, they do not allow for the efficient correction of oxidative DNA damage, which is responsible for spontaneous mutagenesis and apoptosis finally.

All these structural and functional neuronal alterations occurring in a less reactive and poorly anastomosed vascular network make the brain of the elderly particularly sensitive to ischemia and oxidative stress.

32.4   Therapeutic Particularities of the Elderly Subject

The principles of neurointensive care in the elderly are the same as for the young subject. The therapeutic strategy consists in preventing weakly vascularized neurons from necrosis or apoptosis. Due to its low energetic reserves, cerebral neurons are particularly sensitive to ischemia. Peripheral neurons of infarcted zone cease its activity because of insufficient oxygen and nutrient supplies. Neuronal survival in this area of "ischemic penumbra" will depend essentially on good management in avoiding secondary brain injury.

32.4.1   Cerebral Hemodynamics

32.4.1.1   Intracranial Hypertension

Acute intracranial hypertension results from intracranial volume increase. This increase may be related to tissular volume expansion (cerebral edema), to an intracranial expansive process (especially subdural hematomas due to the adhesion of the dura mater to the cranial vault and tumors) or to acute hydrocephalus due to disturbed circulation or reportion of the cerebral spinal fluid. These mechanisms are often intertwined, especially in TBI.

Older adults present different initial clinical presentation compared to younger subjects. The Glasgow Coma Scale (GCS), although the most widely used clinical assessment to determine TBI severity, may be misleading in the elderly. On the one hand, older adults with preexisting dementia may have abnormal GCS at baseline [48]. On the other hand, age-related cerebral modifications leading to atrophy may delay the clinical expression of expanding intracranial hemorrhage and thus the diagnosis of intracranial hypertension. The frequency of brain lesions with paucisymptomatic examination is markedly increased in subjects older than 60 years [49]. Current recommendations suggest treating ICP above 22 mmHg [50]. For the reasons mentioned above, this threshold may be reduced to 18 mmHg in older adults [51].

The treatment of intracranial hypertension relies on good management of secondary brain injuries with a particular attention to the maintenance of the cerebral perfusion pressure (CPP) which is defined by the difference between the mean arterial pressure (MAP) and the intracranial pressure (ICP). Therefore, the optimization of CPP involves the control of MAP and ICP monitoring, which could improve outcome of older adults with severe TBI [52]. The use in the initial phase of osmotherapy to reduce cerebral blood volume and more rarely corticosteroids in certain paraneoplastic edemas, surgical drainage of CSF, or surgical evacuation of a hematoma may allow the control of ICP. The method of surgical intervention may impact outcome. Indeed, a retrospective cohort study that used a propensity score showed that patients who were treated with decompressive craniectomy had worse 6-month outcome compared to those treated with craniotomy [53].

32.4.1.2 Cerebral Autoregulation and Hemodynamic Objectives

The recommended target CCP value for survival and favorable outcomes is between 60 and 70 mmHg [50]. This range has never been clinically validated in older adults. However, the relevance of this objective seems questionable in the elderly because of the physiological changes mentioned above and the frequency of chronic hypertension, which modify the autoregulation of CBF. Moreover, after severe TBI, CBF autoregulation is likely to be altered, making CBF linearly dependent on CPP.

The combination of severe TBI and underlying terrain exposes a coupling between CBF and MAP. Thus, too high MAP therapeutic targets may lead to the development or worsening of intracranial hypertension, especially since atherosclerosis leads to an alteration of the brain-blood barrier. Conversely, too low MAP targets in chronically hypertensive patient expose the risk of a critical decrease in CBF and the extension of ischemic lesions.

In the absence of specific data in the elderly, CPP optimization relies on:

- The control of ICP based on avoiding secondary brain injury and eventually associated with initial osmotherapy to reduce cerebral volume
- The control of MAP based on careful fluid therapy and vasopressors

It seems difficult to fix theoretical MAP and CPP objectives in the elderly. Hence, cerebral monitoring becomes essential and should be, at best, multimodal: ICP monitoring, transcranial doppler (TCD), and eventually advanced cerebral monitors such as microdialysis, jugular venous oxygen monitoring (S_jO_2), cerebral oximetry, and brain tissue oxygen monitoring ($P_{br}O_2$) which allow to monitor cerebral metabolism. Once again, these monitors have not been evaluated in the elderly. Isolated ICP monitoring benefit is limited due to cortical atrophy that lowers ICP. TCD are extremely useful to finely tune MAP and CPP objectives. No study has demonstrated the value of advanced monitoring in the elderly.

32.4.2 Sedation Analgesia in the Elderly

Sedation is an indispensable tool in the management of severe brain injury. It is initiated for the control of intracranial lesions and for the adaptation of the patient to the therapies used (mechanical ventilation, surgery). It allows to decrease the cerebral metabolic consumption and thus to optimize the balance between the needs and the contributions. Classically, patients with severe TBI are sedated during the first 48 hours. The value of continuing sedation or not is then reassessed according to the data of clinical examination and imaging. In practice, the molecules used in neurointensive care for sedation of the elderly differ little from those used for younger patients [54]. The association between propofol and fentanyl/sufentanil is the first-line option for standard sedation and in the case of elevated ICP and status epilepticus. Midazolam is also a good alternative and may be associated with propofol to reduce tissue accumulation of midazolam or to reduce the occurrence of propofol infusion syndrome (PRIS) [55].

In the last ten years, dexmedetomidine, an alpha-2 adrenergic receptor agonist, has been widely evaluated for the prevention of delirium in elderly patients in ICU. In the context of neurointensive care, dexmedetomidine may be a good molecule for the treatment of agitation when weaning off other sedatives; it also allows for a better neurological evaluation including detection of focal neurological defects [56]. Dexmedetomidine provides sedation without inducing unresponsiveness or coma and has analgesic properties without effect on respiratory drive.

The pharmacokinetic and pharmacodynamic particularities of the elderly subject must be taken into account. Indeed, the volume of distribution of hydrophilic substances is reduced by about 25%. The decrease in the concentration of albumin in the blood and the increase of other drug binding proteins such as alpha 1 glycoprotein make it necessary to know the physical and chemical properties of the substances used. Clearance of anesthetics is reduced due to decreased glomerular filtration rate and decreased hepatic function. The titration of sedation becomes an issue to avoid its accumulation which could delay the recovery and the neurological evaluation. Generally speaking, the need for anesthetics is reduced during aging, especially in the context of neurointensive care.

32.5 Outcomes and Ethical Considerations

There is clear evidence that elderly patients with cerebral injury have on average, greater mortality, poorer functional outcomes, and slower cognitive recovery compared to their younger counterparts. While some studies reported a linear relationship between age and outcome [57], some others have reported an inflection point (40–50 years old) at which mortality appears to increase steeply [58, 59]. Whether this increase is linear or not, it still appears that a significant proportion of elderly patients may recover well after cerebral injury [60, 61].

Several elements must be considered when interpreting the neurological outcome of the elderly patient. The first element concerns the role of the caregivers' attitude as well as patient's and family wishes who may be more likely to have life-sustaining therapy withdrawn [62]. Older patients may also have longer delays in obtaining a cerebral imaging, a lower likelihood of being transferred to a neurospecialized center and a lower likelihood of being seen by a senior (versus junior) physician than their younger counterparts [63, 64]. The second element concerns the tools used for outcome assessment. The Glasgow Outcome Scale (GOS) and the GOS extended (GOSE), for example, are the most widely used functional outcome measures in TBI. Neither the GOS nor the GOSE were validated in older adults, and they may not adequately reflect the functional impairment in this population. In a multicenter study, older adults with severe TBI had a significant improvement in physical function over 1 year according to the health-related quality of life measure. This functional improvement was not detected by the GOSE [65].

For all these reasons, age should only be considered in light of other relevant elements of the history that will have an impact on neurological outcome. Consideration of frailty, cognition, previous autonomy, patient wishes, and relatives' opinion are all elements that should be carefully reported in the medical record [2, 66].

Apart from the impact of age on neurological prognosis, the prognosis of neurological injuries is highly dependent on the nature and initial severity of the injury. For example, Kiphuth et al. reported that intracranial hemorrhage, Guillain-Barré syndrome, and myasthenia gravis cerebral neoplasms were associated with a poor vital or neurological outcome in patients admitted to neurointensive care [5].

32.5.1 Mortality

When considering mortality after neurointensive care unit admission, it is important to distinguish between short-term mortality and longer-term mortality. Short-term mortality is high among older adults. For severe TBI, several studies reported in-hospital mortality rates as high as 60–80% in this population [67, 68]. Regarding strokes, ICH is the one associated with the highest 1-month mortality rate (25–61%), which is similar to SAH (26–48%). A better prognosis has been noted for patients with ischemic stroke (9–19%) [14].

In a French monocentric study that looked at the long-term outcome in medical patients aged 80 or over following admission to an intensive care unit, the authors reported a 1-year mortality rate of 60% for patients with coma or neurological admission diagnosis. This mortality rate was not different from that observed for the same causes of admission for all age categories combined (55.5%) [69].

Concerning long-term outcome in acute stroke patients, a multicenter study reported that 1-year mortality for patients requiring mechanical ventilation was dramatically high (77%). Once again, ICH and SAH subtypes presented higher mortality rates with 82.7% and 88.1%, respectively. In the multivariate model, age > 70 years was not a factor significantly associated with 1-year mortality in contrast to the stroke subtype [70].

Several studies have reported higher mortality among older adults versus younger subjects for patients with severe TBI who survive the initial hospitalization. However, this observed increase in mortality may be explained predominantly by the age-related mortality seen in the general aging population [71, 72].

32.5.2 Functional Outcome

The other prognostic approach, which is just as fundamental, concerns the functional outcome, which includes the degree of autonomy expected from the small proportion of patients who will survive the initial phase. Overall, functional outcome of elderly patient admitted to neurointensive care is decreased compared to younger patients.

Concerning TBI, most of the study report that older adults present higher risk of being dependent than younger subjects. Thus, among patients of 60 years old and more who were discharge from ICU with a GOS ≤ 4, Livingston et al. reported that only 37% presented a functional improvement evaluated with the Functional Independence Measure (FIM), while this proportion reached 63–85% in younger subjects [73]. It should be noted that, compared to younger individuals, older adults are at increased risk for post-traumatic epilepsy, stroke, and neurodegenerative disease [74–79]. This increase could largely contribute to the loss of autonomy of elderly subjects after TBI.

In a large Swedish stroke register, Ullberg et al. reported dependency in Activities of Daily Living (ADL) at 12 months for more than 35,000 stroke patients. The proportion of patients of 75 years old and more who were ADL-dependent was significantly increased (from 15–20% to 35–45%) compared to younger subjects [80]. The most predictive factors of being dependent at 12 months were consciousness level at admittance, female sex, a previous stroke history, and ICH stroke.

The functional outcome of aneurysmal subarachnoid hemorrhage is highly influenced by the initial gravity. For poor grade aneurysmal subarachnoid hemorrhage (WFNS 4 and 5), favorable outcome 6 to 12 months (defined as a modified Rankin scale ≤3) were reported for 41.4% of patients aged 60–69 years, 17% of those aged 70–79 years, and only 10% of patients aged 80–90 years ($p = 0.002$) [81].

Finally, Pirracchio et al. reported 1-year functional outcome after neurosurgery for intracranial tumor in elderly patients [82]. At 1 year, 63.6% of the patients were considered as dependent according to Karnofsky Performance Scale and ADL scale.

> **Conclusion**
>
> Once considered futile, the management of elderly patients admitted to neurointensive care has become commonplace. Knowledge of the anatomical and physiological particularities of the elderly should allow a better understanding of the singularities in the presentation of pathologies encountered in neurointensive care. These particularities justify a specific monitoring and treatment strategy in the initial phase. The question of neurological outcome, especially functional outcome, must be addressed taking into account comorbidities, previous autonomy, and the wishes of the patient and his family.

> **Take Home Message**
> - The proportion of elderly patients admitted to neurointensive care is increasing.
> - Management of old patients admitted to neurointensive care differs from younger ones due to variation in physiology.
> - Further work should be done on the specific management of elderly patient with acute neurological conditions.
> - Overall, the outcome of aging patients admitted to neurointensive care units is poor.

References

1. Chibbaro S, Di Rocco F, Makiese O, Mirone G, Marsella M, Lukaszewicz AC, et al. Neurosurgery and elderly: analysis through the years. Neurosurg Rev. 2010;34(2):229–34.
2. Guidet B, de Lange DW, Boumendil A, Leaver S, Watson X, Boulanger C, et al. The contribution of frailty, cognition, activity of daily life and comorbidities on outcome in acutely admitted patients over 80 years in European ICUs: the VIP2 study. Intensive Care Med. 2020;46(1):57–69.

3. Darvall JN, Bellomo R, Paul E, Subramaniam A, Santamaria JD, Bagshaw SM, et al. Frailty in very old critically ill patients in Australia and New Zealand: a population-based cohort study. Med J Aust. 2019;211(7):318–23.
4. Whitehouse KJ, Jeyaretna DS, Wright A, Whitfield PC. Neurosurgical care in the elderly: increasing demands necessitate future healthcare planning. World Neurosurg. 2016;87:446–54.
5. Kiphuth IC, Schellinger PD, Kohrmann M, Bardutzky J, Lucking H, Kloska S, et al. Predictors for good functional outcome after neurocritical care. Crit Care. 2010;14(4):R136.
6. Taylor CA, Bell JM, Breiding MJ, Xu L. Traumatic brain injury-related emergency department visits, hospitalizations, and deaths - United States, 2007 and 2013. MMWR Surveill Summ. 2017;66(9):1–16.
7. Korhonen N, Niemi S, Parkkari J, Sievanen H, Kannus P. Incidence of fall-related traumatic brain injuries among older Finnish adults between 1970 and 2011. JAMA. 2013;309(18):1891–2.
8. Hamill V, Barry SJ, McConnachie A, McMillan TM, Teasdale GM. Mortality from head injury over four decades in Scotland. J Neurotrauma. 2015;32(10):689–703.
9. Hawley C, Sakr M, Scapinello S, Salvo J, Wrenn P. Traumatic brain injuries in older adults-6 years of data for one UK trauma centre: retrospective analysis of prospectively collected data. Emerg Med J. 2017;34(8):509–16.
10. Harvey LA, Close JC. Traumatic brain injury in older adults: characteristics, causes and consequences. Injury. 2012;43(11):1821–6.
11. Dams-O'Connor K, Cuthbert JP, Whyte J, Corrigan JD, Faul M, Harrison-Felix C. Traumatic brain injury among older adults at level I and II trauma centers. J Neurotrauma. 2013;30(24):2001–13.
12. Kumar RG, Juengst SB, Wang Z, Dams-O'Connor K, Dikmen SS, O'Neil-Pirozzi TM, et al. Epidemiology of comorbid conditions among adults 50 years and older with traumatic brain injury. J Head Trauma Rehabil. 2018;33(1):15–24.
13. Virani SS, Alonso A, Benjamin EJ, Bittencourt MS, Callaway CW, Carson AP, et al. Heart disease and stroke statistics-2020 update: a report from the American Heart Association. Circulation. 2020;141(9):e139–596.
14. Bejot Y, Daubail B, Giroud M. Epidemiology of stroke and transient ischemic attacks: current knowledge and perspectives. Rev Neurol (Paris). 2016;172(1):59–68.
15. Reeves MJ, Bushnell CD, Howard G, Gargano JW, Duncan PW, Lynch G, et al. Sex differences in stroke: epidemiology, clinical presentation, medical care, and outcomes. Lancet Neurol. 2008;7(10):915–26.
16. Sen A, Jette N, Husain M, Sander JW. Epilepsy in older people. Lancet. 2020;395(10225):735–48.
17. Porter KR, McCarthy BJ, Freels S, Kim Y, Davis FG. Prevalence estimates for primary brain tumors in the United States by age, gender, behavior, and histology. Neuro-Oncology. 2010;12(6):520–7.
18. Dekaban AS. Changes in brain weights during the span of human life: relation of brain weights to body heights and body weights. Ann Neurol. 1978;4(4):345–56.
19. Manolio TA, Kronmal RA, Burke GL, Poirier V, O'Leary DH, Gardin JM, et al. Magnetic resonance abnormalities and cardiovascular disease in older adults. The cardiovascular health study. Stroke. 1994;25(2):318–27.
20. Resnick SM, Pham DL, Kraut MA, Zonderman AB, Davatzikos C. Longitudinal magnetic resonance imaging studies of older adults: a shrinking brain. J Neurosci. 2003;23(8):3295–301.
21. Habes M, Janowitz D, Erus G, Toledo JB, Resnick SM, Doshi J, et al. Advanced brain aging: relationship with epidemiologic and genetic risk factors, and overlap with Alzheimer disease atrophy patterns. Transl Psychiatry. 2016;6:e775.
22. D'Armiento FP, Bianchi A, de Nigris F, Capuzzi DM, D'Armiento MR, Crimi G, et al. Age-related effects on atherogenesis and scavenger enzymes of intracranial and extracranial arteries in men without classic risk factors for atherosclerosis. Stroke. 2001;32(11):2472–9.
23. Vidal JS, Sigurdsson S, Jonsdottir MK, Eiriksdottir G, Thorgeirsson G, Kjartansson O, et al. Coronary artery calcium, brain function and structure: the AGES-Reykjavik study. Stroke. 2010;41(5):891–7.
24. Uspenskaia O, Liebetrau M, Herms J, Danek A, Hamann GF. Aging is associated with increased collagen type IV accumulation in the basal lamina of human cerebral microvessels. BMC Neurosci. 2004;5:37.
25. Hegedüs K, Molnár P. Age-related changes in reticulin fibers and other connective tissue elements in the intima of the major intracranial arteries. Clin Neuropathol. 1989;8(2):92–7.

26. Moossy J. Pathology of cerebral atherosclerosis. Influence of age, race, and gender. Stroke. 1993;24(12 Suppl):I22–3; i31-2.
27. Michel JB, Heudes D, Michel O, Poitevin P, Philippe M, Scalbert E, et al. Effect of chronic ANG I-converting enzyme inhibition on aging processes. II. Large arteries. Am J Physiol. 1994;267(1 Pt 2):R124–35.
28. Mrak RE, Griffin ST, Graham DI. Aging-associated changes in human brain. J Neuropathol Exp Neurol. 1997;56(12):1269–75.
29. O'Rourke MF. Arterial aging: pathophysiological principles. Vasc Med. 2007;12(4):329–41.
30. Thompson CS, Hakim AM. Living beyond our physiological means: small vessel disease of the brain is an expression of a systemic failure in arteriolar function: a unifying hypothesis. Stroke. 2009;40(5):e322–30.
31. Erdincler P, Tuzgen S, Erdincler UD, Oguz E, Korpinar A, Ciplak N, et al. Influence of aging on blood-brain barrier permeability and free radical formation following experimental brain cold injury. Acta Neurochir. 2002;144(2):195–9; discussion 9-200.
32. Rinkel GJ, Djibuti M, Algra A, van Gijn J. Prevalence and risk of rupture of intracranial aneurysms: a systematic review. Stroke. 1998;29(1):251–6.
33. Vlak MHM, Algra A, Brandenburg R, Rinkel GJE. Prevalence of unruptured intracranial aneurysms, with emphasis on sex, age, comorbidity, country, and time period: a systematic review and meta-analysis. Lancet Neurol. 2011;10(7):626–36.
34. Asllani I, Habeck C, Borogovac A, Brown TR, Brickman AM, Stern Y. Separating function from structure in perfusion imaging of the aging brain. Hum Brain Mapp. 2009;30(9):2927–35.
35. Perez-Denia L, Claffey P, Kenny RA, Finucane C. 75 is cerebral autoregulation altered in ageing? A review. Age Ageing. 2020;49(Supplement_1):i24-i.
36. Bakker SL, de Leeuw FE, den Heijer T, Koudstaal PJ, Hofman A, Breteler MM. Cerebral haemodynamics in the elderly: the Rotterdam study. Neuroepidemiology. 2004;23(4):178–84.
37. Czosnyka M, Balestreri M, Steiner L, Smielewski P, Hutchinson PJ, Matta B, et al. Age, intracranial pressure, autoregulation, and outcome after brain trauma. J Neurosurg. 2005;102(3):450–4.
38. Li N, Kong X, Ye R, Yang Q, Han J, Xiong L. Age-related differences in experimental stroke: possible involvement of mitochondrial dysfunction and oxidative damage. Rejuvenation Res. 2011;14(3):261–73.
39. Li S, Zheng J, Carmichael ST. Increased oxidative protein and DNA damage but decreased stress response in the aged brain following experimental stroke. Neurobiol Dis. 2005;18(3):432–40.
40. Park L, Anrather J, Girouard H, Zhou P, Iadecola C. Nox2-derived reactive oxygen species mediate neurovascular dysregulation in the aging mouse brain. J Cereb Blood Flow Metab. 2007;27(12):1908–18.
41. Peters R. Ageing and the brain. Postgrad Med J. 2006;82(964):84–8.
42. Ota M, Yasuno F, Ito H, Seki C, Nozaki S, Asada T, et al. Age-related decline of dopamine synthesis in the living human brain measured by positron emission tomography with L-[beta-11C] DOPA. Life Sci. 2006;79(8):730–6.
43. Uchida S, Suzuki A, Kagitani F, Hotta H. Effects of age on cholinergic vasodilation of cortical cerebral blood vessels in rats. Neurosci Lett. 2000;294(2):109–12.
44. Jolitha AB, Subramanyam MV, Asha DS. Age-related responses of the rat cerebral cortex: influence of vitamin E and exercise on the cholinergic system. Biogerontology. 2009;10(1):53–63.
45. Segovia G, del Arco A, Mora F. Environmental enrichment, prefrontal cortex, stress, and aging of the brain. J Neural Transm (Vienna). 2009;116(8):1007–16.
46. Rosi S, Ramirez-Amaya V, Hauss-Wegrzyniak B, Wenk GL. Chronic brain inflammation leads to a decline in hippocampal NMDA-R1 receptors. J Neuroinflammation. 2004;1(1):12.
47. Hamilton ML, Van Remmen H, Drake JA, Yang H, Guo ZM, Kewitt K, et al. Does oxidative damage to DNA increase with age? Proc Natl Acad Sci U S A. 2001;98(18):10469–74.
48. Bloch F. Is the Glasgow Coma Scale appropriate for the evaluation of elderly patients in long-term care units? J Eval Clin Pract. 2016;22(3):455–6.
49. Salottolo K, Levy AS, Slone DS, Mains CW, Bar-Or D. The effect of age on Glasgow Coma Scale score in patients with traumatic brain injury. JAMA Surg. 2014;149(7):727–34.
50. Carney N, Totten AM, O'Reilly C, Ullman JS, Hawryluk GW, Bell MJ, et al. Guidelines for the management of severe traumatic brain injury, Fourth Edition. Neurosurgery. 2017;80(1):6–15.
51. Sorrentino E, Diedler J, Kasprowicz M, Budohoski KP, Haubrich C, Smielewski P, et al. Critical thresholds for cerebrovascular reactivity after traumatic brain injury. Neurocrit Care. 2012;16(2):258–66.

52. You W, Feng J, Tang Q, Cao J, Wang L, Lei J, et al. Intraventricular intracranial pressure monitoring improves the outcome of older adults with severe traumatic brain injury: an observational, prospective study. BMC Anesthesiol. 2016;16(1):35.
53. Kinoshita T, Yoshiya K, Fujimoto Y, Kajikawa R, Kiguchi T, Hara M, et al. Decompressive Craniectomy in conjunction with evacuation of intracranial hemorrhagic lesions is associated with worse outcomes in elderly patients with traumatic brain injury: a propensity score analysis. World Neurosurg. 2016;89:187–92.
54. Oddo M, Crippa IA, Mehta S, Menon D, Payen JF, Taccone FS, et al. Optimizing sedation in patients with acute brain injury. Crit Care. 2016;20(1):128.
55. Cremer OL, Moons KGM, Bouman EAC, Kruijswijk JE, de Smet AMGA, Kalkman CJ. Long-term propofol infusion and cardiac failure in adult head-injured patients. Lancet. 2001;357(9250):117–8.
56. Lin N, Han R, Zhou J, Gelb AW. Mild sedation exacerbates or unmasks focal neurologic dysfunction in neurosurgical patients with supratentorial brain mass lesions in a drug-specific manner. Anesthesiology. 2016;124(3):598–607.
57. Mushkudiani NA, Engel DC, Steyerberg EW, Butcher I, Lu J, Marmarou A, et al. Prognostic value of demographic characteristics in traumatic brain injury: results from the IMPACT study. J Neurotrauma. 2007;24(2):259–69.
58. MacKenzie EJ, Rivara FP, Jurkovich GJ, Nathens AB, Frey KP, Egleston BL, et al. A national evaluation of the effect of trauma-center care on mortality. N Engl J Med. 2006;354(4):366–78.
59. Mullins RJ, Mann NC, Hedges JR, Worrall W, Helfand M, Zechnich AD, et al. Adequacy of hospital discharge status as a measure of outcome among injured patients. JAMA. 1998;279(21):1727–31.
60. Merzo A, Lenell S, Nyholm L, Enblad P, Lewen A. Promising clinical outcome of elderly with TBI after modern neurointensive care. Acta Neurochir. 2016;158(1):125–33.
61. McIntyre A, Mehta S, Janzen S, Aubut J, Teasell RW. A meta-analysis of functional outcome among older adults with traumatic brain injury. NeuroRehabilitation. 2013;32:409–14.
62. Turgeon AF, Lauzier F, Simard JF, Scales DC, Burns KE, Moore L, et al. Mortality associated with withdrawal of life-sustaining therapy for patients with severe traumatic brain injury: a Canadian multicentre cohort study. CMAJ. 2011;183(14):1581–8.
63. Kirkman MA, Jenks T, Bouamra O, Edwards A, Yates D, Wilson MH. Increased mortality associated with cerebral contusions following trauma in the elderly: bad patients or bad management? J Neurotrauma. 2013;30(16):1385–90.
64. Munro PT, Smith RD, Parke TR. Effect of patients' age on management of acute intracranial haematoma: prospective national study. BMJ. 2002;325(7371):1001.
65. Haller CS, Delhumeau C, De Pretto M, Schumacher R, Pielmaier L, Rebetez MM, et al. Trajectory of disability and quality-of-life in non-geriatric and geriatric survivors after severe traumatic brain injury. Brain Inj. 2017;31(3):319–28.
66. Guidet B, Vallet H, Boddaert J, de Lange DW, Morandi A, Leblanc G, et al. Caring for the critically ill patients over 80: a narrative review. Ann Intensive Care. 2018;8(1):114.
67. McIntyre A, Mehta S, Aubut J, Dijkers M, Teasell RW. Mortality among older adults after a traumatic brain injury: a meta-analysis. Brain Inj. 2013;27(1):31–40.
68. Brazinova A, Mauritz W, Leitgeb J, Wilbacher I, Majdan M, Janciak I, et al. Outcomes of patients with severe traumatic brain injury who have Glasgow Coma Scale scores of 3 or 4 and are over 65 years old. J Neurotrauma. 2010;27(9):1549–55.
69. Roch A, Wiramus S, Pauly V, Forel JM, Guervilly C, Gainnier M, et al. Long-term outcome in medical patients aged 80 or over following admission to an intensive care unit. Crit Care. 2011;15(1):R36.
70. de Montmollin E, Terzi N, Dupuis C, Garrouste-Orgeas M, da Silva D, Darmon M, et al. One-year survival in acute stroke patients requiring mechanical ventilation: a multicenter cohort study. Ann Intensive Care. 2020;10(1):53.
71. Harrison-Felix C, Kreider SE, Arango-Lasprilla JC, Brown AW, Dijkers MP, Hammond FM, et al. Life expectancy following rehabilitation: a NIDRR Traumatic Brain Injury Model Systems study. J Head Trauma Rehabil. 2012;27(6):E69–80.
72. Flaada JT, Leibson CL, Mandrekar JN, Diehl N, Perkins PK, Brown AW, et al. Relative risk of mortality after traumatic brain injury: a population-based study of the role of age and injury severity. J Neurotrauma. 2007;24(3):435–45.
73. Livingston DH, Lavery RF, Mosenthal AC, Knudson MM, Lee S, Morabito D, et al. Recovery at one year following isolated traumatic brain injury: a Western Trauma Association prospective multicenter trial. J Trauma. 2005;59(6):1298–304. discussion 304

74. Annegers JF, Hauser WA, Coan SP, Rocca WA. A population-based study of seizures after traumatic brain injuries. N Engl J Med. 1998;338(1):20–4.
75. Albrecht JS, Liu X, Smith GS, Baumgarten M, Rattinger GB, Gambert SR, et al. Stroke incidence following traumatic brain injury in older adults. J Head Trauma Rehabil. 2015;30(2):E62–7.
76. Kowalski RG, Haarbauer-Krupa JK, Bell JM, Corrigan JD, Hammond FM, Torbey MT, et al. Acute ischemic stroke after moderate to severe traumatic brain injury: incidence and impact on outcome. Stroke. 2017;48(7):1802–9.
77. Fleminger S, Oliver DL, Lovestone S, Rabe-Hesketh S, Giora A. Head injury as a risk factor for Alzheimer's disease: the evidence 10 years on; a partial replication. J Neurol Neurosurg Psychiatry. 2003;74(7):857–62.
78. Perry DC, Sturm VE, Peterson MJ, Pieper CF, Bullock T, Boeve BF, et al. Association of traumatic brain injury with subsequent neurological and psychiatric disease: a meta-analysis. J Neurosurg. 2016;124(2):511–26.
79. Jafari S, Etminan M, Aminzadeh F, Samii A. Head injury and risk of Parkinson disease: a systematic review and meta-analysis. Mov Disord. 2013;28(9):1222–9.
80. Ullberg T, Zia E, Petersson J, Norrving B. Changes in functional outcome over the first year after stroke: an observational study from the Swedish stroke register. Stroke. 2015;46(2):389–94.
81. Goldberg J, Schoeni D, Mordasini P, Z'Graggen W, Gralla J, Raabe A, et al. Survival and outcome after poor-grade aneurysmal subarachnoid hemorrhage in elderly patients. Stroke. 2018;49(12):2883–9.
82. Pirracchio R, Resche-Rigon M, Bresson D, Basta B, Welschbillig S, Heyer L, et al. One-year outcome after neurosurgery for intracranial tumor in elderly patients. J Neurosurg Anesthesiol. 2010;22(4):342–6.

32

Postoperative Patients: Planned Surgery

Gabriella Bettelli

Contents

🎓 Learning Objectives

- This chapter investigates problems and management principles related with ICU admission after elective surgery in the very old patient. Being this issue part of the global surgical path, the interconnections with the pre-, intra-, and postoperative phases are discussed.
- The aim of this chapter is to make readers familiar with the role exerted by advanced age on surgical risk, circumstances of ICU admission, principles of appropriate care, management of the most common postoperative complications requiring ICU admission, and criteria for discharge.
- Surgeries after which ICU admission is most frequent are analyzed, together with principles of optimal care to follow, in order to make the most appropriate choice when deciding what kind of postoperative treatment to apply, in accordance with patients' needs, functional status (FS) before surgery, foreseeable outcomes, and expected postoperative quality of life (QoL). Special needs of older patients admitted to ICU are analyzed, and clinical outcomes reported in the literature and side effects of ICU stay are also dealt with.
- Finally, organizational issues useful to obtain the best possible clinical outcome, optimize cost/effects ratio, and minimize the biological cost of ICU stay are discussed.

33.1 Overview: ICU Admission Is Part of a Global Clinical Path (See ◘ Table 33.1)

Available data show that the enormous increasing of the geriatric population registered in the last decades has widely impacted with the daily practice in surgery, anesthesia, and intensive care [1]. Not only the volume of surgical interventions performed on older patients and the age at which patients are fit enough to undergo surgery has dramatically increased worldwide, but also, due to both the expanding of the clinical practice and the accumulation of research work, surgical operations today performed on the elderly include a wide spectrum of long-lasting and invasive procedures [2], many of which may require postoperative admission to the ICU. This poses a number of clinical, organizational, economic, and ethical problems.

ICU admission after non-emergent surgery can be planned in advance, on the basis of patient's preoperative clinical conditions and expected need for close monitoring or vital functions support, either can be decided at the end of the surgery (due to unforeseen events occurred intraoperatively, or to a delay on postoperative recovery precluding the transfer to the surgical ward), or in the postoperative days, due to an unexpected deterioration in vital functions.

Whenever feasible, postsurgical ICU should be planned in advance, taking into account the kind of surgical procedure, the patient's clinical conditions, and the reasonable expectations in terms of outcome.

Triage criteria are difficult to define, given the low levels of evidence medical literature provides (great variability in patients' health and FS, clinical outcome and other variables considered in the studies protocols, etc.), the differences in resources availability among institutions, and the coexistence of diverging ethical approaches.

Table 33.1 The ICU admission as a part of the surgical path

When/where	What to do	How to proceed
Preoperative assessment	Assess clinical history and physical examination Perform CGA Assess frailty Assess risk factors for POD	Establish the need for direct ICU admission
Intraoperative management	Preserve normothermia Careful patient positioning Appropriate ventilation Avoidance of too deep anesthesia plans Maintain hemodynamic equilibrium Minimize surgical stress (analgesia, ERAS strategies)	In case of intraoperative unexpected events in pts for whom ICU admittance was not planned, reevaluate the need for IC Careful handover with the ICU team inform the family about intraoperative course and plans for postoperative care
In the ICU	Implement the appropriate level of care Avoid BZDP for sedation Check daily for delirium Ensure adequate pain control, Environment comfort and a minimum of relational exchanges	Start treatment and observe results Reevaluate patient's clinical condition with the whole IC team Decide whether continue or withdraw the IC Inform the family
At the moment of discharge from ICU	Plan postoperative care in accordance with patient's needs	Individuate the right setting of care (intermediate care intensity, surgical ward, transitional care or other) Careful handover with the care team

33

Adequate preoperative evaluation is a pivotal factor in managing postoperative care on the basis of the specific needs older patients present in terms of medical treatment, complication management, and minimization of functional impairment. Data collected before surgery through Comprehensive Geriatric Assessment (CGA), frailty assessment, and risk of postoperative delirium (POD) are essential to plan appropriate ICU care.

Intraoperatively, it is fundamental that the basal measures aimed to preserve homeostasis in geriatric surgical patients are carefully implemented. Among them, accurate positioning on the surgical table in order to prevent respiratory insufficiency (mostly when Trendelenburg position or long-lasting end-expiratory positive pressure are required), use of not too high tidal volumes [3], measures to reduce the surgical stress response [4], avoidance of too deep anesthesia levels, control of hemodynamic balance and fluid intake, normothermia, and early detection of signs of POD are crucial. Before ICU admission, it should be ascertained whether the patient expressed in his/her anticipate directives the refusal toward intensive care and, in case, his/her willingness respected.

The level of care to apply should be discussed inside the team and with the family members, in the light of the objective chances of recovery, the expected outcome, and available resources. Once the patient has been admitted to the ICU, the highest level of physical, cognitive, and emotional comfort should be ensured in accordance with the patient's vigilance and mental status, the need for sedation, and for invasive treatment such as tracheal intubation.

As soon as possible, conditions should be created aimed to offer at least minimal interpersonal exchange with the family members or the caregivers. Signs of POD should be checked every day using validated tools (see below), and, in case, appropriate treatment should be promptly implemented [5]. Malnutrition and muscle atrophy or damage should be avoided ensuring adequate nutritional support and promoting active (whenever possible) or at least passive mobilization. Nursing issues are pivotal to prevent pressure sores, positional pain, and depression and to allow early re-establishment of interpersonal communication and relational processes.

After a few days and in absence of signs of recovery, a team-based discussion on how to proceed in terms of intensity of vital support is appropriate; this step should involve the family members and respect patient's willingness. Discharge from the ICU should be planned on the base of the clinical recovery and the available resources in terms of intermediate care areas, type of postoperative wards, and hospital services.

After discharge, postoperative care should be planned on the basis of patient's physical, cognitive, and functional status, without neglecting the need for FKT treatment, psychological support, and relational exchanges; visual and hearing support should be continuously available.

From the organizational point of view, the anesthesia-surgery-ICU team should share in advance some basic methodological issues (what data to collect before surgery, who is in charge for collecting these data) in order to define a reliable patient risk and functional profile, including data on FS and QoL. In the case of older surgical patients, the European Society of Anaesthesia guideline on preoperative evaluation in noncardiac surgery [6] recommends that data from CGA, frailty scoring, and risk of POD are collected and registered. Regretfully, these principles are not yet routinely implemented in the clinical practice. Adequate handover at any shift, and transfer from different hospital wards, are integrated part of the care process.

33.2 Postoperative Morbidity and Mortality in the Very Old Surgical Patient

33.2.1 Surgical Risk and Risk of Postoperative Complications in the Elderly

It is generally assumed that surgery and anesthesia represent major challenges for older patients, due to aging processes that deteriorate organ functions and reduce FS, and associated conditions [7]. It is also assumed that patients undergoing high-risk procedures represent a major share of ICU admissions [8]. However, a reliable estimation of the role exerted by age itself in increasing surgical risk remains difficult [9].

First, defining the risk linked to an invasive treatment that it is hard to interpret separately from all the other risk factors (patient physical status, surgical team experience in treating older persons, available resources, and organizational aspects) is intrinsically impossible. Even though a number of single-center studies investigating surgical risk and postoperative complications in cardiac, orthopedic, or cancer surgery reported long-term morbidity and mortality in the elderly compared with those collected in younger patients, these conclusions cannot represent a guiding principle; in fact, a small number of older surgical patients undergoing elective surgery are a selected population, not comparable with the general one.

Secondly, wider studies conducted on greater patients' groups such as register-based studies often don't take into account comorbidity, and this is the main reason why such studies do not provide reliable conclusions [10, 11]. Last but not least, despite advancements in surgery and anesthesia, in many countries the majority of older persons neither receive appropriate preoperative assessment and optimization, nor they benefit from suitable geriatric perioperative care [12–14].

As for the surgical procedure, evidence exists that the risk increases in long-lasting, invasive ones, with the highest risk in cardiac [15], thoracic [16], cancer surgery [17], and hip fracture repair [18].

33.2.2 Is Age the Main Risk Factor?

Large studies [19–23], agree that geriatric patients have higher postoperative mortality rate and experience considerable perioperative morbidity when compared to younger subjects undergoing surgery. Nevertheless, age per se doesn't seem to play a critical role. In many cases, the general preoperative conditions and patient-related factors proved to be more important than the type of surgery in predicting mortality. More specifically, severe systemic diseases associated with older age showed to be useful preoperative predictors of ICU admission and adverse outcome, such as complications and 30-day mortality rate. Two recent prospective cohort studies investigating the role of frailty in patients >80 years admitted to ICU [24, 25] reported that this condition negatively impacted on ICU and 30-day mortality; both studies concluded that, being frailty assessment able to predict short-term mortality in these patients, this condition should be systematically evaluated in this patients' group.

33.3 How to Decide About ICU Admission in the Elderly

33.3.1 Lack of Guidelines and Specific Triage Criteria

In comparison with emergent surgery, postoperative morbidity and mortality after planned surgery are lower, and patients are generally more fit and in better conditions [26]. Despite this, deciding what patients should receive postoperative IC after planned surgery and quantifying the advantages offered by ICU admission remains a challenging task.

Age by itself never represents a criterion on which to take the decision, being chronological age unable to describe the patient's conditions and being biological age difficult to define. Scoring systems such as SAPS II, APACHE, or SOFA do not capture any of the specific conditions older patients may present, such as cognitive impairment, depression, cachexia, or frailty. On the other side, it is well known that the elderly population not only presents its own clinical specificities and needs but also shows a wide interpersonal variability both in general conditions and functional profile.

In its guideline issued in 1994, the European Society of Intensive Care Medicine (ESICM) recommended that patients presenting unstable conditions or at risk of severe complications should be admitted to ICU; however these recommendations, issued 25 years ago in a totally different demographic situation, basically refer to a general population and do not take into account the specificities of the geriatric population.

No specific guidelines are available so far, and none of the scoring systems actually in use aimed to predict clinical outcome has showed to be a reliable predictor. A recent review [27] of risk factors for unplanned admission to ICU after major surgery reported that—due to heterogeneity in the studies design—a comparative, quantitative analysis of the admission criteria was not feasible. The authors concluded that further research is needed to test both sensitivity and specificity of three independent risk factors identified in the United States, the United Kingdom, Asia, and Australia (age, body mass index, comorbidity extent), in order to ascertain whether they can be adopted as a guide to plan critical care admission and reduce unplanned admissions rate.

33.3.2 Basic Principles for Appropriate Triage

Even though reliable, evidence-based triage criteria for ICU admission of older surgical patients are not available, some guidance principles can be found on the basis of clinical experience, information on patients' FS, and ethical principles (see ◘ Table 33.2).

◘ **Table 33.2** Principles for appropriate triage

Consider as predictors of ICU admittance	Age>=85 Multimorbidity Heart failure High ASA Class Recent need for hospital admission Major surgery
Assess FS and presurgical QoL	Level of independence Cognition Emotional status Nutritional status Family support Subjective QoL Advance directives
Assess frailty	Fried Index (phenotype theory) Rockwood (deficit accumulation)
Assess risk factors for POD	See ESA Guidelines on POD [5]
Involve the family in the final decision	Clear information about expected results Pursue genuine dialog and mutual confidence

However, these elements are not systematically collected in all the institutions, because the practice of implementing CGA and FS assessment in the preoperative anesthesia consultation is still poorly practiced. Nevertheless, even though often neglected in many cases and in many institutions, these elements become of pivotal importance after some days of treatment, when a reassessment of the care plan is needed on the basis of the obtained results.

It should never be neglected, to conclude, that in the triage process, together with the care-team members (anesthetists, surgeons, intensivists) and the patient himself, family members too play an important role: clearly informing them about expected results, dialoging with them in a genuine way will help in acting in an atmosphere of mutual confidence, and avoiding refusal by principle of ICU admission.

### 33.3.3	Liberal Versus Restrictive Attitude: How This Element May Influence the Choice

The pressure on ICUs in growing everywhere due to many reasons, and that exerted by older patients is continuously increasing [28]. Facing a worldwide diffuse shortage of resources, the patients' group toward which the principle of reserving the best care to those who have the greatest chances of survival is most frequently invoked and is the geriatric population.

Balancing between a restrictive attitude (with the risk of denying ICU admission to some patients who could benefit from the treatment) and a liberal one (admitting older patients without any restriction criteria, with the risk of facing shortly after a bed ICU shortage that would exclude from intensive treatment a patient with higher probability of surviving) is one of the hardest tasks for the intensivist team. As the recent Covid-19 pandemic has dramatically showed, the problem is made even more challenging by the overall limited availability of IC beds observable in many countries and in many institutions. Last but not least, the attitude of intensivists, their ethical orientation, and the cultural background of the country where the process takes place further influence the final choice.

This dilemma is probably more acute when discussing about ICU admission after emergent surgery or due to medical reasons; however deciding about ICU admission in frail, compromised or multimorbid surgical patients over 80 years is a circumstance that doesn't occur only in exceptional cases, being planned surgery the main reason for critical care admission of older patients aged 80 years and more.

Useful principles to manage such situations are represented by optimal communication both inside the care team and between the care team and the patient's family members. Optimal communication among the care team members aims to increase the interpersonal cohesion, the feeling of working within a well-organized group, and avoiding internal discrepancies that ultimately would impact on the quality of care provided. Excellent, systematic communication between the care team and the patient's family will be essential in understanding their attitude toward the risk of escalating the care and in discussing potential risks related with the ICU admission (exposure to nosocomial infections, delirium, increased LOS, restrictive visiting hours).

These ethical issues represent a main aspect in the ICU clinical practice. They are excellently analyzed in a review by Nguyen et al. [29] and in an interview to B. Guidet [30].

33.3.4 Advantages and Risks of ICU Admission

Results reported in the literature about the effectiveness of ICU admission after surgery in the elderly in terms of improved outcome and reduced mortality are very difficult to analyze, due to the great inhomogeneity among the various studies. Globally considering these results and overlooking the role exerted by advanced age, one could argue that ICU admission after surgery can reduce mortality trough early recognition of vital functions deterioration, availability of deep monitoring, respiratory and cardiovascular support, and higher staff density in comparison with surgical wards.

Nevertheless, weighing up pros and cons—and resources availability apart—ICU admission is unavoidably accompanied by elements such as reduced mobility, risk of infectious complications, possible fluid overload, vascular events, or delirium [31], either occurring as a postoperative complication or as a collateral damage of ICU admission, that are extremely dangerous for the older persons. Mostly, delirium in the elderly is a severe risk factor for further non-cognitive complications, adverse outcomes, and mortality. Moreover, in case of survival, permanent cognitive damage with loss of QoL and need for institutionalization are highly probable [5].

33.4 Circumstances for ICU Admission

33.4.1 The Decision Is Taken Before Surgery (Direct Admission)

The preemptive decision to admit to ICU an older surgical patient immediately after surgery is usually carried out in subjects who are expected to need organ support, close monitoring, and high nurse/patient ratio, or it occurs in accordance with established clinical practice, as it is the case of the cardiac surgery [32]. Other factors suggesting ICU admission after planned surgery are high 30-day mortality risk, age >80 years, comorbidity, and long-lasting and invasive surgical procedures [33, 34].

The decision to admit an older patient to ICU after planned surgery can also occur following unexpected events occurring in the post-anesthesia care unit (PACU) or during the postoperative stay in the surgical ward.

33.4.2 The Decision Is Taken in the PACU

At the end of surgery, circumstances that suggest the opportunity of ICU admission are represented by unexpected intraoperative events such as massive hemorrhage, arrhythmia (mostly tachycardia [35, 36],), need to prolong surgery due to unexpected anatomic conditions, severe hypo- or hypertension resistant to medical treatment, hemodynamic instability, respiratory insufficiency, and abnormal delay in recovering from anesthesia. In order to allow an early detection of this fearsome complication, a first check for POD—to be made in the PACU as soon as the patient recovers from anaesthesia [5]—should be made using both validated scores such as CAM or Nu-Desc and RASS Score. In those patients who show only signs of POD and no other, or minor, troubles in vital functions, ICU admission requires a careful pros and cons evaluation, as this event may increase per se disorientation, confusion, and stress.

33.4.3 The Decision Is Taken in the Surgical Ward (Indirect or Intermediate Admission)

The occurrence of major postoperative cardiac, respiratory, renal, or septic complications in the early postoperative period is the main cause of intermediate transfer from the surgical ward to the ICU. These events are more frequent in multimorbid, functionally impaired and frail patients undergoing long-lasting and invasive surgery and find their main causative factors in difficulties in performing appropriate triage, poor internal process organization, and resource limitation. Some evidence exists that, in comparison with indirect admission, direct ICU admission after surgery is accompanied by better outcome; however, a number of studies found significant variability in postoperative mortality, length of stay, or cost/benefit ratio. Moreover, in many cases the choice is determined by expert consensus, and the way the risk is estimated is not specified.

33.4.4 Critical Considerations

There are no data describing the entity of this phenomenon in global terms, and a great variability exists among countries and institutions [37] in this area of clinical practice. Following some studies [36, 38], indirect admission to ICU after surgery seems to increase mortality risk in comparison to direct admission, and this is beyond the consequences of comorbidities, age, gender, type of surgery, and emergency status. This could be due to different factors: lack of perioperative geriatric care, difficulties in performing appropriate triage, ICU bed availability, clock time and poor evaluation of the patient's status (i.e., by phone [39]), or occurrence of unexpected perioperative events. These findings confirm that there is a great need to improve perioperative care in older patients.

33.5 Postoperative Complications and ICU Admission

The most frequent perioperative complication requiring ICU admission registered in the older surgical patients includes cardiovascular (arrhythmia, myocardial infarction), respiratory (atelectasis, respiratory failure, pneumonia), acute kidney injury, sepsis, and delirium. Following the literature, their frequency widely varies due to different case mix or different study protocols, and it is likely influenced by the adoption of preventive strategies implemented before surgery in order to promote preoperative patients' optimization, such as prehabilitation, correction of malnutrition, medication reconciliation, or management of predisposing risk factors for POD.

33.5.1 Cardiac Complications

Cardiac complications are common among older, critically ill patients, mostly after cardiac and major noncardiac surgery [40]. The main patient-related risk factor is represented by preexisting cardiac conditions (angina, coronary artery disease, congestive heart failure mostly when in active phase [41], arrhythmia, hypertension), which all have high prevalence among older patients. Intraoperative hypotension unresponsive to treatment is a predictor of postoperative cardiac complications and death.

Diastolic dysfunction is frequent in patients undergoing cardiac surgery and is associated with poor outcomes in cardiovascular surgery [42, 43]. Female patients seem to have higher degree of diastolic dysfunction and present more adverse outcome, prolonged ICU, and hospital length of stay [44].

Other important risk factors for cardiac complications are represented by association with coexisting diseases (respiratory, renal, diabetes), long-lasting and invasive procedures eliciting severe surgical stress response [45], intraoperative hypothermia and alterations in the balance between prothrombotic and fibrinolytic factors resulting in increased coronary thrombogenicity [46] (see ▶ Box 33.1).

> **Box 33.1 Independent Predictors and Risk Factors for Postoperative Cardiac Complications**
> - Preexisting cardiac conditions:
>   - Angina
>   - CAD
>   - CHF
>   - Arrhythmia (mostly tachycardia)
> - Diastolic dysfunction
> - Comorbidity
> - Long-lasting and invasive surgery eliciting intense stress response
> - Hypothermia
> - Prothrombotic/fibrinolytic imbalance

In a retrospective study [47] on 255 patients aged 80 years and over admitted to ICU after surgery, the need for vasoactive drugs in the first two ICU stay days was the strongest predictor of hospital mortality.

33.5.2 Respiratory Complications

Advanced age has been consistently identified as a risk factor for postoperative respiratory complications, due to both decline in pulmonary reserve and respiratory function, and higher prevalence of respiratory comorbidity (asthma, COPD, emphysema, smoking-induced conditions) in this patients' group. In addition to those mentioned above, further patient-related risk factors include functional dependence, congestive heart failure, OSA, pulmonary hypertension, malnutrition, and impaired renal function. Procedure-related surgery include long-lasting surgery (>3 h), surgical site (thoracic, abdominal), general anesthesia, hemotransfusion, and residual neuromuscular blockade. Preventive measures (smoking cessation, inspiratory muscle training) and appropriate intraoperative management (lower tidal volume, appropriate PEEP levels, recruitment maneuvers, neuromuscular blockade reversal) are essential to reduce the risk.

The most used risk score for predicting postoperative respiratory complications is the ARISCAT (Assess Respiratory Risk in Surgical Patients in Catalonia) [48] (see ▶ Box 33.2).

Box 33.2   Independent Predictors and Risk Factors for Postoperative Respiratory Complications

ARISCAT (Assess Respiratory Risk in Surgical Patients in Catalonia) 2010
- Advanced age
- Low preoperative $SatHbO_2$ in room air
- Respiratory infection in the 30 days prior surgery
- Preoperative anaemia (Hb < =10 g/dl)
- Surgical site (thoracic, abdominal)
- Duration of surgery
- Emergency surgery

In a recent study [49], postoperative respiratory complications in a geriatric population accounted for 11% of indirect ICU admission within 5 days after major orthopedic surgery. In a prospective, multicenter cohort study [50] involving 63 European hospitals and a total of 5384 patients undergoing surgery under both general or regional anesthesia, postoperative respiratory complications accounted for 4.2%. Among patients who developed respiratory complications, in-hospital mortality was significantly higher. Regression analysis identified seven independent risk factors: low preoperative $SatHbO_2$, presence of at least one respiratory symptom, chronic liver disease, history of CHF, open thoracic/abdominal surgery, procedure lasting more than 2 h, and emergency surgery. The study also individuated three levels of severity for predicting postoperative respiratory failure with an 82% accuracy.

33.5.3 Postoperative Delirium

POD can develop during the first three to five postoperative days and may occur in the PACU (see above), during the post-surgery ICU stay or in the surgical ward. Predisposing and precipitating risk factors for its development as postoperative complication—and ICU issues apart—are widely detailed in a recent ESA guideline quoted above [5]], currently under updating and expected to be published within 2022. POD is more frequent after cardiac [51] and major noncardiac surgery and is associated with increased mortality, morbidity, and long-term cognitive dysfunction

[52, 53]. Older patients developing POD have poorer outcome and are more likely to have prolonged ICU and hospital stay and longer intubation time.

As fully detailed in ▶ Chap. 36, delirium in the critically ill patient has shown to be associated with important clinical outcomes including prolonged mechanical ventilation, LOS, cost of care, long-term cognitive impairment, need for post-discharge institutionalization, and mortality.

Basically, patients at lower cognitive and physical reserve likely possess decreased capacity to maintain normal brain functioning in response to external stressors and are, therefore, at higher risk for delirium. Other factors that contribute to increase POD risk in ICU are prolonged mechanical ventilation, sepsis, medications (benzodiazepine infusion for mechanical ventilation [54], anticholinergics [55], dopamine, steroids) altered night-day rhythm, sensory deprivation, immobilization and fasting, and environmental discomfort (lights, noises).

Validated delirium screening tools for ICU patients (CAM-ICU, ICDSC) have improved diagnosis, and routine delirium assessment is currently recommended as standard of care in the ICU. Measures aimed to prevent POD in the ICU and reduce its duration and severity include pharmacological prophylaxis (agents to reduce systemic inflammation such as steroids or statins, antipsychotics), choice of non-benzodiazepines sedation for mechanical ventilation [56], early mobilization [57], sleep hygiene [58], and sedation bundles [59].

POD treatment in the ICU has not yet found its golden standard, as no evidence supports a single effective pharmacologic approach. Antipsychotics can cause sedation, respiratory depression, and prolonged QT interval. Evidence currently supports the use of dexmedetomidine both for prevention and treatment in a wide variety of ICU patients, but further studies are needed. Best results are expected combining pharmacological treatment with the non-pharmacological measures [60] shown in ▶ Box 33.3.

> **Box 33.3   Non-Pharmacological Measures for Delirium Management**
> - Assess, prevent, and manage pain
> - Choice of targeted, light sedation avoiding benzodiazepines
> - Monitor routinely delirium
> - Sleep hygiene
> - Early mobility and exercise
> - Family engagement and empowerment

33.6 Specific Problems Related to the Different Kinds of Surgery

33.6.1 Cardiac Surgery

A study on 646 octogenarians undergoing cardiac surgery reported a 15% incidence of cardiac complications, high in-hospital mortality (7.4%) and increased both ICU and hospital stay. NYHA Class IV, female sex, and preoperative renal failure resulted to correlate with perioperative morbidity [61].

In another study investigating long-term survival of octogenarians undergoing cardiac surgery, risk factors for hospital death were preoperative renal dysfunction, postoperative myocardial infarction, cardiac failure requiring intra-aortic balloon pumping, acute renal failure, stroke, and ventilatory dependency exceeding 48 hours. Postoperative complications and ICU readmission resulted to be stronger risk factors for hospital deaths, preoperative comorbidities, and procedural variables [62].

Atrial fibrillation is the most common postoperative complication after cardiac surgery in the elderly [63]. Off-pump techniques (OPCAB) have been reported to reduce this risk in comparison with coronary artery bypass surgery (CABPG) [64, 65].

POD is also frequent in older patients undergoing cardiac surgery. Acute kidney injury is another postoperative complication frequently occurring in octogenarians undergoing cardiac surgery. In a retrospective study by Ried [66] on a geriatric population including 598 patients (299 septuagenarians and 299 octogenarians) undergoing elective bypass, valve or combined bypass, and valve surgery with cardiopulmonary bypass, acute kidney injury occurred in 21.7%–21.4% in the two groups, respectively. Greatest degrees of renal injury were associated with a stepwise increase in risk for death, renal replacement therapy, and prolonged stay both in ICU and hospital. Overall 30-day mortality was 6% in septuagenarian and 7.7% in octogenarians.

33.6.2 Abdominal Surgery

Older age and a higher ASA status are recognized as independent variables associated with postoperative complications after abdominal surgery. Accordingly, a number of studies report that older patients undergoing abdominal surgery for cancer frequently develop major postoperative complications that may require ICU admission [67]. This is most frequent for patients presenting high preoperative risk due to associated conditions, poly-medication, decreased physiologic reserves, frailty, and immune system disturbances [68, 69]. Perioperative risk is also increased by the need for long-lasting procedures, significant fluid and blood losses [70], use of colloids, fluids overload, and need for vasopressors. The presence of these risk factors strongly suggests the opportunity to plan direct postoperative ICU admission, mostly in case of frailty.

In one of the few studies investigating this issue [71], observed postoperative complications included respiratory (acute respiratory failure, pneumonia, mechanical ventilation lasting more than 48 hours), cardiovascular (acute myocardial infarction, cardiogenic shock, stroke), infectious complications (septic shock and severe sepsis), acute kidney injury, and surgical complications (anastomosis or wound dehiscence, surgical wound infection, re-operation). Mortality was due to septic shock (pulmonary, abdominal or multiple origin).

Preventing complications in these patients is of primary importance not only because it allows a better outcome and reduces cost; also, complications negatively affect QoL and may delay or preclude further cancer treatment.

Preventive measures include identification of predictive modifiable factors and patient optimization, preoperative anemia correction, use of goal directed therapy to avoid fluid overload or hypovolemia, and whenever possible implementation of ERAS strategies.

33.6.3 Orthopedics

Despite the fact that elective major orthopedic surgery (total knee or hip replacement; shoulder, spine, foot, and ankle surgery) not rarely is performed in older patients with multiple comorbidities, literature analyzing the need for ICU admission after elective orthopedic surgery in the elderly is not abundant. A review by Taylor and Gropper [72] found that pulmonary, embolic, and transfusion-related complications are the most frequent postoperative complications after orthopedic surgery in a general population. A Japanese retrospective study [73] analyzing complications of spine surgery in octogenarians found that perioperative complications occurred in 29% of patients; age > 85, estimated blood loss >500 g and operative time > =180′ were significantly associated with major complications.

After total hip arthroplasty, unplanned ICU admission was needed in 7% of cases in a study enrolling 1259 patients [74]; significant risk factors where age >75, OSA, creatinine clearance<60 mL/min, prior myocardial infarction, ASA class>3, need for vasopressor drugs, and obesity. The high rate of unplanned ICU admission testifies about difficulties and pitfalls in triage processes in this patients' group.

33.7 Discharge

In accordance with the main guidelines on this issue [75], the status of patients admitted to an ICU should be revised continuously to identify patients who may no longer need ICU care. Ideally, the transfer from the ICU occurs when the patient no longer meets the admission criteria and meets the admission criteria for a lower level of care. Despite the illusory simplicity of these statements, patient discharge from the ICU to a medical or surgical ward is one of the most high-risk transitions of care, especially in the case of the geriatric patient; the decision is made difficult by the lack of clear and objective parameters to indicate which patients will continue to benefit from critical care and which won't. Moreover, a great heterogeneity exists in critical care discharge practices, often influenced by institutional factors [76].

Organizational aspects can contribute to make the task challenging. First, an obvious gap exists between the available resources in terms of monitoring and immediate intervention between the ICU and the different types of postoperative settings; secondly, communication barriers among professionals everywhere exist, mostly in great institutions or crowded hospitals; finally, a lack of standardization in patient transfer processes is not infrequent. Unforeseen events may influence the timing of discharge and force toward an "after hours" (nighttime) transfer; however, discharge in the evening, night, or weekend has shown to be an independent risk factor for increased mortality and readmission [77].

33.8 Outcome

Studies suggest that patients aged 80 and older after planned surgery have "reasonable" long-term outcomes. In a large multicenter cohort study form the Australian New Zealand Intensive Care Society [28], in geriatric patients admitted to ICU after planned surgery, global ICU and hospital mortality were, respectively, 12% and 25%, and, among survivors, 72% were discharged home.

A Dutch single-center cohort study [78] found that at one year, three quarters of patients living at home before ICU admission were still living at home; of them, only 10% developed cognitive impairment, even though the reported QoL at a follow-up was significantly lower than in the general population.

A more recent Canadian study [79] reported that the median ICU length of stay in older surgical patients was 3.8 days, hospital length of stay was 20.1 days, ICU mortality was 18.7%, and hospital mortality was 31.6%.

33.9 Final Considerations

The rate of octogenarians is growing quickly, and an increasing number of elderly patients are every day admitted to ICU after planned surgery.

Even though not exhaustive and not enough confirmed by large studies or RCTs, reference points and general criteria have been so far outlined, and what reported in the literature summary here took into account can be considered as a basal guidance. Many issues still deserve further research, from a better definition of the triage criteria to methods to minimize ICU side effects, and from the levels of care to deliver, to criteria for care withdrawal and discharge.

All these issues present problems ranging from the clinical to the organizational, economical, relational, and ethical point of view. A "geriatrization" of anesthesiologists, surgeons, and intensivists is one of the main elements for a substantial improvement in the quality of care to offer our seniors, applying what here reported and following future research results. This requires changes in the study courses, improved hospital organization, and farsighted healthcare management. This view is made even more compelling by the recent pandemics, at which one should look not as at an isolated, tragic event, but as a paradigm of the frailty of the human condition in this historical moment and likely in the future, toward which we should be prepared.

Whereas patients' preferences have a central importance when the discussion concerns the choice about how to close one's own life and to refuse the perspective of ICU admission, on the other hand to all of us healthcare professionals pertains the duty of keeping far from prejudice, preconception, and ageism, proceeding in research, improving our communication standards, and sharpening process organization.

> **Take Home Messages**
>
> **Pillars of Optimal Perioperative Intensive Care After Planned Surgery**
> *Preoperative Evaluation*
> Planning for appropriate ICU care in the elderly surgical patient is a process that starts since the beginning of the surgical path, with optimal, comprehensive preoperative evaluation. In the older patient, this step should include, together with clinical history and physical examination as routinely performed in adults, also data that allow understanding patient's functional status (CGA) and QoL, the presence of frailty and other risk factors for POD, life expectancy, and any advance directive.

Data Sharing and Co-management

Knowing these data, pivotal in targeting the right surgical approach, will also help intensivists in tailoring the level of intensive care, communicating with relatives, and balancing between the need to offer the better chances of survival and the avoidance of aggressive treatment.

Indeed, the availability of these data is just one of the ingredients that allow the medical team to optimally operate: other crucial issues are preoperative patient optimization (correction of nutritional deficits, medication reconciliation, cardiac and respiratory prehabilitation, treatment of depression), appropriate communication, and motivation, together with implementation of team-based strategies such as co-management of the care processes, not only with surgeons and anesthesiologists but also with nurses [80] and geriatricians [81].

Prevention of ICU Admission-Related Side Effects

Forced immobility, prolonged sedation, indwelling catheters, altered sleep-wake rhythm, isolation, and environmental discomfort are just the main sources of adverse effects the ICU admission implies [82, 83]. Strategies to reduce ICU-related side effects are many, from delirium prevention to optimal nursing, including cognitive stimulation, mobilization [28], and occupational therapy [84]. The American College of Critical Care Medicine updated the Clinical Practice Guidelines for the management of pain, agitation, and delirium in IC, focusing on the "ABCDEF" bundle [85]. This set includes the following measures:

A. *Assess and manage pain*
B. *Breathing trials and spontaneous awakening*
C. *Choice of sedative*
D. *Daily delirium monitoring*
E. *Early mobility*
F. *Family engagement and empowerment*

References

1. Blot S, Cankurtaran M, Petrivic M, et al. Epidemiology and outcome of nosocomial bloodstream infection in elderly critically ill patients: a comparison between middle-aged, old and very old patients. Crit Care Med. 2009;37(5):1634–41.
2. Suskind AM, Finlayson E. Thinking beyond age for post-acute care after major abdominal surgery. JAMA Surg. 2016;151(8):766–7.
3. Futier E, Constantin JM, Paugam-Burtz C, et al. A trial of intraoperative low-tidal-volume ventilation in abdominal surgery. N Engl J Med. 2013;369:428–37.
4. Millan M, Espina-Perz B, Caro-Tarrago A, et al. ERAS programs in the elderly patients: is there a limit? Int J Color Dis. 2018;33:1313.
5. Aldecoa C, Bettelli G, Bilotta F, et al. European Society of Anaesthesiology evidence-based and consensus-based guidelines on postoperative delirium. Eur J Anaesthesiol. 2017;34:192–214.
6. De Hert S, Staender S, Fritsch G, et al. Pre-operative evaluation of adults undergoing elective non-cardiac surgery. Updated guideline from the European Society of Anaesthesiology. Eur J Anaesthesiol. 2018;35:407–65.
7. Strom C, Rasmussen LS. Challenges in anaesthesia for elderly – review. Singap Dent J. 2014;35:23–9.

8. Nathanson BH, Higgins TL, Brennan MG, et al. Subgroup mortality probability models: are they necessary for specialized intensive care units? Crit Care Med. 2009;37:2375–86.

9. Ausset S, De Saint-Maurice G, Donat N, et al. Morbidité et mortalité postopératoire du patient âgé. In: Anesthésie, analgésie et réanimation du patient âgé. Rueil-Malmaison: Arnette; 2008.

10. Peterson ED, Cowper PA, Jollis JC, et al. Outcomes of coronary artery bypass graft surgery in 24.461 patients aged 80 years or older. Circulation. 1995;92:1185–91.

11. Finlyson E, Fan Z, Birkmeyer, et al. Outcomes in octogenarians undergoing high risk cancer operation: a national study. J Am Coll Surg. 2007;205:729–34.

12. Partridge JS, Collingridge G, Gordon AL, et al. Where are we in perioperative medicine for older surgical patients? A UK survey of geriatric medicine delivered services in surgery. Age Ageing. 2014;43:721–4.

13. Bettelli G, Maggi S. Risk prediction instruments in geriatric surgery are available but often ignored. Eur J Anaesthesiol. 2017;34(9):634–5.

14. Bettelli G. Perioperative care of older persons: where are we? Acta Biomed. 2020;11,91(2):376–8.

15. Rahman IA, Kendall S. Cardiac surgery in the very elderly: it isn't all about survival. Br J Cardiol. 2020;27:5–7.

16. Allen MS. Thoracic surgery in older patients. Curr Ger Rep. 2017;6(2):1–5.

17. Farrington N, Richardson A, Bridges J. Interventions for older people having cancer treatment: a scoping review. Ger Oncol. 2020;11(5):769–83.

18. Huette P, Abou-Arab O, Djebara AZ, et al. Risk factors and mortality of patients undergoing hip fracture surgery: a one-year follow-up study. Sci Rep. 2020;10:9607.

19. Fogaça de Souza AM, Oliveira Leme FC, Dalla Vecchia Grassi L, et al. Perioperative complications and mortality in elderly patients following surgery for femoral fracture: prospective observational study. Rev Bras Anestesiol. 2019;69(6):569–79.

20. Turrentine B, Wang H, Simpson VB, et al. Surgical risk factors, morbidity and mortality in elderly patients. J Am Coll Surg. 2007;203(6):865–77.

21. Eamer G, Al-Amoodi M, Holroyd-Leduc J, et al. Review of risk assessment tools to predict morbidity and mortality in elderly surgical patients. Am J Surg. 2018;216:585–94.

22. Pelavski A, De Miguel M, Garcia-Tejedor A, et al. Mortality, geriatric and nongeriatric surgical risk factors among the eldest old: a prospective observational study. Anesth Analg. 2017;125(4):1329–36.

23. St-Louis E, Sudarshan M, Al-Habboubi, et al. The outcomes of the elderly in acute care general surgery. Eur J Trauma Emerg Surg. 2016;42:107–13.

24. Flaaten H, De Lange DW, Morandi A, et al. The impact of frailty on ICU and 30-day mortality and the level of care in very elderly patients (>=80 years). Intensive Care Med. 2017;43(12):1820–8.

25. Guidet B, De Lange DW, Boumendil A, et al. The contribution of frailty, cognition, activity of daily life and comorbidity on outcome in acutely admitted patients over 80 years in European ICUs: the VIP2 study. Intensive Care Med. 2020;456(1):57–69.

26. Jung C, Wernly B, Muessig JM, et al. A comparison of very old patients admitted to intensive care unit after acute versus elective surgery or intervention. J Crit Care. 2019;52:141–8.

27. Onwochei DN, Fabes J, Walker D, et al. Critical care after major surgery: a systematic review of risk factors for unplanned admission. Anaesthesia. 2020;75(Suppl. 1):e62–74.

28. Bagshaw SM, Webb SA, Delaney A, et al. Very old patients admitted to intensive care in Australia and New Zealand: a multi-centre cohort analysis. Crit Care. 2009;13(2):R45.

29. Nguyen YL, Angus DC, Boumedil A, et al. The challenge of admitting the very elderly to intensive care. Ann Int Care. 2011;1:29–36.

30. Guidet B (Interview to) Elderly care in the ICU. ICU Management & Practice, 2014–15; 4: 39–40 https://healthmanagement.org/c/icu/issuearticle/elderly-care-in-the-icu-professor-bertrand-guidet.

31. Mahanna-Gabrielli E, Schenning KJ, Eriksson LI, et al. State of the clinical science of perioperative brain health: report from the American Society of Anaesthesiologists Brain Health Initiative Summit. Br J Anaesth. 2019;123(4):464–78.

32. Guidet B, Vallet H, Boddaert J, et al. Caring for the critically ill patient over 80: a narrative review. Ann Intensive Care. 2018;8:114.

33. The Royal College of Surgeons of England and Department of Health. The higher risk general surgical patients: toward improved care for a forgotten group. 2011. https://www.rcseng.ac.uk/library-and-publications/rcs-publications/docs/the-higher-risk-general-surgical-patient/.

34. Smith G, Nielsen M. ABC of intensive care: criteria for admission. Br Med J. 1999;318:1544–7.

35. Reich DL, Bennet Guerrero E, Bodian A, et al. Intraoperative tachycardia and hypertension are independently associated with adverse outcome in noncardiac surgery of long duration. Anesth Analg. 2002;95:273–7.
36. Hartmann B, Iunger A, Rohrig R, et al. Intraoperative tachycardia and perioperative outcome. Langenbeck's Arch Surg. 2003;388:255–60.
37. Jerat A, Laupacis A, Austin PC, et al. Intensive care utilization following major noncardiac surgical procedures in Ontario, Canada: a population-based study. Intensive Care Med. 2018;44(9):1427–35.
38. Gillies MA, Harrison EM, Pearse RM, et al. Intensive care utilization and outcomes after high-risk surgery in Scotland: a population-based cohort study. Br J Anaesth. 2017;118:123–31.
39. Garrouste-Orgeas M, Montuclard M, Timsit JF, et al. Predictors of intensive care unit refusal in French intensive care units: a multiple-center study. Crit Care Med. 2005;33:750–5.
40. Poldermans D, Bax JJ, Boersma E, et al. Guidelines for preoperative cardiac risk assessment and perioperative cardiac management in noncardiac surgery: the Task Force for Preoperative Cardiac Risk Assessment and Perioperative Cardiac management in noncardiac surgery of the European Society of Cardiology and endorsed by the European Society of Anaesthesiology. Eur J Anaesthesiol. 2010;27:92–137.
41. Baquero G, Rich MW. Perioperative care in older adults. J Geriatr Cardiol. 2015;12(5):465–9.
42. Vaccarino V, Badimon L, Corti R, et al. Presentation, management and outcomes of ischemic heart disease in women. Nat Rev Cardiol. 2013;10:508–18.
43. Flu WJ, van Kuijk JP, Hoeks SE, et al. Prognostic implications of asymptomatic left ventricular dysfunction in patients undergoing vascular surgery. Anesthesiology. 2010;112:1316–24.
44. Ferreira RG, Worthington A, Huang CC, et al. Sex differences in the prevalence of diastolic dysfunction in cardiac surgical patients. J Card Surg. 2015;30(3):238–45.
45. Neupane I, Arora RC, Rudolph JL. Cardiac surgery as a stressor and the response of the vulnerable older adult. Exp Gerontol. 2017;87(Pt B):168–74.
46. Vetta F, Locorotondo G. Cardiovascular complications. In: Bettelli G, editor. Perioperative care of the elderly: clinical and organizational aspects. Cambridge University Press, Cambridge; 2017.
47. Ford PN, Thomas L, Cook TM, et al. Determinants of outcome in critically ill octogenarians after surgery: an observational study. Br J Anaesth. 2007;99:824–9.
48. Canet J, Mazo V. Postoperative pulmonary complications. Minerva Anest. 2010;76:138–43.
49. Urban MK, Mangini Vendel L, Lymann S, et al. The need for a step-up in postoperative medical care is predictable in orthopedic patients undergoing elective surgery. HSSJ. 2016;12:59–65.
50. Canet J, Sabate S, Mazo V, et al. Development and validation of a score to predict postoperative respiratory failure in a multicentre European cohort: a prospective, observational study. Eur J Anaesthesiol. 2015;32:458–70.
51. Koftis K, Szylinska A, Listewnik M, et al. Early delirium after cardiac surgery: an analysis of incidence and risk factors in elderly (>=65 years) and very elderly (>=80 years) patients. Clin Interv Aging. 2018;13:1061–70.
52. McPherson JA, Wagner CE, Bohem LM, et al. Delirium in the cardiovascular ICU. Crit Care Med. 2013;41:405–13.
53. Bettelli G, Neuner B. Postoperative delirium: a preventable complication in the elderly surgical patient. Monaldi Arch Chest Dis. 2017;87(2):842.
54. Riker RR, Shebabi Y, Bokesch PM, et al. Dexmedetomidine vs midazolam for sedation of critically ill patients: a randomized controlled trial. JAMA. 2009;301:489–99.
55. Steinberg BE, Sundman E, Terrando N, et al. Neural control of inflammation: implications for perioperative and critical care. Anesthesiology. 2016;124:1174–89.
56. Barr J, Fraser GL, Puntillo K, et al. American College of Critical Care M Clinical practice guidelines for the management of pain, agitation, and delirium in adult patients in the intensive care unit. Crit Care Med. 2013;41:263–306.
57. Schweickert WD, Pohlman MC, Pohlman AS, et al. Early physical and occupational therapy in mechanically ventilated, critically ill patients: a randomized controlled trial. Lancet. 2009;373:1874–82.
58. Flannery AH, Oyler DR, Weinhouse GL. The impact of interventions to improve sleep on delirium in the ICU: a systematic review and research framework. Crit Care Med. 2016; Epub Aug 9
59. Morandi A, Brummel NE, Ely EW. Sedation, delirium and mechanical ventilation: the "ABCDE" approach. Curr Opin Crit Care. 2011;17:43–9.

60. Bannon L, McGaughey J, Verghis R, et al. The effectiveness of non-pharmacological interventions in reducing the incidence and duration of delirium in critically ill patients: a systematic review and meta-analysis. Intensive Care Med. 2019;45:1–12.
61. Shurr P, Boeken U, Litmathe J, et al. Predictors of postoperative complications in octogenarians undergoing cardiac surgery. Thorac Cardiovasc Surg. 2010;58(4):200–3.
62. Zingone B, Gatti G, Rauber E, et al. Early and late outcomes of cardiac surgery in octogenarians. Ann Thorac Surg. 2009;87(1):71–8.
63. Nisanoglu V, Erdil N, Aldemir M, et al. Atrial fibrillation after coronary artery bypass grafting in elderly patients: incidence and risk factors. Thorac Cardiovasc Surg. 2007;55(1):32–8.
64. Athanasiou T, Aziz O, Mangoush O, et al. Do off-pump techniques reduce the incidence of postoperative atrial fibrillation in elderly patients undergoing coronary artery bypass grafting? Ann Thor Surg. 2004;7785:1567–74.
65. Knapik P, Hirnle G, Kowalczuk-Wieteska A, et al. Off-pump versus on-pump coronary artery surgery in octogenarians (from the KROK Registry). PLoS One. 2020;15(9):e0238880. https://doi.org/10.1371/journalpone.0238880.
66. Ried M, Puehler T, Haneya A, et al. Acute kidney injury in septua-and octogenarians after cardiac surgery. BMC Cardiovasc Dis. 2011;11:52.
67. Al-Refaie WB, Parsons HM, Henderson WG, et al. Major cancer surgery in the elderly: results from the American College of Surgeons National Surgical Quality Improvement Program. Ann Surg. 2010;251:311–8.
68. Masoomi H, Kang CY, Chen A, et al. Predictive factors of in-hospital mortality in colon and rectal surgery. J Am Coll Surg. 2012;215:255–61.
69. Law S, Wong KH, Kwok KF, et al. Predictive factors for pulmonary complications and mortality after esophagectomy for cancer. Ann Surg. 2004;240:791–800.
70. Pearse RM, Moreno RP, Bauer P, et al. Mortality after surgery in Europe: a 7day cohort study. Lancet. 2012;380:1059–65.
71. Simões CM, Carmona MJ, Hajjar LA, et al. Predictors of major complications after elective abdominal surgery in cancer patients. BMC Anesthesiol. 2018;18:49.
72. Taylor JM, Gropper MA. Critical care challenges in orthopaedic surgery patients. Crit Care Med. 2006;34(9 Suppl):S191–9.
73. Kobayashi K, Imagama S, Ando K, et al. Complications associated with spine surgery in patients aged 80 years or older: Japan Association of Spine Surgeons with Ambition (JASA) Multicenter Study. Global Spine J. 2017;7(7):636–41.
74. Kamath AF, McAuliffe CL, Baldwin KD, et al. Unplanned admission to intensive care unit after total hip arthroplasty. J Arthroplast. 2012;27(6):1027–32.
75. Nates JL, Nunnally M, Kleinpell R, et al. ICU admission, discharge and triage guidelines: a framework to enhance clinical operations, development of institutional policies and further research. Crit Care Med. 2016;44(8):1553–602.
76. Heidegger CP, Treggiari MM, Romand JA, et al. A nationwide survey of intensive care unit discharge practices. Intensive Care Med. 2005;31:1676–82.
77. Singh MY, Nayyar V, Clark PT, et al. Does after-hours discharge of ICU patients influence the outcome? Crit Care Resusc. 2019;12:156–61.
78. De Rooij SE, Govers AC, Korevaar JC, et al. Cognitive, functional and quality of life outcomes of patients aged 80 and older who survived at least 1 year after planned or unplanned surgery or medical intensive care treatment. J Am Geriatr Soc. 2008;56(5):816–22.
79. Ball IM, Bagshaw SM, Burns KE, et al. Outcomes of elderly critically ill medical and surgical patients: a multicentre cohort study. Can J Anest. 2017;64:260–9.
80. Mick DJ, Ackerman MH. Critical care nursing for older adults: pathophysiological and functional consideration. Nurs Clin North Am. 2004;39(3):473–93.
81. Brummel NE, Ferrante LE. Integrating geriatric principles into critical care medicine: the time is now. Ann Am Thorac Soc. 2018;15(5):518–22.
82. Modrykamien AM. The ICU follow-up clinic: a new paradigm for intensivists. Resp Care. 2012;57(5):764–72.

83. Shigeaki I, Hatakeyama J, Kondo Y, et al. Post-intensive care syndrome: its pathophysiology, prevention and future directions. Acute Med Surg. 2019;6:233–46.
84. Costigan FA, Duffet AM, Harris JE, et al. Occupational therapy in the ICU. Am J Occup Ther. 2019;63(2):191–1986.
85. Devlin J, W, Skrobik Y, Gélinas C., et al. Clinical practice guidelines for the prevention and management of pain, agitation/sedation, delirium, immobility and sleep disruption in adult patients in ICU. Crit Care Med. 2018;46(9):e825–73.

Postoperative Patients: Urgent Surgery

Sara Thietart, Margaux Baqué, Judith Cohen-Bittan, Lorène Zerah, and Jacques Boddaert

Contents

34.1 Introduction

The population of patients over 65 years increases disproportionately [1] and is projected to rise by 15.5% in 2035, comparatively with 2010 [2]. Aging of population has an impact on the demand for healthcare services, including surgery. Between 40% and 50% of patients undergoing surgery are aged 65 years or more [3]. Additionally, surgical demand is expected to increase in the following decades: vascular and cancer surgery are predicted to increase, respectively, by 72% and 56% by 2035 [4–6]. The proportion of emergency surgery procedures increases with age, comparatively with elective surgery. Proportion of urgent procedures can reach up to 72% of surgical procedures in patients of 90 years or older [7].

Mortality after urgent surgery is high and varies depending on the type of surgery. A first study on 6968 patients of 85 years and over found that 1-month mortality was 13% after urgent surgery [8]. In another study including Medicare beneficiaries of patients >65 years who underwent urgent abdominal surgery, 1-month postoperative mortality was 20% and 34% 1 year after surgery [9]. Half of the deaths occurred during hospitalization and 90% in the six first months after surgery [9]. In this study, factors associated with mortality were having an age over 85 years, comorbidities (chronic kidney disease, chronic heart failure, dementia), a previous hospitalization 6 months prior to surgery and occurence of postoperative complications [9]. Finally, in a US retrospective cohort of 32,135 injured older adults, 1-year mortality was more than 40% in groups of patients with serious injury (defined using ICISS score), or with high degree of comorbidity or functional decline [10]. These results highlight the add-on effect of comorbidities and functional status on mortality.

Postoperative complications are more frequent in older adults than in younger patients. They are estimated between 16% and 50% in patients of 80 years and older [11]. Older adults undergoing emergency procedures have higher complication rates than those undergoing elective surgery [12]. The most frequent complications are bleeding requiring transfusions, pneumonia, myocardial infarction, wound infections, sepsis, and respiratory failure [8]. Since occurrence of postoperative complications is a known factor influencing mortality [9], prevention, quick screening, and treatment are major challenges to optimize short- and long-term mortality.

Postoperative care is therefore a key factor that influences outcome. As an example, we shall use hip fracture surgery to illustrate this point.

34.2 Hip Fracture Surgery

Hip fracture is a common and serious injury, with an annual worldwide incidence of 1.6 million [13]. It is responsible for a high mortality and morbidity rate. According to studies, 6-month mortality rate varies from 13% to 23%, and 13% of patients need a total assistance to walk 6 months after surgery [10, 14]. Considering all factors encountered during hip fracture perioperative period in older patients, we recently showed that baseline characteristics could explain 62.4% of 6-month mortality, perioperative factors 12.3% and severe postoperative complications 11.9% [15]. Thus, optimization of care pathways, prevention, and management of complications are cornerstones of hip fracture management.

34.2.1 Orthogeriatric Care: Improving Hip Fracture Outcomes

Most postoperative complications are identifiable and reversible. Prevention, early screening, and quick treatment could ameliorate outcome of patients after hip fracture surgery. The aims of postoperative care management are detailed in ▶ Box 34.1.

Box 34.1 Goals of Treatment of the Orthogeriatric Care Models

Immediate management

Early mobilization: armchair within 24 h and walking within 48 h

Pain management: emphasize on regional anesthesia, prescribe morphine and acetaminophen

Prevention and detection of delirium: avoid benzodiazepine withdrawal, regular screening using the confusion assessment method scale

Detect and prevent stool impaction and urinary retention

Pressure ulcer prevention: detect high risk patients using Braden scale, nutrition, and use air-filled mattresses if needed

Aspiration pneumonia prevention: screen for swallowing disorders and adapt food texture

Detection of anemia and acute kidney injury and correction

Intermediate management

Identify etiology of the fall (often multiple):

- Search for predisposing factor(s)
- Search for triggering factor(s)

Evaluate the patient's prescription:

- Initiate and titrate disease-modifying therapy according to patient comorbidities
- Evaluate risk/benefit of each medication
- Remove medication which increases risk of falls
- Remove inappropriate medication according to Beer's Criteria [16].

Treatment of malnutrition: nutritionist follow-up

Intensive physiotherapy and rehabilitation

Initiate and titrate disease-modifying therapy according to comorbidities

> **Predischarge and long-term management**
> Organize an evaluation by a social worker if needed
> Elaborate a discharge plan:
> - Correct selection of discharge setting: recovery unit or at home
> - Increase help at home permanently or temporarily
> - Organize follow-up of patient
>
> Adapt environment at home
> Give to patient and family recommendations about mobilization, nutrition, and medication
> Prevent early readmission

34.2.1.1   Models of Orthogeriatric Interventions

Models of combined care, integrating both medical and surgical care, have been proposed [17]. These models vary from orthopedic care with geriatric consultation to integrated comprehensive orthogeriatric models, as shown in ◘ Fig. 34.1.

Model 1: Routine Orthogeriatric Consultation Models   In this model, the care takes place in the orthopedic ward, where surgeons are in charge of their treatment. A systematic daily geriatric consultation is performed, sometimes associated with physiotherapists, social workers, and nurses experienced in geriatrics. The main limitation of this model is the absence of control of adherence of the orthopedic team on following the geriatrician's recommendations, which varies between 57% and 77% [18, 19].

Model 2: Postoperative Geriatric Ward Models   The care takes place in the geriatric ward, with the surgeon doing punctual consultations [20]. Geriatricians working in this ward have an expertise in orthopedic postoperative care.

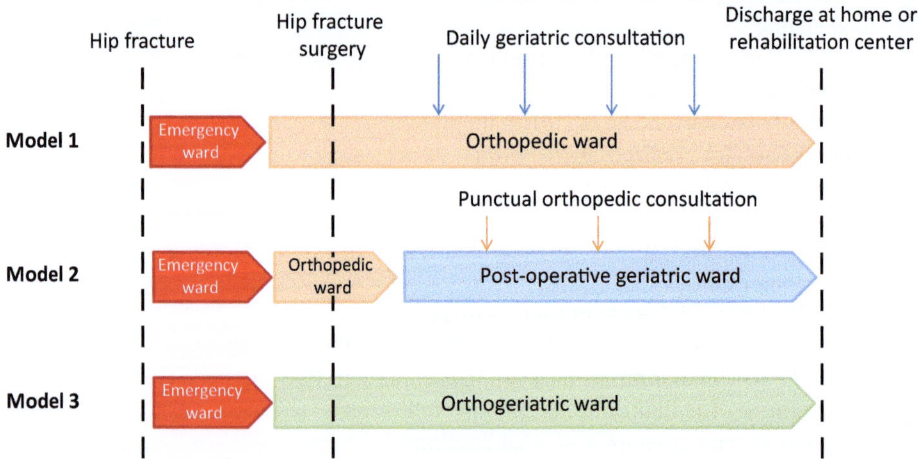

◘ **Fig. 34.1**   The three models of orthogeriatric interventions

Model 3: Comprehensive Shared Orthogeriatric Models In this model, the patient is hospitalized in a specific ward with both orthopedic surgeons and geriatricians [21]. Both protagonists share responsibility on the patient's care [22].

34.2.1.2 Outcome After Integrated Orthogeriatric Care

Many studies evaluating orthogeriatric models have been published, with heterogeneous results. This heterogeneity is due to the variability in the evaluated orthogeriatric model, the differences in patient characteristics, outcome, and in the method of randomization. Most studies are described as having a high risk of bias [23]. A systematic review evaluating the three orthogeriatric models was limited by the high variability between the different studies [17]. In this meta-analysis, routine geriatric consultation did not significantly reduce in-hospital and long-term mortality, nor time to surgery, although length of hospital stay was shorter. The geriatric ward model had a shorter length of stay, but the high variability of the studies made analysis on mortality impossible [17]. Therefore, there is insufficient data to robustly conclude whether these orthogeriatric interventions globally impact outcome. However, it is possible that some models may be more efficient than others, as some models have shown decreased long-term mortality and morbidity [20, 24, 25].

34.2.1.3 Which Is the Best Model?

It is unclear which is the best model, as few studies have compared the models between them.

Clinical trials evaluating routine orthogeriatric consultation models did not result in a significant reduction of postoperative mortality or morbidity [19, 26]. However this model could decrease incidence of postoperative delirium and cognitive decline [18, 27].

The postoperative geriatric care model has shown that it ameliorated mobility 4 months after hip surgery (using short physical performance battery) in a randomized trial comparing it with hospitalization in an orthopedic ward [28]. In a prospective study of 203 patients with hip fracture hospitalized in a postoperative geriatric ward, 6-month mortality was decreased by 40%, 6-month readmission decreased by 50%, and proportion of patients who lost ability to walk decreased by 70%, in comparison with 131 patients hospitalized in an orthopedic ward [20]. To finish, a meta-analysis evaluating the effect of implementing the postoperative geriatric model on 1072 patients found that it reduced mortality risk with an odds ratio of 0.62 (95% confidence interval 0.48–0.80) [25].

The comprehensive integrated orthogeriatric care model seems more efficient than the orthogeriatric consultation model [29]. It has been shown that this model decreases time to surgery (an important factor influencing outcome), length of hospital stay, and incidence of complications [30]. Middleton et al. compared a consulting geriatrician model with a comprehensive orthogeriatric ward model and found that the orthogeriatric intervention decreased 30-day mortality by 22% and length of stay by 23% [24].

34.2.2 Postoperative Geriatric Complications

Medical complications occur more frequently than surgical complications: Three to five complications will occur in older patients hospitalized for hip fracture surgery, whereas surgical revision or infection will occur in less than 2% of patients [15].

- **Delirium**

Delirium incidence greatly varies according to methodology. In older patients undergoing hip fracture surgery, delirium occurs in 30–40% of patients aged 75 years and older [31]. Postoperative delirium is independently associated with 6-month mortality, and each additional day with postoperative delirium is associated with increased mortality [31]. Postoperative delirium is also associated with morbidity, longer length of hospital stay, increased risk of postoperative cognitive disorders, and limitations in activities of daily living [3, 11].

In order to prevent poor outcome, early screening by using the Confusion Assessment Method several times daily and immediate treatment are key features of postoperative care [3, 32]. A clinical trial evaluating the effect of a multicomponent intervention to prevent delirium in 426 hospitalized patients with a mean age of 80 years showed a decreased risk of delirium with an odds ratio of 0.60 (95% CI 0.39–0.92). Although this trial was not performed specifically in postoperative patients, one could also use this intervention after hip fracture surgery [33]. To help the clinician, guidelines on prevention and treatment of postoperative delirium have been published by the European Society of Anaesthesiology [3].

- **Loss of Functional Status**

Prevention of loss of functional ability should be a priority when managing hospitalized older patients. It is a frequent (almost systematic) severe and costly complication and is highly related to previous functional status. Patients which suffer postoperative functional decline have higher rates of hospital readmission, length of stay, and live less often at home 30 days after the procedure [11]. Among patients who were independent before the fracture, only 66% required help in at least one activity of daily living 1 year after the fracture [34].

The most crucial interventions to prevent loss of functional status are to allow early mobilization and walking recovery after surgery. This should be performed daily and involves patients, physicians, nurses, and physiotherapists. Early mobilization is part of the enhanced recovery after surgery protocol, which is a multimodal, multidisciplinary approach that is shown to decrease length of stay, complications, readmission rates, and costs [35, 36]. Then, one must optimize anemia, hydration, and pain management and adapt medication in order to prevent orthostatic hypotension or other drug-related complications.

- **Pain Management**

Pain can be underdiagnosed, as some patients will not spontaneously declare it. Communication disorders due to cognitive impairment, deafness, aphasia, or dysarthria are barriers to detecting pain. Poor pain management is associated with increased risk of delirium and slower recovery [37]. Postoperative pain management should emphasize on regional anesthesia, multimodal analgesia including nonpharmacological measures, cautious morphine administration, and acetaminophen [38]. No association has been found between morphine consumption and postoperative delirium, even among patients with preoperative dementia [39].

■ Other Complications

Constipation can result in paralytic ileus and fecal impaction, resulting in nausea and vomiting. It occurs in up to 40% of patients after hip fracture surgery [40]. It is associated with poor outcome after hip fracture surgery. Postoperative urinary retention is a risk factor of delirium and occurs in 25% of patients undergoing hip fracture surgery [40].

Pressure ulcers are frequent after hip fracture surgery and can occur in up to 12% of patients [41]. They occur particularly among patients with low albumin levels and with comorbidities. Pressure ulcers were associated with higher risk of 6-month mortality [41].

34.3 Generalization of the Postoperative Geriatric Model: An Unmet Need

The use of a geriatric model of care in postoperative situations is recommended by the guidelines from American, Australian, English, French, Irish, and New Zealand societies [38, 42–47].

According to their complexity, management of older patients must be based on a structured care pathway: from the emergency room, to operating room, postoperative unit, and rehabilitation unit, with close collaboration for management of comorbidities, complications, and treatments. Efforts should be made in order to generalize the orthogeriatric postoperative model to other types of surgery, such as cardiac, abdominal, or urological surgery. Bundles of care including preoperative, intraoperative, and postoperative care for urgent abdominal surgery are under evaluation [48]. Use of enhanced recovery after surgery programs after colorectal surgery in older patients decreased incidence of postoperative complications, duration of hospital stay, and hospital costs [36, 49]. However these programs did not include a systematic geriatric expertise.

Conclusion

To conclude, older patients often undergo urgent surgery. Postoperative complications are frequent but are often easily identifiable and reversible. The use of postoperative orthogeriatric care models in orthopedic surgery has proven efficacy in decreasing mortality, complications, and length of stay and ameliorating mobility. There is a need to generalize postoperative care models to other kinds of surgery where incidence of complications and mortality is high.

Practical Implications

Clinicians should be aware that urgent surgery among older patients is burdened with a high risk of complications and death. This knowledge implies that:

1. Early screening of postoperative complications using: daily evaluation of delirium using the Confusion Assessment Method, regular pain evaluation, close monitoring of hemoglobin level, kidney function, acute cardiac failure, constipation, urinary retention, and aspiration pneumonia.
2. Early rehabilitation should be performed in order to prevent loss of functional status.
3. Caregivers of all specialties should acknowledge patient comorbidities and polypharmacy, decide on continuing or temporarily discontinuing medication, and precociously evaluate the risk/benefit of all medication.
4. After hip fracture surgery, patient care should take place in a postoperative geriatric ward or in a comprehensive orthogeriatric ward.
5. Postoperative geriatric wards for other kinds of surgery are missing, and there is a need for creating and organizing such structures.
6. For other kinds of urgent surgery, patients should benefit of recovery programs and geriatric expertise, either with regular geriatric consultations or by transferring the patient in a geriatric ward.

Take-Home Messages

- At least 40% of patients undergoing surgery are 65 years old or over. Among those performed after the age of 90 years, at least 70% are emergency procedures.
- Postoperative mortality and complications are high after urgent surgery in the geriatric population.
- The main postoperative geriatric complications are: delirium, loss of functional status, pain, constipation, urinary retention, and pressure ulcers. These complications are associated with an increased risk of mortality and a longer length of stay.
- Some postoperative orthogeriatric care models decrease mortality and morbidity.
- There is a need to generalize the postoperative geriatric care models to other kinds of surgery.

References

1. GBD. Demographics collaborators (2020) global age-sex-specific fertility, mortality, healthy life expectancy (HALE), and population estimates in 204 countries and territories, 1950-2019: a comprehensive demographic analysis for the global burden of disease study 2019. Lancet. 2019;396:1160–203.
2. THE NEXT FOUR DECADES The Older Population in the United States: 2010 to 2050. 16.
3. Aldecoa C, Bettelli G, Bilotta F, et al. European Society of Anaesthesiology evidence-based and consensus-based guideline on postoperative delirium. Eur J Anaesthesiol. 2017;34:192–214.
4. Jim J, Owens PL, Sanchez LA, Rubin BG. Population-based analysis of inpatient vascular procedures and predicting future workload and implications for training. J Vasc Surg. 2012;55:1394–9; discussion 1399-1400

5. Ellison EC, Pawlik TM, Way DP, Satiani B, Williams TE. The impact of the aging population and incidence of cancer on future projections of general surgical workforce needs. Surgery. 2018;163:553–9.
6. Etzioni DA, Liu JH, Maggard MA, Ko CY. The aging population and its impact on the surgery workforce. Ann Surg. 2003;238:170–7.
7. Blansfield JA, Clark SC, Hofmann MT, Morris JB. Alimentary tract surgery in the nonagenarian: elective vs. emergent operations. J Gastrointest Surg. 2004;8:539–42.
8. Maurer LR, Chetlur P, Zhuo D, El Hechi M, Velmahos GC, Dunn J, Bertsimas D, Kaafarani HMA. Validation of the AI-based predictive OpTimal Trees in Emergency Surgery Risk (POTTER) calculator in patients 65 years and older. Ann Surg. 2020. https://doi.org/10.1097/SLA.0000000000004714.
9. Cooper Z, Mitchell SL, Gorges RJ, Rosenthal RA, Lipsitz SR, Kelley AS. Predictors of mortality up to 1 year after emergency major abdominal surgery in older adults. J Am Geriatr Soc. 2015;63:2572–9.
10. Fleischman RJ, Adams AL, Hedges JR, Ma OJ, Mullins RJ, Newgard CD. The optimum follow-up period for assessing mortality outcomes in injured older adults. J Am Geriatr Soc. 2010;58:1843–9.
11. Zhang LM, Hornor MA, Robinson T, Rosenthal RA, Ko CY, Russell MM. Evaluation of postoperative functional health status decline among older adults. JAMA Surg. 2020;155:950–8.
12. Cooper Z, Scott JW, Rosenthal RA, Mitchell SL. Emergency major abdominal surgical procedures in older adults: a systematic review of mortality and functional outcomes. J Am Geriatr Soc. 2015;63:2563–71.
13. Johnell O, Kanis JA. An estimate of the worldwide prevalence and disability associated with osteoporotic fractures. Osteoporos Int. 2006;17:1726–33.
14. Hannan EL, Magaziner J, Wang JJ, Eastwood EA, Silberzweig SB, Gilbert M, Morrison RS, McLaughlin MA, Orosz GM, Siu AL. Mortality and locomotion 6 months after hospitalization for hip fracture: risk factors and risk-adjusted hospital outcomes. JAMA. 2001;285:2736–42.
15. Zerah L, Hajage D, Raux M, Cohen-Bittan J, Mézière A, Khiami F, Le Manach Y, Riou B, Boddaert J. Attributable mortality of hip fracture in older patients: a retrospective observational study. J Clin Med. 2020; https://doi.org/10.3390/jcm9082370.
16. By the 2019 American Geriatrics Society Beers Criteria® Update Expert Panel. American Geriatrics Society 2019 updated AGS beers criteria® for potentially inappropriate medication use in older adults. J Am Geriatr Soc. 2019;67:674–94.
17. Grigoryan KV, Javedan H, Rudolph JL. Orthogeriatric care models and outcomes in hip fracture patients: a systematic review and meta-analysis. J Orthop Trauma. 2014;28:e49–55.
18. Marcantonio ER, Rudolph JL, Culley D, Crosby G, Alsop D, Inouye SK. Serum biomarkers for delirium. J Gerontol A Biol Sci Med Sci. 2006;61:1281–6.
19. Deschodt M, Braes T, Broos P, Sermon A, Boonen S, Flamaing J, Milisen K. Effect of an inpatient geriatric consultation team on functional outcome, mortality, institutionalization, and readmission rate in older adults with hip fracture: a controlled trial. J Am Geriatr Soc. 2011;59:1299–308.
20. Boddaert J, Cohen-Bittan J, Khiami F, Le Manach Y, Raux M, Beinis J-Y, Verny M, Riou B. Postoperative admission to a dedicated geriatric unit decreases mortality in elderly patients with hip fracture. PLoS One. 2014;9:e83795.
21. Adunsky A, Arad M, Levi R, Blankstein A, Zeilig G, Mizrachi E. Five-year experience with the "Sheba" model of comprehensive orthogeriatric care for elderly hip fracture patients. Disabil Rehabil. 2005;27:1123–7.
22. Friedman SM, Mendelson DA, Kates SL, McCann RM. Geriatric co-management of proximal femur fractures: total quality management and protocol-driven care result in better outcomes for a frail patient population. J Am Geriatr Soc. 2008;56:1349–56.
23. Buecking B, Timmesfeld N, Riem S, Bliemel C, Hartwig E, Friess T, Liener U, Ruchholtz S, Eschbach D. Early orthogeriatric treatment of trauma in the elderly: a systematic review and metaanalysis. Dtsch Arztebl Int. 2013;110:255–62.
24. Middleton M, Wan B, da Assunçao R. Improving hip fracture outcomes with integrated orthogeriatric care: a comparison between two accepted orthogeriatric models. Age Ageing. 2017;46:465–70.
25. Moyet J, Deschasse G, Marquant B, Mertl P, Bloch F. Which is the optimal orthogeriatric care model to prevent mortality of elderly subjects post hip fractures? A systematic review and meta-analysis based on current clinical practice. Int Orthop. 2019;43:1449–54.
26. Naglie G, Tansey C, Kirkland JL, Ogilvie-Harris DJ, Detsky AS, Etchells E, Tomlinson G, O'Rourke K, Goldlist B. Interdisciplinary inpatient care for elderly people with hip fracture: a randomized controlled trial. CMAJ. 2002;167:25–32.

27. Deschodt M, Braes T, Flamaing J, Detroyer E, Broos P, Haentjens P, Boonen S, Milisen K. Preventing delirium in older adults with recent hip fracture through multidisciplinary geriatric consultation. J Am Geriatr Soc. 2012;60:733–9.

28. Prestmo A, Hagen G, Sletvold O, et al. Comprehensive geriatric care for patients with hip fractures: a prospective, randomised, controlled trial. Lancet. 2015;385:1623–33.

29. Pioli G, Giusti A, Barone A. Orthogeriatric care for the elderly with hip fractures: where are we? Aging Clin Exp Res. 2008;20:113–22.

30. Friedman SM, Mendelson DA, Bingham KW, Kates SL. Impact of a comanaged geriatric fracture Center on short-term hip fracture outcomes. Arch Intern Med. 2009;169:1712–7.

31. Bellelli G, Mazzola P, Morandi A, et al. Duration of postoperative delirium is an independent predictor of 6-month mortality in older adults after hip fracture. J Am Geriatr Soc. 2014;62:1335–40.

32. Inouye SK, van Dyck CH, Alessi CA, Balkin S, Siegal AP, Horwitz RI. Clarifying confusion: the confusion assessment method. A new method for detection of delirium. Ann Intern Med. 1990;113:941–8.

33. Inouye SK, Bogardus ST, Charpentier PA, Leo-Summers L, Acampora D, Holford TR, Cooney LM. A multicomponent intervention to prevent delirium in hospitalized older patients. N Engl J Med. 1999;340:669–76.

34. Magaziner J, Hawkes W, Hebel JR, Zimmerman SI, Fox KM, Dolan M, Felsenthal G, Kenzora J. Recovery from hip fracture in eight areas of function. J Gerontol A Biol Sci Med Sci. 2000;55:M498–507.

35. Wainwright TW, Gill M, McDonald DA, Middleton RG, Reed M, Sahota O, Yates P, Ljungqvist O. Consensus statement for perioperative care in total hip replacement and total knee replacement surgery: Enhanced Recovery After Surgery (ERAS®) society recommendations. Acta Orthop. 2020;91:3–19.

36. Ljungqvist O, Scott M, Fearon KC. Enhanced recovery after surgery: a review. JAMA Surg. 2017;152:292–8.

37. Vaurio LE, Sands LP, Wang Y, Mullen EA, Leung JM. Postoperative delirium: the importance of pain and pain management. Anesth Analg. 2006;102:1267–73.

38. Mohanty S, Rosenthal RA, Russell MM, Neuman MD, Ko CY, Esnaola NF. Optimal perioperative management of the geriatric patient: a best practices guideline from the American College of Surgeons NSQIP and the American Geriatrics Society. J Am Coll Surg. 2016;222:930–47.

39. Sieber FE, Mears S, Lee H, Gottschalk A. Postoperative opioid consumption and its relationship to cognitive function in older adults with hip fracture. J Am Geriatr Soc. 2011;59:2256–62.

40. Teng M, Zerah L, Rouet A, Tomeo C, Verny M, Cohen-Bittan J, Boddaert J, Haddad R. Fecal impaction is associated with postoperative urinary retention after hip fracture surgery. Ann Phys Rehabil Med. 2020;64(6):101464.

41. Magny E, Vallet H, Cohen-Bittan J, Raux M, Meziere A, Verny M, Riou B, Khiami F, Boddaert J. Pressure ulcers are associated with 6-month mortality in elderly patients with hip fracture managed in orthogeriatric care pathway. Arch Osteoporos. 2017;12:77.

42. Overview. Hip fracture: management. Guidance. NICE. https://www.nice.org.uk/guidance/cg124. Accessed 13 Apr 2021.

43. Fracture de l'extrémité supérieure du fémur – La SFAR. Société Française d'Anesthésie et de Réanimation. 2017.

44. Association of Anaesthetists of Great Britain and Ireland, Griffiths R, Alper J, et al. Management of proximal femoral fractures 2011: Association of Anaesthetists of Great Britain and Ireland. Anaesthesia. 2012;67:85–98.

45. New Zealand Guidelines Group. Acute management and immediate rehabilitation after hip fracture amongst people aged 65 years and over. Wellington: New Zealand Guidelines Group; 2003.

46. Hip Fracture Clinical Care Standard. Australian Commission on Safety and Quality in Health Care. https://www.safetyandquality.gov.au/publications-and-resources/resource-library/hip-fracture-clinical-care-standard. Accessed 13 Apr 2021.

47. Orthogériatrie et fracture de la hanche. In: Haute Autorité de Santé. https://www.has-sante.fr/jcms/c_2801173/fr/orthogeriatrie-et-fracture-de-la-hanche. Accessed 13 Apr 2021.

34

48. Burcharth J, Abdulhady L, Danker J, et al. Implementation of a multidisciplinary perioperative protocol in major emergency abdominal surgery. Eur J Trauma Emerg Surg. 2019. https://doi.org/10.1007/s00068-019-01238-7.
49. Launay-Savary M-V, Mathonnet M, Theissen A, Ostermann S, Raynaud-Simon A, Slim K, GRACE (Groupe francophone de Réhabilitation Améliorée après Chirurgie). Are enhanced recovery programs in colorectal surgery feasible and useful in the elderly? A systematic review of the literature. J Visc Surg. 2017;154:29–35.

Delirium

Silvia Giovannini, Fabrizio Brau, and Vincenzo Galluzzo

Contents

> **Learning Objectives**
> - Learn the relevance of delirium in terms of epidemiology, prognosis, and mortality, particularly after hospital admission and during the intensive care unit (ICU) stay
> - Understand the pathophysiological basis of delirium, including the importance of risk and precipitant factors
> - Recognize the clinical features of delirium, especially on elderly, and the major differential diagnoses
> - Appropriately investigate the causes of delirium and identify specific treatments
> - Learn the differences between nonpharmacologic and pharmacologic management of delirium

35.1 Introduction

Delirium represents a common medical condition which affects the old and very old patient in a hospital setting, particularly with cognitive impairment. It is characterized by disorganized thinking, inattention, and an altered level of consciousness. Delirium shows a fluctuating course during the acute phase. It might be underdiagnosed, due to the variability of its clinical features. In fact, it can manifest as an overactive or as an underactive form. Physicians could also observe a mixed form.

The onset of a confusional state in hospitalized older people is derived by the interruption of their daily routine, environmental modifications, and loss of orientation. Sleep deprivation, untreated pain, drugs, and medical devices, including bladder catheters, are precipitating factors for delirium.

Considering the complicated assessment of all risk and precipitating factors and the consequent delay of its resolution, delirium can lead to a longer stay and a higher risk of mortality [1], particularly on ICU.

Preventing delirium should be a fundamental goal for clinicians who approach this issue. Early mobilization, reduction of physical restraints, use of hearing and visual aids, and environmental actions to avoid sleep deprivation could represent some strategies in the nonpharmacological management of delirium.

Pain assessment is an important step in the process of care. Finally, treatment with neuroleptic drugs is often mandatory in the acute phase of delirium.

35.2 Definition and Classification

Delirium could be imagined as a cerebral insufficiency, with a fluctuating course, that occurred to people affected by an acute clinical illness, especially with cognitive disorders.

According to fifth edition of the Statistical Manual of Mental Disorders (DSM-5), delirium is based on:
- Disturbance in attention (i.e., reduced ability to direct, focus, sustain, and shift attention) and awareness (reduced orientation to the environment). The disturbance develops over a short period of time (usually hours to few days), represents an acute change from baseline attention and awareness, and tends to fluctuate during the course of a day.
- An additional disturbance in cognition (e.g., memory deficit, disorientation, language, visuospatial ability, or perception).

The disturbances are not better explained by another preexisting, established, or evolving neurocognitive disorder and do not occur in the context of a severely reduced level of arousal, such as coma.

There is evidence from the history, physical examination, or laboratory findings that the disturbance is a direct consequence of a medical condition.

Delirious patients also present behavioral disorders. Although not essential criteria for the diagnosis of delirium, psychomotor activities, emotional disturbances, and sleep interruption are common features of a confusional state. The two delirium phenotypes are the hyperactive patient and the hypoactive one [2].

The hyperactive delirious patient shows euphoria and agitation, with psychomotor manifestations. He is not collaborating and does not respond easily to medications. This kind of confusional state is associated with hospitalization, environmental modification, untreated pain, and medical devices.

The hypoactive delirious patient tends to exhibit lowers levels of attention, even if he is awake. It is usual to see daytime sleepiness. The typical trait is the exhausted ability to react to external stimuli. Hypoactive delirium derives from an acute illness. It does not require medications, but the management of the underlying acute disease is fundamental for the resolution of delirium, especially because this form of confusional state is associated with higher risk of mortality.

The mixed form includes both positive and negative symptoms. Emotional manifestations concern hallucinations, fear, and delusions.

35.3 **Epidemiology**

Confusional states are mainly observed during hospitalization. Delirium determines a longer stay than usual and consequent increase of the costs [3]. Potentially, all hospitalized patients present high risk of delirium, especially after surgery [4]. Among very old patients admitted at hospital, one third of them might develop confusion during the stay. The incidence of delirium on elderly changes from 25% after major elective surgery to 50% after hip fracture repairing surgery or other high-risk procedures [2]. Approximately, 10–15% of older persons presenting to emergency departments manifest delirium in association to the main illness [5]. The rate of delirium mostly increases in the intensive care unit (ICU), and this issue often persists during the ICU stay [6]. Moreover, delirium in the ICU is associated with worse short-term outcomes [7] and three-times increased risk of death both during and after the ICU stay [8].

About long-term care, such as post-acute and end-of-life care settings, in which the majority of patients are frail, delirium is a frequent and very frequent complication, respectively.

35.4 **Pathogenesis**

The pathophysiology of delirium is partially clear, but there are some theories concerning the etiology of this issue. We can explain how delirium develops with three mechanisms: alteration in neurotransmission, inflammation, and the connection between risk and precipitating factors.

Neurotransmitters act both on subcortical and cortical brain areas. Neuroimaging and somatosensory evoked potentials have shown the role of subcortical zones (such as pontine reticular formation, basal ganglia, and thalamus) in the onset of confusional state. In fact, attention and arousal are mediated by truncus encephali. Moreover, persons affected by clinical conditions associated with lesions on subcortical areas, like Parkinson disease or subcortical stroke, are susceptible for delirium. On the other side, electroencephalography (EEG) shows that delirium is associated with altered cortical function, that is, the slowdown of the dominant alpha rhythm and the onset of slow-wave activity, which is not physiological. Attention is governed by cortical functions, particularly in the frontal lobes. Thus, we can suppose that delirious patients with inattention might have altered pathways on these regions.

Acetylcholine seems to participate in the pathogenesis of delirium. We know how this neurotransmitter plays a fundamental role in Alzheimer disease, in which there is loss of cholinergic neurons. Some neuroleptic and cardiovascular medications, such as clozapine, olanzapine, and atropine, exhibit anticholinergic activity; at therapeutic doses, their serum concentration on elderly is likely to increase [9]. These considerations might explain why polymedicated older people affected by Alzheimer disease are at high risk to manifest delirium. Moreover, in some precipitating conditions for delirium, such as hypoxia and hypoglycemia, the acetylcholine synthesis decreases. Nevertheless, anticholinergic inhibitors do not prevent delirium [10].

The altered serum concentrations of other neurotransmitter, such as dopamine, gamma-aminobutyric acid (GABA), glutamate, melatonin, somatostatin, endorphins, serotonin, histamine, and norepinephrine, have been seen. Drugs that act against these molecules can develop delirium-like symptoms. The most described pathophysiological mechanisms for these neurotransmitters are: increased synthesis of dopamine, glutamate, or norepinephrine; reduced melatonin availability; and excess or deficiency, depending on symptoms presentation, of GABA, serotonin, and histamine concentration [11].

None of these altered pathways might develop the clinical manifestation of delirium alone. It is more reasonable that more than one abnormal mechanism is involved in the pathogenesis of delirium.

Inflammation develops in specific clinical situations, such as infections, cancer, surgery, or after falls. The interleukins and tumor necrosis factor-alpha levels increase during the onset of delirium, especially with hyperactive forms. Moreover, inflammation may alter the blood-brain barrier, and consequently it can promote the activity of cytokines and drugs on central nervous system.

Different clinical factors can participate in the pathogenesis of confusional states. At first, we must consider those *risk factors* (▶ Box 35.1) which expose patients to major vulnerability. The most common chronic diseases associated with delirium are dementia, other cerebral disorders, and advanced cancer. Among acute illnesses, we must mention stroke, hip fracture, and dehydration. Depression, drugs, and alcohol addiction represent other risk factors for confusional states. Advanced age, if interested with multimorbidity and polypharmacy, makes a person more prone to complications. Malnutrition and sarcopenia can worsen the functional state. Generally, frail people present reduced tolerance to exogenous factors, which determines adverse health outcomes, including delirium.

Risk factors, if connected with precipitating factors, cause the onset of delirium. In ▶ Box 35.2 we can mention all the recognized precipitating factors among very older people, both out or during the hospital stay. Drugs represent the most common reason for the onset of delirium. Antipsychotics are effective in the resolution of acute psychomotor disorders, but they can also increase the risk of delirium. Sedative-hypnotics, skeletal muscle relaxers, and opioids can cause confusional states. Generally, the risk of delirium increases as much as the number of prescribed medications augments. Among acute disorders, we can include fever, infections, heart failure, hypoxemia, and electrolyte disorders. If pain is untreated or undertreated, it might precipitate delirium. Hospitalization exposes to alteration in daily routine, particularly for people with reduced autonomy and cognitive impairment. Environmental modifications are fundamental in the onset of delirium. Sharing room with other patients and sleep deprivation should be considered. Finally, but not less important, physical restraints and all medical devices, such as urinary catheters, nasogastric tubes, central and peripheral venous catheters, oxygen devices, and tracheostomy, precipitate delirium.

Box 35.1   Risk Factors for Delirium

Aging

Cerebral disorders

Dementia

Brain cancer

Stroke

Multimorbidity

Polypharmacy

Reduced functional state

Malnutrition

Sarcopenia

Frailty

Advanced cancer

Hip fracture

Dehydration

Depression

Drugs or alcohol addiction

Box 35.2   Precipitating Factors for Delirium on Very Old Patient

Drugs

Analgesics (opioids, NSAIDs)

Antibiotics and antivirals (cephalosporins, penicillins, fluoroquinolones, linezolid, metronidazole, aminoglycosides, isoniazid, rifampin, sulfonamides, acyclovir)

Anticonvulsants (carbamazepine, levetiracetam, phenytoin, valproate)

Antidepressants (mirtazapine, selective serotonin reuptake inhibitors, tricyclic antidepressants)

Antihistamines

Antipsychotics

Cardiovascular drugs (atropine, beta blockers, antiarrhythmics, clonidine, digoxin, diuretics)

Corticosteroids

Diphenhydramine

Dopamine agonists (levodopa, pramipexole, ropinirole, amantadine)

Gastrointestinal drugs (antiemetics, loperamide, scopolamine, histamine-2 receptor blockers)

Hypoglycemics

Sedative-hypnotics (barbiturates, benzodiazepines)

Skeletal muscle relaxers

Other drugs (lithium, disulfiram, phenothiazines, cholinesterase inhibitors)

Drugs side effects

Hyperammonemia from valproic acid

Serotonin syndrome

Drugs of abuse and poisons

Ethanol

Hallucinogens

Heroin

Others (carbon monoxide, methanol, ethylene glycol)

Pain

Fever

Infections

Pneumonia

Urinary tract infections

Sepsis

Encephalitis

Meningitis

Abdominal infections

Hypoxemia

Electrolyte disorders

Hypoglycemia

Hypovolemia

Myocardial infarction

Acute organ failure

Head injury

Major trauma

Hospitalization

Hip surgery

Major surgery

Environmental modifications

Sleep deprivation

Physical restraints

Medical devices

Urinary catheters

Peripheral venous catheters

Central venous catheters

Nasogastric tubes

Oxygen devices

Tracheostomy

Monitoring devices

Urinary retention

Fecal impaction

35.5 Clinical Presentation

The diagnosis of delirium is not self-evident, due to the complex variety of presentation, as it can manifest in different ways, and often requires an experienced clinician. Among younger people, an underlying illness is more likely to be found; on elderly, an acute disease might not manifest itself except for behavioral disorders. As discussed before, delirium can manifest with hypoactive or hyperactive form [12]. The first one is the most common phenotype on very old people, and it is characterized by lethargy, inability to be alert when awake, and reduced psychomotor functions. These alterations can be confused with depressed mood or fatigue; for this reason, it is often not recognized. On the other side, the hyperactive form manifests itself with symptoms of agitation, increased alertness, and often hallucinations. Moreover, patients may fluctuate from the hypoactive to the hyperactive phenotype (mixed motor type). The mixed form represents a critical diagnostic challenge for physician, to differentiate it from psychotic illnesses and mood disorders. The hallmarks of delirium are the acute onset and the disturbance of attention. One of the first manifestations of delirium is an altered level of consciousness and the inability to maintain attention (e.g., easy distractibility). However, assessing the delirious patient's attention is not simple, especially if the cognitive status before the acute event is unknown. The role of caregivers is often necessary, to assess what the patient's functional level was before delirium has started. The onset of this confusional state is generally abrupt, occurring within hours or days. A critical aspect is the fluctuating course, with symptoms having significant variations within 24 hours, with alternating moments of lucidity and severe exacerbation of delirium. The worst moments for the onset of symptoms are the evening or nighttime hours, while during daily hours a normal and lucid state is typical. These fluctuations do not help the clinician during the assessment of delirium. A delirious patient also shows easily distraction, fails to perform complex tasks, and does not follow the thread of a conversation. He may present with disorganization of thought, which evolve into non-fluent, incoherent, and disorganized speech. Other signs might include temporospatial disorientation, memory alterations, psychomotor agitation, perceptual alterations, sleep-wake cycle alterations, and emotional instability. Perceptual alterations might be visual, auditory, or somatosensory hallucinations, with little insight or misinterpretations of objects or people (i.e., mistaking one person or an object for another). Delirium can be often preceded by a prodromal phase, including easy irritability, mood alterations, restlessness, alterations in sleep-wake rhythm, and hypersensitivity to sound or light.

35.6 Diagnosis

Detecting the clinical history of delirium is fundamental in the process of diagnosis. During the first evaluation, preexisting cognitive status and changes of mental status must be investigated. It is critical to search for a possible cause of delirium and evaluate every acute reported symptom, such as pain or dysuria. It is important to investigate those symptoms/signs appeared during the last hours or days, medications or their recent changes, and the previous history, evaluating any previous episode and comorbidities. In an estimated 70% of cases, the clinician does not recognize delirium. The diagnosis of delirium is primarily clinical, and it is often difficult to do a history collection and a careful cognitive assessment. Evaluation scales might help on this phase.

35.6.1 Physical Examination

The physical examination will investigate any detectable causes, such as signs of infection, dehydration, focal neurologic changes, or thermal changes. It may be complex to make a completely objective assessment in a patient who is poorly cooperating. Furthermore, it is important to pay attention on the physiological changes among elderly, which might alter the clinical presentation of common diseases. Some examples are infections, such as sepsis, which can manifest with a temperature lower than 38.5°, acute coronary syndrome that might arise without chest pain, or pneumonia with any auscultatory or radiographic changes. Moreover, older persons with delirium are unable to report pain. Neurological objective examination, although it may be altered and tainted by the presence of inattention and altered consciousness, may reveal focal neurological signs of new onset, such as cranial nerve or visual field alterations, or multisegmental disorders, such as myoclonus or tremor. Some specific signs, such as multifocal myoclonus, asterixis, or postural action tremor, are usually associated with a metabolic/toxic cause of delirium.

35.6.2 Evaluation Scales

In order to obtain a correct diagnosis, the various aspects of delirium must be considered. For this purpose, the use of evaluation scales can be helpful. There are several assessment scales, both for identification of delirium and identification of its severity. Among identification scales, the most known one is the Confusion Assessment Method (CAM) [13], of which some variants have been validated depending on the setting where it is performed (e.g., CAM-ICU in the intensive care unit, CAM-ED and B-CAM in emergency rooms, and NH-CAM in nursing homes). The 3D-CAM takes 3 min to perform it and evaluates the cardinal and accessory clinical features of delirium. Another quick and simple test is the 4AT scale that is based on four items, and its purpose is to identify the presence of delirium. Tools for assessing the severity of delirium include the Delirium Index, the Memorial Delirium Assessment Scale, and the Delirium Rating Scale. Each scale has strengths and limitations, so it is important that the choice of a scale is made by experienced clinicians.

35.6.3 Searching for Precipitating Factors

As part of the initial evaluation of a patient with delirium, it is critical to search potential causes of delirium. It is important to identify life-threatening conditions and exclude confounding factors or possible alternative diagnoses. The most common causes of delirium are postoperative status, infections (e.g., respiratory inflammation, urinary tract infection), pain syndromes, alterations in hydro-electrolyte balance, metabolic disorders (e.g., hypoglycemia, uremia, liver failure), hypoperfusion states such as shock, and withdrawal or toxicity of certain medications.

35.6.4 Laboratory and Instrumental Tests

Nowadays, there is no specific diagnostic test for delirium. The choice to perform specific tests depends on clinical picture. They might be useful to identify the underlying cause of delirium. We can mention some common laboratory and instrumental tests, usually performed to achieve the diagnosis of the underlying illness: complete blood count; renal, liver, and pancreatic function; serum electrolytes; blood glucose; inflammatory markers; chest x-ray; electrocardiogram (EKG); urinalysis; and arterial blood gas test. Culture tests should be requested only in the suspicion of an ongoing infectious state. Other blood tests should be considered patient by patient, and they might include vitamins (e.g., B12), thyroid and adrenal hormones, blood ammonium, plasma drug assays, and screening for specific infectious diseases (e.g., syphilis). In selected cases, such as a patient with febrile delirium or neurologic signs, some tests like brain imaging, lumbar puncture, or electroencephalogram (EEG) might be performed.

	Table 35.1 Main clinical differences between delirium and dementia	
	Delirium	**Dementia**
Onset	Acute (hour/days)[a]	Progressive, insidious (months/years)
Attention	Impaired (fluctuating)[a]	Stable
Orientation	Impaired (but fluctuating)	Normal until late stage (less fluctuating)
Course in a day	Fluctuating	No major changes
Consciousness	Variable, from lethargic to hyperalert	Normal until late stage
Hallucination	Visual (auditory)	Sometimes
Memory	Impaired commonly	Prominent impairment
Speech	Disorganized, illogical, incoherent	Aphasia, anomia
Delusions	Common	Common

[a]Hallmark of delirium

35.7 Differential Diagnosis

It is not easy to differentiate a chronic confusional state, as dementia can be, from delirium alone or delirium superimposed on dementia. However, delirium differs from dementia in some clinical features (■ Table 35.1). Cognitive impairment has a more progressive and insidious onset, where fluctuations are, if present, very nuanced. The Lewy body dementia has more pronounced fluctuations in attention, but visual hallucinations (especially animal images) are more frequent and typical. Some psychiatric disorders might enter in differential diagnosis with delirium, such as acute psychosis or depressive disorder. A particular phenomenon, still poorly understood, is sundowning, typical of patients with dementia, in which the deterioration occurs in the evening hours and it can be confused with delirium.

35.8 Prevention

Prevention is a fundamental aspect to avoid the onset of delirium, particularly for very old people, admitted on hospital setting. A wide set of nonpharmacologic measures and individualized approaches might reduce the risk of confusional state. These strategies aim to provide supportive and regenerative care, prevent cognitive and physical decline, and minimize or eliminate precipitating factors. Some of the interventions that can help to reduce the risk of delirium are descripted below, and they can be applied also during the ICU stay.

Several procedures are specific to hospitalized patients which include reducing the length of stay in the emergency room, preventing falls in patients with a reduced functional state, and creating specialized spaces for hospitalized patients with delirium (delirium room). Furthermore, the activation of geriatric counseling in some contexts (e.g., postoperative states after hip fracture surgery) could be important in the process of recovery. No medications have shown to prevent delirium. Currently, several classes of drugs could be effective in preventing delirium. Some of these include antipsychotics, dexmedetomidine, melatonin and melatonin agonists, gabapentinoids, and cholinesterase inhibitors. Nevertheless, we suggest focusing on multicomponent, nonpharmacologic interventions to modify risk factors and reduce the incidence of delirium [14].

> **Practical Implications**
>
> To prevent delirium, we can suggest some strategies:
> - Try to avoid exposure to some instrumental devices that may contribute to the development of delirium (e.g., indwelling bladder catheters)
> - Remove precipitating factors, physical restraints, indwelling catheter, conditions of impaired visual or auditory function, and treat pain as soon as possible
> - Limit immobilization as much as possible (as in postoperative bedding), encouraging early mobilization (even from the first postoperative day), with the activation of motor rehabilitation services
> - Limit sleep deprivation and promote physiological sleep, particularly in hospitalized patients, by limiting medical and nursing interventions at night and reducing noise and any source of sleep disturbance
> - Avoid or monitor closely categories of drugs or substances that may facilitate the onset of delirium (e.g., benzodiazepines, opioids, antidepressants, dopamine agonists)
> - Ensure adequate hydration
> - Promote moderate cognitive stimulation through regular family visits, especially for patients with cognitive impairment (but overstimulation is not recommended)
> - Use reorientation procedures, such as providing tools like clocks and calendars
> - Ensure the availability and easy access to non-threatening personal effects

35.9 Management

The management of delirium consists into two main components that happen simultaneously: supportive therapy and assessment of the underlying cause.

35.9.1 Etiological Treatment

Once the potential cause of delirium is identified, therapy is needed. The treatment of the underlying condition might be pharmacologic or nonpharmacologic, and that is specific to each hypothesized cause, such as analgesics for pain, antibiotic therapy for infections, fluid replacement for dehydration, drug removal, or antidote for drug toxicity.

35.9.2 Supportive Therapy: Nonpharmacological Treatment

Nonpharmacologic treatment is the first-line choice in the management of delirium itself. This type of intervention includes reorientation and behavioral practices, for example, allowing as soon as possible family members to be close to the patient, or showing calendars, clocks, objects from the patient's home. It is important that the patient with hearing or visual impairments has hearing aids or glasses. Communication with the delirious patients is also critical: reassure and calm them, attempt reorientation, and explain where they are and what is happening. These patients could be able to appreciate specific aspects of the communication: a calmly and quietly speech, nonverbal language, sitting close to the patient, maintaining eye contact, smiling, and appearing friendly. On the other hand, superficial, hostile, hasty, heedless, or surly attitudes will most likely be counterproductive. Temporary use of physical restraints is allowed if they are the only available way to ensure the patient's safety. Therefore, it is advisable to promote the patient's mobility and autonomy as much as possible, reducing bedridden time and placing personal belongings. Other relevant factors to consider are good ambient illumination, preferably natural, during daylight hours, whereas it is important to limit light sources and noise during nighttime hours. Other strategies to improve sleep quality in a nonpharmacological way are music and bright light therapy. To achieve these objectives, "delirium rooms" are increasingly common and specifically created for this type of patient. Although there are conflicting data, it seems that nonpharmacological interventions can reduce the duration and occurrence of delirium [14, 15].

35.9.3 Supportive Therapy: Pharmacological Treatment

Pharmacologic management is based on symptomatic treatments (■ Table 35.2). Drugs need to be administered in the hyperactive delirium. On hypoactive delirious patients, there is no agreement on the use of antipsychotics or psychostimulants.

■ ■ Antipsychotic Medications

The use of these medications for the treatment of delirium is off-label. This class of drugs is effective in delirium and psychomotor agitation to prevent the patient from harming themselves. The most frequently used drug is haloperidol [16], which can be administered orally or parenterally, either intramuscularly or intravenously; however, the latter is to be reserved in patients in whom the rapid onset of drug effect is required, paying attention to the risk of polymorphic ventricular tachycardia and sudden death. The initial haloperidol dose must be low (0.25–10.5 mg), repeatable every 30 min, until sedation is achieved or up to a maximum of 5 mg per day. However, older patients never treated with antipsychotic treatment require a maximum initial daily dosage of 3–5 mg. A maintenance dose, corresponding to half of the loading dose, should be administered in the course of the next 24 h. Then, it might be scaled up over the next 48 h as agitation resolves.

Continuous or prophylactic administration of haloperidol is not advisable. In any case, the time of haloperidol administration should be as short as possible

Table 35.2 Main antipsychotic medications for delirium in older adults

Pharmacological treatment	Dose	Mechanism of action	Focus on	Geriatric considerations
Haloperidol	**PO**: Initial 0.5–0.1 mg (may repeat every 30 min) **IM/IV**: 0.125–0.25 mg (may repeat every 30 min) Max: 5 mg/day **Maintenance dose**: Half loading dose in multiple doses over the next 24 h, with subsequent tapering in 48–72 h	**Blockade of brain dopamine receptor D2**	Extrapyramidal syndrome (dystonia, dyskinesia, parkinsonism, akathisia, dysphagia) is dose related QT prolongation, cardiac arrhythmia, and cardiac arrest Pneumonia Leukopenia and thrombocytopenia Neuroleptic malignant syndrome Seizures Glycemic and lipid parameters and weight gain Electrolytes (hyponatremia/SIADH) Sexual dysfunction Hypothermia *Not indicated in Parkinson disease and Lewy body dementia*	Beers criteria: High risk medication (increased risk of cerebrovascular accident, cognitive decline, and mortality)
Risperidone	**PO**: 0.5–1 mg every 4 h, max 2–3 mg/day	**Antagonism of 5-HT2, dopamine-D2, alpha 1, alpha 2 adrenergic and histaminergic receptors** Low affinity for 5-HT1a, 5-HT1c, 5-HT1d and dopamine-D1	Extrapyramidal syndrome (dystonia, dyskinesia, parkinsonism, akathisia, dysphagia) is dose related QT prolongation, cardiac arrhythmia, and cardiac arrest Pneumonia Leukopenia and thrombocytopenia Neuroleptic malignant syndrome Angioedema Glycemic and lipid parameters and weight gain Orthostatic hypotension, syncope, falling Sexual dysfunction Hypothermia	Beers criteria: High risk medication (increased risk of cerebrovascular accident, cognitive decline, and mortality)

■ **Table 35.2** (continued)

Pharmacological treatment	Dose	Mechanism of action	Focus on	Geriatric considerations
Quetiapine	**PO/nasogastric tube**: Initial 12.5–25 mg once/twice daily. Increase gradually based on response	**Antagonism of 5-HT2, dopamine-D2, alpha 1, alpha 2 adrenergic, histaminergic receptors, dopamine-D1**	Extrapyramidal syndrome (dystonia, dyskinesia, parkinsonism, akathisia, dysphagia) is dose related QT prolongation, cardiac arrhythmia, and cardiac arrest Leukopenia and thrombocytopenia Neuroleptic malignant syndrome Orthostatic hypotension, syncope, falling Sexual dysfunction Glycemic and lipid parameters and weight gain Anticholinergic syndrome (constipation, urinary retention, xerostomia, blurred vision)	Beers criteria: High risk medication (increased risk of cerebrovascular accident, cognitive decline, and mortality) May be used with more safety in Parkinson's disease
Olanzapine	**PO/IM**: 2.5 mg once daily	**Strong antagonism of 5-HT2a, 5-HT2c, dopamine-D1–4, histamine H1, alpha1-adrenergic receptors. Moderate antagonism 5-HT3, muscarinic M1–5**	Extrapyramidal syndrome (dystonia, dyskinesia, parkinsonism, akathisia, dysphagia) is dose related QT prolongation, cardiac arrhythmia, and cardiac arrest Leukopenia and thrombocytopenia Neuroleptic malignant syndrome Orthostatic hypotension, syncope, falling Sexual dysfunction Glycemic and lipid parameters and weight gain Anticholinergic syndrome (constipation, urinary retention, xerostomia, blurred vision) Hypersensitivity reactions	Beers criteria: High risk medication (increased risk of cerebrovascular accident, cognitive decline, and mortality)

because of the increased risk of mortality and stroke in patients with dementia. Strong antipsychotics, such as haloperidol, expose to an increased risk of extrapyramidal effects and acute dystonia. These effects are dose-dependent and occur for doses greater than 4–5 mg per day. In addition, especially in elderly patients, this drug can accumulate on the body, and side effects can develop with submaximal doses. Also, its use in patients with Parkinson's disease is not recommended. Atypical antipsychotics such as quetiapine, risperidone, and olanzapine have been shown to have fewer side effects and similar efficacy [17]. However, haloperidol remains the most widely used drug because of the greater clinical experience with its use [18]. Some evidence, however, seems to indicate that antipsychotics might prolong the duration of delirium.

■■ Benzodiazepines

This class of drugs is not recommended as a first-line therapy for delirium. Benzodiazepines, such as lorazepam, have a rapid onset of pharmacologic effects. However, they can cause worsening delirium, paradoxical agitation, and excessive sedation, particularly on elderly. An exception is delirium caused by alcohol or drug withdrawal, seizures, or when antipsychotics are contraindicated. In this case, we suggest to consider low-dose lorazepam (0.5 mg). It is important to remember that benzodiazepines are chronically used by older patients, and we need to pay attention to the risk of withdrawal syndrome when modifying such therapy.

■■ Others

Other drugs have been studied in the past, such as cholinesterase inhibitors, propofol, dexmedetomidine, selective serotonin reuptake inhibitors, and clonidine. Studies conducted have shown conflicting results, and there is no consensus on their use in delirium treatment.

35.9.4 Special Circumstances: End-Life Patients

Delirium in palliative care is common; more than 80% of terminally ill patients develop delirium, either in the hyperactive or hypoactive form. It is essential to involve both patient and family on establishing the goals of treatments, assessing the needs of the patient and his family, and discussing together the intensity and appropriateness of possible medical treatments. As already mentioned, the cause of delirium is often identifiable and removable, but in some cases, particularly in palliative care settings, it may result in the practice of invasive procedures. Nonpharmacological treatment is the first-line recommended approach also on these patients [19]. Sedation should be considered, but it will affect the interaction with family members. Medications used in this context are primarily antipsychotics, especially haloperidol. If sedation is required, lorazepam is the first-line agent, with a starting dose of 0.5–1 mg, either orally or parenterally, which is short-acting and easily titrated.

35.10 **Prognosis**

Older and very older adults are highly susceptible to worse outcomes from delirium: increased risk for mortality, cognitive decline, institutionalization, and prolonged hospitalization. Delirium appears to be an independent marker of mortality at 6–12 months after hospitalization [20]. In addition, delirium sequelae may persist for a long time. Some studies have shown that some degree of cognitive dysfunction was present even at 12 months, especially if an underlying cognitive impairment was present. Furthermore, although delirium has always been considered a transient and reversible condition, in some cases, delirium can persist for a prolonged time, even for months, while some studies indicate that about 20% of patients have complete resolution of symptoms within the first few months after the acute event. Finally, a clear correlation between the severity of the clinical picture and outcomes has not yet been demonstrated. However, a report indicated that patients with severe delirium following femoral fracture surgery have a higher mortality rate and a subsequent admission to a nursing home [21].

Conclusion

Delirium represents a common complication for the elderly patient with an acute disease. It is associated with worse outcomes and higher risk of mortality. Older and very older persons are more susceptible to delirium due to the higher incidence of dementia, reduced functional state, or multimorbidity. Preventing delirium among people with those risk factors for the onset of confusional state should not be underestimated. All the probable precipitating factors for the onset of delirium must be investigated to perform an appropriate approach to this issue. Some interventions to reduce the risk of delirium can be applied in every hospital department, including ICU. Management of delirium concerns the resolution of precipitating factors and the treatment of delirium itself both with nonpharmacological and pharmacological therapies.

Take-Home Messages

- Delirium mainly affects hospitalized older people with previous cognitive impairment.
- Delirium is associated with a longer stay and increased risk of mortality.
- Untreated pain, infections, and major surgery might precipitate delirium. The use of medical devices is less tolerated by vulnerable people.
- Management of the underlying cause is fundamental in the process of care, both for community dwelling and hospitalized patients.
- Treatments with drugs for delirium itself must not be the only strategy for the recovery of old delirious patients.
- Preventing delirium is fundamental for clinicians who approach the old and the very old patient. Environmental actions to facilitate orientation, physiologic sleep, avoiding physical restraints, and promoting early mobilization should be considered, also on ICU.

References

1. Slooter AJ, Van De Leur RR, Zaal IJ. Delirium in critically ill patients. Handb Clin Neurol. 2017;141:449–66. https://doi.org/10.1016/B978-0-444-63599-0.00025-9.
2. Marcantonio ER. Delirium in hospitalized older adults. N Engl J Med. 2017;377(15):1456–66. https://doi.org/10.1056/NEJMcp1605501. PMID: 29020579; PMCID: PMC5706782.
3. Caplan GA, Teodorczuk A, Streatfeild J, Agar MR. The financial and social costs of delirium. Eur Geriatr Med. 2020;11(1):105–12. https://doi.org/10.1007/s41999-019-00257-2. Epub 2019 Dec 21
4. Schubert M, Schürch R, Boettger S, Garcia Nuñez D, Schwarz U, Bettex D, Jenewein J, Bogdanovic J, Staehli ML, Spirig R, Rudiger A. A hospital-wide evaluation of delirium prevalence and outcomes in acute care patients - a cohort study. BMC Health Serv Res. 2018;18(1):550. https://doi.org/10.1186/s12913-018-3345-x. PMID: 30005646; PMCID: PMC6045819.
5. Elie M, Rousseau F, Cole M, Primeau F, McCusker J, Bellavance F. Prevalence and detection of delirium in elderly emergency department patients. CMAJ. 2000;163(8):977–81. PMID: 11068569; PMCID: PMC80546.
6. McNicoll L, Pisani MA, Zhang Y, Ely EW, Siegel MD, Inouye SK. Delirium in the intensive care unit: occurrence and clinical course in older patients. J Am Geriatr Soc. 2003;51(5):591–8. https://doi.org/10.1034/j.1600-0579.2003.00201.x.
7. van den Boogaard M, Schoonhoven L, van der Hoeven JG, van Achterberg T, Pickkers P. Incidence and short-term consequences of delirium in critically ill patients: a prospective observational cohort study. Int J Nurs Stud. 2012;49(7):775–83. https://doi.org/10.1016/j.ijnurstu.2011.11.016. Epub 2011 Dec 22
8. Ely EW, Shintani A, Truman B, et al. Delirium as a predictor of mortality in mechanically ventilated patients in the intensive care unit. JAMA. 2004;291(14):1753–62. https://doi.org/10.1001/jama.291.14.1753.
9. Chew ML, Mulsant BH, Pollock BG, Lehman ME, Greenspan A, Mahmoud RA, Kirshner MA, Sorisio DA, Bies RR, Gharabawi G. Anticholinergic activity of 107 medications commonly used by older adults. J Am Geriatr Soc. 2008;56(7):1333–41. https://doi.org/10.1111/j.1532-5415.2008.01737.x. Epub 2008 May 26
10. Tampi RR, Tampi DJ, Ghori AK. Acetylcholinesterase inhibitors for delirium in older adults. Am J Alzheimers Dis Other Dement. 2016;31(4):305–10. https://doi.org/10.1177/1533317515619034. Epub 2015 Dec 8
11. Maldonado JR. Neuropathogenesis of delirium: review of current etiologic theories and common pathways. Am J Geriatr Psychiatry. 2013;21(12):1190–222. https://doi.org/10.1016/j.jagp.2013.09.005.
12. Peterson JF, Pun BT, Dittus RS, Thomason JW, Jackson JC, Shintani AK, Ely EW. Delirium and its motoric subtypes: a study of 614 critically ill patients. J Am Geriatr Soc. 2006;54(3):479–84. https://doi.org/10.1111/j.1532-5415.2005.00621.x.
13. Marcantonio ER, Ngo LH, O'Connor M, Jones RN, Crane PK, Metzger ED, Inouye SK. 3D-CAM: derivation and validation of a 3-minute diagnostic interview for CAM-defined delirium: a cross-sectional diagnostic test study. Ann Intern Med. 2014;161(8):554–61. https://doi.org/10.7326/M14-0865. Erratum in: Ann Intern Med. 2014 Nov 18;161(10):764. PMID: 25329203; PMCID: PMC4319978.
14. Hshieh TT, Yue J, Oh E, Puelle M, Dowal S, Travison T, Inouye SK. Effectiveness of multicomponent nonpharmacological delirium interventions: a meta-analysis. JAMA Intern Med. 2015;175(4):512–20. https://doi.org/10.1001/jamainternmed.2014.7779. Erratum in: JAMA Intern Med. 2015 Apr;175(4):659. PMID: 25643002; PMCID: PMC4388802.
15. Kang J, Lee M, Ko H, Kim S, Yun S, Jeong Y, Cho Y. Effect of nonpharmacological interventions for the prevention of delirium in the intensive care unit: a systematic review and meta-analysis. J Crit Care. 2018;48:372–84., ISSN 0883-9441. https://doi.org/10.1016/j.jcrc.2018.09.032.
16. Girard TD, Exline MC, Carson SS, Hough CL, Rock P, Gong MN, Douglas IS, Malhotra A, Owens RL, Feinstein DJ, Khan B, Pisani MA, Hyzy RC, Schmidt GA, Schweickert WD, Hite RD, Bowton DL, Masica AL, Thompson JL, Chandrasekhar R, Pun BT, Strength C, Boehm LM, Jackson JC, Pandharipande PP, Brummel NE, Hughes CG, Patel MB, Stollings JL, Bernard GR, Dittus RS, Ely EW, MIND-USA Investigators. Haloperidol and ziprasidone for treatment of delirium in critical illness. N Engl J Med. 2018;379(26):2506–16. https://doi.org/10.1056/NEJMoa1808217. Epub 2018 Oct 22. PMID: 30346242; PMCID: PMC6364999.

17. Gilchrist NA, Asoh I, Greenberg B. Atypical antipsychotics for the treatment of ICU delirium. J Intensive Care Med. 2012;27(6):354–61. https://doi.org/10.1177/0885066611403110. Epub 2011 Mar 25

18. Inouye SK, Westendorp RG, Saczynski JS. Delirium in elderly people. Lancet. 2014;383(9920):911–22. https://doi.org/10.1016/S0140-6736(13)60688-1. Epub 2013 Aug 28. PMID: 23992774; PMCID: PMC4120864.

19. Clegg A, Siddiqi N, Heaven A, Young J, Holt R. Interventions for preventing delirium in older people in institutional long-term care. Cochrane Database Syst Rev. 2014;1:CD009537. https://doi.org/10.1002/14651858.CD009537.pub2.

20. McCusker J, Cole M, Abrahamowicz M, Primeau F, Belzile E. Delirium predicts 12-month mortality. Arch Intern Med. 2002;162(4):457–63. https://doi.org/10.1001/archinte.162.4.457.

21. Marcantonio E, Ta T, Duthie E, Resnick NM. Delirium severity and psychomotor types: their relationship with outcomes after hip fracture repair. J Am Geriatr Soc. 2002;50(5):850–7. https://doi.org/10.1046/j.1532-5415.2002.50210.x. PMID: 12028171

Logistic Challenges and Constraints in Intensive Care During a Pandemic

Sigal Sviri, Michael Beil, Yoram G. Weiss, Arie Ben-Yehuda, and P. Vernon van Heerden

Contents

H. Flaatten et al. (eds.), *The Very Old Critically Ill Patients*, Lessons from the ICU,
https://doi.org/10.1007/978-3-030-94133-8_36

⚲ Learning Objectives

- To discuss the major challenges hospitals and ICUs are faced with during prolonged periods of increased morbidity and demand.
- To discuss the importance of flexibility in resource allocation during increasing and decreasing demand.
- To understand the importance of prioritization at a national, regional, and institutional level.
- To discuss options for increasing availability of personnel and equipment
- To understand the importance of staff safety, protection, and reducing burnout
- To increase pre and post ICU capabilities
- To improve triage decisions in the elderly population
- To plan for future events based on past experience

36.1 Introduction

We define a "disaster" in the medical sphere as any situation in which the number of casualties or cases exceeds the available resources to deal with them [1]. Twenty victims of a bomb blast on a bus may represent a sudden emergency, while many cases presenting with respiratory failure due to viral pneumonitis caused by COVID-19 may represent a more gradual emergency [2, 3]. Health system planners are very familiar with planning for acute surges in cases as may occur after a natural occurrence (earthquake or flooding) or a terrorist attack, and although such an occurrence may temporarily overwhelm the healthcare system, it is soon over (in a matter of weeks or days) [1, 4]. What we are less used to dealing with, and which we have now unfortunately been schooled in, is planning for and dealing with a situation where medical resources are inundated and indeed overwhelmed for a prolonged period of time (weeks and months) [5]. This chapter will address some aspects of the logistic challenges in the practice of intensive care medicine under pandemic conditions and how they have been dealt with. ◻ Table 36.1 summarizes the major challenges and suggested solutions.

◻ **Table 36.1** Summary of major challenges and suggested solutions

	Challenges	Suggested solutions
Flexibility	Sudden and quick/exponential increases in patient load Fluctuating load according to surges and lockdown measures Changing requirements for equipment and personnel Availability of PPE Extended period of uncertainty	Flexibility in admitting changing number of patients in a short period of time Expanding and decreasing number of dedicated beds and human resources depending on surges **Quick planning by management** and regular multidisciplinary meetings, updates, and overseeing implementation **Integrating new knowledge** about disease mechanisms and evidence (e.g., requirement for invasive interventions, updating treatment protocols)
National prioritization	Protecting the healthcare system	Lockdown measures Vaccination programs

□ Table 36.1 (continued)

	Challenges	Suggested solutions
Regional prioritization	Providing adequate care for Covid-19 and non-Covid-19 patients Adjusting load	Dedicated Covid-19 wards or hospitals Transferring patients to less overloaded centers
Institutional prioritization	Dedicated area for Covid-19 patients Providing adequate care for Covid-19 and non-Covid-19 patients	**Expanding intensive care facilities**, beds, equipment, and personnel Deciding which services to maintain and which to reduce
Equipment	Purchasing and producing a large number of equipment in a short period of time Competing with other centers/countries Costs	Quick decision-making Dedicated funds (government support, national funds, diversion of hospital funds, donations) Planning future needs
Personnel and burnout	Shortage in critical care nurses and doctors Maintaining standard of care Mixed teams having to work together Long working hours Difficult working conditions High patient load High mortality	**Planning additional training programs and continuous updates and refresher courses** (e.g., ESICM online training programs) Mixing ICU nurses with non-ICU nurses Recruiting and training non-ICU physicians and nurses Reducing nurse/patient ratio **Support groups** **Psychological support** Changing teams regularly Childcare arrangements Positive feedback and acknowledgment Overtime and bonuses
Staff safety	High risk for staff and their families Absences due to exposure and fatigue/burnout	Providing constant and adequate PPE **Regular staff PCR testing** Priority in vaccinations
Pre- and post-ICU care	Large patient load in the community Reducing hospitalizations After loading acute care beds	Increased home care capabilities Increased post Covid-19 respiratory and physical rehabilitation programs
Elderly patients	Improving triage to intensive care of elderly patients with uncertain reserve and prognosis	**Incorporating multi-morbidity and frailty in triage decisions** Considering a time-limited trial in the ICU Admission to high dependency units
Limited resources	Increased demand during ICU shortage	**Development and implementation of institutional and national triage guidelines** based on a broad consensus and within established legal and moral frameworks

(continued)

Table 36.1 (continued)

	Challenges	Suggested solutions
Future	Learning from the Covid-19 experience Planning for the next pandemic	Defining successes and failures Implementing conclusions Stressing the importance of intensive care, increasing ICU beds **Increasing pool of trained medical and nursing staff** Regular training programs and refresher courses Public relations work—Limits of what intensive care can achieve

36.2 Flexibility

It is true of any emergency that no amount of planning will foresee all eventualities, as described by the old adage that in times of war the best laid plans do not survive the first bullet fired. One of the first lessons for the healthcare system is to **heed warnings** and to be flexible in the response to the perceived load of cases expected [6, 7]. The warning period may be short (a few hours) in the event of a bomb blast before the cases start arriving at the hospital. It may also be longer, as we have seen during the COVID-19 pandemic, when we were able to see what was happening in the rest of the world and plan accordingly in the areas where we provide services. The healthcare system also needs to accommodate for increasing and decreasing morbidity, as surges come and go and thus be able to expand and reduce resources as required [8, 9].

In the case of the COVID-19 pandemic, we all had weeks to prepare for what was to come. What was uncertain was the scale of what we would have to deal with, especially during the first wave of the pandemic in Spring 2020. This brings us to the second important point—the healthcare system has to be **flexible** to be able to cope with the situation [10, 11]. We may have planned to deal with thousands of ventilated patients and only received hundreds, or vice versa. However, we had to deal with what we got. The uncertainty caused by the unknown morbidity of the disease resulted in, for instance, a run on mechanical ventilators around the world where suppliers were not able to meet the demand and factories were repurposed for the manufacture of these devices in several countries [12–15].

36.3 Prioritization

To provide and plan for the cases during the pandemic, there had to be a system of prioritization. This occurred at all levels. At the national level there had to be a decision to limit the spread of the disease with a system of lockdowns and curfews versus keeping businesses open and the economy vibrant [16]. Strict lockdown measures had severe economic consequences in most countries, especially in countries where citizens work as day laborers and depend on their daily income to feed their families [17]. In some countries this process was politicized, with demonstrations against lockdown measures [18]. Nations also had to deal with issues such as border closures, who to let into the country, and how to deal with new arrivals, such as place and duration of quarantine. Countries that were successful in reducing patient numbers placed their resources in strict lockdowns, limiting entry to the country and extensive "test and trace" procedures to identify cases and their contacts. All of these measures required resources or had an economic cost but resulted in less burden on the healthcare system and less lives lost, these all being economic upsides of this approach [19]. Other countries took a different approach and favored keeping the economy going at the expense of a greater burden on the healthcare system and subsequent greater loss of life.

Another, perhaps less welcome, aspect of national prioritization seen during the pandemic was increased nationalism in the management of resources, such as wealthier nation states paying a premium for medical equipment, such as mechanical ventilators, personal protection equipment (PPE), and vaccines, at the expense of those countries not able to pay high prices. The converse of this was the willingness to transfer critically ill patients from one country (with less available resources) to neighboring countries with more, as was seen with the transfer of cases between France, the Netherlands, and Germany, for instance, at the height of the pandemic.

There have also been excellent examples of resource prioritization on the **international** level, such as the rapid development of vaccines against COVID-19, where huge economic resources were diverted for this purpose, for the benefit of humanity in general.

Regional prioritization concerns planning on the city or state/provincial level, where decisions were made to concentrate resources for the care of COVID-19 patients, that is, not every hospital had to be able to receive patients requiring strict barrier isolation and intensive care services [20]. Some hospitals could be set up as COVID-19 hospitals, with the required equipment and staff to receive high numbers of these cases, while its other services could be moved to nearby hospitals [21]. This approach made the logistics of providing oxygen, medications, and PPE to fewer locations easier but placed a burden on patient transport systems in order to get patients to regional COVID-19 centers from further away. In some instances, new COVID-19 hospitals were set up de novo, such as the example of a 1000 bed hospital being set up in Wuhan, China, in a matter of weeks to deal with COVID-19 cases. The advantage of this approach, besides concentrating resources, is the ability to continue providing regular services at "unaffected" hospitals, this being of benefit to the populace (e.g., not cancelling elective surgery or cancer treatment) and providing ongoing income for the institutions, depending on the funding model.

The focus of this chapter is the local or **institutional prioritization** of resources to deal with the COVID-19 pandemic. There was involvement of hospital management, divisional reorganization and departmental (intensive care) reorganization, and expansion within each institution dealing with COVID-19 patients [22].

Hospital management had two main priorities, deciding on which services to retain during the pandemic and then providing the resources to expand the intensive care services in the hospital. Intensive care services benefited from the recognition they received by hospital management and the general population at large, as being essential to the care of critically ill COVID-19 patients, who require a high degree of monitoring and vigilance, all forms of supplemental oxygen therapy, including mechanical ventilation and extracorporeal membrane oxygenation (ECMO) and additional organ support [23]. Providing the infrastructure, space, beds, and equipment to provide these services was expensive and paid for out of existing funds, diversion of funds from other services, or new budgets provided by funding bodies such as state or national funding bodies [24]. There were many instances of misuse and misappropriation of these funds around the world in health systems usually chronically underfunded and then suddenly having access to "excess" funds. Management also had to oversee many aspects of the clinical management of COVID-19 patients, for example, setting up a committee to specifically review changing information from around the world and advise on current and acceptable therapeutic approaches.

In terms of providing the equipment, such as monitors and mechanical ventilators for newly established intensive care services, besides finding the means to purchase the equipment, hospitals also had trouble finding suppliers able to provide the equipment due to the increased worldwide demand [25]. Purchases also had to be made, not only with the immediate needs in mind but also with some thought to "the day after," that is, how the equipment would be utilized in the future after the pandemic had passed, and so purchase equipment responsibly and not in a panic. It has to be recognized that in many instances ICUs had to be set up de novo or existing ICUs had to be rapidly expanded. This required equipment and manpower.

A common realization at the institutional level, based on personal experience and a survey of European intensive care units (personal communication) was that, once the equipment needs had been satisfied, the major resource missing was trained intensive care nurses. Although nurses used to dealing with acute medical cases (such as recovery room and operating room nurses) were drafted in to help with COVID-19 cases, they were not initially able to provide the same level of service to the critically ill patients as their intensive care-trained colleagues. It took time for their integration into the intensive care therapeutic teams and for them to become familiar with equipment and procedures [26]. This deficit was much more pronounced when non-acute nurses (e.g., from dermatology) were drafted into intensive care units. It was difficult to provide intensive care services at the same level as pre-pandemic times for two more reasons related to nursing staff. Often the number of patients cared for by each nurse at any one was increased (less time per patient, staff exhaustion), and intensive care nurses may have been taken from their regular units to care for COVID-19 patients. This reduced the level of care to non-COVID-19 patients, resulting in so-called "collateral" damage to these patients.

Most hospitals coped with the nursing shortage, in addition to drafting in nurses from other areas and reducing the nurse to patient ratio in the intensive care units (ICUs), by also instituting urgent training schemes (courses and on-the-job training) for non-intensive care nurses, as well as rehiring nurses who had left or retired from the profession. There was also an increased use of support staff to reduce the workload on nurses, such as student nurses and aides [27]. A major realization was the fact that developing teamwork between new intensive care team members takes time before there is smooth functioning of the team, that is, all the elements of the team may be in place, but it takes time until the team works well together. The lesson from this is that nursing staff need to be continuously trained and refreshed in their knowledge of critical care, even in non-pandemic times, so that there is a known reservoir of trained nursing staff that can be called upon in times of emergency/disaster. Between refresher courses, they can be deployed to their usual places of work.

The shortage of intensive care medical personnel was also brought into sharp relief by the pandemic, resulting in longer shifts, more patients per doctor, use of nonspecialist doctors, and more use of support staff, such as medical students. In many institutions resident medical staff from all other specialties were required to work in the intensive care units.

Hospitals had to provide additional support services to medical and nursing staff to cope with the stressful working conditions and high morbidity and mortality among the COVID-19 critically ill patients, such as counseling services for burnout and post-traumatic stress [28–30]. Staff had to cope with a much higher death rate among patients (e.g., 50% of ventilated COVID-19 patients died, many more than regular intensive care patients), often while being exposed to an increased risk of being infected with the virus as well as witnessing their family, friends, and colleagues also getting sick [31].

There was a definite evolution of the use of resources at the institutional level during the pandemic [32], ranging from uncertainty about how many cases would be received and what resources would be needed to deal with them to eventually recognizing that resources supporting frontline staff had to be provided, such as counseling services and other psychological support.

Special areas had to be set up either in existing ICUs or newly established ICUs to be able to care for COVID-19 patients while working with full barrier precautions. Working in full PPE gear for any length of time is challenging for anyone. It also requires additional attention to everyday infection control procedures for non-intensive care trained staff as well as for intensive care doctors and nurses dealing with invasive procedures such as central line insertion and maintenance and tracheal intubation or tracheostomy [26]. It also demanded additional special resources, such as communication equipment to allow communication between the "inside" and "outside" environments of closed COVID-19 intensive care units.

Additional ancillary staff had to be enrolled to deal with the large numbers of critically ill patients and their distressed relatives, such as clergy, social workers, and psychologists [31, 33]. These additional human resources all came at an economic cost and sometimes to the detriment of their regular services. Additional support services such as laboratory personnel, clerical staff, medical engineering staff to deal with medical equipment, respiratory technicians, and others were all unexpected human resources that had to be found and enrolled in the service of patients affected by the pandemic.

All of the human resources mentioned above were subject to sudden and significant absences that had to be managed and covered, either due to illness or due to the need to isolate because of exposure at work or outside of the work environment. This required extreme flexibility in managing the human resources, as well as expending more resources in the regular polymerase chain reaction COVID-19 (PCR) testing of the staff [34, 35].

Several more issues arose from the management of human resources, which were unexpected and difficult to plan for:

- Expecting medical staff from different specialty backgrounds to work together in the care of COVID-19 patients and the time it took to build effective medical teams

- Childcare arrangements, especially for nursing staff who had to work while children were at home due to closure of schools or kindergartens
- The need to recognize the additional hard work of staff, for example, by paying occasional bonuses, such as occurred in several European countries.

The practical day-to-day management of patients in the COVID-19 ICUs was and is a challenge, requiring more time, patience, and resources, for example, obtaining specialist consultations (more time for outside specialists to attend to consultations), or performing bedside investigations such as echocardiography (needing a separate machine or delaying the investigation until the end of the day when the machine could be cleaned and decontaminated).

36.4 Pre- and Post-ICU Care of COVID-19 Patients

The healthcare system as a whole also had to find resources to deal with three other special groups of patients affected by the pandemic:
- Patients who became **sick at home** and who either could not or would not come to the hospital for treatment. Many such patients were cared for by home carers and visited by doctors and nurses at home. They also required resources such as oxygen therapy (supplied via cylinder or oxygen concentrator), medications, and radiology and laboratory tests [36]. It was estimated that at the height of the third wave of the pandemic in Israel, there were more than 1000 such patients being cared for at home.
- Patients who have recovered from acute COVID-19 and required prolonged mechanical ventilation and rehabilitation, either in hospital or dedicated institutions [37, 38].
- The relatively large number of patients who remained extremely hypoxemic despite best-practice mechanical ventilation and were treated with ECMO [39]. This is an extremely resource-intense activity.

None of these groups of patients were anticipated when planning for the pandemic.

Critically ill patients also clearly require support before admission to the ICU and after discharge from the ICU. This treatment falls to the regular wards in the hospital, be they medical or surgical wards, placing an additional burden on them also.

36.5 When Resources Are Limited

This chapter is not focused on the issue of patient triage (see chapter on "ICU decision-making under constraints"); however, the subject warrants a mention in the context of resources. When there is no possibility of increasing resources to meet demand, then in extreme cases the demand has to be reduced to meet the current resources. This is done by instituting a system of triage, where the patients most likely to benefit from intensive care are selected above those with a more limited prognosis [9, 40, 41]. In this light many national institutions or peak bodies in the specialty of intensive care drew up triage guidelines for use during the pandemic [42, 43]. There was some debate in the popular press not to base these guidelines on factors such as age or disability. We await political and legal review of these guidelines.

> ### The Elderly Patient with Uncertain Prognosis
>
> Even in non-pandemic times, the decision whether to admit elderly patients to intensive care is challenging; however, evidence has shown that there may be an increased benefit from intensive care in this population in comparison to younger cohorts [44]. It has also been shown that chronological age in itself is not the most precise predictor to determine benefit from intensive care [45]. Increased age is associated with multi-morbidity which is associated with increased mortality [46]. Frailty is another important parameter for assessing vulnerability and functional reserves during critical illness and is also associated with increased mortality [47–49].
>
> During pandemic times, when resources are limited and younger patients are competing for the last bed, the issues of age, multi-morbidity, and frailty become even more important for triage decisions [50, 51].
>
> A possible solution for such dilemmas may be a time-limited trial, where patients' response to critical care is reassessed at certain time points and the level of further support is then determined accordingly [52].
>
> In periods of severe resource constraints, however, time-limited trials in ICU might not be feasible anymore, and treatment in other units, such as high-dependence units, should be considered.

36.6 "The Day After"

In many jurisdictions, the pandemic is now abating, in some countries due to continued lockdown measures and in some countries due to extensive vaccination. Vaccines are another valuable resource that needs to be managed, for example, prioritizing which sector of the population to vaccinate first, sourcing sufficient vaccines, transportation, and rolling out the vaccination process in each country [53, 54].

Human nature being what it is, it will be tempting to put the pandemic down to a bad experience, which is or soon will be behind us and look to the future. Clearly, this is not the lesson to be learned. We should take the lessons in management and resource allocation of high acuity services as outlined above and plan for the next pandemic, which is inevitable [55].

> ### Take-Home Message
>
> Logistic challenges in the practice of intensive care medicine under pandemic conditions include flexibility of the healthcare system, hospitals, and intensive care units to increasing and decreasing demand, protecting the national and regional healthcare systems, making sure care is provided for both COVID-19 and non-COVID-19

patients and allocating enough equipment and personnel to meet demand. Triage decisions in elderly patients need to include multi-morbidity and frailty. Training and protecting the staff is crucial, and increased burnout must be dealt with. Planning for the future based on past experience is crucial.

References

1. Farmer JC, Carlton PK Jr. Providing critical care during a disaster: the interface between disaster response agencies and hospitals. Crit Care Med. 2006;34(3 Suppl):S56–9.
2. Bauer J, Brüggmann D, Klingelhöfer D, Maier W, Schwettmann L, Weiss DJ, et al. Access to intensive care in 14 European countries: a spatial analysis of intensive care need and capacity in the light of COVID-19. Intensive Care Med. 2020;46(11):2026–34.
3. Yang CJ, Tsai SH, Chien WC, Chung CH, Dai NT, Tzeng YS, et al. The crowd-out effect of a mass casualty incident: experience from a dust explosion with multiple burn injuries. Medicine. 2019;98(18):e15457.
4. Wax RS. Preparing the intensive care unit for disaster. Crit Care Clin. 2019;35(4):551–62.
5. Remuzzi A, Remuzzi G. COVID-19 and Italy: what next? Lancet. 2020;395(10231):1225–8.
6. Coccolini F, Sartelli M, Kluger Y, Pikoulis E, Karamagioli E, Moore EE, et al. COVID-19 the showdown for mass casualty preparedness and management: the Cassandra syndrome. World J Emerg Surg. 2020;15(1):26.
7. Sellers D, Ranse J. The impact of mass casualty incidents on intensive care units. Aust Crit Care. 2020;33(5):469–74.
8. Mangunta VR, Patel D. The era of mass casualty events: perspectives on care paradigms from a critical care Anesthesiologist. Mo Med. 2019;116(1):49–52.
9. Maves RC, Downar J, Dichter JR, Hick JL, Devereaux A, Geiling JA, et al. Triage of scarce critical care resources in COVID-19 an implementation guide for regional allocation: an expert panel report of the task force for mass critical care and the American College of Chest Physicians. Chest. 2020;158(1):212–25.
10. Harris G, Adalja A. ICU preparedness in pandemics: lessons learned from the coronavirus disease-2019 outbreak. Curr Opin Pulm Med. 2021;27(2):73–8.
11. Machi D, Bhattacharya P, Hoops S, Chen J, Mortveit H, Venkatramanan S, et al. Scalable epidemiological workflows to support COVID-19 planning and response. medRxiv. 2021; https://doi.org/10.1101/2021.02.23.21252325.
12. Iyengar K, Bahl S, Raju V, Vaish A. Challenges and solutions in meeting up the urgent requirement of ventilators for COVID-19 patients. Diabetes Metab Syndr. 2020;14(4):499–501.
13. Suzumura EA, Zazula AD, Moriya HT, Fais CQA, Alvarado AL, Cavalcanti AB, et al. Challenges for the development of alternative low-cost ventilators during COVID-19 pandemic in Brazil. Rev Bras Ter Intensiva. 2020;32(3):444–57.
14. Truog RD, Mitchell C, Daley GQ. The toughest triage - allocating ventilators in a pandemic. N Engl J Med. 2020;382(21):1973–5.
15. King WP, Amos J, Azer M, Baker D, Bashir R, Best C, et al. Emergency ventilator for COVID-19. PLoS One. 2020;15(12):e0244963.
16. Alfano V, Ercolano S. The efficacy of lockdown against COVID-19: a cross-country panel analysis. Appl Health Econ Health Policy. 2020;18(4):509–17.
17. Besley T, Stern N. The economics of lockdown. Fisc Stud. 2020;41(3):493–513.
18. Ferraresi M, Kotsogiannis C, Rizzo L, Secomandi R. The 'Great Lockdown' and its determinants. Econ Lett. 2020;197:109628.
19. Di Domenico L, Pullano G, Sabbatini CE, Boëlle PY, Colizza V. Impact of lockdown on COVID-19 epidemic in ?le-de-France and possible exit strategies. BMC Med. 2020;18(1):240.
20. Roadevin C, Hill H. How can we decide a fair allocation of healthcare resources during a pandemic? J Med Ethics. 2021:medethics-2020-106815. https://doi.org/10.1136/medethics-2020-106815.
21. Adam EH, Flinspach AN, Jankovic R, De Hert S, Zacharowski K. Treating patients across European Union borders: an international survey in light of the coronavirus disease-19 pandemic. Eur J Anaesthesiol. 2021;38(4):344–7.

22. Yoram G, Weiss IB, Alon R, Adar Y, Lavi B, Rothstein Z. Long-term hospital management in the presence of COVID-19: a practical perspective. Journal of. Hosp Adm. 2020;9(3):18–23.
23. Emanuel EJ, Persad G, Upshur R, Thome B, Parker M, Glickman A, et al. Fair allocation of scarce medical resources in the time of Covid-19. N Engl J Med. 2020;382(21):2049–55.
24. Bartsch SM, Ferguson MC, McKinnell JA, O'Shea KJ, Wedlock PT, Siegmund SS, et al. The potential health care costs and resource use associated with COVID-19 in the United States. Health Aff. 2020;39(6):927–35.
25. Ranney ML, Griffeth V, Jha AK. Critical supply shortages - the need for ventilators and personal protective equipment during the Covid-19 pandemic. N Engl J Med. 2020;382(18):e41.
26. Bruyneel A, Gallani MC, Tack J, d'Hondt A, Canipel S, Franck S, et al. Impact of COVID-19 on nursing time in intensive care units in Belgium. Intensive Crit Care Nurs. 2021;62:102967.
27. Casafont C, Fabrellas N, Rivera P, Olivé-Ferrer MC, Querol E, Venturas M, et al. Experiences of nursing students as healthcare aid during the COVID-19 pandemic in Spain: a phemonenological research study. Nurse Educ Today. 2021;97:104711.
28. González-Gil MT, González-Blázquez C, Parro-Moreno AI, Pedraz-Marcos A, Palmar-Santos A, Otero-García L, et al. Nurses' perceptions and demands regarding COVID-19 care delivery in critical care units and hospital emergency services. Intensive Crit Care Nurs. 2021;62:102966.
29. Azoulay E, De Waele J, Ferrer R, Staudinger T, Borkowska M, Povoa P, et al. Symptoms of burnout in intensive care unit specialists facing the COVID-19 outbreak. Ann Intensive Care. 2020;10(1):110.
30. Dewey C, Hingle S, Goelz E, Linzer M. Supporting clinicians during the COVID-19 pandemic. Ann Intern Med. 2020;172(11):752–3.
31. Thusini S. Critical care nursing during the COVID-19 pandemic: a story of resilience. Br J Nurs. 2020;29(21):1232–6.
32. Wahlster S, Sharma M, Lewis AK, Patel PV, Hartog CS, Jannotta G, et al. The coronavirus disease 2019 pandemic's effect on critical care resources and health-care providers: a global survey. Chest. 2021;159(2):619–33.
33. Montauk TR, Kuhl EA. COVID-related family separation and trauma in the intensive care unit. Psychol Trauma. 2020;12(S1):S96–s7.
34. Treibel TA, Manisty C, Burton M, McKnight LJ, Augusto JB, et al. COVID-19: PCR screening of asymptomatic health-care workers at London hospital. Lancet. 2020;395(10237):1608–10.
35. Oster Y, Wolf DG, Olshtain-Pops K, Rotstein Z, Schwartz C, Benenson S. Proactive screening approach for SARS-CoV-2 among healthcare workers. Clin Microbiol Infect. 2021;27(1):155–6.
36. Luks AM, Swenson ER. Pulse oximetry for monitoring patients with COVID-19 at home. potential pitfalls and practical guidance. Ann Am Thorac Soc. 2020;17(9):1040–6.
37. McWilliams D, Weblin J, Hodson J, Veenith T, Whitehouse T, Snelson C. Rehabilitation levels in patients with COVID-19 admitted to intensive care requiring invasive ventilation. An observational study. Ann Am Thorac Soc. 2021;18(1):122–9.
38. Candan SA, Elibol N, Abdullahi A. Consideration of prevention and management of long-term consequences of post-acute respiratory distress syndrome in patients with COVID-19. Physiother Theory Pract. 2020;36(6):663–8.
39. Dreier E, Malfertheiner MV, Dienemann T, Fisser C, Foltan M, Geismann F, et al. ECMO in COVID-19-prolonged therapy needed? A retrospective analysis of outcome and prognostic factors. Perfusion. 2021;36(6):582–91.
40. Booke H, Booke M. Medical triage during the COVID-19 pandemic: a medical and ethical burden. J Clin Ethics. 2021;32(1):73–6.
41. Ehni HJ, Wiesing U, Ranisch R. Saving the most lives-a comparison of European triage guidelines in the context of the COVID-19 pandemic. Bioethics. 2021;35(2):125–34.
42. Iacorossi L, Fauci AJ, Napoletano A, D'Angelo D, Salomone K, Latina R, et al. Triage protocol for allocation of critical health resources during Covid-19 pandemic and public health emergencies. A narrative review. Acta Biomed. 2020;91(4):e2020162.
43. Vincent JL, Creteur J. Ethical aspects of the COVID-19 crisis: how to deal with an overwhelming shortage of acute beds. Eur Heart J Acute Cardiovasc Care. 2020;9(3):248–52.
44. Sprung CL, Artigas A, Kesecioglu J, Pezzi A, Wiis J, Pirracchio R, et al. The Eldicus prospective, observational study of triage decision making in European intensive care units. Part II: intensive care benefit for the elderly. Crit Care Med. 2012;40(1):132–8.

45. Daubin C, Chevalier S, Séguin A, Gaillard C, Valette X, Prévost F, et al. Predictors of mortality and short-term physical and cognitive dependence in critically ill persons 75 years and older: a prospective cohort study. Health Qual Life Outcomes. 2011;9:35.

46. Nunes BP, Flores TR, Mielke GI, Thumé E, Facchini LA. Multimorbidity and mortality in older adults: a systematic review and meta-analysis. Arch Gerontol Geriatr. 2016;67:130–8.

47. Guidet B, de Lange DW, Boumendil A, Leaver S, Watson X, Boulanger C, et al. The contribution of frailty, cognition, activity of daily life and comorbidities on outcome in acutely admitted patients over 80 years in European ICUs: the VIP2 study. Intensive Care Med. 2020;46(1):57–69.

48. Fronczek J, Polok K, de Lange DW, Jung C, Beil M, Rhodes A, et al. Relationship between the clinical frailty scale and short-term mortality in patients ≥ 80 years old acutely admitted to the ICU: a prospective cohort study. Crit Care. 2021;25(1):231.

49. Maltese G, Corsonello A, Di Rosa M, Soraci L, Vitale C, Corica F, et al. Frailty and COVID-19: a systematic scoping review. J Clin Med. 2020;9(7):2106.

50. Hussien H, Nastasa A, Apetrii M, Nistor I, Petrovic M, Covic A. Different aspects of frailty and COVID-19: points to consider in the current pandemic and future ones. BMC Geriatr. 2021;21(1):389.

51. Jung C, Flaatten H, Fjølner J, Bruno RR, Wernly B, Artigas A, et al. The impact of frailty on survival in elderly intensive care patients with COVID-19: the COVIP study. Crit Care. 2021;25(1):149.

52. Bruce CR, Liang C, Blumenthal-Barby JS, Zimmerman J, Downey A, Pham L, et al. Barriers and facilitators to initiating and completing time-limited trials in critical care. Crit Care Med. 2015;43(12):2535–43.

53. Herlitz A, Lederman Z, Miller J, Fleurbaey M, Venkatapuram S, Atuire C, et al. Just allocation of COVID-19 vaccines. BMJ Glob Health. 2021;6(2):e004812.

54. Wouters OJ, Shadlen KC, Salcher-Konrad M, Pollard AJ, Larson HJ, Teerawattananon Y, et al. Challenges in ensuring global access to COVID-19 vaccines: production, affordability, allocation, and deployment. Lancet. 2021;397(10278):1023–34.

55. Arabi YM, Azoulay E, Al-Dorzi HM, Phua J, Salluh J, Binnie A, et al. How the COVID-19 pandemic will change the future of critical care. Intensive Care Med. 2021;47(3):282–91.

36

Future Developments

Contents

Future Challenges for Geriatric Intensive Care

Hans Flaatten, Bertrand Guidet, and Hélène Vallet

Contents

© The Author(s), under exclusive license to Springer Nature Switzerland AG 2022
H. Flaatten et al. (eds.), *The Very Old Critically Ill Patients*, Lessons from the ICU,
https://doi.org/10.1007/978-3-030-94133-8_37

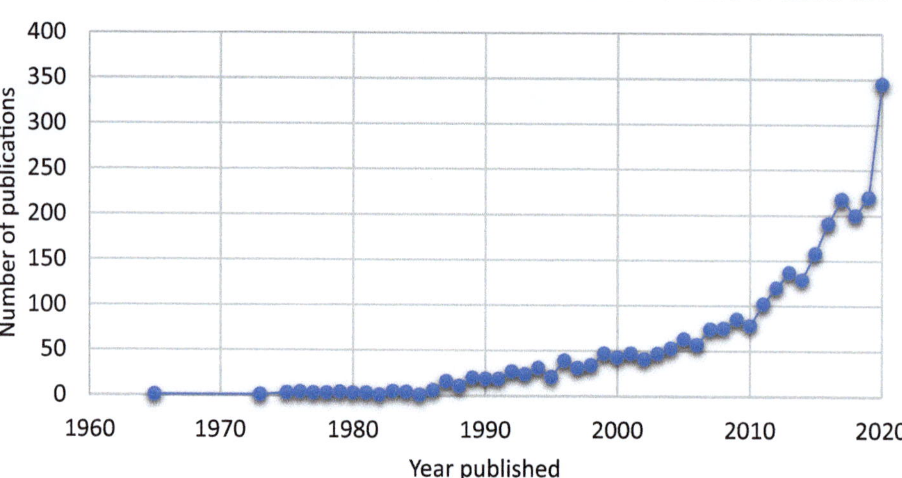

Fig. 37.1 Figure one shows the results from a PubMed search on publications on the very old ICU patients

» We cannot solve our problems with the same thinking we used when we created them.
  –Albert Einstein

37.1 Introduction

There is a rapid growing focus on the old and very old ICU patients, and this is reflected in the number of published papers on the subject. Looking at publications listed in PubMed that includes old and intensive care in title or abstract illustrates a very rapid increase from 2010 and onward (■ Fig. 37.1) demonstrating an exponential increase about this topic.

Naturally not all these publications are pure scientific reports but include all types of publications including editorials, state of the art, and reviews but nevertheless illustrate the increased focus on the very old ICU patients. With increase in the number of elderly ICU patients, it is easy to be a wizard and predict that this trend most likely continues in the coming decades. We still have a lot to learn and improve about providing intensive care in this group.

37.2 Future Organization: Intensive Care for the Very old

At present, care of the critical ill elderly patients is with only few exceptions organized within general intensive care units throughout the world, although there have been published experiences from alternative organization [1]. This discussion was recently raised again, but for many reasons, it is not easy to change current routines to admit the elderly patients to general ICUs since there are not many

Table 37.1 Advantages and disadvantages of different models for geriatric intensive care A traditional ICU, B hybrid ICU, C pure geriatric ICU

Type	Advantages	Disadvantages
A	Well-known Equal competence at all levels Simple solution No reorganization	Suboptimal competences Need external consultation (geriatric physician and nurse) Less focus and development Need a dedicated program for the old patients within the ICU
B	Can be established within existing infrastructure, no separate unit A special competence group of nurses, physicians (including daytime geriatrician), and others may be present at least during day time	Probably not feasible in smaller units (< 20 beds) Need a separate dedicated area within the ICU Vulnerable for lack of competent personnel 24/7 with geriatric competence
C	Can focus on the elderly only Area for both intensivists and geriatricians working together Can be designed solely with the elderly in mind	If only manned by geriatrician, they need training in general intensive care or receive continuous support from intensivists May be less attractive to work in compared to A and B for "traditional" ICU personnel

alternatives in most hospitals [2]. There are several options that can be applied in order to cover the specific requirement this group presents, and separate intensive care units are just one.

◻ Table 37.1 illustrates three different concepts with aims to improve quality of care to this specific group. Type A represents the traditional organization with a total integration within a general adult ICU. Type B illustrates treatment in a "sub-unit" within a general ICU where elderly ICU patients are treated in a dedicated area partly with dedicated personnel. This is probably feasible only in larger units where space and human resources may allow such an organization. Type C is a completely stand-alone geriatric ICU. The table reveals advantages and disadvantages of these three models.

A special consideration must be paid to post-intensive care. Regardless of how intensive care for elderly will be given, there must be a dedicated track for geriatric rehabilitation, probably within an acute geriatric unit. Maybe this development should be priority one if one starts to reorganize geriatric intensive care within a hospital (see ▶ Chap. 28).

We have enough information and knowledge from treating critical ill elderly during the last two decades that a transition from the traditional type A ICUs to either B or C should feasible in most hospitals. Just the share number of elderly patients admitted today and in particular in the coming decades should be an additional reason to initiate such change now. When expansion of ICU capacity is planned within a hospital, maybe a dedicated geriatric ICU could be an attractive option since soon approximately one third of all ICU patients will be above 70.

37.3 Cooperation with Who and When

Intensive care has developed to be a "melting pot" of different areas in medicine. Since the start, often from within anesthesiology and internal medicine, most acute specialities are engaged in these patients, and lately also interventional radiologists have been proven valuable. Formal cooperation with geriatricians is seldomly reported, although in-depth knowledge on how this is solved or not solved within units and across countries is largely missing. This also extends to the inclusion of geriatric nurses and physiotherapists in the ICU. In particular, elderly ICU patients in the end of their ICU stay should have established a contact with a geriatrician while still in the ICU [3]. Regardless of where the rehabilitation is continued, it starts in the ICU, and important guidance for the post-ICU track may be decided before discharge.

Also, from the ICU admission, important contribution to pharmacotherapy in the elderly may be given from geriatricians and pharmacists. Elderly patients frequently are multimorbid and use many medications. Data from the VIP2 study illustrates the burden of comorbidities and number of daily medications prescribed to elderly patients at ICU admission [4]. In that study, 40% had five comorbidities or more, and 68% had five or more drugs prescribed at daily basis illustrating the huge burden of co-existing disease and polypharmacy in this group. This is an area where geriatricians possess specific competency and can be of invaluable help to intensivists.

37.4 Research Agenda from 2017, Where Are We Now?

In 2017, we published a paper on the status of research in this group of patients and found in particular ten areas where high-quality data was poor or missing [5], briefly summarized in ◘ Table 37.2. As can be seen, only frailty and sepsis can be said to be studied in several independent research papers, but the rest have been insufficiently studied and some not studied at all. Hence the list may still guide to important areas for research in the coming decade.

Some of these unanswered research items are indirectly illustrated in ◘ Fig. 37.2, where the trajectories of the very old ICU patient and their caregivers are described as it is usual today and how one could hope it could be in the future. However, very few of these proposed actions are studied in-depth and create a huge opportunity for research in the coming decade.

37.5 Future Changes in Critical Care of the Elderly

We propose a change in how the elderly patients can be treated from pre-ICU until post hospital discharge, a change from usual practice today to future care and hopefully improved care (◘ Fig. 37.2). Shortly, the changes consist of the following:
-	Broad anchored guidelines for ICU admittance, from evidence-based medicine to acceptance in potential patients and caregivers, politicians, and ICU personnel.

Table 37.2   Research areas specified in 2017 [5]

The occurrence of frailty and sarcopenia and effects on outcome	Covered in several studies in particular frailty
The opinion of octogenarians on ICU admission	Not covered
Effects of including geriatricians in assessment and discharge	Not covered
Delirium, effects of non-pharmacological interventions	Poorly covered
The burden of post-intensive care in caregivers	Poorly covered
Development of prognostic tools specifically for the very old	Partially covered
Sepsis in the very old	Covered in several studies
Dementia development post-ICU in survivors	Poorly covered
Sedation and pharmacokinetics in the very old	Poorly covered
End of life trajectories in the very old	Poorly covered

- Increased involvement of caregivers in the admission process.
- Use of time-limited ICU trials in cases of uncertainty.
- Use of specific treatment protocols for critical ill elderly patients.
- Involvement of geriatric competence, at least in the transition from intensive care to ward and rehabilitation.
- Dedicated support for patients and caregivers after hospital discharge.

Many of these steps need to be developed, evaluated, and some also tested in clinical trials and will add to the list previously discussed research items from 2017 (Table 37.2).

In particular, the first bullet point could prove vital in order to really increase the focus on treatment of critical ill elderly in the future. All stakeholders in this "chain" illustrated in Fig. 37.2 need to come together for collaboration in all levels. First and foremost, in the actual treatment of these patients, but as important is the development of multi-professional guidelines in close cooperation with important stakeholders like the potential patients (very old persons), their relatives and caregivers, and politicians. We are far from this goal, and even discussions between intensivists and geriatricians are lacking in most ICUs.

Each of these steps requires much, both with regard to research but also production of guidelines for multi-professional cooperation within this field, and as stated previously we need evidence from different organization models of care.

In summary, we have challenges enough for the next decade and can join a conclusion set forward nearly 20 years ago: *"Critical illness in the elderly remains a fertile area for future research"* [6].

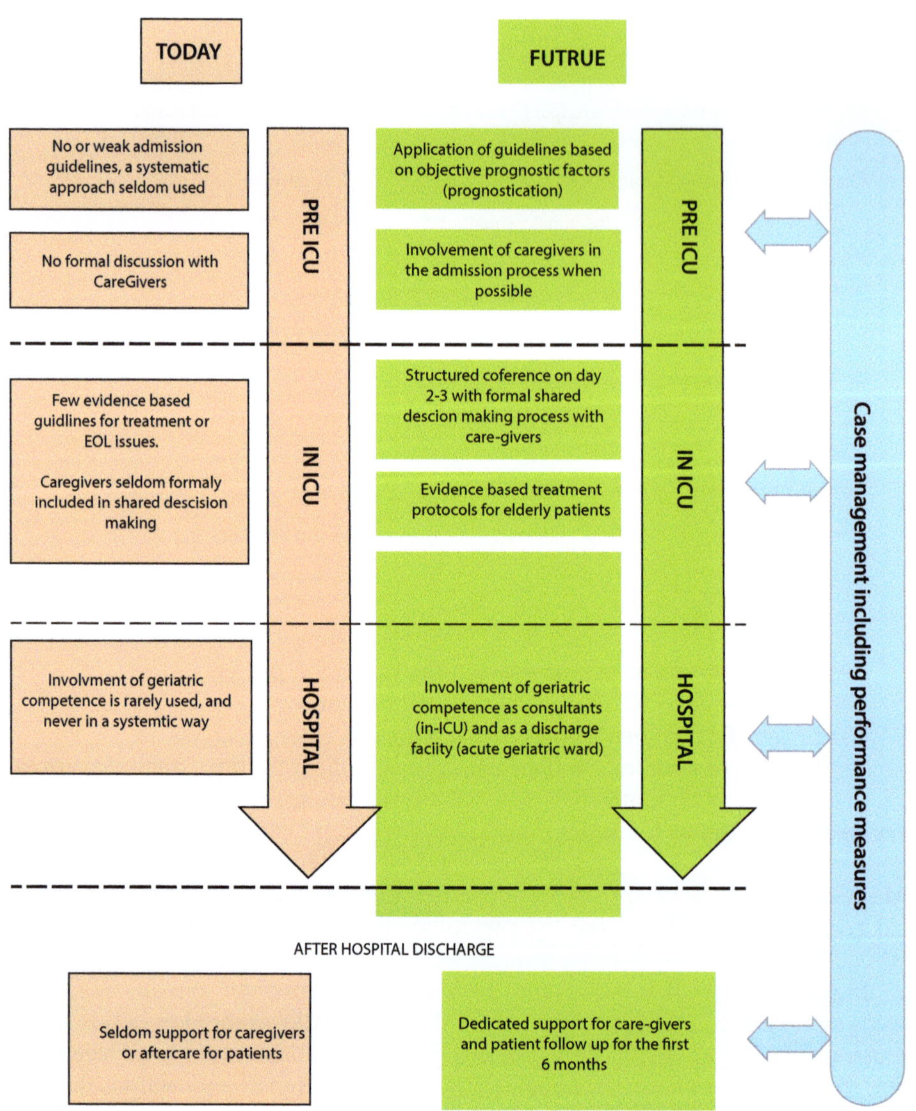

Fig. 37.2   Present and future pathways for the very old critical ill patients

References

1. Zeng A, Song X, Dong J, et al. Mortality in relation to frailty in patients admitted to a specialized geriatric intensive care unit. J Gerontol A Biol Sci Med Sci. 2015;70(12):1586–94.
2. Brummel NE, Ferrante LE. Integrating geriatric principles into critical care medicine: the time is now. Ann Am Thorac Soc. 2018;15(5):518–22.
3. Philp I. The contribution of geriatric medicine to integrated care for older people. Age Ageing. 2015;44(1):11–5.
4. Guidet B, de Lange DW, Boumendil A, et al. The contribution of frailty, cognition, activity of daily life and comorbidities on outcome in acutely admitted patients over 80 years in European ICUs: the VIP2 study. Intensive Care Med. 2020;46(1):57–69.
5. Flaatten H, Lange DW, Artigas A, et al. The status of intensive care medicine research and a future agenda for very old patients in the ICU. Intensive Care Med. 2017;43(9):1–10.
6. Nagappan R, Parkin G. Geriatric critical care. Crit Care Clin. 2003;19:253–70.

If you have any questions about our products,
you can contact us at
Product-Safety@springernature.com
In case a product is not functioning properly,
for returns contact your representative [EC REP]
Springer Nature Customer Service Center GmbH
Kurpalzplatz 3, 69115 Heidelberg, Germany

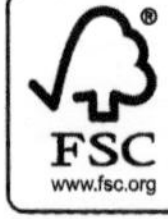